Steps to Successful Regional Anesthesia

Mukesh Kumar Prasad
Sukhminder Jit Singh Bajwa
Editors

Steps to Successful Regional Anesthesia

Challenges and Solutions

Springer

Editors
Mukesh Kumar Prasad
Department of Anesthesiology
Teerthanker Mahaveer Medical College
Moradabad, Uttar Pradesh, India

Sukhminder Jit Singh Bajwa
Department of Anesthesiology &
Intensive Care Medicine
Gian Sagar Medical College & Hospital
Patiala, Punjab, India

ISBN 978-981-97-4097-0 ISBN 978-981-97-4098-7 (eBook)
https://doi.org/10.1007/978-981-97-4098-7

This Springer imprint is published by the registered company Springer Nature Singapore Pte Ltd.
The registered company address is: 152 Beach Road, #21-01/04 Gateway East, Singapore 189721, Singapore

I would like to dedicate this entire effort to my charming wife, Dr. Kanchan, who is the very reason behind the inception of this book. The idea that a book could be planned was there, but I was totally unconvinced I could do it. It was she who made me believe. She stood by me right from the very beginning and propped me throughout, whenever I wavered in intensity. Despite her own busy schedule, she made it a point to ensure that my efforts were fructified by supporting me in ways that cannot be quantified.

I would also like to give a special mention to Master Rohan, my son, who has been a strong motivating force for me throughout the compilation.

Notwithstanding the contribution of all others, nothing would have been possible without their vital roles.

Foreword

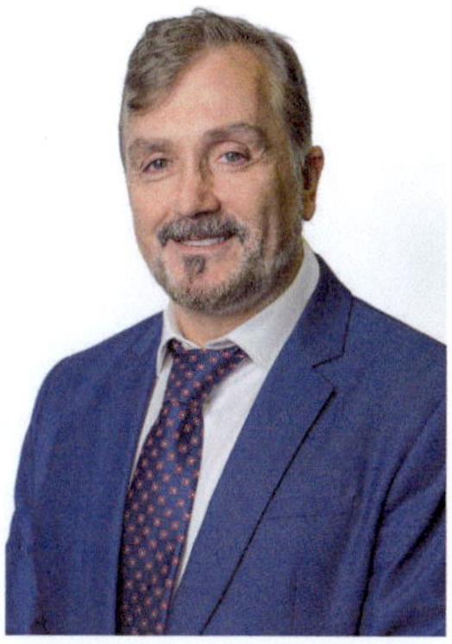

With the introduction of ultrasound into regional anesthesia practice, a general enthusiasm occurred within the anesthesiology community, especially into a generation of new specialists who could see the benefit of visualizing nerves and vessels.

Additionally, this has brought a new angle to point-of-care procedures and a very effective and safe way to provide excellent pain relief to their patients.

Interestingly, the ultrasound machines were complemented with a revitalized learning of anatomy, the practical use of understanding muscles, tendons, nerves, and vessels, and the pathologies like inflammation, impingements, fascial planes, and variations in the distribution of the nerves. The anesthesiologist realized that a broad knowledge of anatomy was not enough and now could target and trace nerves through normal and not so normal scenarios. At the end of the day, anesthesiologists are very practical specialists.

Together to ultrasound-guided techniques, this book makes an effort to present a comprehensive approach to the use of anatomical landmarks and peripheral nerve stimulators with two aims: To increase the success rate and to decrease the occurrence of complications.

In this book, a tremendous amount of work has been done over the years to create texts in all areas of clinical relevance. The number of anatomical descriptions mentioned is endless with personal pearls thoroughly described. This makes it extremely valuable and easy to read. It is definitely a book to keep in our offices for quick consultation of regional blocks.

My dear colleague *Dr. Siva Krishna Kota* requested me to consider introducing this book, and I am pleased to do so, because in my opinion, this book is not only for doctors in anesthesiology but also for emergency doctors, rheumatologists, plastic surgeons, and others like orthopedics, neurosurgeons, neurologists, and rehabilitation doctors, not to forget nurses, including specialized and non-specialized in pain medicine.

Finally, my most sincere congratulations to the authors and Dr. Mukesh Kumar Prasad, who has taken the lead in getting all the contributors under one umbrella. This is an outstanding attempt to come with a comprehensive work on ultrasonography-guided regional blocks, which is complete with all the practical tips and tricks.

I welcome everyone to enjoy this book.

Director of Pain Division, Corniche Hospital
Abu Dhabi, UAE

Rafael Blanco

Preface

Regional anesthesia is among the subspecialties of anesthesiology to have taken enormous leaps to evolve into a distinct entity in its own right. It is harbinger of a new era in the practice of anesthesia, which itself is one of the most recent specialties of modern medicine, almost a wonder of the new age. The enthusiasm of the gen-next of this specialty promises a completely new chapter in patient care encompassing all its aspects be it physiological, psychological, or monetary.

History can vouch for the fact if anything has been difficult, it is to bring about a change in the conventional. And so it is, with regional anesthesia practices. A lot many hurdles are being and will be encountered during the mastering of these techniques, requiring knowledge of core subjects, determination to learn, apply, and practice, and redo the cycle again and again. The attitude to take failures in stride and start all over again toward a singular goal of proficiency in this discipline is integral to success.

It is this very attitude that inspired us to write this book. The enthusiasm of my colleagues, juniors, and students to explore this field for the betterment of patient care has been inescapable. The genuineness of their desire to learn and perfect these techniques, aware that it will greatly enhance patient experience in terms of recovery and perioperative analgesia was the greatest motivation for us.

While we never claim to be the best in business, but I dare say we each of the contributors has had significant success in practicing these nerve blocks over the years in a sizeable number of patients. The improved patient experience and the decreasing morbidity, especially observed in compromised patients were real push to try and fructify our dream of sharing our experiences, observations, judgments not only with the upcoming generations but also with those of our contemporaries who are desirous of having a better grasp of the techniques in regional anesthesia.

Almost all the contributors have spent a significant amount of time practicing this discipline and often, while troubleshooting for a struggling trainee or a comparatively fresh practitioner, one has encountered the same question—"Sir, how did you do this?" While one does explain this in the moment, we reckoned it would be worthwhile to try and harness these years of experience, pepper them with our own flavors of improvisations we may have devised over the years and present them in an organized manner, which might be easy to access and refer to on an "as and when needed" basis.

The fact that we intended to bring together a good number of some of the very good minds in this field promised that all kinds of situations would be addressed, right from the commoner ones to the rarer ones.

We have taken this opportunity to try our level best to present the various techniques of regional anesthesia which will not only include the head, facial, truncal, thorax, central neuraxial, upper limb, and lower limb blocks but also a peek into the relevant equipment and local anesthetics. We have tried to highlight ergonomics of USG and discuss in detail, coagulation issues in regional anesthesia (RA), issues faced with pediatric patients, emerging and re-emerging techniques, and the use of RA in the field of gynecology. There are specially added chapters on the use of RA in limited resource settings, palliative care, and recent advances.

The foremost reason behind putting this book together was to share the real problems the new practitioners in this sphere are most likely to face and provide systematic and efficacious solutions to them. The agenda behind this book was to highlight the real-life scenarios in a simplified way along with all relevant information about a block making it a wholesome package for beginners as well as the established practitioners.

The journey of writing and collection of chapters has been nothing short of a roller-coaster ride, full of discussions, imaginations, passionate arguments, and hundreds of editing sessions all ending up in a hopefully comprehensive and unique textbook touching almost every aspect of regional anesthesia.

With a lifetime of practicing regional anesthesia and considering minutely, all the pros and cons of RA, we have used it in best possible case scenarios to the worst possible ones successfully, thus being encouraged to document all our knowledge and experience carefully, thoughtfully, and responsibly for all our readers, to inspire them, support them, and perhaps, guide them toward the most practicable and effective path toward successful application of blocks.

Here's hoping this book will serve all the needs and clear all the queries of our readers. Looking forward to a great journey ahead for all!

Happy reading!

Happy studying!

Happy Blocks!

Moradabad, Uttar Pradesh, India Mukesh Kumar Prasad

Preface

Regional anesthesia is favored and treasured by every practitioner of anesthesiology. In fact, regional anesthesia techniques are most desired in patients with comorbidities who are on the rise, in all age groups and in most clinical situations. They are a part of the multimodal anesthesia techniques and enhanced recovery after surgery protocols.

There is nothing more pleasant than an optimally acted peripheral nerve block or central neuraxial block with a comfortable anesthesiologist, surgeon/obstetrician, and patient. In the same vein, there is nothing more distressing than those frenzied, confused, and panic-struck chaotic moments when a spinal block fails or when a nerve block given for analgesia just does not work and the anesthesiologist starts cursing the block, blaming the technique, the equipment, and the patient. Feelings of self-guilt and remorse start creeping in at those times, not to forget the operating surgeon's growing doubts in the clinical skills of the anesthesiologist. Who can forget the scene of an anesthesiologist who has just had a failed block, now busy trying to pacify a patient in pain on the operation table and casting sheepish glances at an equally distressed surgeon waiting impatiently with his knife to take the incision? Who can forget the frustration of the anesthesiologist struggling with a difficult spine or a nerve block and attempting repeated punctures only to be unsuccessful? As a practitioner, I have often faced such clinical situations and it is those moments of desperation that inspired me to create this book on *Steps to Successful Regional Anesthesia*.

This book has chapters on how to manage troubleshooting during the administration of neuraxial block and various other nerve blocks including upper limb blocks, lower limb blocks, thoracic blocks, truncal blocks, and scalp, facial, and airway blocks. The methods to administer successful regional nerve blocks in obstetric anesthesia, palliative care, trauma, critical care, and pediatric anesthesia are also described. There are chapters providing strategies on how to administer successful regional anesthesia in challenging situations such as in low-resource settings and in patients with coagulation disorders. Artists can be successful only if they are provided with the correct tools with which they can work comfortably. Similarly, a successful regional anesthesiologist should be equipped with the correct instruments, local anesthetics, and adjuvant drugs. Two chapters in this book provide information on these aspects. Newer technology has now made things easier for us; a chapter in this book provides an update and newer insights on regional anesthesia techniques. Nevertheless, the authors in all the chapters provide tips and tricks and anytime recipes that can improve the success and quality of regional anesthesia. Most of these are evidence-based and based on the authors' rich clinical experiences.

It is said that a mother's lap is the place where you weep, sleep, and find peace; similarly, I am sure that the busy practicing anesthesiologists and budding postgraduate students in anesthesia will find solace and strength in this book that can boost up their clinical confidence in regional anesthesia and help them sail smoothly through difficult perioperative times.

Patiala, Punjab, India Sukhminder Jit Singh Bajwa

Acknowledgements

I am thankful to the Chancellor and Vice-Chairman of Teerthanker Mahaveer University, Moradabad, India, for providing a platform to use our skills to the fullest and provide best possible care to patients.

Here, I would also like to thank Mr. Abhishek Kapoor for providing me constant encouragement throughout the process of writing this book.

I would like to thank Mr. Ajay Garg for guiding me at every step of the publishing process.

I would like to sincerely thank all the contributing authors for sparing their time and expertise in this endeavor. It is much appreciated that they have put in a lot of effort, especially in trying to stick to deadlines, considering the vastness of the scope of this book. It goes without saying that this book would not have been possible without the hard work and support received from all of them. A special thanks to all for allowing editors the liberty to edit the chapters unhindered, to maintain uniformity throughout this book.

Dr. Payal Jain has been an incessant source of support, one of the strongest pillars in the foundation of this book. She has been extensively involved in every aspect, throughout the substantial gestational period of this book. She has considerable knowledge of her subject and has employed it extensively in shaping this book, right from editorial interventions to subject matter contributions wherever required. Her role cannot be overemphasized, and I am grateful to her for taking time out for this venture.

Not to forget a special mention to Dr. Pulak Puneet, a friend and colleague who contributed significantly to the authoring of book chapter besides moral boosting in each and every step in evolution of this book.

I would like to thank Dr. Ankit Verma for helping with and putting together finally, majority of the images. The schematic diagrams drawn with precision go a long way in information accurately. Dr. B Sahithi Charan and Dr. Ankit formed an effective team in presenting visually impactful images with accurate labeling.

I would like to thank the experts Dr. Rohit Varshney and Dr. Shahbaz Alam who took the time and trouble to review the chapters and provide valuable inputs.

I would like to thank Dr. Uday Kiran Gunja and Dr. Pratiksha Gogia for providing their expertise in photography, which was essential while capturing real-time patient scenarios to convey precisely the situations the reader is likely to encounter in day-to-day practice. Also, Dr. Pratiksha's efforts need special mention for her exclusive art of collecting and compiling data on any and every topic assigned to her.

I would also like to thank Dr. Macha Niranjan Reddy, Dr. Shashank Sahu, and Dr. Shashank Jain for compiling the images and ensuring their accurate placement along with final formatting of the document.

I would also like to thank my anesthesiology residents and postgraduate students, especially Dr. Neha, Dr. Divya Arora, Dr. Parampreet Kaur, and Dr. Osho Raag Chowdhury who have been a constant source of support and volunteered to be patient models whenever required.

A special thanks to the editorial team of Springer who have been phenomenal in their support and proactiveness in shaping this project right down to the last detail.

Lastly, it is wonderful to express gratitude to all those who have supported and believed in my vision.

Contents

Editors and Contributors

About the Editors

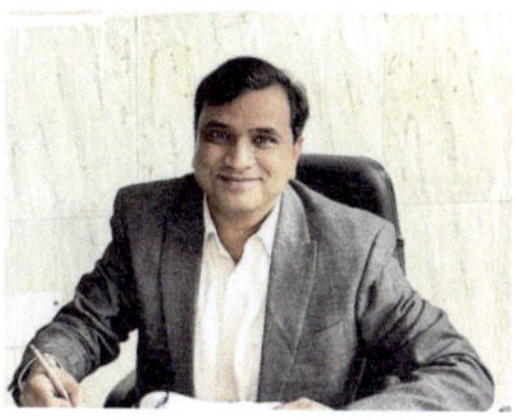

Mukesh Kumar Prasad
(MD, MBA, PGDHHM, and FIPM) has completed his post-graduation in the field of anesthesiology. He is currently working as the Head of Department and Professor in the Department of Anesthesiology, Teerthanker Mahaveer Medical College, Moradabad, India. He has extensive experience working in cardiac, pediatric, neuro, plastic, and general anesthesia. Dr. Mukesh is particularly knowledgeable in the field of regional anesthesia and peripheral nerve blocks, with immense experience in landmark-guided, fluoroscopic-guided, and USG-guided nerve blocks. He has several peer-reviewed national and international publications, serves as a reviewer, and is a member of the editorial boards of many reputable journals. Dr. Mukesh is constantly engaged in teaching faculty members and postgraduate students the techniques to troubleshoot common and uncommon problems encountered during regional anesthesia. Dr. Mukesh also runs a pain clinic within the department and did exemplary work in managing a 100-bed COVID-19 ICU. He has received numerous awards and is a member of several national and international societies.

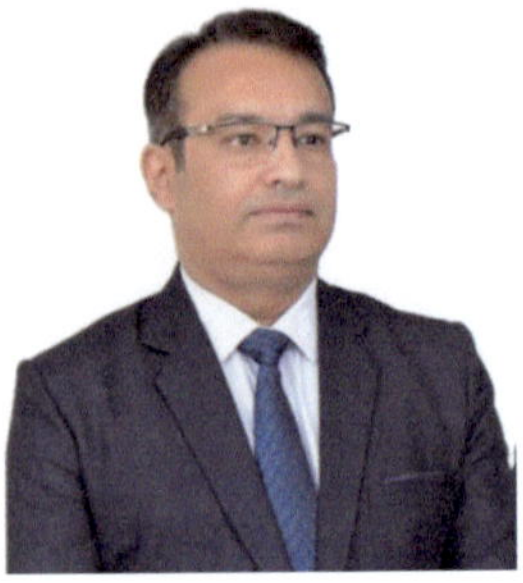

Sukhminder Jit Singh Bajwa

(MD, MBA, ACEE) is currently a Professor and Head in the Department of Anesthesiology and Intensive Care Medicine at Gian Sagar Medical College and Hospital, Banur, Patiala, Punjab, India. He has published more than 400 international and national publications and eight book chapters. Dr. Bajwa serves as editor-in-chief, associate editor, and editorial board member for various national and international journals. He has been honored with several awards, including the Best Young Anesthesiologist Award for 2012, which is the KPR Young Anesthesiologist of India award.

Contributors

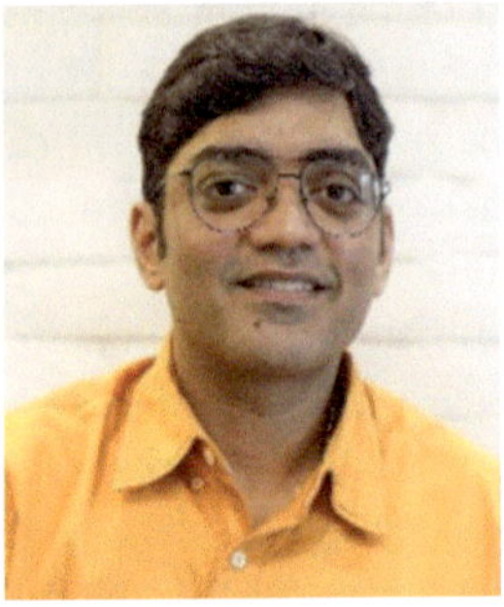

Gaurav Agarwal Department of Anaesthesiology and Pain Medicine, CARE Hospitals, Bhubaneswar, Odisha, India

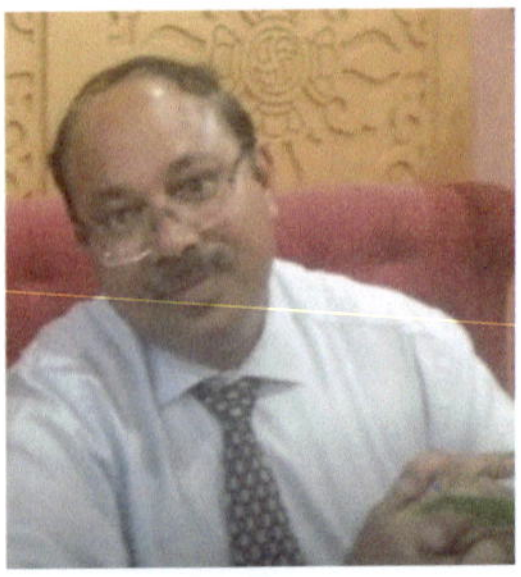

Sanjay Agrawal Department of Anaesthesiology, AIIMS, Rishikesh, Uttarakhand, India

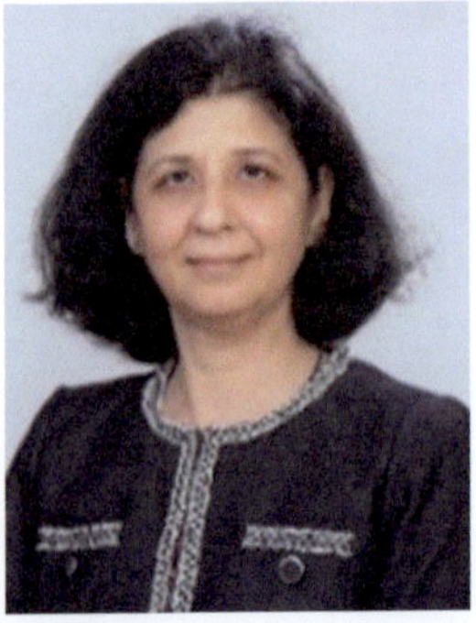

Vanita Ahuja Department of Anaesthesiology and Intensive Care, Government Medical College, Chandigarh, Haryana, India

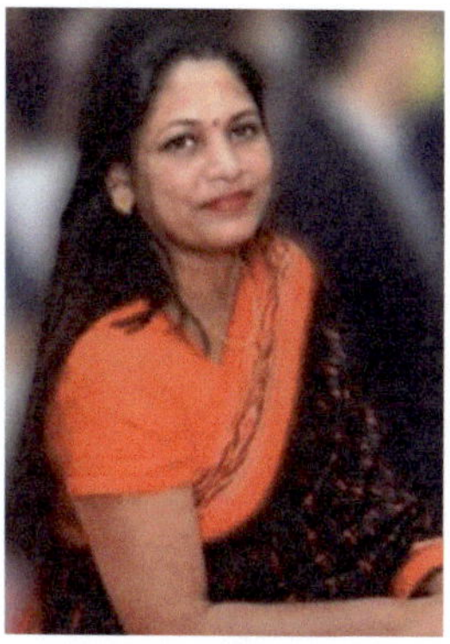

Veena Asthana Department of Anaesthesiology, HIMS, SRHU, Jolly Grant, Dehradun, Uttarakhand, India

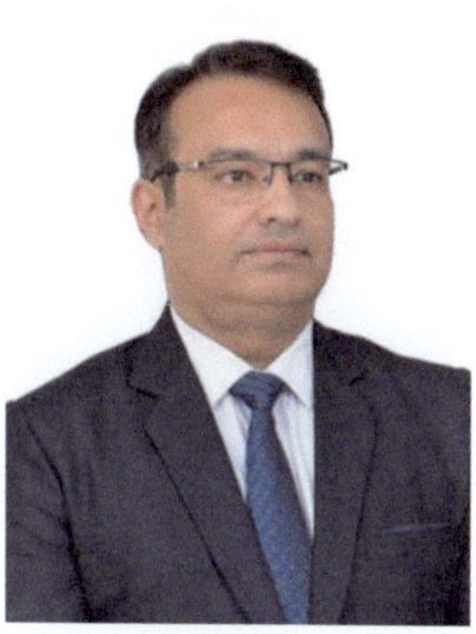

Sukhminder Jit Singh Bajwa Department of Anaesthesiology and Critical Care, Gian Sagar Medical College and Hospital, Patiala, Punjab, India

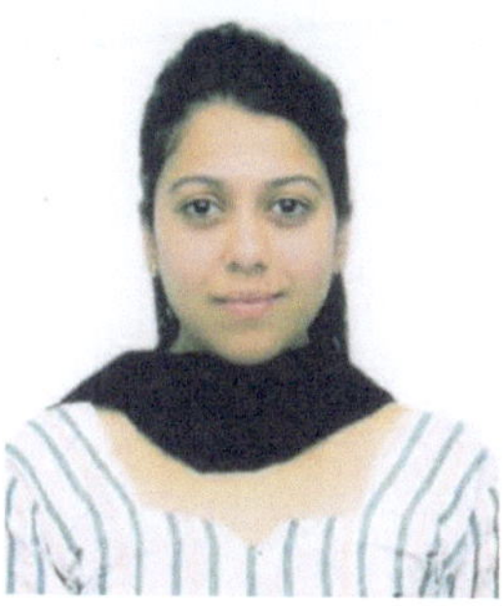

Amrita Banerjee Department of Anaesthesia, AIIMS, Bilaspur, Himachal Pradesh, India

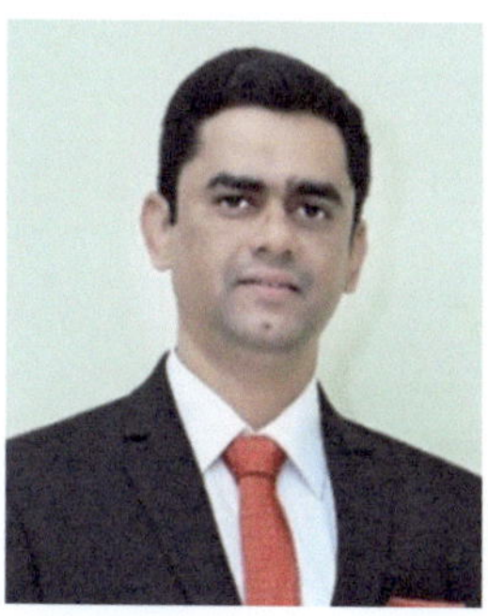

Saurabh M. Barde Faculty at Datta Meghe Medical College and SMHRC, Nagpur, Maharashtra, India

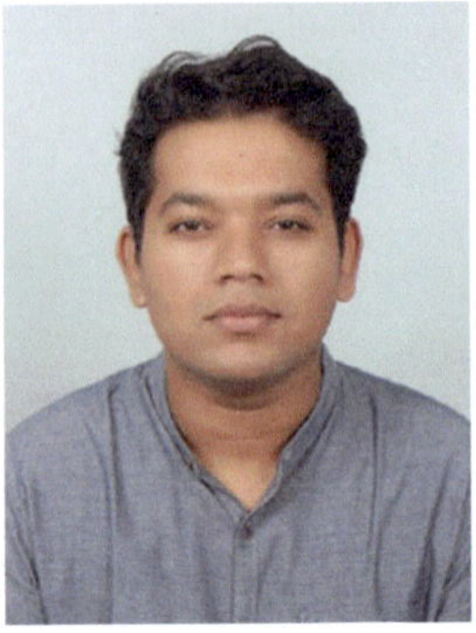

Rohit Hanmanta Bhandari North Middlesex University Hospital, London, UK

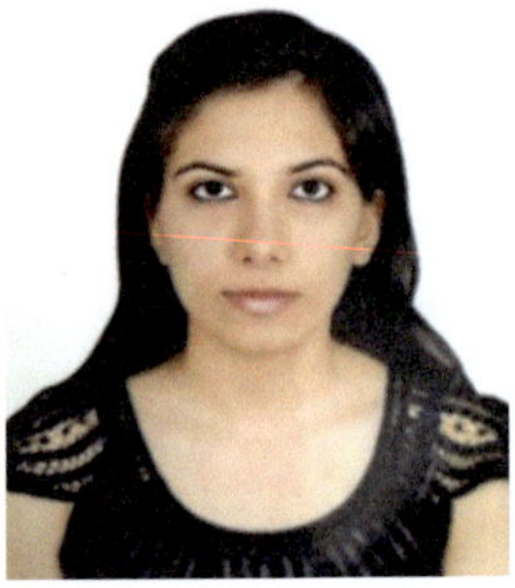

Soumya Bindra Department of Oncoanaesthesia and Palliative Medicine, Dr. B.R.A.I.R.C.H, AIIMS, New Delhi, India

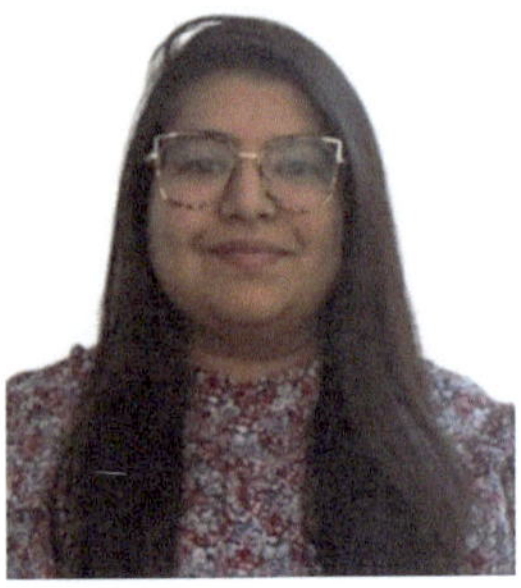

Pratiksha Gogia Department of Anaesthesiology, Teerthanker Mahaveer Medical College and Research Centre, Moradabad, Uttar Pradesh, India

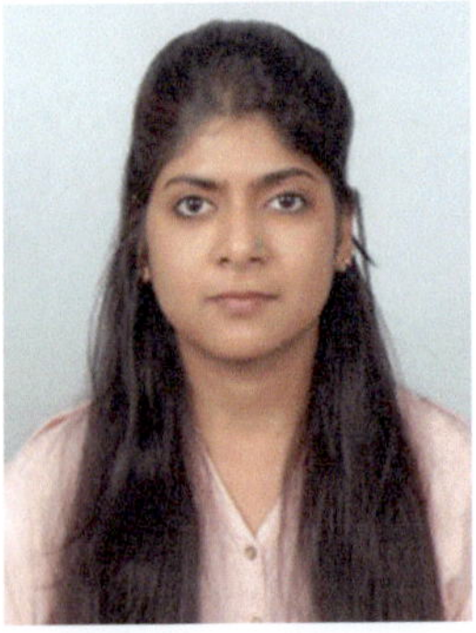

Sonali Gupta North Middlesex University Hospital, London, UK

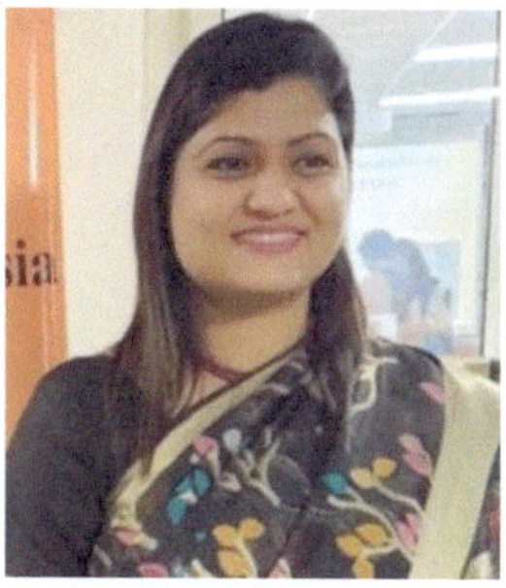

Sana Yasmin Hussain Department of Anaesthesiology, Pain Medicine and Critical Care, AIIMS, New Delhi, India

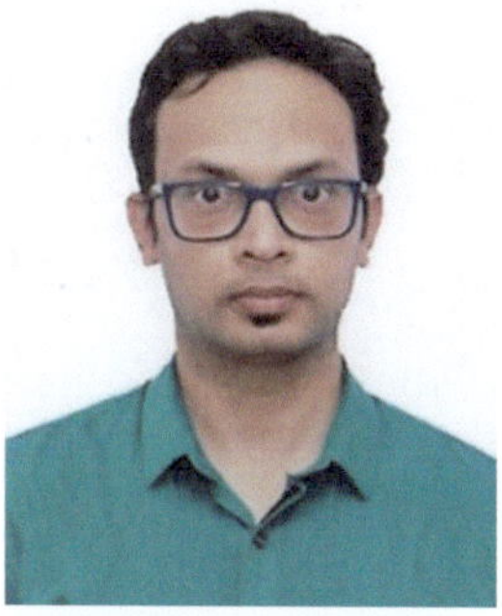

Dhruv Jain Department of Anaesthesiology, Pain Medicine and Critical Care, AIIMS, New Delhi, India

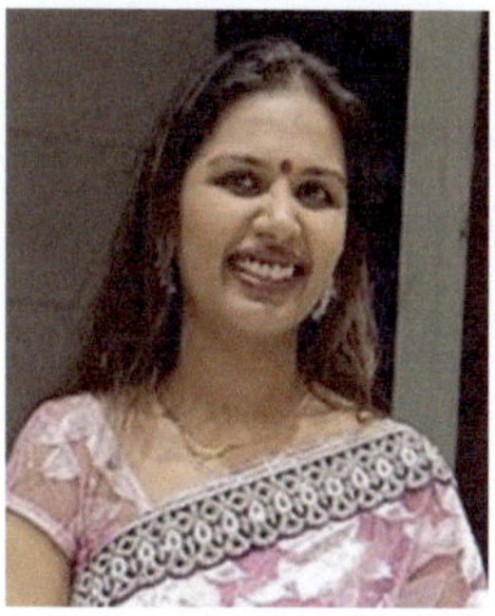

Payal Jain Department of Anaesthesiology, Teerthanker Mahaveer Medical College and Research Centre, Moradabad, Uttar Pradesh, India

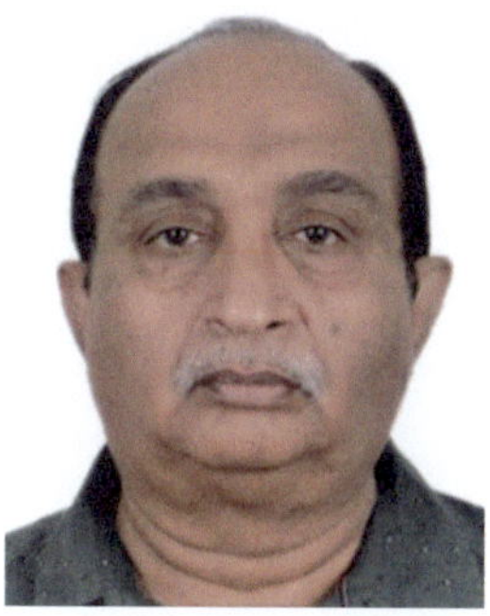

Gurdeep Singh Jheetay Department of Anaesthesiology, Graphic Era University, Dehradun, Uttarakhand, India

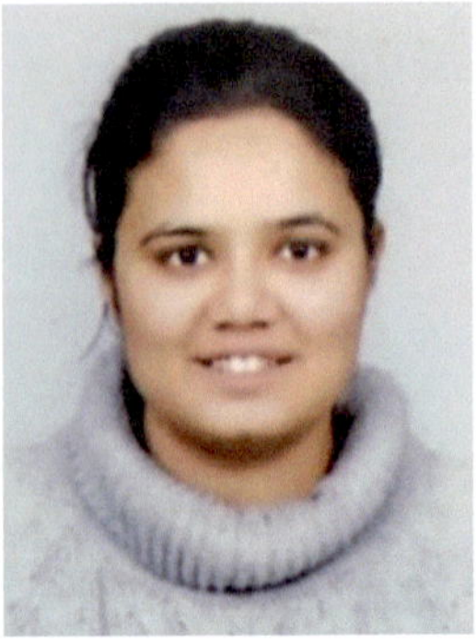

Kali Kapoor Department of Anaesthesiology, Rama Medical College, Kanpur, Uttar Pradesh, India

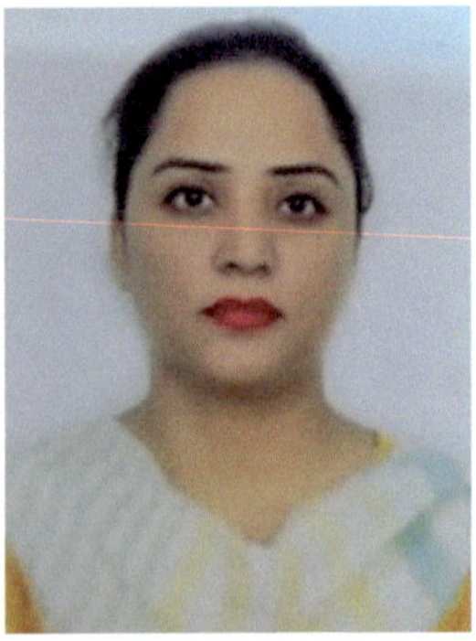

Harkomal Kaur Department of Anaesthesiology, Nalanda Medical College and Hospital, Patna, Bihar, India

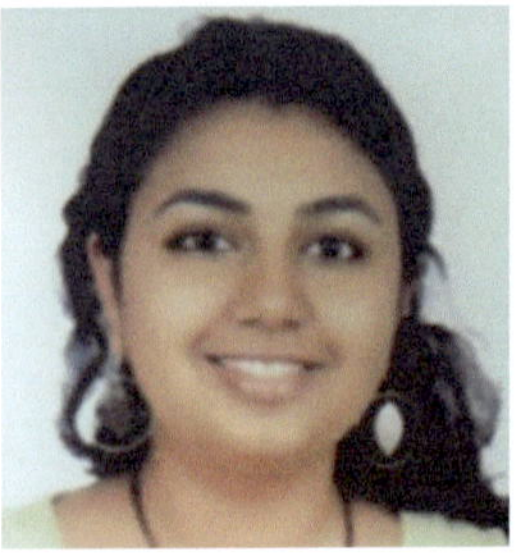

Aditi Khare Department of Anaesthesiology, Global Hospital, Gwalior, Madhya Pradesh, India

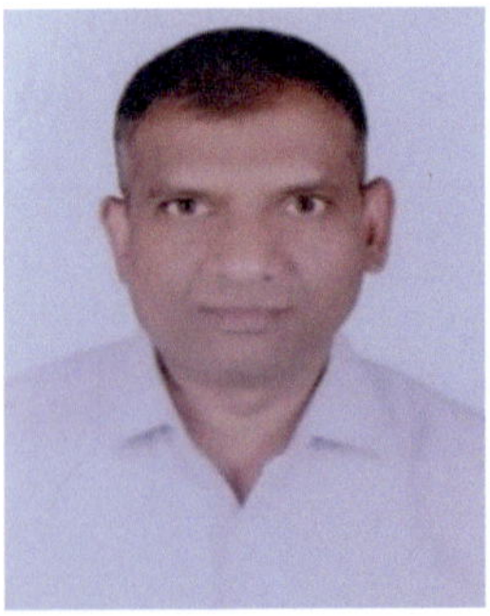

Rajnish Kumar Department of Anaesthesiology, AIIMS, Patna, Bihar, India

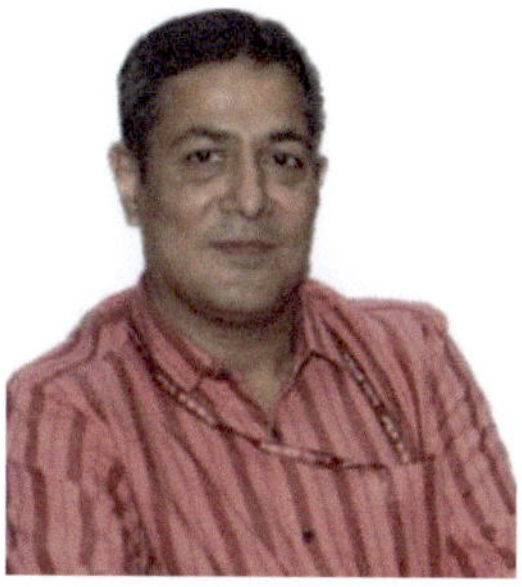

Shailendra Kumar Department of Anaesthesiology, Pain Medicine and Critical Care, AIIMS, New Delhi, India

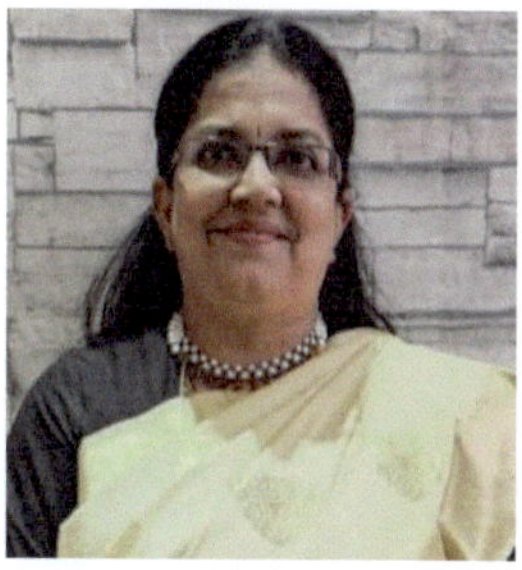

Madhuri S. Kurdi Department of Anaesthesiology, Karnataka Medical College and Research Institute (KMC RI), Hubballi, Karnataka, India

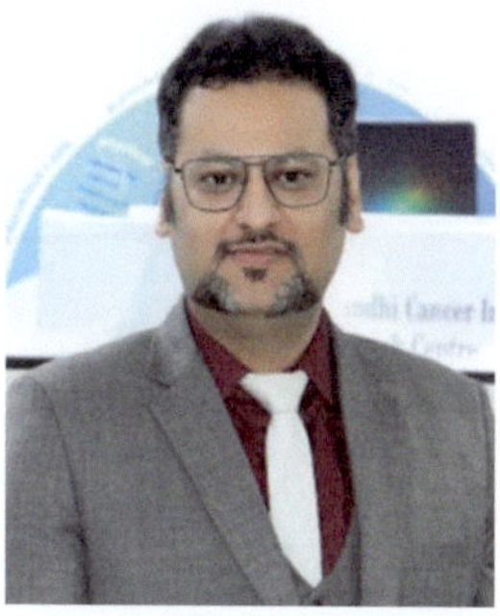

Sunny Malik Department of Pain and Palliative Medicine, Rajiv Gandhi Cancer Institute and Research Centre, New Delhi, India

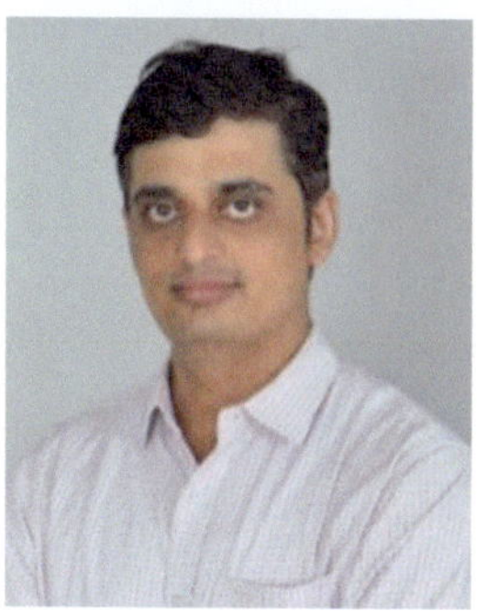

Milon Mitragotri Department of Anaesthesiology, Karnataka Institute of Medical Sciences, Hubballi, Karnataka, India

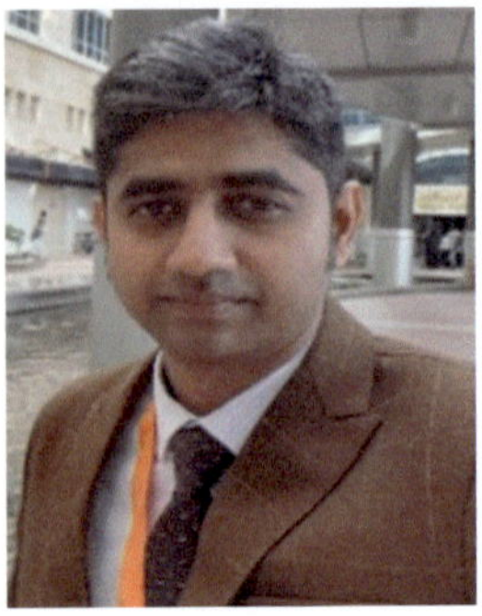

Mohammad Omar Department of Anaesthesiology, Mediclinic Hospital, Abu Dhabi, UAE

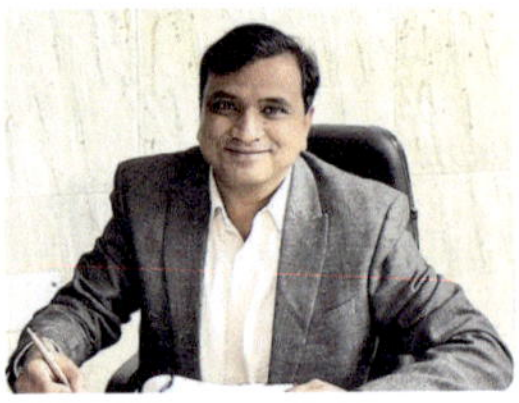

Mukesh Kumar Prasad Department of Anaesthesiology, Teerthanker Mahaveer Medical College and Research Centre, Moradabad, Uttar Pradesh, India

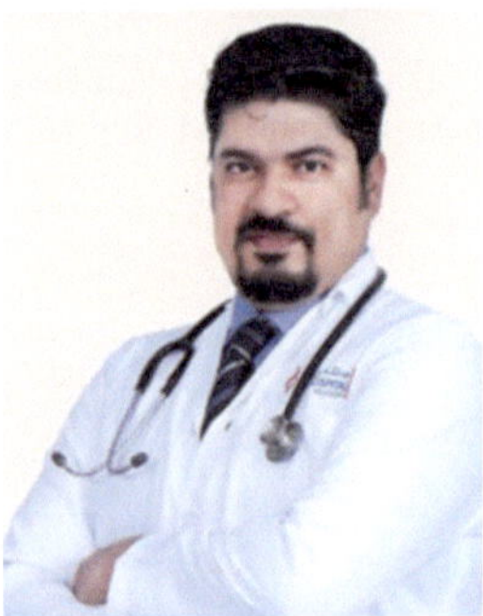

Pulak Puneet Department of Anaesthesiology, Lifecare Hospital, Abu Dhabi, UAE

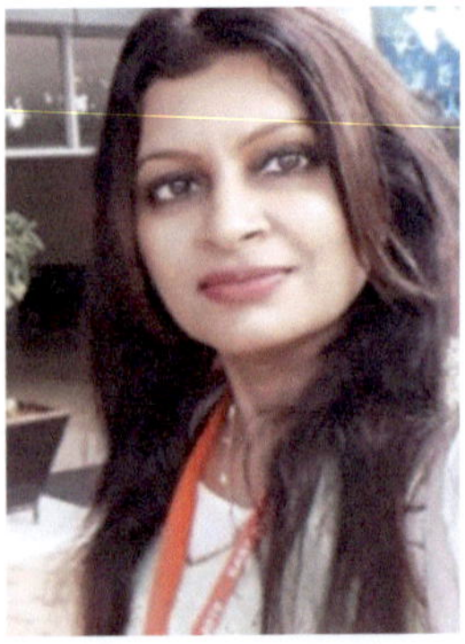

Kanchan Rani Department of Obstetrics and Gynaecology, Teerthanker Mahaveer Medical College and Research Centre, Moradabad, Uttar Pradesh, India

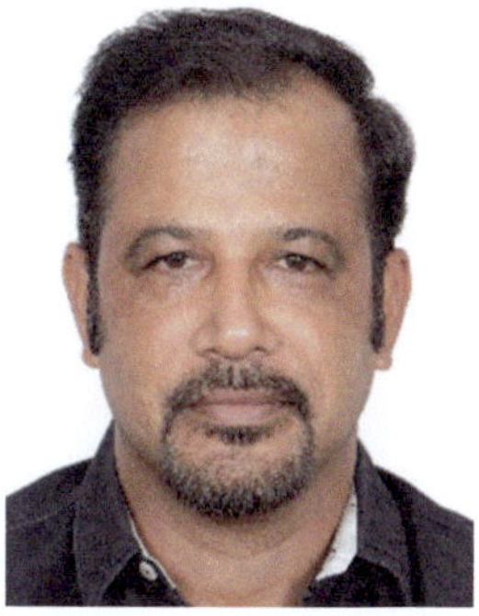

Ritesh Roy Department of Anaesthesiology and Pain medicine, CARE Hospitals, Bhubaneswar, Odisha, India

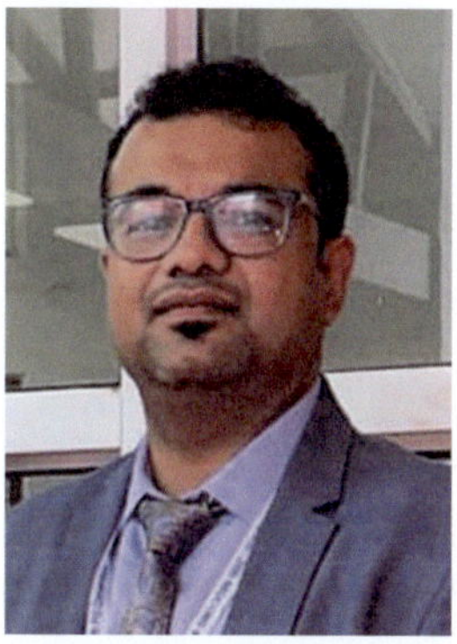

Vibhu Ranjan Sahni Department of Pain and Palliative Medicine, Rajiv Gandhi Cancer Institute and Research Centre, South Delhi, New Delhi, India

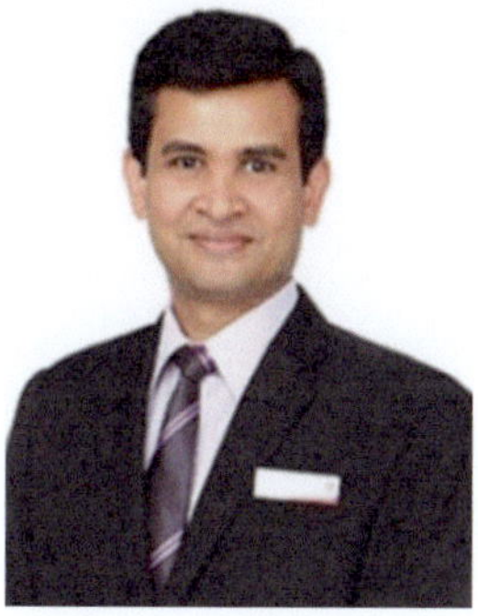

Ashish Ranjan Satapathy Department of Anaesthesiology, Ng Teng Fong General Hospital (NUHS Jurong Campus), Singapore, Singapore

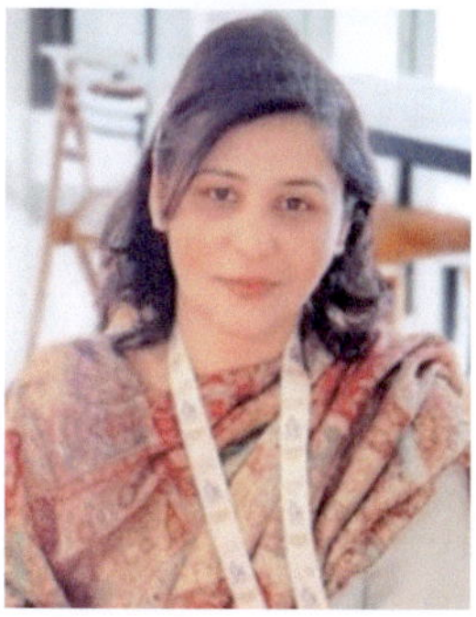

Ridhima Sharma Department of Anaesthesiology and Critical Care, AIIMS, Nagpur, Maharashtra, India

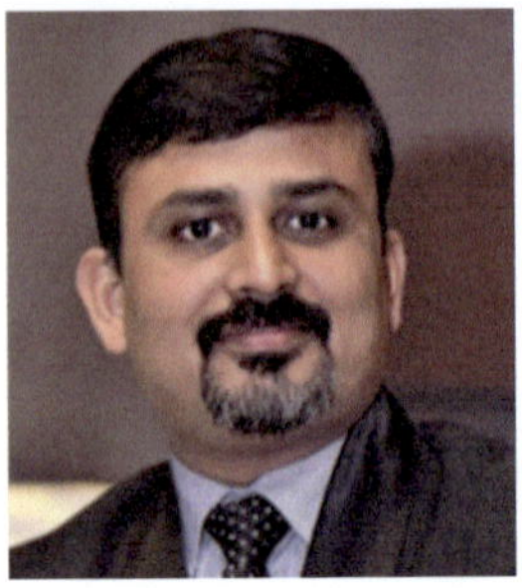

Santosh Kumar Sharma Department of Anaesthesiology, AIIMS, Gorakhpur, Uttar Pradesh, India

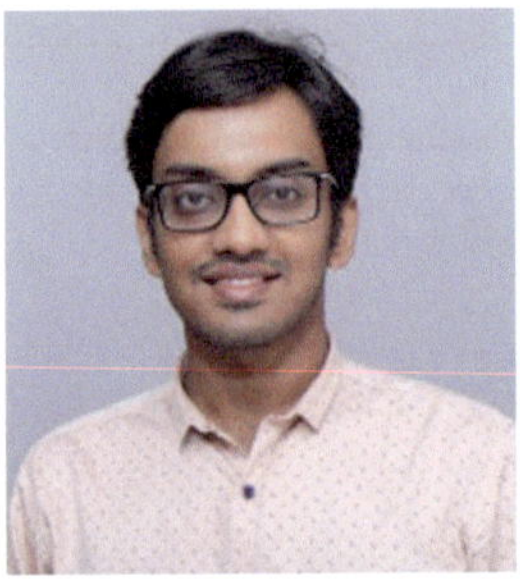

Kaushic A. Theerth Department of Neuronaesthesia and Critical Care, Medical Trust Hospital, MG Road, Ernakulam, Kerala, India

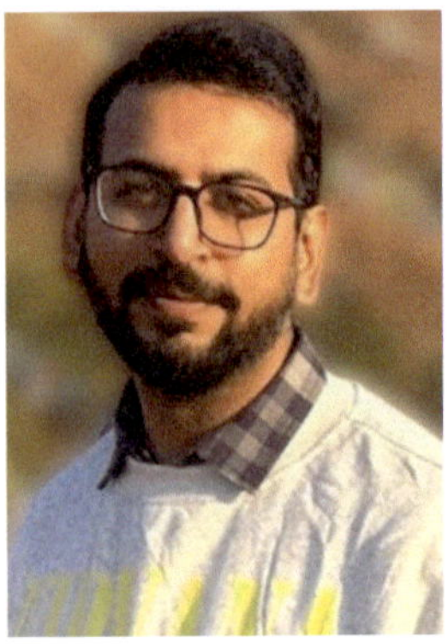

Ankit Verma Department of Anaesthesiology, Teerthanker Mahaveer Medical College and Research Centre, Moradabad, Uttar Pradesh, India

Abbreviations

AA	Axillary artery
ACB	Adductor canal block
ACS	Acute compartment syndrome
ACT	Activated clotting time
AIIS	Anterior inferior iliac spine
AK	Akshu approach
ALP	Alkaline phosphatase
ALT	Alanine aminotransferase
AON	Accessory obturator nerve
AP	Anterior–posterior
aPCC	Activated prothrombin complex concentrate
aPTT	Activated partial thromboplastin time
ARS	Anterior rectus sheath
AS	Anterior scalene
ASA	American Society of Anesthesiologists
ASIS	Anterior superior iliac spine
ASRA	American Society of Regional Anesthesia
AST	Aspartate aminotransferase
ATP	Adenosine triphosphate
AV	Axillary vein
BCRL	Breast cancer-related lymphedema
BF	Biceps femoris
BMI	Body mass index
C	Celsius
CA	Caudal anesthesia
CAIT	Compressed air injection technique
CCBPB	Costoclavicular brachial plexus block
CC	Cardiovascular collapse
cc	Cubic centimeter
CCS	Costoclavicular space
CD	Cesarean delivery
CEI	Continuous epidural infusion
CIPCEA	Computer-integrated patient-controlled epidural analgesia
cm	Centimeters
CNN	Convolutional neural network
COPD	Chronic obstructive pulmonary disorder
CPB	Clavipectoral fascia

CPNB	Continuous peripheral nerve block
CrCL	Creatinine clearance
CRPS	Complex regional pain syndrome
CSA	Continuous spinal anesthesia
CSE	Combined spinal epidural
CSE	Continuous spinal epidural
CSF	Cerebrospinal fluid
CT	Computer tomography
CTG	Cardiotocography
CVP	Central venous pressure
CVS/CNS	Cardiovascular system/central nervous system
D5W	Dextrose 5%
dB	Decibel
DCIA	Deep circumflex iliac atery
DDAVP	Desmopressin
DIC	Disseminated intravascular coagulopathy
DIP	Distal interphalangeal
DPE	Dual puncture epidural
DPN	Deep peroneal nerve
DST	Double space technique
DVPRS	The Defense and Veterans Pain Rating Scale
DVT	Deep venous thrombosis
ECG	Electrocardiogram
EDL	Extensor digitorum longus
eg	Example
EHL	Extensor hallucis longus
EI	External intercostal
EMLA	Eutectic mixture of local anesthetics
EMR	Evoked medial response
EO	External oblique
EOLC	End-of-life care
EOP	External occipital protuberance
EpiM	Epimysium
ERAS	Enhanced recovery after surgery
ESM	Erector spinae muscle
ESPB	Erector spinae plane block
FCU	Flexor carpi ulnaris
FDA	Food and Drug Administration
FDP	Flexor digitorum profundus
FFP	Fresh frozen plasma
FIB	Fascia iliaca block
FICB	Fascia iliaca compartment block
FN	Femoral nerve block
FOB	Fiberoptic bronchoscope
FXa	Factor Xa
G	Gauge
GA	General anesthesia
GAN	Greater auricular nerve

Gm	Gluteus maximus
GON	Greater occipital nerve
GPN	Greater petrosal nerve
GPS	Global positioning system
GT	Greater trochanter
HELLP	Hemolysis, elevated liver enzymes, and low platelets
HNC	Head and neck cancer
HR	Heart rate
Hrs	Hours
Hz	Hertz
IC	Iliac crest
ICB	Intercostobrachial
ICBPB	Infraclavicular brachial plexus block
ICN	Intercostal nerve
ICTD	Intercostal chest tube drainage
IDC	Indwelling catheter
IDDS	Intrathecal drug delivery system
IEA	Inferior epigastric artery
II	Internal intercostal
IIIH	Ilioinguinal and iliohypogastric nerve
IM	Intramuscular
Inj.	Injection
INR	International normalized ratio
IO	Internal oblique
IOP	Intraocular pressure
iPack	Infiltration between popliteal artery and posterior capsule of knee
IPE	Iliopubic eminence
IT	Intrathecal
IT	Ischial tuberosity
IU	International unit
IUFD	Intrauterine fetal death
IV	Intravenous
Kg	kilogram
KHz	Kilohertz
LACN	Lateral antebrachial cutaneous nerve
LA anesthetics	Local
LAST	Local anesthetic systemic toxicity
LAX	Long axis view
LC	Longus colli
LCD	Liquid crystal display
LDI	Low dose infusion
LDM	Latissimus dorsi muscle
LDM	Low dose mixture
LFCN	Lateral femoral cutaneous nerve
LIFT	Lateral interfascial triangle
LMWH	Low molecular weight heparin

LON	Lesser occipital nerve
LOP	Limb occlusion pressure
LOR	Loss of resistance
LORT	Loss of resistance technique
LP	Lumbar plexus
LP	Lumbar puncture
LPN	Lateral pectoral Nerve
LS	Linea semilunaris
LSB	Lumbar sympathetic block
LTN	Long thoracic nerve
MACN	Medial antebrachial cutaneous nerve
mA	Milliamperes
MAP	Mean arterial pressure
MAST	Military antishock trousers
MaxL	Midaxillary line
MBCN	Medial brachial cutaneous nerve
mcg	Microgram
MCNA	Medial cutaneous nerve of arm
MCNF	Medial cutaneous nerve of forearm
mEq	Milliequivalent
MFC	Medial femoral condyle
Mg	Milligram
MHz	Megahertz
min	Minute
MIPSI	Minimally invasive pain and spine interventions
ml	Milliliters
MLAC	Minimum local anesthesia concentration
MM	Medial malleolus
mm	Millimeters
mmHg	Millimeters of mercury
MPE	Malignant pleural effusion
MPN	Medial pectoral nerve
MPS	Myofascial pain syndrome
MS	Middle scalene
MVA	Manual vacuum aspiration
NIBP	Noninvasive blood pressure
NMDA	N-Methyl-D-aspartate
NPO	Nil per oral
NRS	Numerical rating scale
NSAID	Nonsteroidal anti-inflammatory drug
NVM	Nerve to vastus medialis
OCIM	Obliquus capitis inferior muscle
ON	Obturator nerve
OOP	Out of plane
ORAEs	Opioid-related adverse effects
OT	Operation theater
PACN	Posterior antebrachial cutaneous nerve

PACSLAC	Pain Assessment Checklist for Seniors With Limited Ability to Communicate
PART	Pressure, alignment, rotation tilt
PBI	Posterior border of Ischium
PCC	Prothrombin complex concentrate
PCEA	Patient-controlled epidural analgesia
PCNL	Percutaneous nephrolithotomy
PDPH	Postdural puncture headache
PE	Pulmonary embolism
PEA	Pediatric epidural analgesia
PEC	Pectoral
PEG	Percutaneous electrode guiding
PENG	Pericapsular nerve group
PeriT	Peritoneum
PIEB	Programmed intermittent epidural boluses
PIP block	Parasacral ischial plane block
PIP	Proximal interphalangeal
pKa	Kilopascals
PL	Pulse length
Pm	Piriformis muscle
PNS	Peripheral nerve stimulator
PNVB	Pudendal neurovascular bundle
pO2	Partial pressure of oxygen
POE	Point of entry
PONV	Postoperative nausea and vomiting
PPF	Pterygopalatine fossa
PPG	Pterygopalatine ganglion
PRF	Pulse repetition frequency
PRS	Posterior rectus sheath
PS	Psoas major
psi	Pound square inch
PSIS	Posterior superior iliac spine
PT	Prothrombin time
PT	Pubic tubercle
PVCs	Preventricular complexes
PVS	Paravertebral space
QL	Quadratus lumborum muscle
RA	Regional anesthesia
RAM	Rectus abdominis muscle
RF	Radiofrequency
RLB	Retrolaminar block
ROTEM	Rotational thromboelastometry
RPF	Retroperitoneal fat
RR	Respiratory rate
RSB	Rectus sheath block
RS	Respiratory system
SAM	Serratus anterior muscle
SAX	Short axis view

SAYGO	Spray as you go technique
SC	Sacral cornua
SC	Subcutaneous tissue
SCM	Sacrococcygeal membrane
SCM	Sternocleidomastoid
SCM	Subcostal margin
SCUT	Supraclavicular upper trunk
SDGA	Saphenous branch of descending geniculate artery
SEA	Superior epigastric artery
Sec	Second
SENs	Sequential electric nerve stimulation
SFA	Superficial femoral artery
SGB	Stellate ganglion block
SH	Sacral hiatus
SHPB	Superior hypogastric plexus block
SN	Sciatic nerve
SP	Spinous process
SPG	Sphenopalatine ganglion
sPO2	Saturation of oxygen
SsCM	Semispinalis capitis muscle
SSN	Suprascapular nerve block
SSS	Single shot spinal
SST	Single space technique
STK	Streptokinase
sTP	Superficial transverse perineal muscle
SubC	Subcoastal margin
SWG	Standard wire gauge
TAA	Thoraco-acromial artery
TAA	Transversus abdominis aponeurosis
TAP	Transversus abdominis plane
TDN	Thoracodorsal nerve
TEA	Thoracic epidural analgesia
TEG	Thromboelastography
TENS	Transcutaneous electrical nerve stimulation
TFP	Transversalis fascia plane
TGC	Time gain compensation
THA	Total hip arthroplasty
THRIVE	Transnasal humidified rapid insufflation ventilatory exchange
TKA	Total knee arthroplasty
TL	Tulgar approach
TLF	Thoracolumbar fascia
TLIP	Thoracolumbar interfascial plane block
TP	Transverse process
t-PA	Tissue plasminogen activator
TPB	Transversus plane block
TPVB	Thoracic paravertebral block
TSGB	Thoracic sympathetic ganglion block
TT	Thrombin time

TTMPB	Transversus thoracic muscle plane block
UFH	Unfractionated heparin
UMB	Umbilicus
US	Ultrasound
USB	Universal serial bus
USG	Ultrasonography
VAS	Visual analog scale
VATS	Video-assisted thoracic surgery
VCH	Vertebral canal hematoma
VIB	Vertical infraclavicular block
VKA	Vitamin K antagonist
vWD	Von Willebrand disease
vWF	Von Willebrand factor
WBC	White blood cell
WFH	World Federation of Hemophilia
WRMD	Work-related musculoskeletal disorder
μg	Microgram

A Peek into Regional Anaesthesia Instruments

1

Payal Jain, Kali Kapoor, and Pratiksha Gogia

Abstract

Regional anaesthesia has stood the test of time. Since its introduction till date it has helped anaesthetists to tide over major obstacles and challenges incurred in day-to-day practice. The beauty of these techniques lies in the diversity it offers in anaesthetizing the complex neural structure created by the Mighty One rendering us all bewildered at the power of a petite needle.

Thus, with ever increasing advancement in regional anaesthesia techniques their is constant improvement in regional anaesthesia equipments as well. In this chapter we have tried to cover the central neuraxial block, peripheral nerve block instruments starting from conventionally basic ones to advanced ones.

Keywords

Equipment · Spinal · Regional anaesthesia · Nerve blocks · Advance

1.1 Introduction

Regional anaesthesia is the cornerstone of today's practice. With ever evolving newer techniques and complexity of cases the need for proper understanding of sophisticated equipment has become the need of the hour.

The tools needed for a neural blockade procedure will change depending on the anaesthetic technique being used. However, advice on the most basic equipment may be helpful to most and can be tailored to the process, patient, and practitioner needs. This chapter will be a journey from past to present and future of the equipment used in central neuraxial block as well as peripheral nerve block.

1.2 Central Neuraxial Anaesthesia Equipment

Central neuraxial anaesthesia is a collective word used for spinal, epidural and caudal spaces anaesthesia. Spinal anaesthesia started way back in 1800. First spinal anaesthesia was administered by August Bier in 1898. Since the last century lots of development & changes have happened in central neuraxial equipment like needle material, diameter, and tips geometry.

P. Jain (✉) · P. Gogia
Department of Anaesthesiology, Teerthanker Mahaveer Medical College and Research Centre, Moradabad, India

K. Kapoor
Department of Anaesthesia, Rama Medical College, Kanpur, India

M. K. Prasad, S. J. S. Bajwa (eds.), *Steps to Successful Regional Anesthesia*,
https://doi.org/10.1007/978-981-97-4098-7_1

1.2.1 Spinal Needle

Hypodermic needle originated in 1859 (Greek origin: "hypo" meaning under and derma, meaning skin).

1.2.1.1 Material

Most spinal needles are made up of stainless-steel alloys, a combination of iron, carbon and chromium.

1.2.1.2 Parts of Needle

Spinal needle has a tip, bevel, orifice, shaft, hub and an introducer needle (Fig. 1.1). These days we use a transparent polycarbonate hub for easier visualization.

Interest in needles has focused primarily on patient safety and comfort, speed of injection, angle of bevel, and the role of needle size in nerve trauma and association with the incidence of Post-Dural Puncture Headache (PDPH). The incidence of PDPH, as well as technical aspects of reliably performing the dural puncture is directly related to needle design.

1.2.1.3 Size

Spinal needle is available in various sizes from 16 to 30 G.

1.2.1.4 Types

Atraumatic needles cause less of PDPH as they slice the fibres of meninges, allowing less leakage of CSF and promoting faster healing (Table 1.1 and Fig. 1.2).

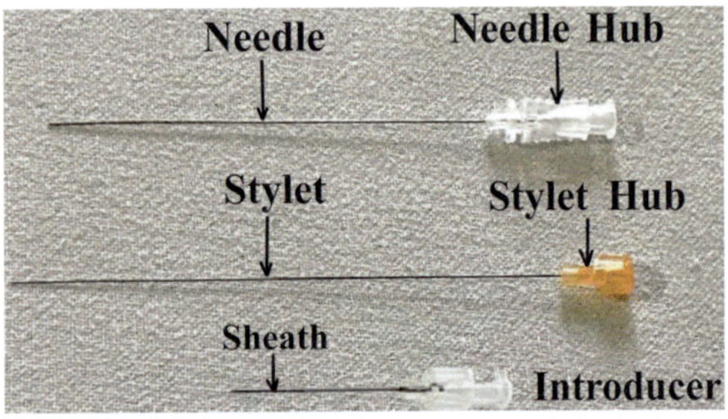

Fig. 1.1 Parts of spinal needle

1.2.1.5 Variations

- **Atraucan needle**—Double bevelled with sharp point for incision and blunt end for dilation.
- **Ball pen**—Pencil point needle with a stylet forming tip.
- **Double orifice pencil point tip by Eldor**—More rapid CSF flow and better distribution of injectate, decreased risk of deformation.
- The distance (1 mm) between the tip and the orifice location of pencil point needles versus cutting needle has been hypothesized to result in a higher incidence of paraesthesia due to deeper needle insertion and the potential to contact the spinal roots or cord.

1.2.1.6 Gauge of Spinal Needle and Colour Coding

Spinal Needle Diameter Spinal needle drives its measure from Standard Wire Gauge (SWG), a guide to measure electrical wires. Currently, accepted gauges were standardized using measuring instruments developed by Holzapffel and Stubs in 1847. As per the approximation taken gauges are multiples of 4/1000 of an inch, with gauge inversely proportional to diameter. The most common gauges of spinal needles used are (Fig. 1.3).

Nomenclature of Spinal Needle—28 G ½ (Number, Gauge Symbol, Length in Inches).

Standard spinal needle is Quincke-Babcock needle. It consists of small hub, medium bevel length with sharp edges, sharp tip, and end injection. The hub consists of a Luer-lock connector.

Tip

1. Needle gauge is inversely proportional to the diameter, more gauge leads to smaller puncture, lesser CSF leakage and reduced incidence of PDPH.
2. Needle bending and deviation (physical flexibility) are more common with lesser diameter needle (lesser deviation is observed when the bevel of the needle is placed 180° to bevel of introducer).

Table 1.1 Comparison between different types of spinal needles

Property	Whitacre (atraumatic)	Quincke (traumatic)	Greene (atraumatic)	Sprotte (atraumatic)	Pitkin (traumatic)
Tip of needle	Solid end drawn to pencil point. Conical elliptical shaped (22–27 G) (length 90–119 mm)	Sharp point (18–27 G) (length 89 mm)	Rounded tip (20–26 G)	Pencil point Elongated tip (20-27G). Conical elliptical tip	Sharp point (20–22 G)
Bevel type	Non-cutting bevel	Cutting bevel	Non-cutting medium-length bevel with matching stylet	Side injection	Short, blunted bevel with matching stylet with 45° taper
Opening of bevel (orifice location)	Side of the needle; 2–4 mm proximal to tip of needle	Tip of the needle (lesser chances of failed spinals)	Tip of needle (end injection)	Lateral large size orifice	End injection
Advantages	Less likely to injure vessels and nerves Tissue separating Less chance of PDPH	Loss of tissue triggering inflammatory reaction Cuts through the tissues and ligaments—insertion easier and smooth	Separate dural fibres, less incidence of PDPH	Larger orifice provides faster CSF and injectate flow Less chance of PDPH	Cuts through the tissues and ligaments—insertion easier and smooth
Disadvantages	Can require more force to puncture tissues and lack the steering ability, which consequently increases procedure time	Higher incidence of PDPH Less tactile feedback Increased risk of nerve damage Increased chances of tip occlusion	Spinal nerve injury (accidental needle-tip contact)	Does not puncture the skin freely. Incomplete block due to loss of drug in subdural space	Dura cutting needle, traumatic

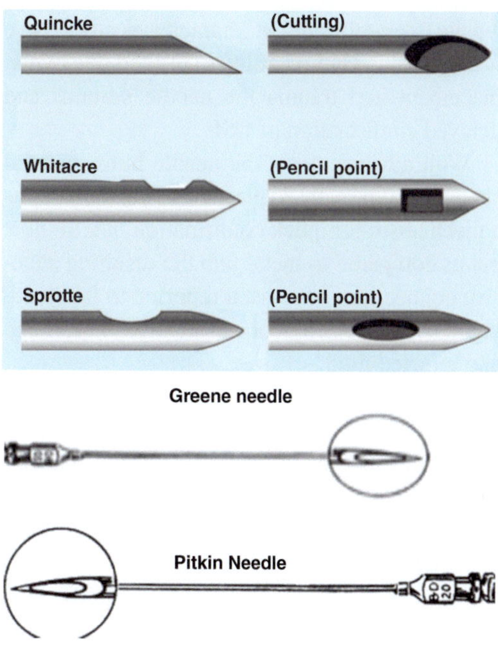

Fig. 1.2 Different kinds and tips of spinal needle

3. Deflection is more seen with cutting tip needles with increased tip angles.
4. One should be careful while using the long-bevel disposable needles. The metal with which these needles are made is too soft, thus when such a needle strikes bone, the tip develops hook or barb which causes extensive damage to the tissue it passes through. Frequent observation and wiping of the tip of the needle across sterile gauze will allow recognition of this problem. Moreover, as a dictum needles that are bent or otherwise deformed should be discarded for a neural blockade procedure and a new needle should be used.
5. Smaller needles have slow rate of fluid from them.
6. The use of a needle with a security bead at its proximal shaft has been advocated to preclude loss of broken needles.

Fig. 1.3 Different gauges of spinal needle

OD (mm)	GAUGE	COLOR & CODE	90mm
0.40	27G	Grey	
0.45	26G	Brown	
0.50	25G	Orange	
0.55	24G	Purple	
0.60	23G	Blue	
0.70	22G	Black	
0.80	21G	Green	
0.90	20G	Yellow	
1.10	19G	Cream	
1.20	18G	Pink	

Nomenclature of Spinal Needle- 28 G ½ (Number, Gauge Symbol, Length in Inches).

7. Needle should be close fitting with removable stylet, preventing skin and adipose tissue from blocking needles and possibly entering the subarachnoid block.
8. Bevel of needle should be redirected longitudinally to decrease the incidence of PDPH.
9. The commonly used smaller needles are passed through a large gauge introduce, and have an obturator which should always be in place when the needle is advanced, as it confers structural rigidity, which reduces the chance of tip shearing.
10. Orifice size has to be smaller so not to compromise tip stability and possibility of orifice straddling the epidural and spinal spaces simultaneously. Like Gertie Marx needle which has appropriate size orifice in comparison with Sprotte and Whitacre.

1.2.1.7 Spinal Needle Length

Accurate selection of LP needle is important to optimize patient care. Selecting a needle that is too short subjects the patient to unnecessary trauma with an excessive number of attempts and duration of procedure. Selecting a needle that is too long increases the technical difficulty of the procedure. There are four formulas derived for the same.

Bonadio et al—Depth of LP (cm) = 0.77 cm + 2.56*BSA (m^2).

Craig et al—LP depth (cm) = height (cm)*0.03.

Henretig and King—Premature infants and term newborns to 2 years old—1.5 in. needles.

3–12 years—2.5 in.

>12 years—3.5 in.

Abe formula-LP depth (cm) = 1 + 17 * weight/height.

1.2.1.8 Material

Most spinal needles in current use are made of stainless-steel alloys, a combination of iron, carbon, and chromium, and since the 1960s were designed to be single use. Due to improvement in tensile strength smaller diameter needles have been produced but its utility is limited due to displacement and trauma the needle sustains and delayed confirmation of CSF.

With advancements the needle hubs material changed from metal to plastic (polycarbonate) as a mechanism for quick confirmation of CSF flow but as compared to metal hub the resulting adhesive connections have been reported to fail, leading to needle detachment and leakage of aspirated and injected fluid.

Comparative effects of spinal needle

1. As needle gauge increase, shaft diameter decreases.

   Pros—smaller puncture, less CSF leakage and a reduced PDPH chance.

   Cons—Increased technical difficulty, higher failure rate, needle shaft deviation and bending is more.

1.2.2 Spinal Catheters

Intrathecal therapy allows releasing drugs directly into the cerebrospinal fluid eluding first pass metabolism and Blood Brain Barrier Filter, leading to reduction in doses as well as limited interaction with systemic receptors. (Fig. 1.4).

1.2.2.1 Indications

Cancer pain, chronic pain (failed back surgery syndrome, lumbar post laminectomy syndrome, complex regional pain syndrome 1 and 2), severe spasticity (IT Baclofen).

1.2.2.2 Contraindications

Refusal by patient, coagulopathies, immunodepression, limited life expectancy (<3 months), epidural metastases, heart disease, cerebrovascular disease, poor efficacy against headaches and facial pains.

1.2.2.3 Drugs

Morphine, ziconotide and baclofen are approved by FDA for intrathecal administration. However, hydromorphone, fentanyl, sufentanil, bupivacaine, clonidine used alone or in combination have been recommended by Polyanalgesic Consensus Conference.

1.2.2.4 Device

Programmable pump: It contains and infuses drug via a dedicated software and algorithm. It is a mechanical pump.

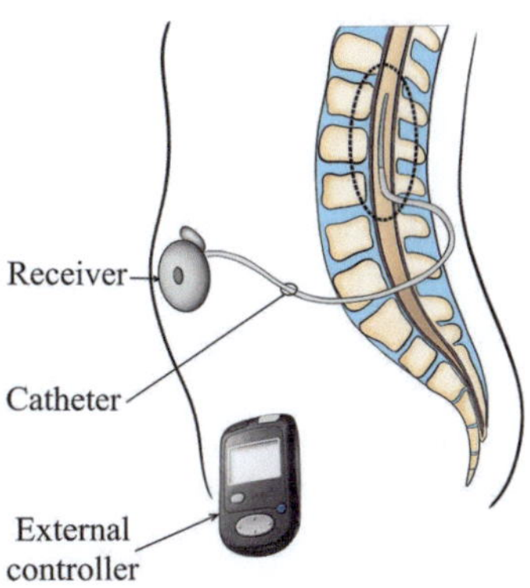

Fig. 1.4 Spinal catheter with programmer

1.2.2.5 Catheter

Positioned in intrathecal space like a 24-gauge epidural catheter through a 19-gauge Tuohy needle; a 28-gauge microcatheter through a 22-gauge spinal needle; a 22-gauge spinal catheter over a 27-gauge spinal needle through an epidurally placed 18-gauge Crawford needle.

1.2.2.6 External Device (Programmer)

It allows an extra dosage of medication when needed.

The pump is powered by a lithium battery with an average life span of 5–7 years. It is a mechanical pump equipped with an antenna allowing communication to programmer via computer. Pump has a drug reservoir with capacity of 20–40 mL and the reservoir can be refilled with a thin needle introduced through the skin. The reservoir should be refilled every 6 months (FDA recommendation). The pump has different drug delivery modes:

(A) Continuous (fixed) mode—Delivers drug continuously for 24 h.
(B) Flexible infusion mode—Clinician can change the daily dose as per requirement.
(C) Patient controlled analgesia—Patient can administer "on demand" prefixed dose in addition to continuous dose.

1.2.3 Broken Spinal Needle (Fracture Spinal Needle)

1.2.3.1 Choice of the Needle

1. There is higher likelihood of damage with smaller needles during insertion. Needle shaft, tip deviation, bending and trauma are all common with smaller needles.

   (Tip—Needles are less likely to get damaged if manufacturer specified introducer is used).
2. Atraumatic needles are more likely to be chipped or roughened whereas Quincke needle is likely to bend. It is extremely important because on withdrawal of needle from subarachnoid space, a damaged tip can lead to jagged tear in dura, increasing the risk of postdural puncture headache.

1.2.3.2 Technique

1. Commonest reason for spinal needle breakage is due to impact on bone or resistance due to rigid ligaments/capsules.
2. Needle redirected without withdrawal to superficial tissues.
3. Manipulation of needle after stylet has been removed.

Tip

1. While repositioning the needle, stylet, introducer, and spinal needle should all be withdrawn as one unit to superficial tissue.
2. Keep stylet inside the needle while manipulation as it makes needle function as solid metal shaft, making it resistant to fracture.
3. The spinal needle via epidural needle technique can be used for more support of the spinal needle.
4. Ensure patient's optimal position, if difficult spinal landmarks USG use is recommended.
5. If difficult spinal puncture consider using atraumatic smaller gauge needle with larger diameter, that are less vulnerable to breakage.
6. Never manipulate or reposition spinal needle through the introducer without mobilizing it.
7. Always advance small diameter needle with stylet in situ.
8. If more attempts needed, replace the needle for a new one.
9. Don't continue the puncture if abnormal resistance or a bone contact.

1.2.4 Epidural Needle

1.2.4.1 History

The first intentional administration of epidural anaesthesia began when two French physicians, Jean Anthanase Sicard and Fernand Cathelin injected drug through sacral hiatus to treat severe intractable sciatica pain in patients.

1.2.4.2 Types of Epidural Needles

1. **Tuohy (1945) needle** (Fig. 1.5): A curved bevel needle tip was created by renowned American anaesthesiologist Edward Boyce Tuohy. This made it easier to insert catheters in the epidural space in either a caudal or cephalic manner. It is a hollow hypodermic needle.

   The most common epidural needle used for punctures and insertion of catheters is the Tuohy epidural needle. It is available in 16 G and 18 G, 10 cm long and 15 cm long, blunt level tip to help push away the dura and gentle curve at 15–30° for insertion of catheter. It has calibrated marking for depth insertion, 3 cm from tip and then 1 cm each five markings (Lee centimetre markings). Thus, it is 11 cm long with 8 cm needle length and 3 cm hub assembly. It is a thin-walled needle to allow insertion of catheter. Its tip is known as Huber tip. It is provided with stylet for introduction and has wings (Macintosh wings) at its hub for better control and handling.

   In combined spinal technique 26 G spinal needle of length 12 cm is used along with 16 G Tuohy's needle. The disadvantage of the tip is that a catheter that has been passed beyond this needle tip cannot be withdrawn without the risk of being sheared off.

   *A 19 G needle of 5 cm for paediatric use has 0.5 cm surface markings. A 21 G catheter can now pass because of this.

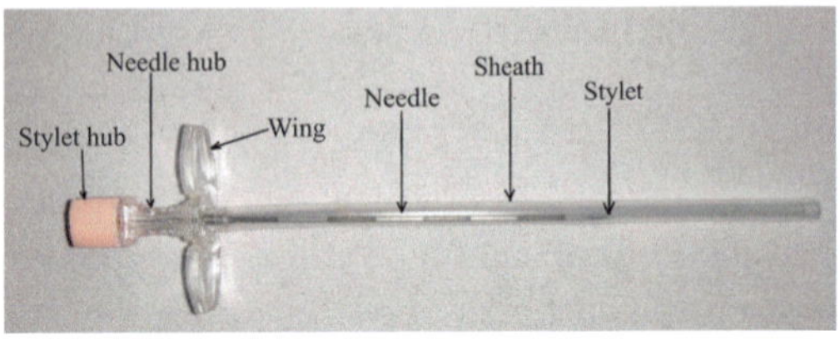

Fig. 1.5 Tuohy needle

2. **Sprotte (1989) atraumatic epidural Tip**: It has conical tip needles to conduct the continuous epidural procedure. In order to guide the catheter through the lateral hole, a plastic edge to the needle's inner distal face was added.
3. **Crawford:** It is a straight needle, which is thin walled with short conventional bevel with smooth edges (Fig. 1.6). It is sometimes used for paramedian approach, as it slides off the lamina easily and a catheter can thread if an

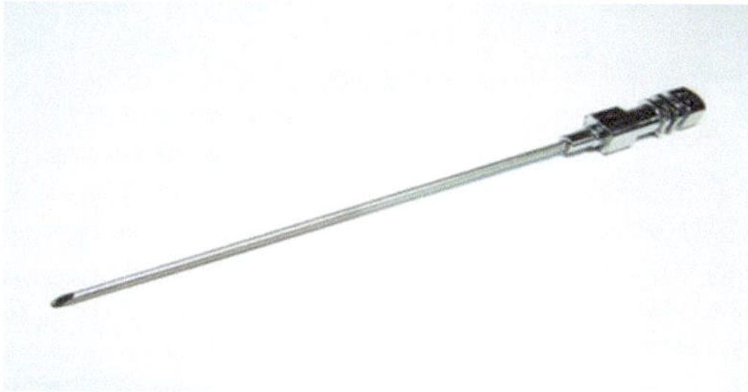

Fig. 1.6 Crawford needle

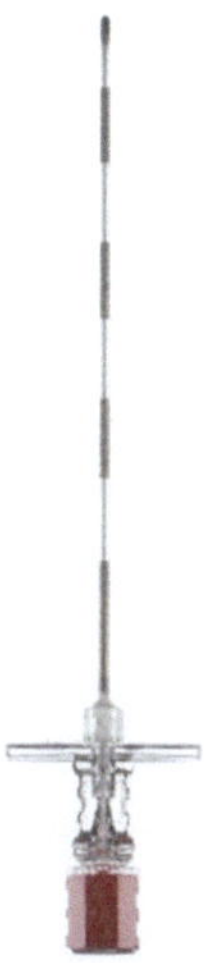

Fig. 1.7 Hustead needle

angle of 45–60° is used to enter the space. It is a thin-walled needle with higher incidence of dural puncture.

4. **Hustead needle:** Further modifications of Tuohy needle with needle opening not exceeding 2.7 mm in length. Needle tip is bent at an angle of 12–15° (Fig. 1.7). The heel of the needle bevel was smoothened to reduce the danger of epidural catheter cutting while withdrawing.
5. **Weiss needle:** It is a newer disposable epidural needle with Tuohy Huber configuration, it has metal wings to improve the hand grasp (Fig. 1.8).
6. **Portex needles:** Available in sizes 16G (light blue) and 18G (dark blue). (Fig. 1.9).

All epidural needles are supplied with closed fitted stylet made up of plastic to prevent tissue entering the lumen on insertion.

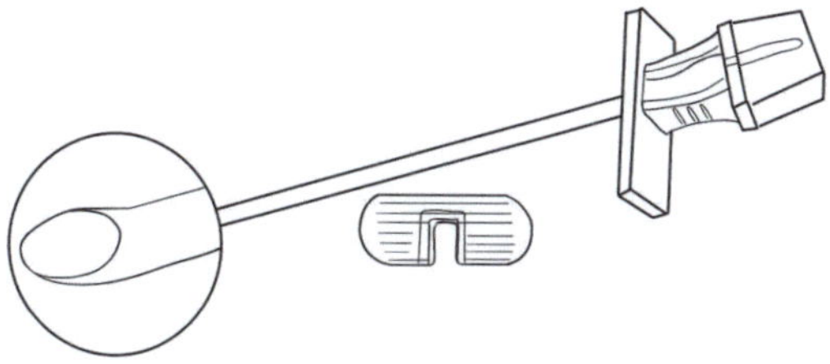

Fig. 1.8 Weiss needle

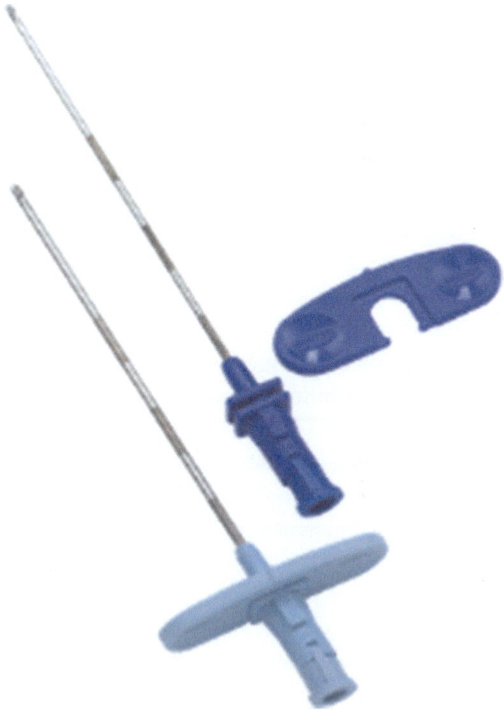

Fig. 1.9 Portex needle

1.2.5 Epidural Catheter

- Epidural catheters can be passed via the epidural needles because of their design. It was first described by Flowers et al. in 1949.
- It is radio opaque constructed from polytetrafluoroethylene—extremely low coefficient of friction that facilitates catheter placement, a high melting point minimizing thermolability and a great tensile strength and is biologically inert (Fig. 1.10).
- Tip is rounded, atraumatic, and has lateral apertures (3*120° eyes) in addition to a closed end (to avoid dural trauma).

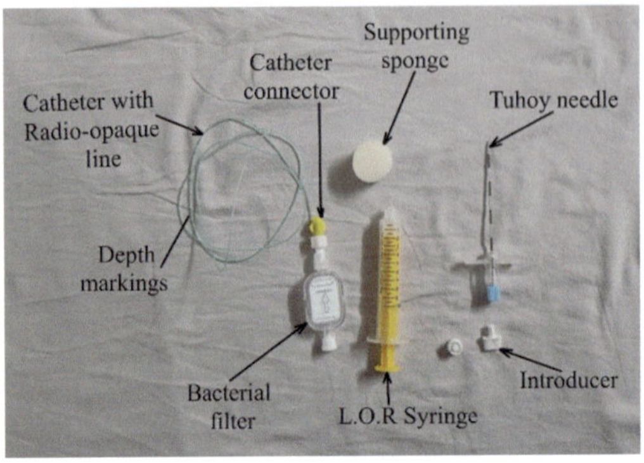

Fig. 1.10 Epidural set with catheter

- It is 90–100 cm long malleable and transparent catheter with marks at 5, 6, 7, 8, 9, 10, 15, and 20 cm from the tip.
- Available catheter sizes include 16 G, 18 G, 19 G, and 20 G, which can be introduced in corresponding larger gauge needle.
- Micron mesh filter is attached to proximal end for bacteria and foreign body, 0.22 μm in size and is hydrophilic. It should be replaced every 24 h.
- Luer-lock cap is present on the connector.
- 3–5 cm should be the maximum amount of catheter advancement into the epidural space.
- The catheter may transect if the catheter is removed after it has past the Tuohy needle's bevel. Therefore, it is safe to remove the catheter and needle concurrently.

1.2.5.1 Wire-Reinforced Catheters

Wire-reinforced catheters are most recent technological advancement in epidural catheter design. The inner wire coil is designed to provide sufficient columnar strength for insertion, lumen patency and kink resistance, surrounded by either a polyurethane or nylon blend catheter. These are designed with fewer coils in the distal tip to confer greater flexibility to minimize paraesthesias and perforations of the dura and epidural vessels.

A low friction syringe made up of plastic, glass or combined glass and metal is used to aid in the identification of epidural space using loss of resistance technique.

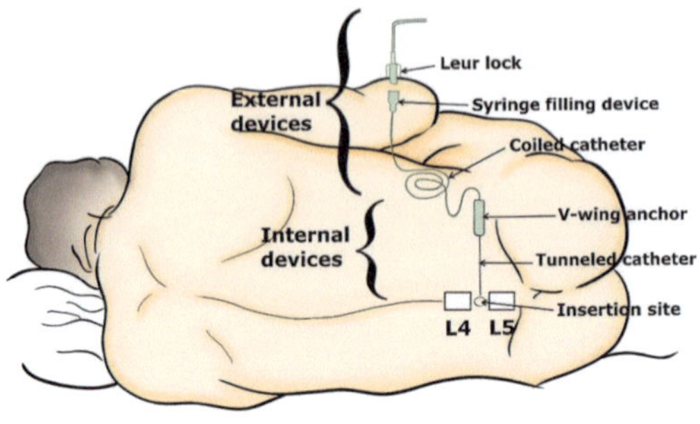

Fig. 1.11 Continuous epidural catheter

1.2.5.2 A Continuous Epidural Catheter

Continuous epidural catheter is also used especially in chronic pain management or for postoperative analgesia (Fig. 1.11).

1.2.6 Types of Combined Spinal-Epidural Needles

*There are two techniques of giving CSE: (a) Single space technique (SST), (b) Double space technique (DST).

1.2.6.1 Conventional Set

A 16 G Tuohy needle through which 26 G spinal needle (12 cm) can pass through (needle-through-needle technique, SST) or 18 G epidural needle (1.2 cm longer than the spinal needle) and a 27 G (Whitacre spinal needle-through-needle) needle, with an epidural catheter of 20 G (Fig. 1.12).

It may lead to several complications: Rotation of the Tuohy needle to increase the distance between the dural puncture site and the insertion of the epidural catheter may lead to dural tear by the Tuohy needle.

Friction between two metal needles can damage the point of the spinal needle and generate metal fragments, which may be introduced epidurally or spinally.

1.2.6.2 Double-Lumen Needles

A Tuohy needle is equipped with a parallel tube that acts as a guide for a thinner spinal needle.

There are two types:

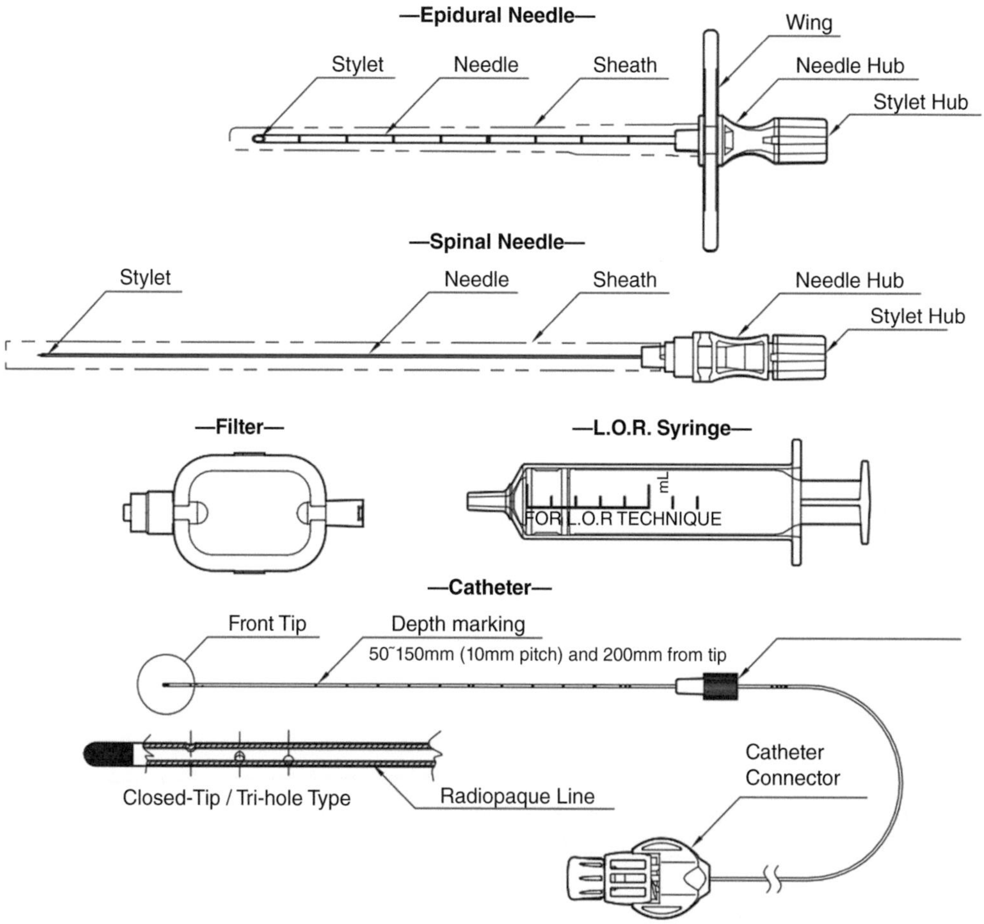

Fig. 1.12 CSE set

1. **A bent parallel tube**—It consists of a curved 20- to 22-gauge spinal needle of the same length as the Tuohy needle (Fig. 1.13).
2. **The straight tube** is fixed on the side of a Tuohy needle; the point of the guide is situated 1 cm behind the eye of the Tuohy needle (Fig. 1.14).

Advantages

(a) It allows insertion of the epidural catheter before positioning the spinal needle. Thus, rotation of the Tuohy needle in situ is unnecessary, and the possibility for a spinal placement of the catheter is diminished.
(b) Avoidance of bending of the spinal needle when it leaves the eye of an ordinary Tuohy needle.

Disadvantage

Friction between the two needles, especially when the bent introducer is used.

1.2.6.3 *Portex "Secure" CSE Needle

This epidural needle includes marks on its hub that start at 0 and go up to 15 mm in 0.5 mm increments. On the marks are written even numerals. The hub of the spinal needle has similar notches. It contains a locking mechanism on its hub to stop spinal needle displacement during medication injection, preventing failure or patchy block (Fig. 1.15),

1.2.6.4 CSE Tuohy Needles with Additional Aperture

It involves the use of a 17-gauge Tuohy needle with an additional aperture situated at the end

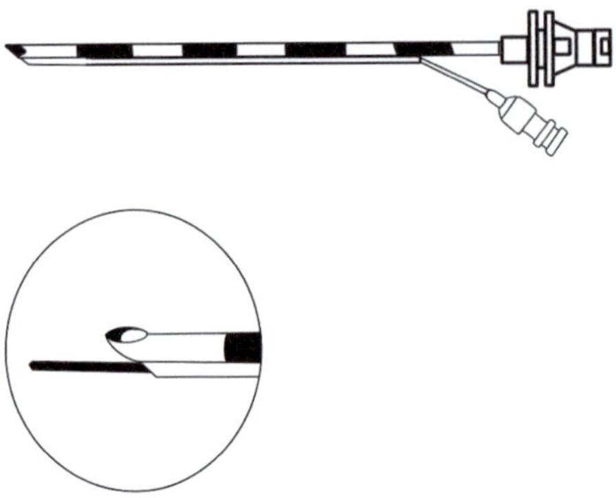

Fig. 1.13 Double-lumen Tuohy needle with curved tube. A 22-gauge needle welded to an 18-gauge Tuohy needle. The guiding needle allows introduction of a 27-gauge spinal needle. The epidural catheter can be inserted before dural puncture

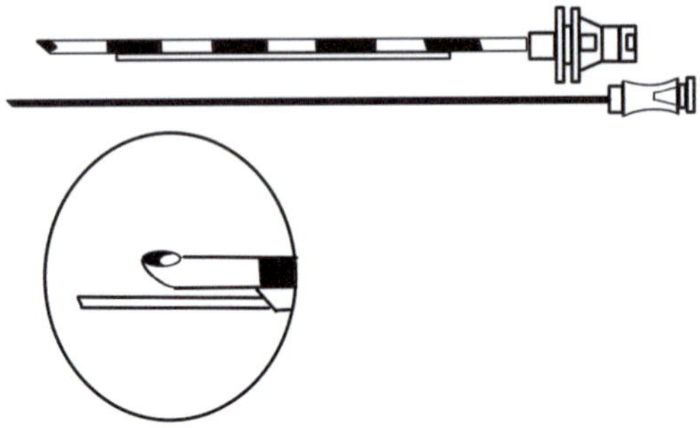

Fig. 1.14 Double-lumen Tuohy needle with straight tube. A short 20-gauge guide tunnel welded onto the lateral side of an 18-gauge Tuohy needle. A 25-gauge spinal needle can be inserted through the guide. The epidural catheter can be inserted before dural puncture

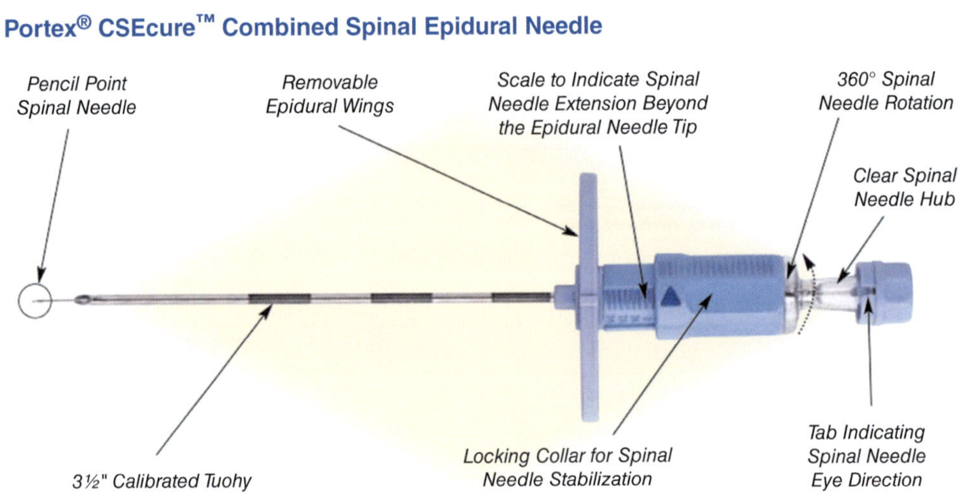

Fig. 1.15 Long 25-gauge spinal needle inserted through a 17-gauge Tuohy needle previously placed in the epidural space. The spinal needle leaves the Tuohy needle through the Huber aperture

of the longitudinal axis (back eye) through which spinal needle can be introduced facing the same way as the Huber opening of the Tuohy needle. After dural puncture, the spinal needle is withdrawn and the epidural catheter introduced through the usual Huber opening. (Fig. 1.16).

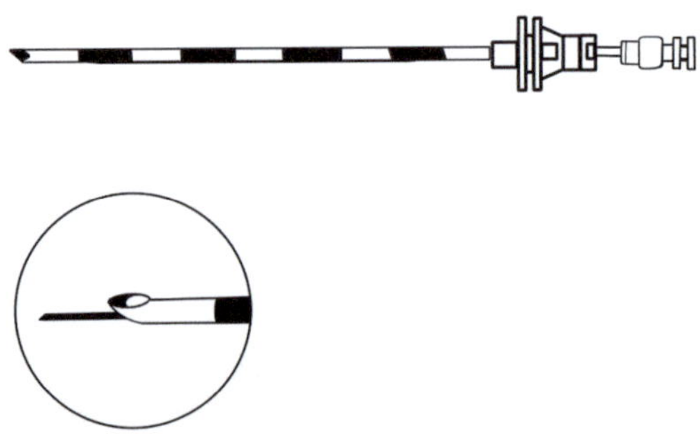

Fig. 1.16 Tuohy needle with additional aperture ("back eye"). A 17-gauge Tuohy needle modified with an aperture in the distal curve, allowing passage of a 26-gauge spinal needle. The epidural catheter leaves the Tuohy needle through the Huber aperture

Advantages

(a) Suitable introducer for even the thinnest spinal needle, as kinking and friction in the Huber eye of the Tuohy needle is avoided.

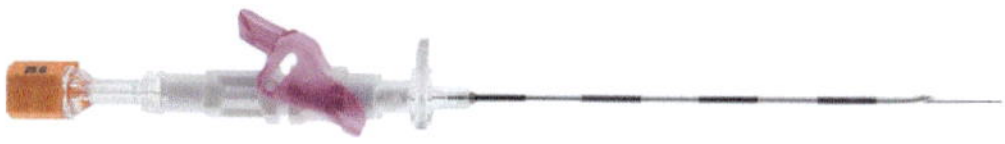

Fig. 1.17 EpiSpin lock

1.2.7 EpiSpin Lock

It is a CSE kit using atraumatic Sprotte needle and continuous epidural catheter placement using the Tuohy needle. The unique feature is the integrated locking mechanism that stabilizes the spinal needle while reducing the risk of a needle displacement (Fig. 1.17).

1.3 Peripheral Nerve Blockade Equipment

1.3.1 Peripheral Nerve Stimulators

(Fig. 1.18)

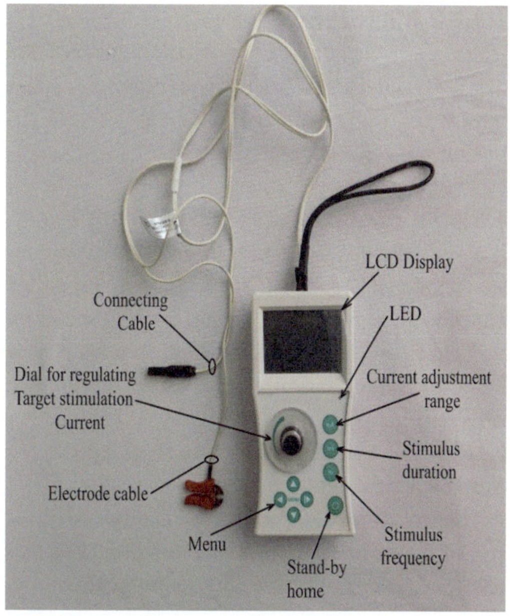

Fig. 1.18 Peripheral nerve stimulator

1.3.2 Ideal Electrical Characteristics of a Peripheral Nerve Stimulator

1.3.2.1 Constant Current Generator

The current between the anode and cathode of the nerve stimulator is kept constant regardless of the impedance or resistance of the tissue surrounding the nerve since nerve stimulators are made to be constant current generators.

1.3.2.2 Current Waveform

Use should be made of a current square wave that is monophasic and has a rapid ascent. Current only moves in one direction.

1.3.2.3 Pulse Width

With a small pulse width, such as 50–100 s, alpha fibre chronaxies are induced, which results in muscle twitches rather than pain. The perfect combination for activating a nerve with a motor response that is not painful for the patient is low intensity current with a short pulse width.

1.3.3 Safety Features

It should be possible to receive notifications for malfunction, low battery, impedance, and circuit disconnection. To prevent confusion about which lead is the cathode and which is the anode, leads should be clearly identified. Stimulators in contemporary machines can only be connected to the cathode of nerve stimulators. If a constant current nerve output stimulator is employed, it is irrelevant where on the patient's skin the anode is attached. It is preferable to use stimulators that can only produce low-output stimulation and cannot detect neuromuscular blockage. This is due to the fact that stimulators made for neuromuscular monitoring operate at currents that are significantly greater than necessary and are not advised for localizing peripheral nerves. The existence of this characteristic can greatly increase confusion.

1.3.4 Nerve Stimulator Components

1.3.4.1 Clock Reference

The nerve stimulator's synchronization system serves as the clock reference. A crystal oscillator generates a precise, high-frequency clock signal.

1.3.4.2 Microcontroller

It serves as the most crucial component of the nerve stimulator. A low power microcontroller must be chosen because the majority of stimulators are powered by batteries.

1.3.4.3 Constant Current Generator

It is also known as the reference current. No matter what impedance (or resistance) load is attached to a constant current source, it should still produce the same amount of current. A perfect continuous current source is not feasible in real-world applications.

1.3.4.4 Controls

A common nerve stimulator typically has three sets of controls: frequency, pulse width, and current. Every control, whether analogue or digital, raises or lowers the value of the controlled parameter.

1.3.4.5 Current Reference Generator

It is based on a low tolerance digital potentiometer that is controlled by the microcontroller using a series of command pulses that direct it to increase or decrease the value, as well as a precisely known voltage source.

1.3.4.6 Display

Standard liquid crystal displays (LCDs) are more common than light emitting diode displays because they consume less current and are more adaptable. The majority of displays display the current, frequency, and pulse width values. Additionally, some models might also have displays that show aberrant impedance, needle disengagement, and low battery levels.

1.3.5 Clinical Pearls While Using a Nerve Stimulator

The best skin electrodes ought to be used. To make sure the conducting gel is present and hasn't dried up, the skin electrode needs to be visually and physically inspected.

When the circuit is finished, there is typically an indicator (a flashing light or auditory sound). To confirm this and that the set current is being delivered, one should periodically check the LCD indicator while administering the block.

1.3.6 Recent Developments in Nerve Stimulation

Recent developments like percutaneous electrode guiding (PEG) and sequential electric nerve stimulation (SENSe) may be able to address some of the drawbacks of traditional nerve stimulators.

1.3.6.1 Sequential Electric Nerve Stimulation

The majority of nerve stimulators work with fixed pulse durations (0.1 ms or 0.2 ms). There are new neural stimulators that can change the pulse duration, but you can only use one set pulse duration at once. Conventional electrical stimulation has been done by continuous adjustment of current amplitude at a single, set pulse duration (conventionally, 0.1 ms). It is a novel technique for nerve location by utilization of a peripheral-nerve stimulator (PNS) programmed to deliver sequential electrical nerve stimuli (SENS).

1.3.7 Transcutaneous Nerve Mapper

A nerve-mapping pen (Fig. 1.19) can be used to locate superficial nerves (up to a maximum depth of approximately 3 cm) with transcutaneous nerve stimulation before the nerve block needle is inserted especially for teaching purpose or

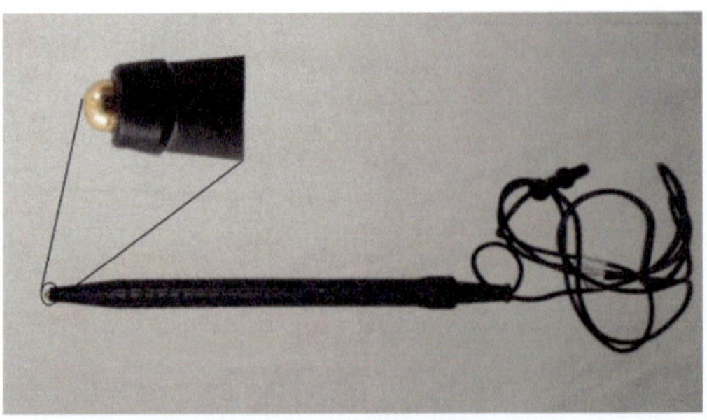

Fig. 1.19 Nerve mapper (transcutaneous)

patients with difficult anatomy. It should be noted that longer stimulus duration (e.g.-1 ms) is needed to accomplish transcutaneous nerve stimulation, as larger energy is required to elicit a motor response from the neural structures transcutaneously, (5 mA at minimum, 12 kΩ output load). The electrode tip of the pen should have an atraumatic, ball-shaped tip. The conductive tip diameter should not be larger than approximately 3 mm to provide sufficient current density and spatial discrimination, which may not be the case with larger tip diameters.

1.3.7.1 Percutaneous Electrode Guidance

Percutaneous electrode guidance combines transcutaneous nerve stimulation (nerve mapping) with nerve block needle guidance. It consists of a small aiming device mounted and locked on a conventional peripheral block needle. Once the best response is obtained, the needle is advanced through the skin in the usual fashion, and the remainder of the apparatus continues to stabilize the needle and guide it towards the target. The device also allows the operator to make indentations in the skin and tissue so that the initial distance between the needle tip at the skin level and the target nerve is reduced, and the nerve block needle has less distance to travel through tissue. The technique allows for prelocation of the target nerve(s) prior to skin puncture (Fig. 1.20).

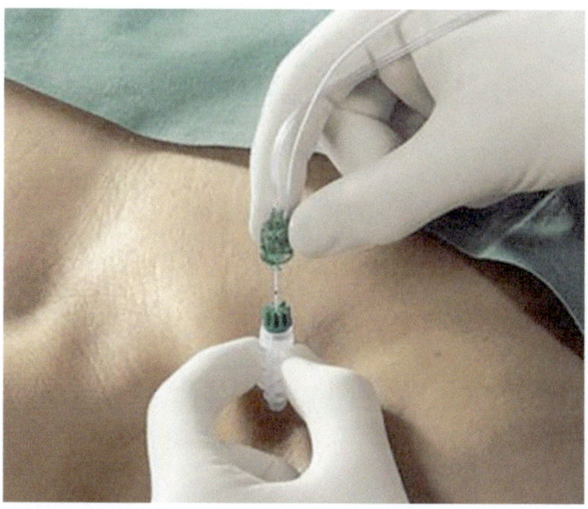

Fig. 1.20 Percutaneous nerve guidance

1.3.8 Regional Block Needles

Insulated needles were first used for peripheral nerve blocks by Pearson.

Montgomery and associates showed that uninsulated common needles could potentially also be utilized to pinpoint increased current in the nerves.

Insulated needles are coated throughout, with the exception of the tip, with a layer of nonconducting material (such as silicon or polytetrafluoroethylene). There are needles with pin-point electrode tips where the shaft and bevel are both coated and just the tip conducts current, improving localization accuracy.

Commercially available needles for single-shot nerve blocks usually come with pre-attached extension tubing to facilitate aspiration and injection of D5W or local anaesthetics and feature a female attachment for connection to a nerve stimulator (Fig. 1.21), One should note that the Luer-lock for the attached tubing may occasionally be loose, which can lead to leakage of injected local anaesthetic as well as air on aspiration.

1.3.8.1 Needle Designs

The practitioner's choice of needle depends on the type of block used, the patient's size, and personal preference.

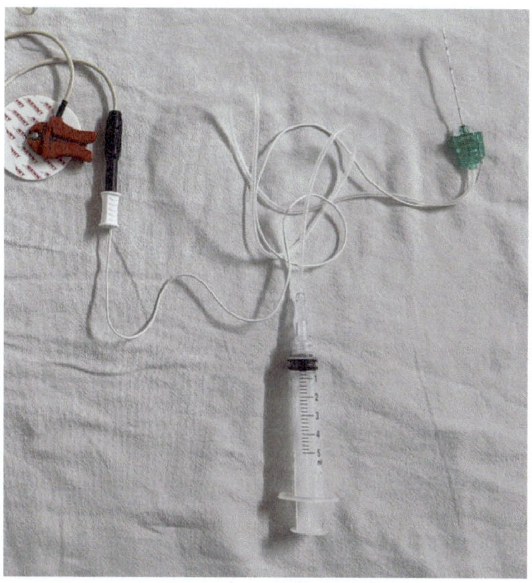

Fig. 1.21 Peripheral block needle

1.3.8.2 Parts of the Insulated Needles

A pleasant finger grip is placed at the needle's proximal end, and a wire connecting the needle to the stimulator is attached to the shaft, which is insulated save for the tip.

This wire contains a suitable connector for the nerve stimulator and is attached to the needle shaft.

The needle normally has a bevel ranging from 15° to 45° with different brands and manufactures; this helps the injection of local anaesthetics and also allows for the early identification of blood.

Centimetre markings on the needles make it easier to gauge the distance between the needle and the skin.

1.3.8.3 Needle Tip

The pencil-point or short, blunt-bevel needle designs are the most popular needle-tip designs because they are said to result in fewer damage during nerve blocks.

Workers still make arguments for choosing between long bevel (cutting, sharp) and short bevel (blunt, pencil-point) needles despite the research.

1.3.8.4 Needle Length

The choice of needle length depends on the type of block, ultrasound can help to judge the trajectory of the needle to the nerve to be blocked.

Needles should have depth markings for monitoring of the depth of penetration into the tissue.

The correct needle length (shortest possible) will allow for better handling and manipulation.

1.3.8.5 Needle Gauge-22

Gauge needle is the most commonly used. Larger Gauge needles tend to cause more tissue injury but can be directed easily whereas smaller gauge needles have more chances of intrafascicular injury and bend easily and also it takes longer time for blood to get aspirated.

Whether the block is single shot or continuous, the patient's profile and availability all affect the needle gauge choice.

1.3.8.6 Echogenic Needles

Echogenic needles reflect ultrasound beams through a variety of mechanisms, including a special coating that traps micro-air bubbles, grooves near the needle tip, or echogenic "dots" made by "cornerstone" reflectors. Needles with enhanced echogenicity may reduce visualization time during ultrasound-guided procedures (Figs. 1.22 and 1.23).

1.3.9 Continuous Catheter Assemblies

Catheter-over-needle assemblies have been gaining popularity for delivering continuous regional anaesthesia and analgesia more than catheter through needle design.

With catheter-through-needle assemblies, a gap is left between the skin and the catheter on the removal of the needle. In contrast, withdrawal of the needle in the catheter-over-needle assembly does not affect the snug fit of the catheter in the skin because the needle is housed inside the

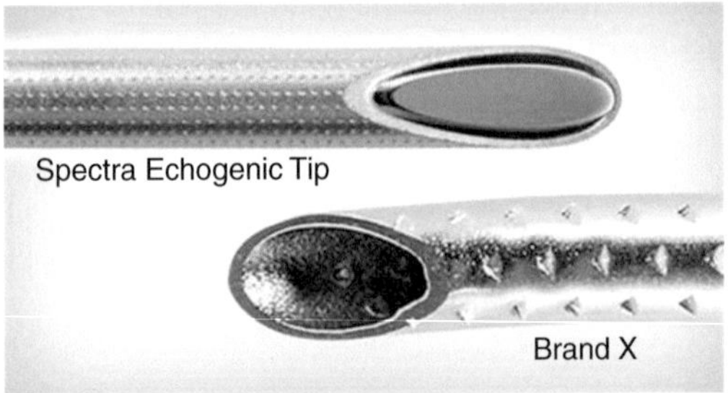

Fig. 1.22 Serrated echogenic needles

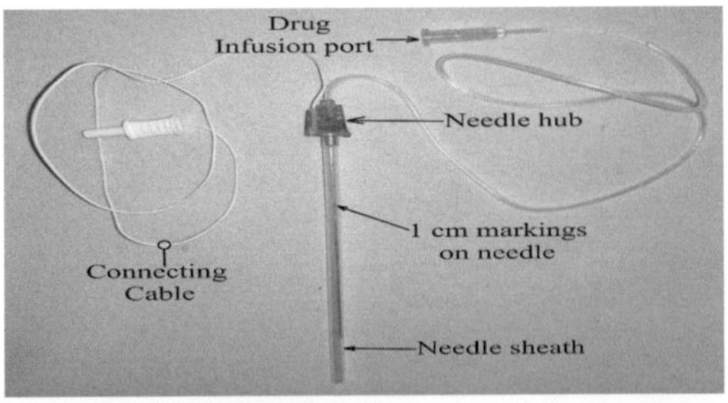

Fig. 1.23 Echogenic needles

catheter, thus decreasing the chances of leakage and migration (Fig. 1.24).

Another recently introduced variation is the E-Cath catheter within catheter design, which features two components, the outer catheter sheath, and the flexible inner catheter, that create a non-kinkable unit.

Several advantages of the catheter-over-needle design include potential:

- Simple to use with an insertion technique compared to that of a single-shot nerve block
- Less leakage from the catheter insertion site, for example, during shoulder surgery when the patient is in a sitting position with potential for surgical field contamination
- Less risk of dressing adhesive disruption
- Fewer steps and less risk of dislodgement
- Easy visualization of the catheter, especially the catheter tip

1.3.10 Injection Pressure Monitoring

Monitoring injection pressure can help distinguish needle-tip location in the perineural tissue versus the needle-nerve contact or intrafascicular needle placement (i.e., perineural vs. intraneural-interfascicular).

High opening injection pressure (≥15 psi)—the pressure that must be overcome before injection can commence—may be indicative of intraneural needle placement, it is important to monitor injection pressure carefully during local anaesthetic injection. Furthermore, high injection pressure can also cause undesired neuraxial spread during certain regional blocks close to the neural axis, for example, lumbar plexus block or brachial plexus block.

Methods of monitoring injection pressure include the following: syringe feel, inline pressure manometer, and compressed air injection technique (CAIT).

1.3.10.1 A Subjective "Syringe Feel"

A subjective "syringe feel" technique has been used to assess resistance to injection of local anaesthetic and is performed by the anaesthesiologist or assistant while the anaesthesiologist maintains the correct needle position.

1.3.10.2 Inline Pressure Manometer

The main principle behind the use of an injection pressure monitor is that a certain amount of injection pressure (opening pressure) must be reached before the injection (the flow of the anaesthetic) can commence. The critical opening pressure necessary to inject local anaesthetic when the needle is in contact with the nerve or is intrafascicular has been estimated in several studies to be more than 15 psi. Therefore, if the injection is halted before the opening pressure is reached and the flow of anaesthetic is initiated, injection in vulnerable needle–nerve interaction can be avoided. Example—Bsmart, Epiguard (Fig. 1.25).

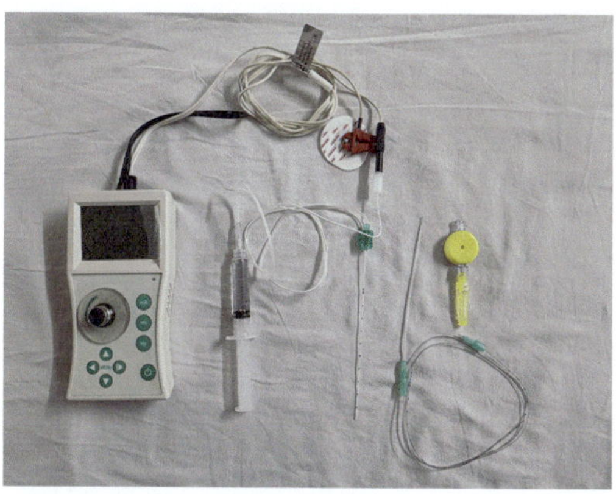

Fig. 1.24 Continuous catheter set

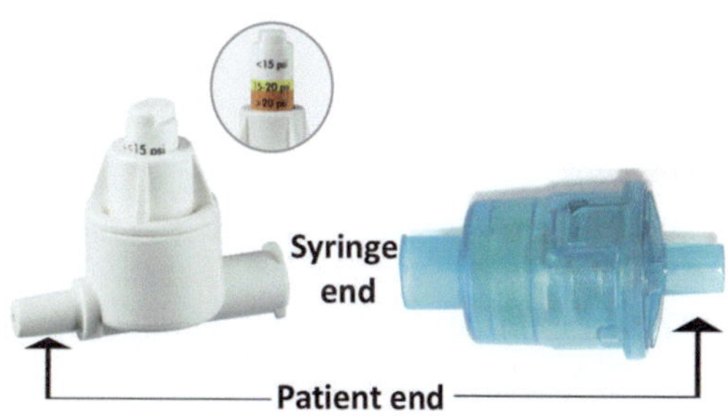

Fig. 1.25 Injection pressure monitors

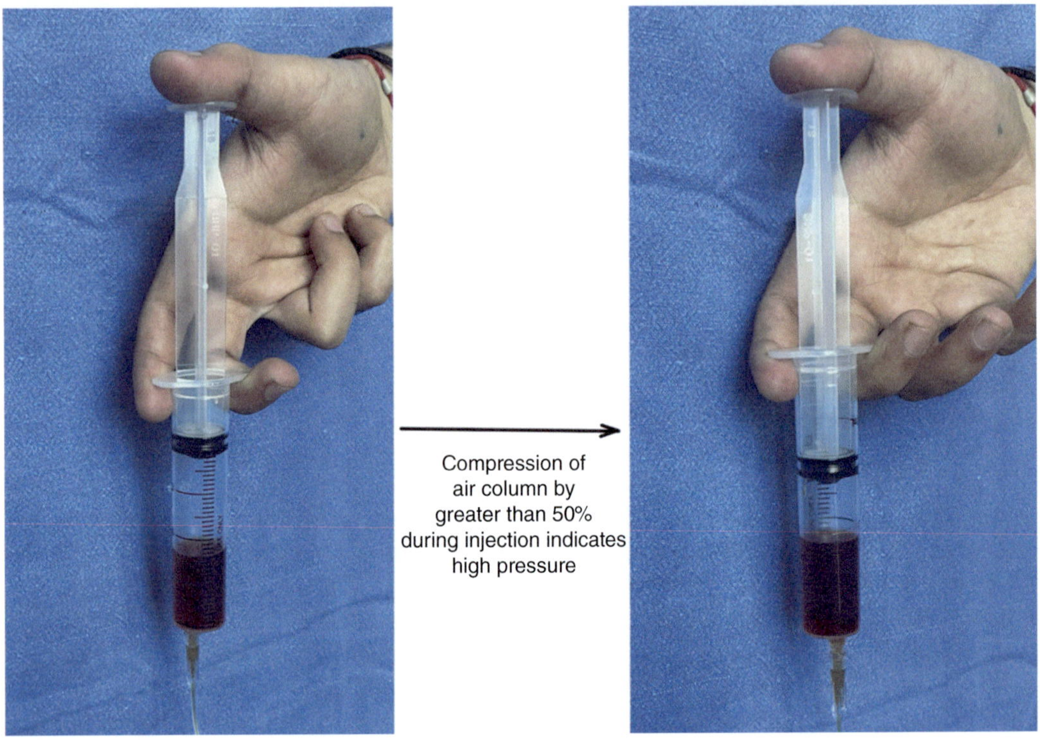

Fig. 1.26 Compressed air injection technique

1.3.10.3 Compressed air injection technique

This is the clinical application of Boyle's law (Pressure × Volume = Constant). At a constant temperature, a set volume of gas (air) varies inversely with the pressure. Technique involves aspirating a set amount of air above a volume of injectate within a syringe. During injection, the volume of air is compressed and maintained at a certain percentage. It involves aspirating a set amount of air above a volume of injectate within a syringe. During injection, the volume of air is compressed and maintained at a certain percentage. (Fig. 1.26).

Advantages

1. It reduces the speed of injection, which in turns.
2. Decreases the risk of intrafascicular injection.
3. Siphoning the local anaesthetic to unwanted tissue planes.
4. The pressures generated by CAIT are stable throughout the injection period. This is likely due to the "cushioning" effect from the volume of air, which dampens the initial high pressure.

1.4 Block Assessment Tools

Tools and scales used to assess sensory and motor block vary greatly and offer subjective feedback on the degree to which a nerve block is achieving its desired goal.

Pain scales or scores are used to indicate a patient's comfort level; as with block-monitoring tools, these scales and scores provide a more objective and reproducible means to assess the severity of pain.

1.4.1 Sensory (Dermatome) Testing

These stimuli are usually temperature based (ice, alcohol swab), but a graded filament can also be used to measure diminishing and returning cutaneous sensation

1.4.2 Temperature/Infrared Recording

The studies showed that infrared thermography of the digits had high positive predictive value for block success following brachial plexus anaesthesia, because of the increase in the temperature (due to vasodilation).

1.4.3 Current Perception Threshold

Current perception threshold (CPT) is a means of applying electrical current via a percutaneous electrode connected to a specialized current generator (e.g., Neurometer) to test sensory level, i.e. if the current required to elicit a sensory response was greater over time than the baseline (pre block or unblocked region) current, this was an indicator of block progression.

1.4.4 Pain Assessment

The numeric rating scale (NRS) and visual analogue scale (VAS) are validated pain rating scale. The Defense and Veterans Pain Rating Scale (DVPRS) has facial cartoons that can be used to obtain feedback on pain severity from individuals with limited communication ability. For elderly patients, the Pain Assessment Checklist for Seniors With Limited Ability to Communicate (PACSLAC) can be used to assess pain in individuals with dementia or cognitive impairment and who have trouble communicating.

1.4.5 Motor Block Assessment

The most common motor assessment tool is the Bromage score, a 4-point scale ranging from 0 (full movement) to 3 (complete block/no movement). Another more objective method that can assess the onset of and recovery from a nerve block is strength testing. This can be performed with a portable force transducer.

Some modern force transducers come equipped with a universal serial bus (USB) stick that, along with a portable computer, allows force data to be collected wirelessly in real time.

1.4.6 Maintenance of Regional Anaesthesia

Regional anaesthesia practice has relied on infusion pumps to provide continuous delivery of local anaesthetic through a perineural catheter.

1.5 Continuous Peripheral Nerve Blocks (CPNB)

It provides a number of advantages in the perioperative period.

1. flexibility to prolong intraoperative and postoperative anaesthesia/analgesia.
2. avoiding the risks and side effects of general anaesthesia.
3. reduced opioid consumption and decreased opioid-related side effects.
4. less hypotension, urinary retention, pruritus, and mobility restrictions.

CPNBs have beneficial effect on postoperative sleep patterns and cognitive function as well as early rehabilitation. CPNBs have historically been relatively underused. This early lack of popularity was multifactorial; however, inadequate CPNB equipment likely contributed.

1.5.1 Continuous Peripheral Nerve Block Equipment Typically Includes the Following

(Figure 1.27)

(a) An insulated, large-bore needle except uninsulated pinpoint area at its most distal tip. (i.e. Tuohy tip) with an integrated stimulating wire to allow nerve stimulation.

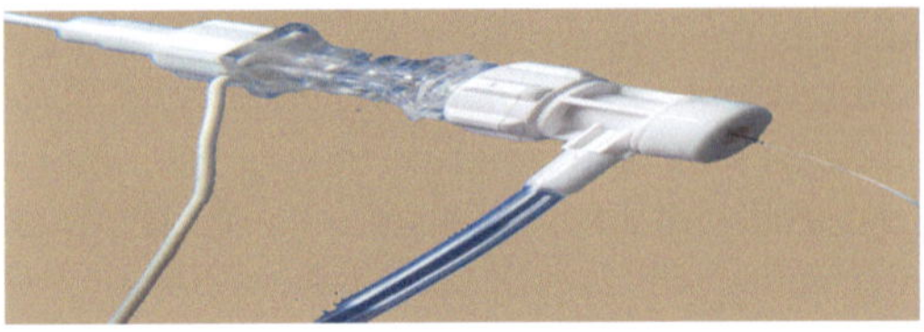

Fig. 1.27 Continuous peripheral nerve catheter

(b) A flexible, atraumatic 20 G multi-orifice (closed distal tip and three distal openings—0.5, 1.0, and 1.5 cm from the tip) catheter that is threaded through the needle into a perineural location.
(c) Some versions incorporate an adapter with a Luer-lock head and a haemostatic valve fitted to the proximal end of the needle. The adapter has a central diaphragm that allows passage of a catheter.
(d) Clear, flexible extension tubing that can be attached to the side arm of the adapter for continuous aspiration of blood and injection of drug.

Tips

1. Catheter used for epidural can be used as they are flexible, non-irritating and provide minimal friction on passage through the needle.
2. These catheters have graduated markings, thus help in deciding the insertion depth and are radio-opaque in nature, thus future visualization can be done.

1.5.2 Stimulating Catheters

A stimulating catheter can confirm perineural location and in comparison with non-stimulating catheters for CPNB it is associated with lower local anaesthetic consumption and reduced requirement for rescue analgesia but it may be more technically challenging to place under ultrasound guidance. The basic mechanism of functioning of stimulating catheter is its ability to conduct current to their distal end.

Use—They were developed as a tool to assess the proximity of the catheter's distal tip to the neural structures and to reduce the likelihood of secondary block failure.

Various Models of Stimulating Catheters Have Been Developed Till Date

Sutherland et al. employed a ureteral catheter (Portex-Boots, Kent, UK) with a metal stylet. The distal tip of the catheter was cut back by 50 mm, and the metal stylet was rethreaded such that it barely protruded. In order to make it easier to connect electrically to the nerve stimulator, the proximal portions of the style and catheter were folded together.

The use of a wire-reinforced epidural catheter was described by another author. They employed a nonferromagnetic stainless steel stylet (Fig. 1.28) (Arrow Theracath®) and a polyurethane (Tecothane®) thermoplastic catheter with an inner steel spring reinforcement for continuous block delivery. A portion of the outer catheter was also removed. A later modification involved the addition of an insulated needle with an inner metal stylet to the set (Fig. 1.29) (StimuCath®, Arrow International). Further revisions resulted in the addition of an alligator clip to allow direct connection to a nerve stimulator.

Kick et al. created a different stimulating catheter (Fig. 1.30) (Stimulong) with a 405-mm indwelling detachable conducting stylet and a 20-gauge, single-hole, 400-mm polyamide catheter. With the exception of the distal 0.3 mm, the metal wire stylet was coated in Teflon insulation the entire way around. A plug on the proximal end allowed attachment to a nerve stimulator.

Many manufacturers have incorporated echogenic features into their CPNB equipment. B. Braun incorporates laser reflectors into the needle of their Contiplex Ultra series (Figs. 1.31 and 1.32). Pajunk catheters are wire reinforced and contain radiocontrast strips at their distal end for better visualization of equipment inserted under ultrasound guidance.

Fig. 1.28 Wire-reinforced epidural catheter with a nonferromagnetic stainless steel stylet

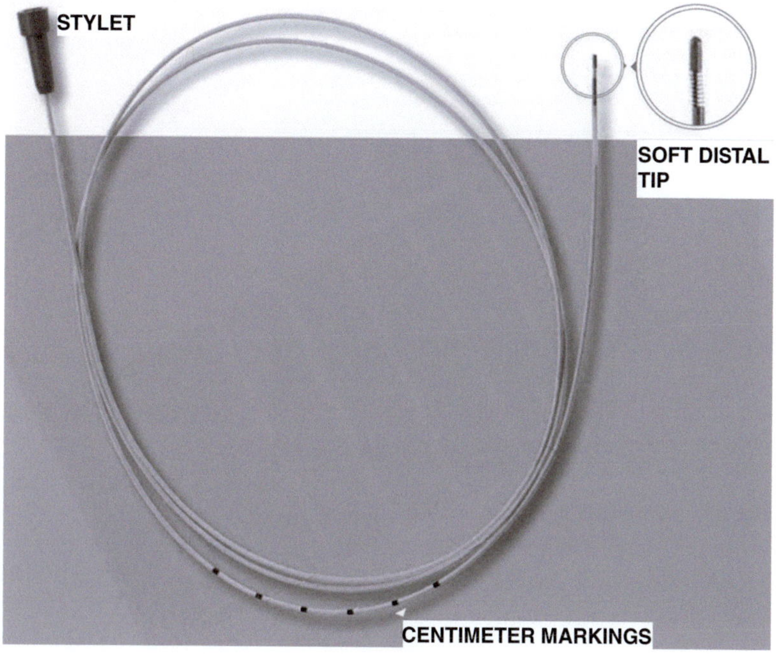

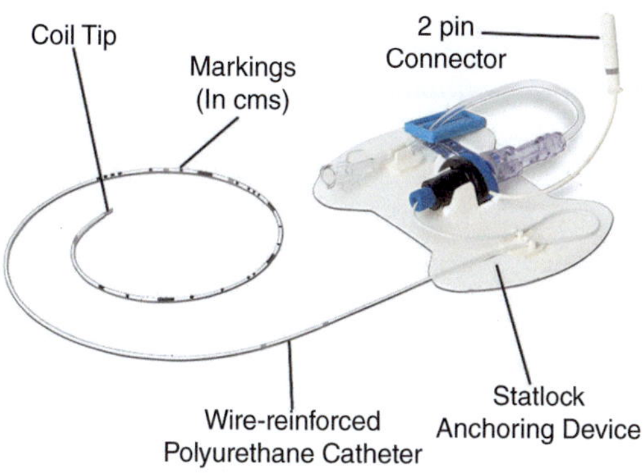

Fig. 1.29 Wire-reinforced epidural catheter with insulated needle and an inner metal stylet

Fig. 1.30 Stimulating catheter with indwelling detachable conducting stylet and a polyamide catheter

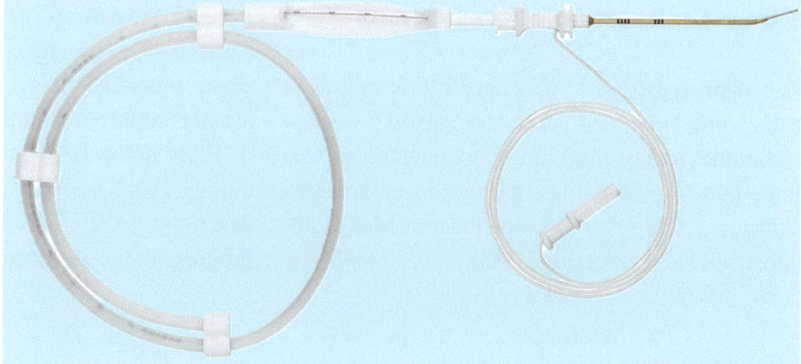

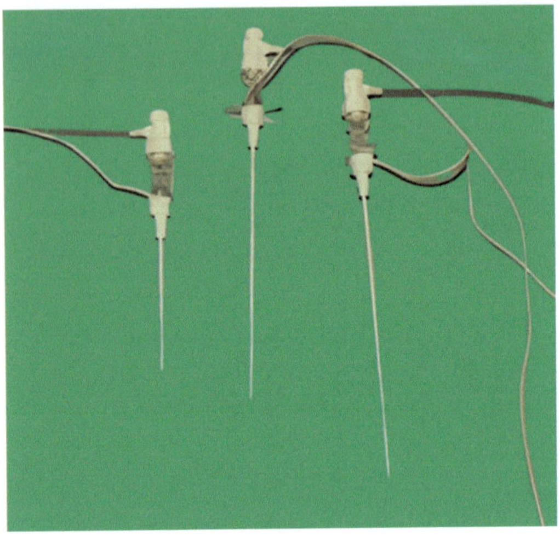

Fig. 1.31 Contiplex Ultra series

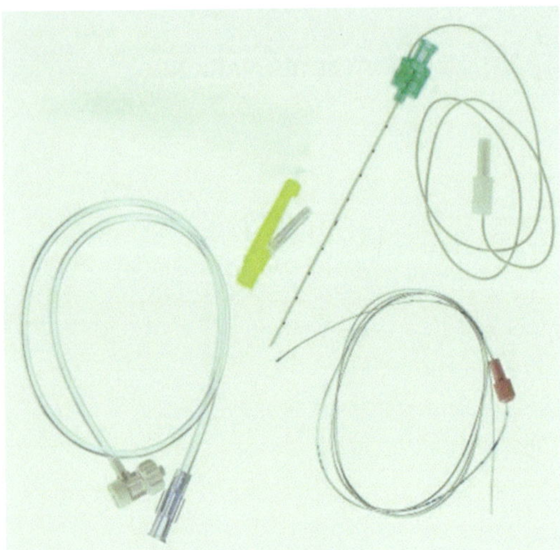

Fig. 1.32 Contiplex peripheral nerve block catheter system

1.6 Catheter Fixation Systems

The main reason for secondary block failure is catheter dislodgement, in order to avoid it various techniques can be used like subcutaneous tunnelling, adhesive dressings fixing the catheter to skin, i.e., Epi-Guard (Copenhagen Med Lab, Glostrup, Denmark) (Fig. 1.33).

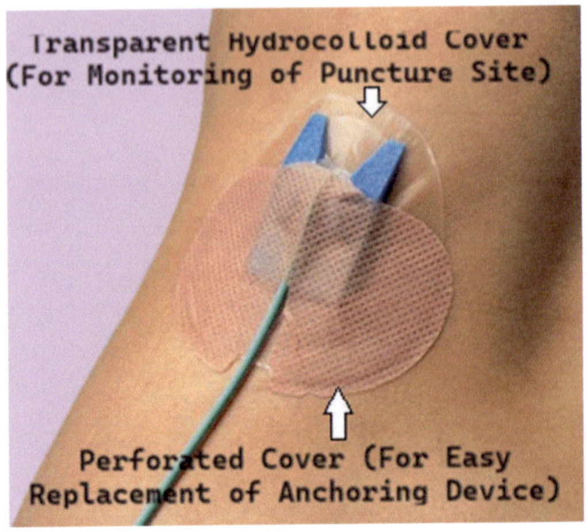

Fig. 1.33 Epiguard fixation device

1.7 Nerve Localization System

Nerves to be blocked can be identified using nerve stimulators, ultrasound, fluoroscopy, fascial clicks and paraesthesia. One of the newest nerve localization techniques involves the use of a global positioning system (e.g., SonixGPS, Ultrasonix, Richmond, BC, Canada). Both the needle and the ultrasound probe contain sensors. As a result, the ultrasound screen displays the predicted needle trajectory and the location where the needle will intersect with the ultrasound beam.

1.8 Ultrasound-Guided Blocks

A very old and well-researched area of anaesthesia is regional anaesthesia. Many years before local anaesthetic was really utilized, in 1848 James Young Simpson examined its advantages. Even before his time, others tried peripheral nerve blockage using antiquated methods like nerve compression and ligation.

Early in the 1970s, the use of ultrasound technology for peripheral nerve blocking was described. As USG technology continued to progress in the 1990s, there was a greater interest in and use of USG guided nerve blocks. The brachial plexus nerve block with various methods and lower extremity nerve blocks like femoral and popliteal nerve blocks are the two most prevalent USG-guided nerve blocks that will be the subject of this chapter.

1.8.1 Basic Principles and Physics of Ultrasound

Piezoelectric Effect

Quartz is one naturally occurring crystal that displays the piezoelectric action. In it, electrical energy is converted reversibly into mechanical energy and vice versa.

When the appropriate electric potentials are applied across many piezoelectric crystals in the transducer of an ultrasonic machine, they enlarge and shrink. They lead to the production of mechanical sound waves that travel through the human tissues as alternating compression and rarefaction zones. The piezoelectric crystals in the transducer vibrate as a result of the reflected sound waves, converting mechanical energy into electric energy, which is then used to produce the image on the ultrasound screen.

1.8.1.1 Characteristics of Ultrasound

Ultrasound is a form of mechanical sound energy that travels through a conducting medium (e.g., body tissue) as a longitudinal wave producing alternating compression (high pressure) and rarefaction (low pressure). (Fig. 1.34).

The frequency of medical ultrasound is in the 2.5–15 MHz range. The speed of sound is assumed to be 1540 m/sec (constant) for most human soft tissues.

The speed of sound (c) = wavelength (λ) × frequency (f). Thus, sound with a high frequency has a short wavelength and vice versa.

Ultrasound waves are generated in pulses (intermittent trains of pressure waves) and each pulse commonly consists of 2 or 3 sound cycles of the same frequency.

Pulse length (PL) It is the distance travelled per pulse.

Pulse Repetition Frequency (PRF) It is the rate of pulses emitted by the transducer (number of pulses per unit time). The PRF for medical imaging ranges from 1 to 10 kHz (Fig. 1.35).

Generation of Ultrasound Image

The pulse wave emitted from the transducer is transmitted into the body, reflected off the tissue interface and the transducer waits to receive the returning wave (i.e. echo, mechanical energy) after each pulsed wave. Then it transforms the mechanical energy into an electrical signal which is processed and eventually displayed as an image on the screen.

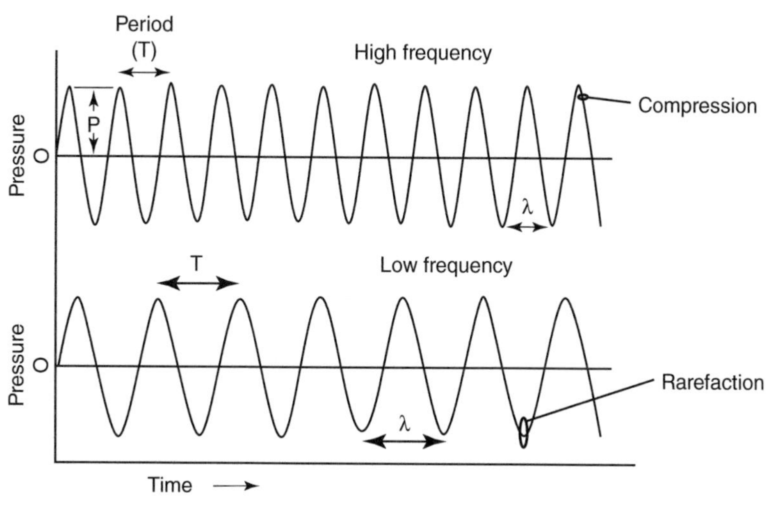

Fig. 1.34 Pressure versus time graph

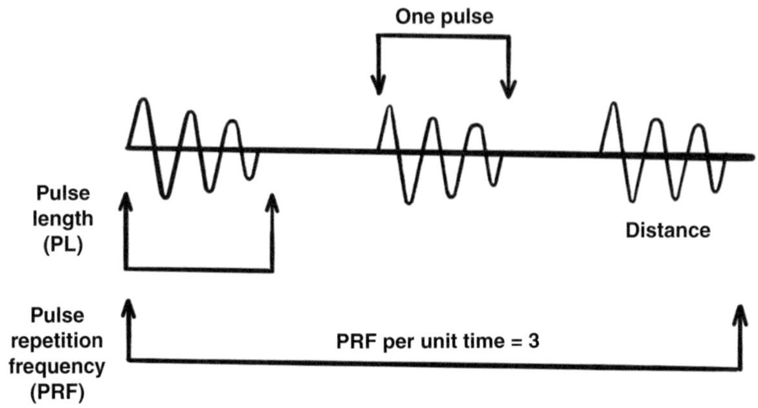

Fig. 1.35 Pulse repetition frequency

The image can be displayed in a number of modes:

1. **Amplitude (A) mode**—It is used to judge the depth of an organ or otherwise assess an organ's dimensions.
2. **Brightness (B) mode**—It is the display of a 2D map of B mode data, the display is called the greyscale.
3. **Motion (M) mode**—It is used for analysing moving body parts commonly in cardiac and foetal cardiac imaging.
4. **Real-time mode (B mode dynamic)**—It is a phased array transducer, most often used to scan abdomen and to check the foetus in pregnant women.
5. **The Doppler mode—**Among the 3 modes, the B mode is most commonly used for ultrasound-guided regional anaesthesia.

Ultrasound Tissue Interaction

The amplitude of the original signal becomes attenuated (energy loss) as the depth of penetration of wave increases. The degree of attenuation varies directly with the frequency of the ultrasound wave and the distance travelled.

Attenuation is due to

1. absorption (conversion of acoustic energy to heat),
2. reflection,
3. scattering at interfaces.

The higher the attenuation coefficient, the more attenuated the ultrasound wave is by the specified tissue, thus limiting the penetration.

In a nutshell- ↑ Frequency = ↑ Attenuation; ↑ Attenuation = ↓ Penetration.

Compensation for attenuation is done by amplifying only the return signals called as the gain. An increase in the overall gain will increase brightness of the entire image.

Preferably, the time gain compensation (TGC) is adjusted to selectively amplify the weaker signals returning from deeper structures to avoid amplification of background noise in return signals.

1.8.2 Machine and Knobology

1.8.2.1 Transducer

It is the ultrasound machine's most crucial component. It establishes the ultrasound image's frequency and resolution. Piezoelectric crystals are present in the transducer in which the piezoelectric action is visible.

Different types of transducers are used for scanning (Fig. 1.36):

1. **Linear:** These are high-frequency transducers and they provide high resolution of the superficial structures. The propagation of the sound wave is in a linear fashion parallel to the surface of the transducer.

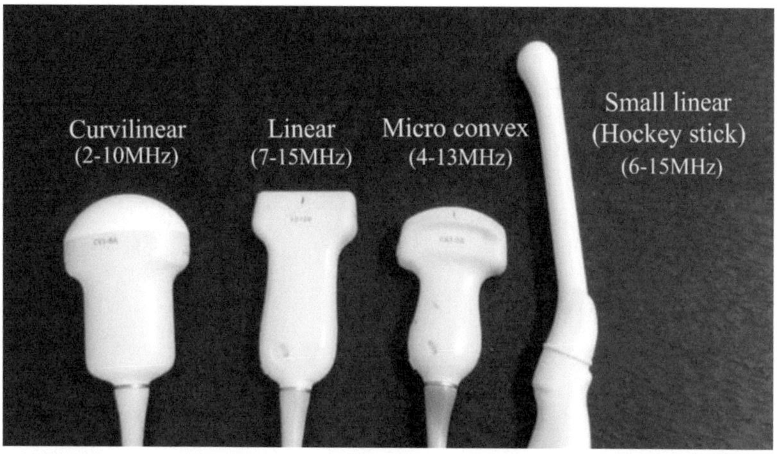

Fig. 1.36 Different types of transducers

2. **Curvilinear:** These are low-frequency transducer which is designed to good resolution of the deeper structures. The propagation of the sound wave is in a divergent fashion so there is an increased field of vision.
3. **Hockey Stick:** These are high-frequency transducer with a small footprint. They are best for visualizing small areas.

1.8.3 Holding the Transducer

It should be held in the dominant hand of the operator, between the thumb and the index fingers. The patient's body should be supported by the little and ring fingers (Table 1.2).

1.8.4 Movements of the Transducer

The transducer can be adjusted in the ways listed below to align the beam perpendicular to the reflective acoustic border and lessen anisotropy artefacts.

Heel-Toe Manoeuvre
It is angling the transducer along its long axis.
Toggling
It is angling the transducer from side to side.

1.8.5 Knobology

1.8.5.1 Frequency

The frequency knobs control the frequency of the emitted sound wave from the transducer.

High Frequency: used to visualize the superficial structures.
Low frequency: used to visualize the deeper structures.

1.8.5.2 Depth

On the left side of the ultrasound machine's screen, it is displayed. Limiting the empty space beneath the image and properly visualizing the intended structure should be changed.

1.8.5.3 Greyscale Gain

The brightness of the image is adjusted using the greyscale gain knob. Without impacting the image's overall resolution, changing the greyscale gain makes the image brighter and changing it darker makes the image darker.

1.8.5.4 Time Gain Compensation (TGC)

Numerous knobs on it can be slid in either the right or left direction. Each knob corresponds to its location on the ultrasound screen relative to another, and the brightness can be individually

Table 1.2 Different types of probe and there application in anaesthesia

Probe	Transducer array and typical size	Frequency	Nominal field depth (max.)	Resolution	Blocks
Linear	Linear 38 mm	6–12 MHz	6 cm	0.5 mm axial 1 mm lateral	Brachial plexus, abdominal wall, femoral and distal sciatic, peripheral nerves, vascular access
Hockey stick	Linear 25 mm	6–15 MHz	6 cm	As above but paediatric applications (small footprint)	
Curved	Curved 60 mm	2–7 MHz	30 cm	2 mm axial 3 mm lateral	Neuraxial, lumbar plexus, proximal sciatic

adjusted at various depths. The image is brighter when all the knobs are moved to the right, and darker when all the knobs are moved to the left.

1.8.5.5 Focus

The focus knob is used to limit the lateral resolution. It is indicated on the side of the screen where depth is indicated by either a small symbol or colour dot. It should be positioned at the same level as the target of interest so that the divergence of the beam is minimized at that particular point.

1.8.5.6 Tissue Echogenicity

The amplitude of reflected echo is represented by the degree of brightness (i.e. echogenicity) of a dot on the display. Combination of all the dots forms the final image.

Hyperechoic—Strong reflections, i.e. increased brightness than surrounding tissues.

Hypoechoic—Weaker lesser echoes thus darker than the surrounding tissues.

Anechoic—No reflections thus producing darker dots.

1.8.6 Appearance of Different Structures in Ultrasound

1.8.6.1 Skin

The superficial and deep layers of the skin appear hyperechoic.

1.8.6.2 Subcutaneous Layer

Due to the hyperechoic connective tissue septa and fat lobules present, it seems to be hypoechoic.

1.8.6.3 Muscle

In ultrasound, muscle displays a hypoechoic with hyperechoic pattern. The surrounding connective tissue, or perimysium, appears hyperechoic, while the muscle fibres in between appear hypoechoic.

1.8.6.4 Tendon

The longitudinal arrangement of the tightly packed collagen fibrils gives tendons a fibrillar appearance. Predominantly hyperechoic if technical artefact (hypoechoic).

1.8.6.5 Nerve

Hypoechoic and hyperechoic echotexture characterizes the nerve. The epineurium is hyperechoic (amount of connective tissue within a nerve), whereas the nerve fascicles are hypoechoic. Nerves below the clavicle and in the lower limbs are predominantly hyperechoic and have a honey comb appearance.

Anisotropy refers to a change in echogenicity of tissues (e.g., tendon and nerve) as a result of transducer angle. A hyperechoic nerve structure can appear hypoechoic when the angle of incidence is changed from 90° to 45°.

1.8.6.6 Bone

The bone has an acoustic shadow and seems hyperechoic. We can spot osteophytes, spurs, and disruptions in the bony cortex with the aid of ultrasound.

1.8.6.7 Veins

When using a transducer to apply light pressure, they appear as an anechoic structure that is nonpulsatile, compressible, and devoid of steady flow.

Vein thrombosis results in the loss of anechoic appearance, incapacity to compress, and loss of flow.

1.8.6.8 Arteries

By using a transducer to apply mild pressure and a Doppler to measure steady flow, they appear as anechoic structures that are pulsatile, non-compressible, and anechoic.

1.8.6.9 Colour Doppler

Colour Doppler is an instrument to characterize blood flow. There is an apparent change in the returning echoes due to the relative motion between the sound source (Blood flowing, RBC) and the receiver (stationary transducer). Colour Doppler detection is worst when the transducer is perpendicular to the vessel and best when the transducer is parallel to the blood flow.

1.8.7 For Image Optimization, the Following Points Should Be Kept in Mind

- Frequency of the Transducer, Depth adjustment, Gain, Focus, Compound imaging use (Fig. 1.37).

1.8.8 Needling Technique

The Ultrasound beam travels in a straight line, like a thin sheet, perpendicular to the probe.

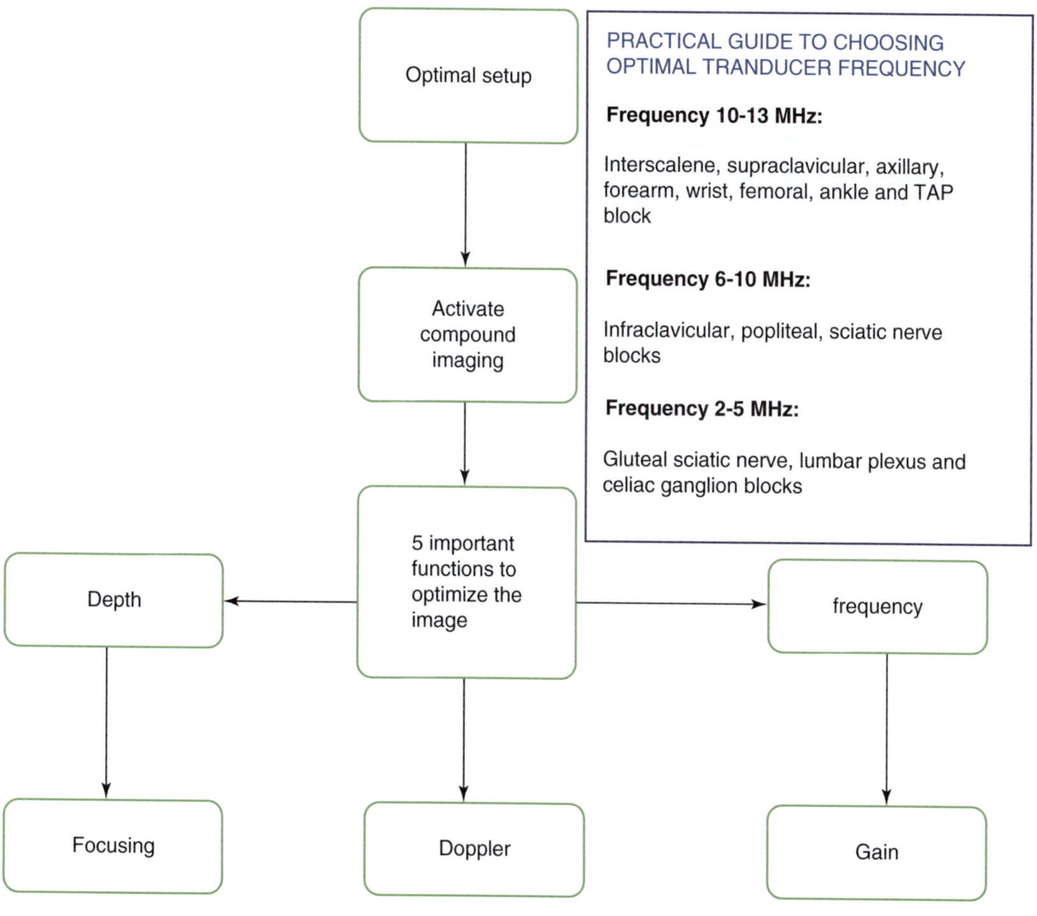

Fig. 1.37 For USG image optimization

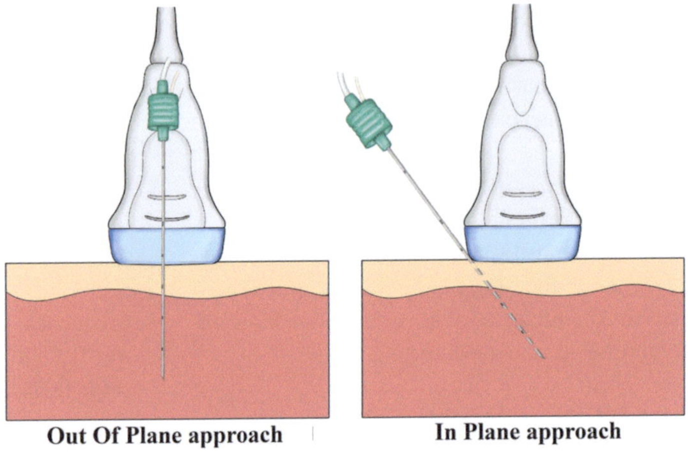

Fig. 1.38 Needle orientation with respect to transducer

1.8.8.1 In Plane

The needle is placed parallel to the transducer. The needle shaft and tip are both visible. This approach is safe and easy to learn but is difficult to practice in deeper blocks. Flatter the angle (acute angle), the better is the image.

1.8.8.2 Out of Plane

The needle is placed perpendicular to the transducer probe. Only tip is visible thus, echogenic needles are preferred. One should see the displacement of the tissue as pseudo marker for needle advancement (Fig. 1.38).

1.8.9 Summary of USG

Knowledge of ultrasound physics is needed for image optimization. The key understandings are:

- Appropriate transducer selection
- Gain settings
- Depth settings
- Tissue echo characteristics
- Ultrasound artefacts

For optimal imaging, it is important to adjust the pressure, alignment, rotation and tilt (PART) of the probe.

1.9 Conclusion

Regional anaesthesia has developed from an "art" done by a small number of people to a "science" that, with the right education and expertise, may be used by many. There are a few essential rules that must be followed to ensure safe and effective regional anaesthetic, regardless of who is administering the block or where it is being performed. It is critical that there be a defined space, and that all medications and equipment are easily accessible. Every institution's standard process should be thorough block procedure documentation. In order to prevent nerve damage, adequate patient monitoring is necessary. This monitoring should include routine ASA monitoring as well as objective ultrasound-nerve stimulator and injection pressure monitoring. Needling will be simpler and more accurate when the right tools are used, including the right needle length and gauge. The shortcomings of conventional catheter-through-needle designs can be lessened by new catheter-over-needle assemblies if a continuous block is desired, and recent advancements in long-term local anaesthetic delivery techniques, such as intermittent bolus and remote control, represent worthwhile alternatives.

In summary, a variety of techniques, tools, and monitoring technology are used in current regional anaesthetic practice. These techniques and instruments are essential for ensuring that the regional block is carried out in the safest and most efficient manner possible at every stage of the procedure, even though some of them take some time to become adequately proficient with.

A more recent technique, ultrasound-guided peripheral nerve blocks, has revolutionized the nerve block method. It has been demonstrated that USG-guided nerve blocks reduce the amount of local anaesthetic needed and increase block success rates, onset times, and duration.

Further Reading

American Society of Anesthesiologists, House of delegates. Standards for basic intraoperative monitoring. Park Ridge: ASA; 1986 Oct 21, amended October 13, 1993.

Brull R, Macfarlane AJ, Tse CC. Practical knobology for ultrasound-guided regional anesthesia. Reg Anesth Pain Med. 2010;35:S68–73.

Capdevila M, Choquet O, Saporito A, Djanikian F, Swisser F, Marques M, Bringuier S, Capdevila X. Injection pressure monitoring during peripheral nerve blocks: from bench to operating theatre. Anaesth Crit Care Pain Med. 2020;39(5):603–10.

Craig D, Carli F. Bromage motor blockade score – a score that has lasted more than a lifetime. Can J Anaesth. 2018;65(7):837–8.

Deiling B, Mullen K, Shilling A. Continuous catheter techniques. Clin Sports Med. 2022;41:317–28.

Ford DJ, Pither C, Raj PP. Comparison of insulated and uninsulated needles for locating peripheral nerves with a peripheral nerve stimulator. Anesth Analg. 1984;63:925.

Gadsden J. Current devices used for the monitoring of injection pressure during peripheral nerve blocks. Expert Rev Med Devices. 2018;15(8):571–8.

Gaudreault F, Drolet P, Fallaha M, Varin F. The reliability of the current perception threshold in volunteers and its applicability in a clinical setting. Anesth Analg. 2015;120(3):678–83.

Guo S, Schwab A, McLeod G, Corner G, Cochran S, Eisma R, Soames R. Echogenic regional anaesthesia needles: a comparison study in Thiel cadavers. Ultrasound Med Biol. 2012 Apr;38(4):702–7.

Klein SM, Melton MS, Grill WM, Nielsen KC. Peripheral nerve stimulation in regional anesthesia. Reg Anesth Pain Med. 2012;37(4):383–92.

Neuburger M, Schwemmer U, Volk T, Gogarten W, Kessler P, Steinfeldt T. Lokalisation peripherer Nerven. Erfolg und Sicherheit mit elektrischer Nervenstimulation [Localization of peripheral nerves. Success and safety with electrical nerve stimulation]. Anaesthesist. 2014;63(5):422–8.

Nightingale R, Chieng R, Bell D, et al. Ultrasound transducer. Reference article. Radiopaedia.org. Accessed on 31 Jan 2023.

Paqueron X, Gentili ME, Willer JC, Coriat P, Riou B. Time sequence of sensory changes after upper extremity block: swelling sensation is an early and accurate predictor of success. Anesthesiology. 2004;101:162–8.

Sharma S, Philip J, Lacour T, Perez B, Slaymaker E, Weidner C, Wiley J, Yamanouchi K, Sidawi J, Wallace D. Comparison of commonly used spinal needles. Anesth Analg. 1999;88(2S):266S.

Solodiuk J, Curley MA. Pain assessment in nonverbal children with severe cognitive impairments: the Individualized Numeric Rating Scale (INRS). J Pediatr Nurs. 2003;18(4):295–9.

Souki FG, Zbeidy R. Efficacy and ease of use of a newly designed pencil-point epidural needle compared to conventional Tuohy epidural needle: a randomized single-blind pilot study. Cureus. 2022 Oct 19;14(10):e30473.

Suksompong S, von Bormann S, von Bormann B. Regional catheters for postoperative pain control: review and observational data. Anesth Pain Med. 2020 Feb;10(1):e99745.

Toledano RD, et al. Epidural catheter design – history, innovations, and clinical implications. Anesthesiology. 2014;121(1):9–17.

Tsui BC, Li LX, Pillay JJ. Compressed air injection technique to standardize block injection pressures. Can J Anaesth. 2006;53(11):1098–102.

Urmey WF, Grossi P. Percutaneous electrode guidance: a noninvasive technique for prelocation of peripheral nerves to facilitate peripheral plexus or nerve block. Reg Anesth Pain Med. 2002;27:261–7.

Urmey WF, Grossi P. Percutaneous electrode guidance and subcutaneous stimulating electrode guidance: modifications of the original technique. Reg Anesth Pain Med. 2003;28:253–5.

Voepel-Lewis T, Malviya S, Tait AR, Merkel S, Foster R, Krane EJ, Davis PJ. A comparison of the clinical utility of pain assessment tools for children with cognitive impairment. Anesth Analg. 2008;106(1):72–8.

Walker KJ, McGrattan K, Aas-Eng K, Smith AF. Ultrasound guidance for peripheral nerve blockade. Cochrane Database Syst Rev. 2009;7(4):CD006459.

Yoshimura M, Shiramoto H, Koga M, et al. Skin temperature changes after ultrasound-guided supra-inguinal fascia iliaca block: a prospective observational study. JA Clin Rep. 2021;7:31.

Revisiting Local Anaesthesia Use in Regional Anaesthesia

2

Milon V. Mitragotri
and Sukhminder Jit Singh Bajwa

Abstract

Local anaesthetics (LA) play a pivotal role in the success of any regional anaesthesia procedure. LA blocks nerve impulse transmission in the peripheral and central nervous systems without causing central nervous system depression or altered mental status. The duration of action of LA can range from 30 min to 12 h or more. The range depends on the location of the block (e.g. high blood supply equals shorter duration), the specific local anaesthetic used, adjuvant used and its preparation. Hence, it's imperative that we understand all about LA and their individual properties.

Keywords

Local anaesthetics · LAST · Mixtures · Adjuvant

M. V. Mitragotri (✉)
Department of Anaesthesiology, Karnataka Institute of Medical Sciences, Hubballi, India

S. J. S. Bajwa
Department of Anaesthesiology & Critical Care, Gian Sagar Medical College & Hospital, Patiala, Punjab, India

2.1 History

Local anaesthetics didn't see the dawn of the day till Zophar Jayne invented the hypodermic needle in 1841, Niemann isolated cocaine from coca leaves in 1856 and till Karl Koller used it as LA for eye surgery. Dentists were the main proponents of local anaesthesia in those days considering that they were in contact in patients in pain. In 1903, Henrich Braun started adding adrenal gland hormone to cocaine for decreasing side effects while Halstead and Hall introduced the concept of conduction block after their success in blocking the supraorbital and infraorbital nerve.

In 1905, the first synthetic LA was born, i.e. Procaine also called Novocaine, introduced by Alfred Einhorn. However, it was noted that it was weak and needed high amounts of adrenaline for infiltration procedures. In 1943 to 1946, Lofgren and Lunquist synthesized an amide-based LA, Lidocaine. Thereafter, many amide-based LAs were synthesized which are being used currently.

M. K. Prasad, S. J. S. Bajwa (eds.), *Steps to Successful Regional Anesthesia*,
https://doi.org/10.1007/978-981-97-4098-7_2

2.2 Structure and Physical Properties of Clinically Useful LAs

2.2.1 Structure of Local Anaesthetics

Local anaesthetics have a hydrophobic aromatic ring and a hydrophilic amide end connecting them is either ester linkage (Ester LAs) or amide linkage (Amide LAs) (Fig. 2.1). The lipid solubility determines the potency of the drug which is decided by the aromatic ring and its substitutions along with the tertiary amines whereas the intermediate chain determines the elimination pathway.

2.3 Mechanism of Action

All LAs are believed to work in the same way, that is, block voltage-gated sodium channels, which prevents sodium influx into the cell and blocks impulse transmission (Fig. 2.2).

LA binding and blocking is stereospecific, concentration-dependent and brings in a conformational change in the sodium channels (Fig. 2.3). The binding of LA to the sodium channels is dependent on the number of sodium channels in activated open state. Higher the rate of depolarization, more are the sodium channels open leading to increased LA binding. This is known as *frequency-dependent block, use-dependent or phasic block*. Based on the type of connecting chain, LA is stated as an ester or an amide LA.

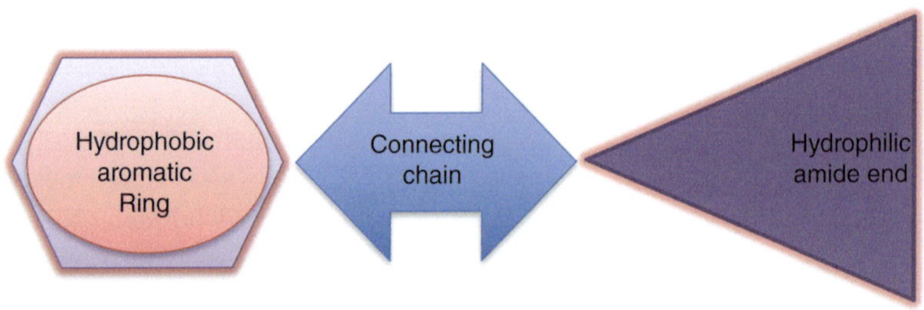

Fig. 2.1 The molecular structure of LAs

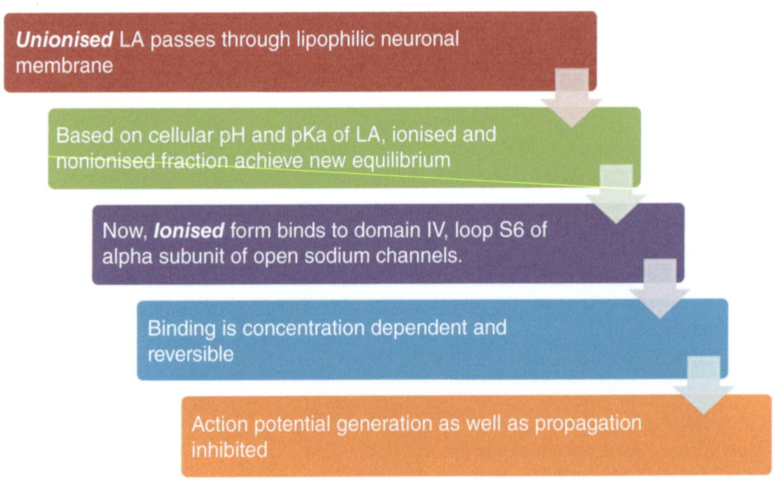

Fig. 2.2 Mechanism of action of local anaesthetics

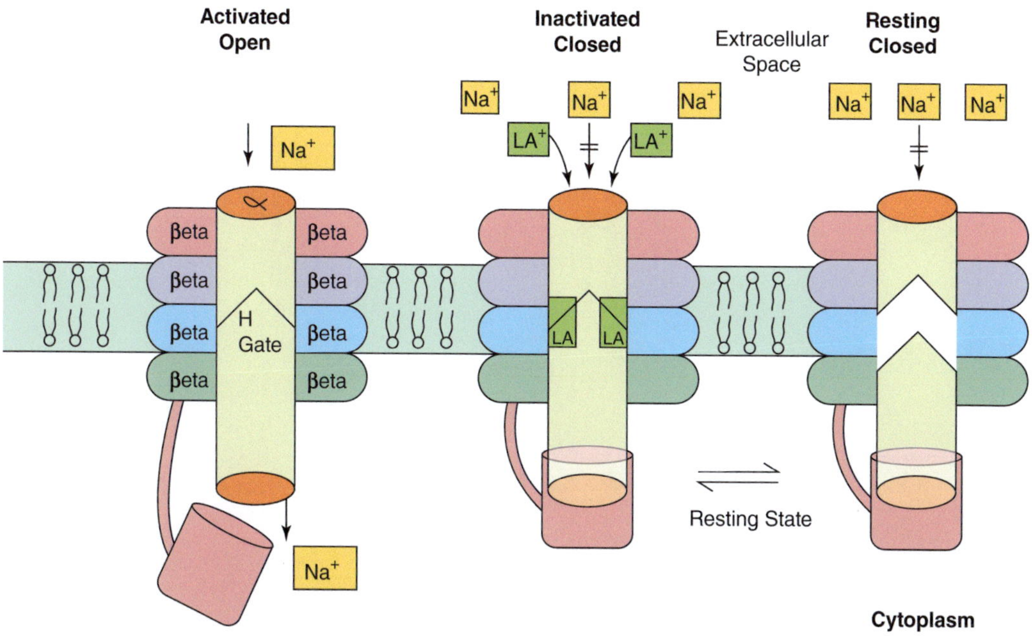

Fig. 2.3 Representative diagram depicting mechanism of action of LA on the sodium channels. (three types—activated open, inactivated closed and resting closed). LA binding acts on the inner H-gate of the alpha pore when sodium channels are in the inactivated closed state, preventing entry of sodium and hence propagation of action potential

2.4 Comparative Pharmacology of LA

Comparative pharmacology of LA (Table 2.1).

2.4.1 Stereochemistry of LA

Bupivacaine, Ropivacaine and Levobupivacaine are all pipecoloxylidide local anaesthetics classified as chiral compounds because they possess an asymmetric carbon atom. Bupivacaine is a 50:50 racemic mixture of R and S enantiomers. The R enantiomer is well known to be more cardiotoxic and neurotoxic than S enantiomer. Hence, levobupivacaine and ropivacaine have been developed as pure S enantiomers.

Table 2.1 Comparative pharmacology of LA

Local anaesthetic (common concentrations)	Type	pKa	Protein binding	Lipid solubility	Onset (min)	Duration (min)	Max. dose (mg/kg)	Max. dose (mg/kg)with adrenaline	Metabolites
Esters									
Procaine (1% 2%, 10%)	Short acting	8.9	6	Low	5	45–60	8	10	Paraaminobenzoic acid diethyaminoethanole
Tetracaine (1%)	Intermediate acting	8.2	76	High	7	60–180	2	2	NA
Chloroprocaine (1%, 2%, 3%)	Short acting	8.7	–	High	5–6	30–45	10	15	
Amides									
Lignocaine (2%)	Intermediate	7.9	70	Intermediate	2–4	60–120	5	7	Mono ethylglycinexylidide
Prilocaine	Intermediate	7.9	55	Intermediate	2	60–120	7	8	
Bupivacaine (0.25%, 0.5%)	Long-acting	8.1	95	High	5–8	240–480	2	2.5	N-debutylbupivacaine
Levobupivacaine (0.25%, 0.5%)	Long-acting levo isomers	8.1	97	High	5–8	240–480	2.5	3	NA
Ropivacaine (0.5%, 0.75%)	Long-acting levoisomers of bupivacaine	8.1	94	High	5–8	240—480	3	3	2,6-pipecoloxylidide and 3-hydroxyropivacaine

NA not available

2.5 Drug Distribution, Metabolism and Elimination After Regional Anaesthesia

Pharmacokinetics of Drugs After RA (Table 2.2).

2.6 Potency/Efficacy of LA

2.6.1 Factors Affecting Action of LAs (Table 2.3)

Table 2.2 Pharmacokinetics of drugs after RA

Absorption	Depends on multiple factors including the intrinsic vasodilator property, the use of adrenaline, site of injection, dose used, etc.
Distribution	LA bind to both albumin and alpha1 acid glycoprotein (ACGP) but more strongly to ACGP. Due to lack of ACGP in neonates and albumin in pregnancy, there is increased risk of systemic toxicity Cardiac output is an important determinant for the redistribution of the LA to other organs Tissue distribution depends on tissue/partition coefficient of LA, mass and perfusion of the tissue
Metabolism	Ester-based LAs are metabolized rapidly by cholinesterases while amide-based LAs are metabolized slowly by the liver by aromatic hydroxylation and N-dealkylation. The rate-limiting step of metabolism of LA is hepatic perfusion which may be hampered in critical illness leading to accumulation of LA
Elimination	Mainly hepatic with minimal renal elimination of unchanged drug minimal
Placental transfer	LA readily cross the placenta by simple diffusion and factors influencing are mainly the degree of ionization, characteristics of LA, concentration in maternal blood and properties of placenta. Any hemodynamic fluctuation will affect the placental transfer and prolonged administration of LA can lead to foetal accumulation

Table 2.3 Factors affecting action of LAs

Factors	
Type of LA	1. The onset depends on two properties—pKa (the pH at which ionized and non-ionized fraction are at equilibrium) and lipid solubility. Lower the pKa and higher the lipid solubility, faster the onset 2. The duration depends on protein binding capacity. Higher the protein binding, the longer the duration of LA 3. Amide LA undergoes first pass pulmonary extraction and this is dose-dependent especially with bupivacaine. Pulmonary uptake rapidly gets saturated and this is blocked if the patient has received propranolol
Dose of the drug used	The minimum effective concentration or minimum local analgesic concentration (MLAC) is the concentration of LA required to be effective in 50% of subjects. The 'up-and-down' sequential allocation of LA to subjects is used to estimate MLAC (9). MLAC again depends on the LA used and the site of RA. For example, 0.11% ropivacaine was found to be MLAC for caudal block in children
Concentration and volume used	Discussed further
Site of injection	The order of peak plasma concentration after a single dose of LA depends on the vascularity of the site. i.e., intrapleural > intercostal > lumbar epidural > brachial plexus > subcutaneous > sciatic > femoral
Sensitivity of nerve fibres	Myelinated fibres > unmyelinated fibres Sympathetic (B fibres) > A gamma > A-delta > C fibres This leads to *differential block* with sympathetic fibres most easily blocked with lowest concentration of LA followed by temperature and pain. Proprioception and motor fibres are last to get blocked(5) Studies have noted that diabetic nerve fibres are more sensitive to effects of LA but concerns have been raised regarding the susceptibility to neurotoxic potential too
Adjuvant and vasoconstrictor used	Discussed further
Baricity of the LA	Baricity refers to the density of the LA in comparison with the density of the CSF at 37° C (CSF density 1.0003–1.0006). Hyperbaric solutions tend to pool in the direction of gravity while hypobaric solution vice versa. Isobaric solutions as the name suggests remain the site of injection irrespective of gravity. LAs are made hyperbaric by adding dextrose or hypobaric by adding pure water. The duration of analgesia can't correlate with the baricity

2.7 Uses of LA

1. EMLA and Amethocaine cream—These two creams of local anaesthetics are used to minimize the pain of venipuncture and other superficial painful procedures. EMLA, more commonly used, is an eutectic mixture of local anaesthetics, i.e. 2.5% lignocaine and 2.5% prilocaine in an oil- and water-based emulsion. To be effective, EMLA cream should be applied at least 1 h prior to intervention. EMLA has been used for laser treatment, skin harvesting, paediatric urological procedures and shock wave lithotripsy (12).
2. Topical anaesthesia—LAs like benzocaine, procaine, tetracaine **are** used for topical purposes in cataract surgeries and dental procedures. They are used for analgesic purposes.
3. Tumescent anaesthesia—Here very dilute concentrations of local anaesthetics are infiltrated into the subcutaneous tissue to make firm and tense. Doses of 55 mg/kg of lignocaine are used for liposuction and doses of 4.5 mg/kg and 7 mg/kg (with adrenaline) are used for infiltration purposes in dermatology and plastic surgery. Use of such high volumes can increase risk of LAST many hours after the procedure. Bupivacaine has not been used for this purpose due to limited experience and cardiovascular toxicity.

   Klein's solution is commonly used which is prepared by mixing 50 mL of lignocaine, 1 mL of adrenaline (1:1000) with 1 L of normal saline. This solution has a concentration of 0.05% lignocaine and 1:1000000 adrenaline. 10 mEq of sodium bicarbonate is added to the solution to prevent stinging during injection and to increase non-ionized fraction.
4. Regional anaesthesia.
5. Anti-arrhythmia drug—Preservative-free lignocaine is classified as class 1B antiarrhythmic drug in doses of 2 mg/kg when given intravenously to treat ventricular tachyarrhythmias.
6. Postoperative analgesia—Systemic lignocaine infusion is used perioperatively for its analgesic, anti-hyperalgesic and anti-inflammatory properties. It has also found a role in enhanced recovery protocols and chronic pain.

2.8 Adverse Effects

1. Allergy
2. Local anaesthetic systemic toxicity
3. Local anaesthetic neurotoxicity
4. Local anaesthetic myotoxicity.

2.8.1 Allergy

LAs are considered to be hypoallergenic and are rarely known to cause allergy (4). Ester LAs are more frequently associated with allergy because of their metabolism by esterases into para-amino benzoic acid. Hypersensitivity due to para-benzoic acid, preservatives like methylparaben may result in **an** anaphylaxis type response or a vasovagal response. A patient with known allergy to ester LA can be switched to amide LA and vice versa making sure the preparation is preservative free.

2.8.2 Local Anaesthetic Systemic Toxicity (LAST)

Summarize LAST (Table 2.4).

2.8.3 LA Myotoxicity

There are high chances of accidental LA injection in the muscle or spillage of LA in the substance of muscle after high volume LA injections especially after the widely popular ultrasound-guided fascial plane blocks. The incidence is not yet known and needs further study.

Table 2.4 Summarize LAST

What is LAST?	Inadvertent intravascular injection or administration of supra therapeutic levels of LA leading to absorption into the circulation can trigger LAST. All LAs are invariably toxic in a dose- and time-dependent manner on all tissues, including nerves and muscles
Incidence	1 in 1000
Predictive and risk factors	LA type, dose and volume, site of injection and co-morbidities, extremes of age, pregnancy, cardiac disease, renal or hepatic disease, sepsis, current medications, cholinesterase deficiency, foetal acidosis influence rate of absorption and hence LAST CVS/CNS ratio is ratio of the dose of LA needed to cause cardiac signs compared to neurotoxic effects. Bupivacaine has been found to have lower CC ratio and hence more cardiotoxic With the use of ultrasound, though the incidence of LAST has decreased, the occurrence of delayed onset of LAST especially with fascial plane blocks has increased
Mechanism	The mitochondrial metabolism—Important clinical target. Heart and brain are highly intolerant of anaerobic metabolism and hence easily susceptible Reducing LA content at tissue site can only salvage the condition
Symptoms	Usually of central nervous system (CNS) first followed by cardiovascular *Prodromal symptoms* start 1–5 min after injection, which include oral numbness, metallic taste, drowsiness and disorientation *Excitatory phenomena* like slurred speech, restlessness, vertigo, tinnitus, muscles twitches and generalized tonic-clonic seizures occur initially Followed by *CNS depression* including coma based on the systemic concentration of LA *Cardiovascular signs* like severe vasodilatation and myocardial depression ensue at higher concentration Accidental IV injection of bupivacaine can cause solitary CVS signs without neurological signs like premature ventricular contractions (PVC), broad QRS complexes and ventricular tachycardia
Toxic levels	Lidocaine and prilocaine demonstrate effects on the CNS at plasma concentrations of 5 to 10 μg/mL. The typical plasma concentration of bupivacaine associated with seizures is 4.5 to 5.5 μg/mL. The threshold for cardiotoxic effect of bupivacaine is decreased in the presence of medications decreasing conduction like beta blockers, calcium channel blockers, digitalis, etc.
Treatment	*Key elements*—Immediate diagnosis and treatment include airway and resuscitation, administration of intralipid, prevention of hypoxia, hypercarbia and acidosis which can further accentuate LAST Stop LA Administration ↓ Call for help ↓ Airway management with resuscitation and circulatory support with 100% oxygen ↓ *Intralipid* *Mechanism*—Rescue measure as mechanism is not known and it doesn't work as an antidote. It acts as a 'shuttle' removing the positively charged lipophilic LAs from the organs into the negatively charged lipid sink then redistributing them into the other vascular-rich organs like liver for elimination *Dose* Initial bolus of 1.5 mL/kg of 20% lipid over 2–3 min (approximately 100 mL in a 70 kg adult patient)→ Infusion of 0.25 mL/kg/min (approx. 1000 mL/h for 70 kg patient) until 10 min after stability is achieved (average total dose approximately 2.8 mL/kg).→ If stability is not regained, a further bolus followed by increasing the infusion rate (e.g. 0.5 mL/kg/min) can be considered (max total dose of 10–12 mL/kg) *Adverse effects*—minor
Points to remember	Propofol is not a substitute for lipid emulsion due to its potent cardio-depressant effects and the high doses needed for sequestration of LA Avoid hypercarbia or hypocarbia Benzodiazepines for control of convulsions rather than propofol or thiopentone Muscle relaxants if tonic-clonic convulsions are refractory Arrhythmias are usually refractory and calcium channel blocker, beta blockers and lidocaine being cardiac depressant in nature should not be used Adrenaline in doses less than 1 μg/kg as it is known to be arrhythmogenic Vasopressin is contraindicated Cardiopulmonary bypass and extracorporeal membrane oxygenation if all the above measures fail

2.8.4 LA-Induced Neurotoxicity

Use of LA can result in damage to nerve fibres which are dependent on the concentration or mass of LA used.

2.9 Effect of LA Concentration and Volume on Peripheral Nerve Block

The search of the ideal dose, minimum effective LA volume (MEAV) and concentration are still on.

Effect of LAs concentration and volume on peripheral nerve block (Table 2.5).

Table 2.5 Effect of LA concentration and volume on peripheral nerve block

Dose	Smaller doses associated with incomplete nerve block Higher doses associated with risk of LAST
Concentration	Higher concentration associated with neurotoxicity as well as LAST Success of RA depends on length of the nerve exposed to LA mass rather than concentration
Volume	Higher dose and concentration of LA associated with longer duration of sensory and motor block but not higher volume 4 mL of 2% lidocaine with epinephrine produced upper limb anaesthesia in adults undergoing upper limb surgery using axillary approach

2.10 Role of USG in Regional Anaesthesia

Advantages and disadvantages of USG (Table 2.6).

2.11 Mixture of LA

Advantages and disadvantages of mixture LA (Table 2.7).

Table 2.6 Advantages and disadvantages of USG

Advantages	Disadvantages
Dose reduction	Unwanted reduction in duration of analgesia
Fascial plane block	Local anaesthetic myotoxicity due to spillage of LA in the muscle
Incidence of LAST decreased	Delayed LAST especially in patients receiving fascial plane blocks

Table 2.7 Advantages and disadvantages of mixture LA

The use of LA mixtures is a very common practice with its effects being unpredictable. Most commonly short-acting LAs are mixed with long-acting LAs to hasten onset, prolong duration and decrease side effects and LAST	
Disadvantages	1. The efficacy, compatibility, safety and pharmacokinetics are not yet tested. This may render them ineffective and potentially harmful 2. Lignocaine is mixed commonly with bupivacaine; however, such a mixture will neither hasten onset nor provide an effective duration of block because mixtures of these LA cause decreased/halving of concentration of individual LA resulting in decreased delivery LA mass at the nerve fibres 3. In one study, plain bupivacaine without the addition of lignocaine gave longest duration compared to any other mixture 4. LA toxicity here is more additive than synergistic
Advantage	Addition of lignocaine to bupivacaine to speed up the onset should be done only if suboptimal duration is acceptable

2.12 Adjuvants to LA in Regional Anaesthesia

Adjuvants are medications used to prolong the duration of LA from the conventional maximal duration of 8–14 h. Though continuous nerve catheters have been able to circumvent this problem of duration, they still need precision of placement of catheters, technical expertise, cost-intensive and need to follow-up. An ideal adjuvant should be able to prolong the duration of analgesia without motor blockade, with no or minimal side effect and no neurotoxic after effects. Of the several adjuvants studied, perineural dexamethasone and dexmedetomidine are the only ones found to reliably increase the mean duration of analgesia.

2.12.1 Adjuvants Are of Two Types

Classification of adjuvants (Table 2.8).

However, midazolam, fentanyl, neostigmine, morphine, tramadol, ketamine are no longer recommended either due to lack of efficacy or due to evidence of neurotoxicity.

Table 2.8 Classification of adjuvants

Name and doses commonly used	Mechanism	Remarks
A. Those that increase the efficacy of LA itself		
1. Adrenaline (100–300 μg)	Alpha1-mediated vasoconstriction which adds efficacy also by preventing LAST and decreasing dose of LA used	Perineural adrenaline was able to prolong LA duration by 66 min ASRA recommends caution due to concerns of nerve ischaemia and neurotoxicity occurring due to prolonged exposure to LA (reduced clearance) resulting especially in those with new-onset peripheral neuropathy
2. 8.4% sodium bicarbonate (0.1–4 mL)	Alkalinization of the LA solution increasing the pH closer to the pKa of LA	Studies haven't been able to confirm its efficacy
3. Hyaluronidase (15 U/L)	Used in cataract and other ophthalmic surgeries.	
B. Those that work by direct actions on nerve		
1. Buprenorphine (0.1, 0.15, 0.2 and 0.3 mg)	Blocks Na+ channels and μ receptors at the unmyelinated C fibres of axons	Prolongs the duration of analgesia up to 8 h with no neurotoxic effects Risk of significant postoperative nausea and vomiting
2. Dexamethasone (4–8 mg)	Acts on glucocorticoid receptors with increased expression of inhibitory potassium channels	Dexamethasone(4 mg) prolongs the duration of nerve blockade, both sensory as well as motor block Hyperglycaemia risks delayed wound healing and systemic infection No significant neurotoxic potential
3.Dexmedetomidine (50–60 μg)	Alpha 2 blocker Maintains the hyperpolarized state of neuron channels by blocking the hyperpolarization-activated nucleotide-gated channels (32) Differential prolongation of sensory action compared to motor by acting more on A-delta and C fibres	Prolongs the duration of sensory analgesia by 264 min and motor block by 192 min Hypotension, bradycardia and sedation Optimal dose with minimal side effects is 50–60 μg Neurotoxic potential debatable
4. Clonidine	Similar to dexmedetomidine	
5. Magnesium	Magnesium increases LA's capacity to boost A-beta fibre excitation threshold while reducing peripheral nerve excitability	In a dose of 50 mg it prolongs the effect of intrathecal and epidural LA block in labour. However, high dose has been reported to be associated with neurological toxicity In peripheral nerve block it prolongs the duration of analgesia and hastens onset of sensory and motor blockade in various doses (125, 250, 500 mg)

Researchers are now comparing the perineural versus intravenous administration of adjuvants to analyse whether the effects are the same with intravenous administration. This will also serve the purpose of avoiding the potential neuro-active actions of these drugs. Dexamethasone in doses of 0.1–0.2 mg/kg has been found to be ideal in providing good analgesia in patients with moderate pain even in those cases with no nerve blockade.

2.13 Future Perspectives

Newer Development in LA (Table 2.9).

Table 2.9 Newer development in LA

LA action on tumour mitogenesis	Recent evidence that LAs are pleomorphic and bind to many molecular proteins (channel as well as non-channel proteins) rendering surrogate effects like anti-inflammatory, anti-thrombotic and immunomodulatory activities. These effects are linked to beneficial effects they provide in prevention of cancer mitogenesis, chronic pain, chronic inflammation and chronic functional disorders
Newer LA	1. *Liposomal bupivacaine*—long-acting sustained released preparation of bupivacaine marketed as Exparel. It's an encapsulated micro vesicular liposomal preparation providing extended release of bupivacaine up to 96 h. Off-label use for peripheral nerve blocks has shown equivocal results and it needs further study 2. *Hyperbaric preparations of ropivacaine and levobupivacaine*—these are not available in the Indian market now. Now found to be equally efficacious to bupivacaine especially for gynaecological procedures, more studies needed to confirm its efficacy for other higher level procedures and the optimal dosing 3. *SABER bupivacaine*—is a depot preparation of bupivacaine which is still under study needing FDA approval 4. *HTX-011 marketed as ZYNRELEFTM* is US-FDA approved for treating acute postoperative pain by infiltration at the surgical site. It's an extended-release, fixed formulation of bupivacaine and meloxicam providing analgesia for up to 3 days 5. *Neosaxitoxin*—is a phycotoxin which has more affinity to block sodium channels of nerves compared to myocardium. This favourable pharmacodynamic profile assists in prolonging the analgesic effect of LA. It still awaits FDA profile for clinical use
New subtype-specific sodium channel blockers	Search is on to find specific LAs which do not bind to the sodium channels of the heart and the brain
2-chloroprocaine	Renewed interest in shorter acting LA for rapid recovery
Phentolamine	Non-selective alpha antagonist used as LA reversal agent in dentistry

Further Reading

Albrecht E, Kern C, Kirkham KR. A systematic review and meta-analysis of perineural dexamethasone for peripheral nerve blocks. Anaesthesia. 2015 Jan;70(1):71–83.

Almasi R, Rezman B, Kriszta Z, Patczai B, Wiegand N, Bogar L. Onset times and duration of analgesic effect of various concentrations of local anesthetic solutions in standardized volume used for brachial plexus blocks. Heliyon. 2020 Sept 2;6(9):e04718.

Antel R, Ingelmo P. Local anesthetic systemic toxicity. CMAJ. 2022 Sept 26;194(37):E1288.

Desai N, Kirkham KR, Albrecht E. Local anaesthetic adjuncts for peripheral regional anaesthesia: a narrative review. Anaesthesia. 2021a;76(S1):100–9.

Desai N, Kirkham KR, Albrecht E. Local anaesthetic adjuncts for peripheral regional anaesthesia: a narrative review. Anaesthesia. 2021b Jan;76(Suppl 1):100–9.

Fenten MGE, Schoenmakers KPW, Heesterbeek PJC, Scheffer GJ, Stienstra R. Effect of local anesthetic concentration, dose and volume on the duration of single-injection ultrasound-guided axillary brachial plexus block with mepivacaine: a randomized controlled trial. BMC Anesthesiol. 2015 Sept 30;15:130.

Garmon EH, Huecker MR. Topical, local, and regional anesthesia and anesthetics [Internet]. StatPearls [Internet]. StatPearls Publishing; 2022 [cited 2022 Dec 23]. Available from: https://www.ncbi.nlm.nih.gov/books/NBK430894/

Gitman M, Fettiplace MR, Weinberg GL, Neal JM, Barrington MJ. Local anesthetic systemic toxicity: a narrative literature review and clinical update on prevention, diagnosis, and management. Plast Reconstr Surg. 2019 Sept;144(3):783.

Grage SL, Culetto A, Ulrich AS, Weinschenk S. Membrane-mediated activity of local anesthetics. Mol Pharmacol. 2021 Nov 1;100(5):502–12.

Jason C, Liane G, Alan CS. Obstetric regional anaesthesia, [Internet]. Nysora; 2023 [cited 2023 Sept 7]. Available from: https://www.nysora.com/topics/sub-specialties/obstetric/obstetric-regional-anesthesia/

Kim JE, Kim JY, Lee HS, Seok S, Kil HK. Analgesic effect of trigger point injection and EMLA for shoulder pain in patients undergoing total laparoscopic hysterectomy: A randomized controlled study. Medicine (Baltimore) [Internet]. 2019 Jan [cited 2023 Feb 3];98(2). Available from: https://www.ncbi.nlm.nih.gov/pmc/articles/PMC6336620/

Macfarlane AJR, Gitman M, Bornstein KJ, El-Boghdadly K, Weinberg G. Updates in our understanding of local anaesthetic systemic toxicity: a narrative review. Anaesthesia. 2021;76(S1):27–39.

Nathan J, Asadourian L, Erlich MA. A brief history of local anesthesia. Int J Head Neck Surg. 2016;7(1):29–32.

Neal JM, Barrington MJ, Brull R, Hadzic A, Hebl JR, Horlocker TT, et al. The second ASRA practice advisory on neurologic complications associated with regional anesthesia and pain medicine: executive summary 2015. Reg Anesth Pain Med. 2015;40(5):401–30.

Nestor CC, Ng C, Sepulveda P, Irwin MG. Pharmacological and clinical implications of local anaesthetic mixtures: a narrative review. Anaesthesia. 2022 Mar;77(3):339–50.

Schnabel A, Reichl SU, Zahn PK, Pogatzki-Zahn EM, Meyer-Frießem CH. Efficacy and safety of buprenorphine in peripheral nerve blocks: a meta-analysis of randomised controlled trials. Eur J Anaesthesiol. 2017 Sept;34(9):576–86.

Soto G, Naranjo González M, Calero F. Intravenous lidocaine infusion. Rev Esp Anestesiol Reanim. 2018 May;65(5):269–74.

Taylor A, McLeod G. Basic pharmacology of local anaesthetics. BJA Educ. 2020 Feb;20(2):34–41.

Themes UFO. Local anesthetics [Internet]. Anesthesia key. 2016 [cited 2023 Jan 7]. Available from: https://aneskey.com/local-anesthetics-16/

Tschopp C, Tramèr MR, Schneider A, Zaarour M, Elia N. Benefit and harm of adding epinephrine to a local anesthetic for neuraxial and locoregional anesthesia: a meta-analysis of randomized controlled trials with trial sequential analyses. Anesth Analg. 2018 July;127(1):228–39.

Vorobeichik L, Brull R, Abdallah FW. Evidence basis for using perineural dexmedetomidine to enhance the quality of brachial plexus nerve blocks: a systematic review and meta-analysis of randomized controlled trials. Br J Anaesth. 2017 Feb;118(2):167–81.

Regional Anesthesia: General Considerations

3

Payal Jain and Pulak Puneet

Abstract

Regional anesthesia is fast becoming an integral part of anesthesiologist practice. Successful practice of it depends not only on the expertise of the practitioner but also on precise and proper preparation of the patient, equipment as well as the provider. For this it is extremely important to follow certain protocols, guidelines to minimize the failure rates as well as harm not only to the patient but also to decrease the incidence of work-related disorders for the anesthesiologist. In this chapter we have covered the general considerations with the objective to put emphasis on proper preparation of every aspect of Regional Block, pondering over the need, contraindications of block and above all the use of ergonomics while placement of Ultrasound guided blocks to heightened the percentage of success and keeping in mind the well-being of provider too.

Keywords

Ergonomics · Contraindications · Ultrasound · Regional anesthesia

3.1 Introduction

It is now an established fact that Regional Anesthesia is not only becoming an important part of an Anesthesiologist's armamentarium, its importance and relevance is expected to grow even more in the future.

As with any intervention with the human body, the practice of anesthesia should have some basic objectives which can be shortlisted for ready reference:

- The objective of the intervention should be clear and justified.
- The intervention should have a clear plan or roadmap of action steps.
- The methodology should be tailored to have the potential for maximum accuracy and efficiency and minimum potential for harm or side effects.

To achieve this, it is important that the practitioner draws up a protocol which he can follow every time. It's important that this protocol be methodical, sequential and includes every step

P. Jain (✉)
Department of Anaesthesiology, Teerthanker Mahaveer Medical College and Research Centre, Moradabad, India

P. Puneet
Lifecare Hospital, Abu Dhabi, UAE

M. K. Prasad, S. J. S. Bajwa (eds.), *Steps to Successful Regional Anesthesia*,
https://doi.org/10.1007/978-981-97-4098-7_3

that is essential and covers some common but unexpected circumstances.

3.2 "Well Prepared Is Half Done."

They can be further elaborated as follows:

3.2.1 Patient Related

(a) Meticulous preoperative assessment, with particular emphasis on any possible contra-indications (relative or absolute), e.g. ongoing oral anticoagulation treatment.
(b) Choosing the most appropriate regional anesthesia and establishing its relevance and benefits.
(c) Discussing with and counseling the patients/bystanders regarding the appropriateness of the proposed anesthetic technique.
(d) Ensuring the presence of a written and informed consent for the anesthetic technique.
(e) Documented NPO status.
(f) Working, secure IV access.
(g) Appropriate use of sedation as suitable.
(h) Site and side re-confirmed and marked.

3.2.2 Procedure Related

(a) Monitoring equipment as per ASA recommendations.
(b) Working ultrasound machine with linear and curvilinear probes, sterile sleeve, and gel.
(c) Peripheral nerve stimulator.
(d) Sterile gloves, marking pen, and surface electrodes.
(e) Sterile procedure set including sterile draping towels and gauze pieces. Sterile towels and 4 × 4 inch gauze packs.
(f) Sterile syringes—one 5 cc and four 10 cc.
(g) Local anesthetic for skin and subcutaneous infiltration, commonly Inj Lidocaine 2%.
(h) Sterile needles—one 4 cm long 25 G for skin infiltration and one 5 cm/10 cm long, 21 G/22G, short beveled insulated stimulating needle.
(i) Injection pressure monitor.
(j) Site and side of the proposed block to be confirmed and marked.

A definite plan for positioning of the USG machine and operator keeping in mind the laterality of the block site and handedness. This leads to the procedure being carried out most ergonomically, thus maximizing the accuracy and efficiency. (An example would be—for a right-handed operator performing a supraclavicular block on the left side of the patient, the most ergonomic arrangement would be for him to stand by the side of the patient's left hand and the USG machine be placed at the head end of the patient so that the injection site and the monitor of the USG machine both can be in his direct line of sight, making it easier for him to orient his movements)

3.2.3 Emergency/Adverse Event Related

(a) Source of uninterrupted oxygen supply.
(b) Emergency crash cart, including all emergency resuscitation drugs and airway management equipment.
(c) A working defibrillator.
(d) Sufficient amount of Inj. Intralipid availability to counteract local anesthetic toxicity.

3.3 Contraindications

It would be pertinent to mention here, commonly encountered contraindications to regional anesthesia administration. The contraindications are more or less similar for every block. Given below is enlisted the common C/I to all the blocks.

1. Absolute:
   (a) Patient refusal.
   (b) Known allergy to local anesthetics
   (c) Infection at the proposed injection site.
2. Relative:

(a) Patient receiving ongoing anticoagulation therapy or suffering from bleeding diathesis.
(b) Neuromuscular disease/damage in contralateral limb in ambulatory patient.
(c) Lack of expertise.

3.4 Induction and Block Room

This area can be in the operating room or as a separate block room, with proper lighting and enough area to ensure safe and efficient ergonomics for anesthetist, on the one hand, and enhancement of the conditions for patient's safety as well successful block placement, on the other. There should be provision for emergency resuscitation cart with proper monitoring (ASA standards) with easy access is of paramount importance.

3.5 Monitoring

Routine cardio-respiratory monitoring should consist of pulse oximetry, non-invasive blood pressure, electrocardiogram, respiratory rate and mental status. Local anesthesia has a biphasic pattern of action (a) During and immediately after the injection (seen after intravascular injection) (b) 10 to 30 mins (due to typical absorption and peak effect), therefore patients should be continuously monitored for minimum of 30 min for signs of local anesthetic toxicity.

3.6 Block Trays

Anesthesiologists have witnessed a progressive improvement in the quality and reliability of disposable, commercially prepared nerve block trays (Fig. 3.1). "Custom trays" tailored to the specific needs and preferences of the department are frequently used, which have virtually eliminated the use of internally prepared nerve block trays in most centers.

Drugs packaged in commercially prepared, disposable trays have been sterilized, usually with ethylene oxide. It is important, however, that 24–72 h be allowed for the extrusion of ethylene oxide if it is used to sterilize the entire block tray.

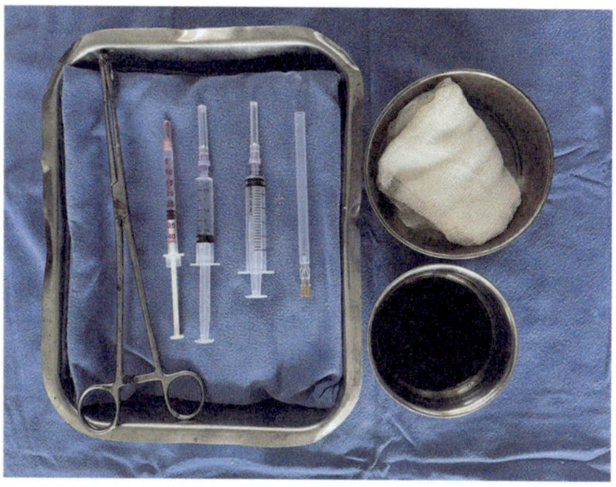

Fig. 3.1 Block tray

To improve the success rate of neural blockade or to make it possible in very difficult cases or extreme circumstances, special devices, needles, and pieces of equipment have been advocated or introduced.

3.6.1 Clinical Use of Peripheral Nerve Stimulation

The following are a few important aspects for successful electro-localization of the peripheral nerves using PNS:

- Use only a nerve stimulator specifically manufactured for nerve blocks.
- Use insulated nerve stimulation needles.
- Use high-quality skin electrodes with a low impedance.
- Some lower-priced ECG electrodes can have very high impedance/resistance.
- Before starting the procedure, check for the proper functioning of the nerve stimulator and the connecting cables.
- During the procedure, check frequently to assure that the current is being delivered and leads disconnect does not occur.
- The design of the connectors should prevent a faulty polarity connection.
- Connect the nerve stimulation needle to the nerve stimulator (which should be turned on) and set the current amplitude and duration to the desired levels.
- For superficial blocks, select 1.0 mA as a starting current intensity.
- For deep blocks, select 1.5 mA as a starting current intensity.
- Select between 0.1 and 0.3 ms of current duration for most purposes.
- With ultrasound guidance, select the current as 0.5 mA; it is rarely necessary to change the current as motor response with ultrasound guidance is not sought. However, when unexpectedly elicited, it warns the operator that the needle is in the immediate vicinity of the nerve or intraneurally placed.

3.7 Ergonomics for Ultrasound Use

Ergonomics is a scientific discipline of paramount importance for anesthesiologists working in the field of peripheral nerve blocks of which ultrasound has become an integral part.

Use of ultrasound has a long learning curve which can be divided into mastering the two aspects of it—Optimal Imaging structures in plane of section especially the target nerve and most importantly guiding the needle to the target.

Hereby in this section the tips /techniques to increase the efficiency and competency of an anesthesiologist while working with an ultrasound for peripheral nerve blocks will be discussed.

The parts of body most commonly affected as a result of poor posturing leading to tendinitis and tenosynovitis are the shoulders (76%), neck (74%), wrists (59%), back (58%), and hands (55%).

In addition to reduction in injuries, the whole drill of increasing the productivity and reduction of quality issues, errors and failures can be addressed via keeping in mind certain simple things

3.7.1 Optimization of visual spatial neuroprocessing and cognitive ability

It requires ability to balance the visual and sensory cues along with the orientation to direct the needle tip to the desired location and accurate decision making for success.

Tips

(a) Choose appropriate transducer/frequency.
(b) Understand underlying anatomic relationships.
(c) Basic knowledge of recognition of 3D anatomy.

3.7.2. Optimal posture and position to reduce fatigue and decrease the failures to balance the needle tip control.

3.7.3. Optimal strategy to achieve needle beam alignment for optimal needle visualization to select an effective strategy to facilitate injection of local anesthetic to the target nerve.

Tips

PART In order to optimize the ultrasound image, Pressure, Alignment, Rotation, and Tilting (PART) is recommended.

(a) *Pressure*—In order to compress the underlying subcutaneous tissue to decrease the distance to the target nerve.
(b) *Alignment*—Positioning of the transducer with respect to nerve to be visualized (longitudinal or transverse axis).

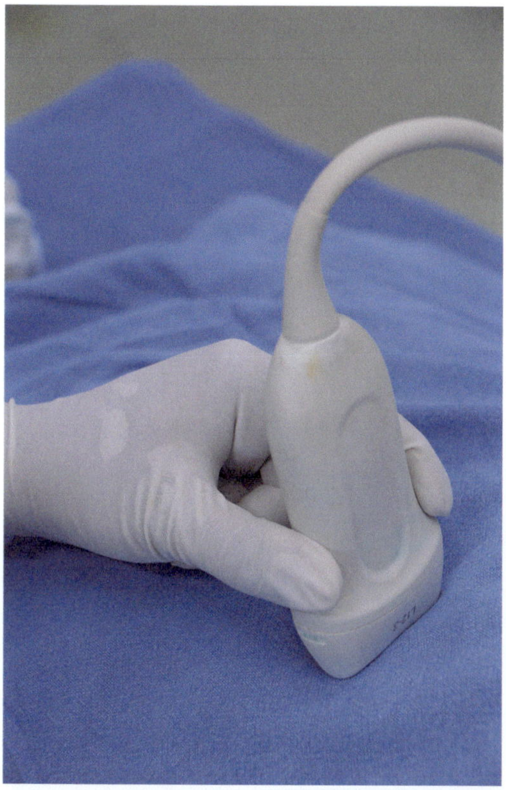

Fig. 3.2 Pincer Grasp

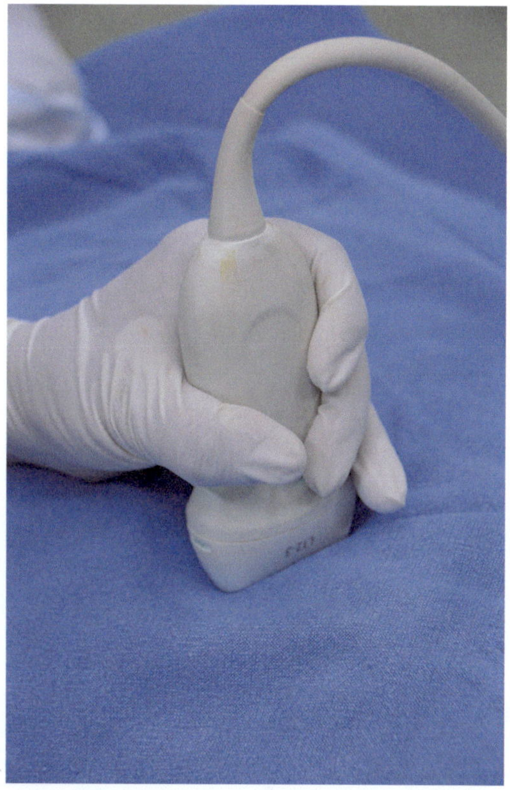

Fig. 3.3 Volar Grasp

(c) *Rotation*—Probe is rotated in order to fine-tune the image.
(d) *Tilting*—It brings the transducer face perpendicularly to the target in order to maximize the return echoes to have the best possible view.

3.7.4. Best position of the monitor is in front of the operator, at the level of hands allowing gaze-down viewing and in order to reduce transducer wandering keep the needle and probe alignment with the viewing axis.

3.7.5. Hold the block needle in the dominant hand for optimal fine motor control and better competence. Assume neutral wrist position while holding the probe or the block needle. Maintain a firm palmar (volar) grip rather than pinch grip on the probe (Figs. 3.2 and 3.3).

3.7.6. Ensure the screen adjustment so that the needle movements are displayed correspondingly on the monitor screen.

3.7.7. US monitor should be straight in front of operator with a slight 15–20 °C neck flexion while performing the block to avoid excessive neck movements (> 45° turn) and protraction and rotation of cervical spine (Fig. 3.4).

3.7.8. Organizational aspect also plays an extremely important role, comfortable OT/Block room environment is essential—keeping the temperature at least 20–23 °C with relative humidity between 20% and 60%.

3.7.9. Adjustable indirect lightning with respect to proper visualization of screen should be done.

3.7.10. Noise levels should be minimized between 40 db and 80 db that too for short periods, preferably to keep silence around.

3.7.11. OT should be minimal of the size 400–600 square feet with adequate air exchanges of 20 air changes/hour.

3.7.12. Asepsis should be maintained throughout the procedure.

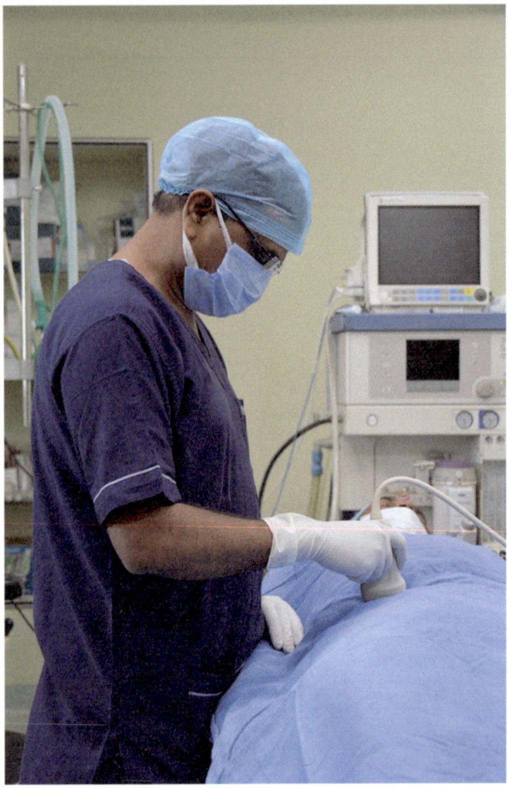

Fig. 3.4 Flexion at head and neck joint

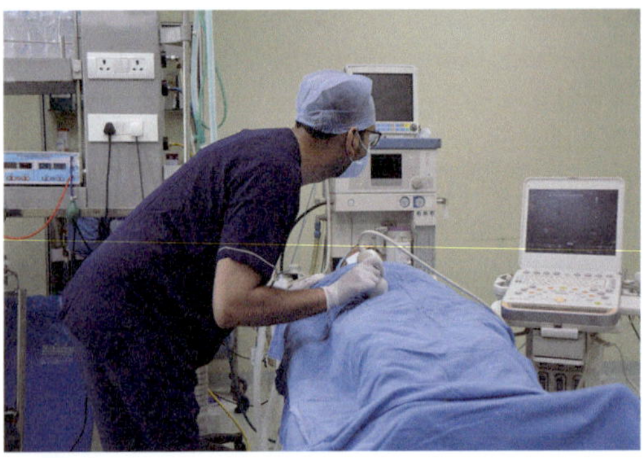

Fig. 3.5 Flexion of body

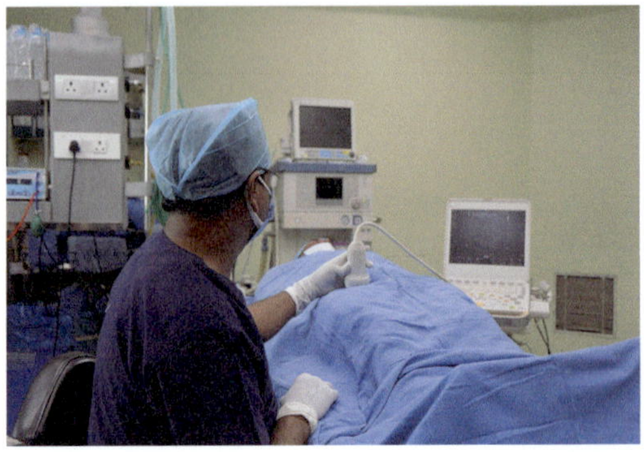

Fig. 3.6 Torso twisting

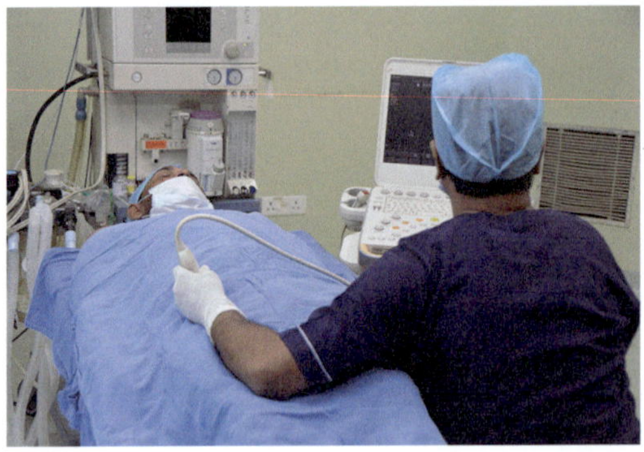

Fig. 3.7 Hyperabduction of arm

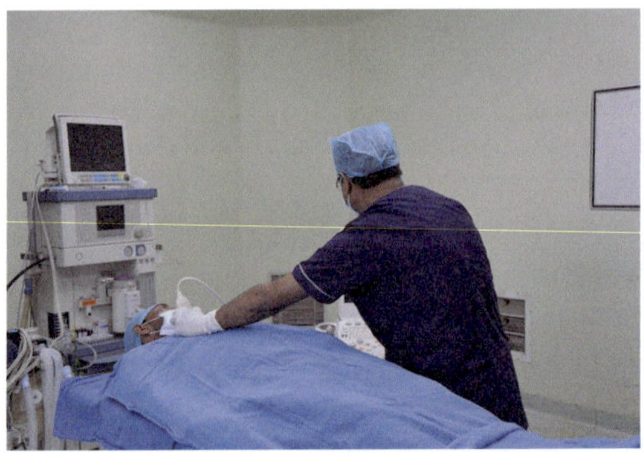

Fig. 3.8 Hyperextension of arm

3.7.13. Ideally other than operator, two assistants are required—One for injecting drug while monitoring the needle hub for blood and observing the expansion of the space around the nerve. The assistant should be standing on the dominant side of the operator. Second assistant is required for communication, reassurance, and patient positioning, most importantly for keeping track of unusual pain/paresthesia during nerve block.

3.7.14. Work-related musculoskeletal disorder (WRMD) has an incidence of 84–90% incidence among the ultrasound users. To mini-

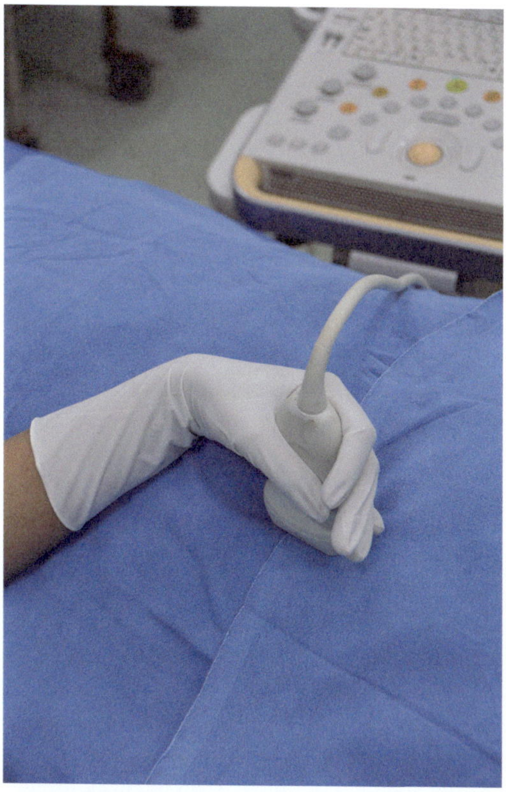

Fig. 3.9 Flexion at wrist

mize WRMD maintain a neutral position, i.e. posture balanced around operator's center of gravity. If feasible work from a sitting position with arm supported on bed.

3.7.15. Excessive forward bending and torsion of torso can be avoided by adjusting the height of the patient bed, trolley, or operating table in order to align the ultrasound and patient to same visual axis (Figs. 3.4, 3.5, and 3.6).

3.7.16. Move the patient closer to operator (table with lateral retractile supports) to avoid arm abduction greater than 30 degree and over-reaching the patient (Figs. 3.7 and 3.8).

3.7.17. Patient should be comfortable, safe and in the best possible position while giving the block.

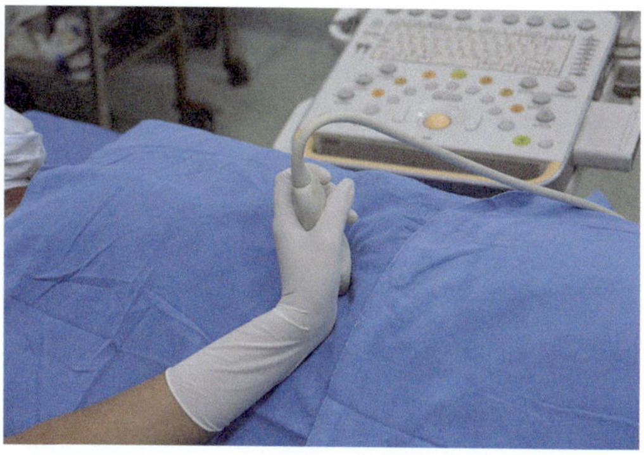

Fig. 3.10 Extension at wrist

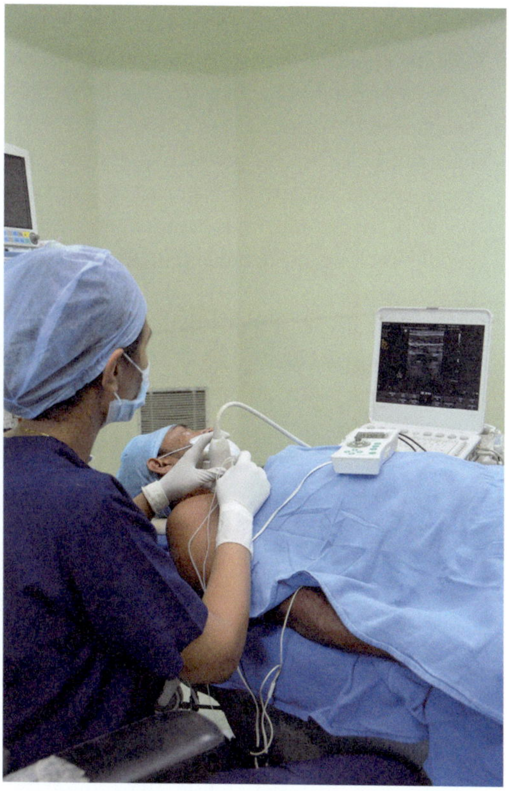

Fig. 3.11 Visual axis aligned

3.7.18. Regional anesthesia cart should be on the dominant side of the provider for easy handedness and avoiding cumbersome outreaching for the equipment.

3.7.19. Patient should be comfortable and appropriately covered with privacy maintained. The best possible safe, pain free position must be maintained.

3.7.20. Operator should rest the hand on the patient to reduce fatigue which can eventually lead to compromised needle transducer alignment. Avoid excessive flexion and extension at the wrist joint (Fig. 3.9 and 3.10).

3.7.21. The visual axis and the monitor screen should be aligned with each other (Fig. 3.11).

3.7.22. To enhance needle visualization various advancements have come up like echogenic needles (with serrations to enhance the scattering of USG beam), needle recognition software, needle guides (laser guidance and GPS system), hydro-location, augmented reality, needle tracking, electromagnetic tracking, and magnetism.

3.7.23. Vertically adjustable articulating monitors can help achieving the ideal position, plus rolling chair with adjustable height for the operator.

3.8 Pointers for Successful USG Blocks

1. For beginners recognition of the nerve is easier in short axis (probe face perpendicular to target), i.e. transducer is held in transverse direction across the long axis of the arm or leg. The nerves are hypoechoic on ultrasound imaging, while the connective tissue between fascicles is hyperechoic, thus nerves appear as dark nodules (honeycomb appearance).
2. Taking anatomic and technological considerations into being needle can be imaged in two planes.
   (a) *In plane*—Needle is parallel to the probe (Advantage—Whole length of needle is visible, Disadvantage—Technically challenging).
   (b) *Out of plane*—Needle is perpendicular to probe (Advantage—Easier to practice, Disadvantage—Only cross section of needle is seen as a hyperechoic dot).
3. During In-Plane approach needle beam angle should be greater than 55 degrees for better visualization. In reference to visual axis, it is always better to introduce the needle along the visual axis, i.e., parallel.
4. Tendons and nerves may be difficult to distinguish from each other especially when viewed in short axis.

   TIP—Operator to follow course of structure caudad to cephalad, tendons will eventually disappear into the muscle of origin or insert into bones.
5. Pre-block scan—Before actual needling of the patient, one should plan the route of needle and do a pre-block scan to check for any vulnerable structures such as blood vessel, pleura, etc.
6. Doppler mode should be used in order to identify the vessels, which can be taken up for nerves especially in short axis view. It is useful to locate vessels whose lumen gets obliterated with normal transducer pressure thus, decreasing the chances of LAST.
7. To enhance the image the needle should be inserted slightly further away from the probe at lesser acute angle, keeping it as parallel to the face of probe as possible to maximize the reflected echoes.

   TIP—Take a longer needle for this (10 cm).
8. Heeling—Transducer edge opposite the side of the needle insertion site is pressed to enhance the parallel alignment of the probe face with the needle.
9. When fascial plane just abuts the nerve, needle should be guided in a tangential fashion

to avoid impaling the nerve when fascia releases the needle, advance slowly awaiting a pop.

Tips

(a) Avoid unintended advancement of needle.
(b) Review the image optimization (inadvertent redirection of needle) due to forward thrusting of needle.
(c) Steepening the needle angle permits easy control of passage at expense of clear image.

10. Reoptimize the image of needle tip after passing through the fascia, do not advance until tip is located.

    TIP—In order to avoid nerve injury, ascertain that nerve doesn't move with the needle, indicating breach of epineurium, keep the tip adjacent to the nerve, not at its center.
11. For fascial plane block longitudinal spread of drug along the sheath should be the target whereas for nerves deposit the LA circumferentially around it (Donut /Halo).
12. Concomitant use of peripheral nerve stimulator along with USG is for safety monitoring rather than block efficacy.

Tip

(a) Motor movements at 0.4 mA should warn of intra-fascicular injection.
(b) If neural structures are difficult to visualize due to anatomical challenges like depth or osseous interference.
(c) PNS is an invaluable tool to identify individual nerves.

13.
    (a) Drug delivery should be in small aliquots of 3–5 ml preceded by aspiration.
    (b) Opening injection pressure should be <15 psi.
    (c) Stop injecting the drug if patient complains of continuous pain or paresthesias.
    (d) Inject drug under visualization, failure to do so suggests that tip of needle either is out of plane or is in the lumen of a vessel.

Thus, adoption of appropriate ergonomics leads to dual beneficial effect—first block success secondly potentially good health.

Further Reading

Chakraborty A, Ashoka B. Safety and ergonomics of ultrasound-guided regional anaesthesia. Singapore: Springer; 2021.

Folino TB, Mahboobi SK. Regional anesthetic blocks. Stat Pearls Publishing; 2023.

Hadzic A. Textbook of regional anaesthesia and acute pain management. McGraw Hill Professional; 2009.

Hadzic A. Hadzic's peripheral nerve blocks and anatomy for ultrasound-guided regional anesthesia. 3rd ed. New York: McGraw-Hill; 2022.

Kaye AD, Urman RD, Vadivelu N. Essentials of regional anaesthesia. Cham: Springer; 2018.

Marhofer P. Safe performance of peripheral regional anaesthesia: the significance of ultrasound guidance. Anaesthesia. 2017;72:427–38.

Morgan GE, Mikhail MS, Murray MJ. Peripheral nerve blocks. In: Morgan GE, et al., editors. Clinical anesthesiology. New York: Lange Medical Books; 2006.

Approach and Troubleshooting to Scalp, Facial, and Airway Blocks

4

Kaushic A. Theerth and Mukesh Kumar Prasad

Abstract

Head and neck area has a rich nerve supply from the branches of the fifth cranial nerve and the cervical spinal nerves. The use of regional anaesthesia has been commonplace for ophthalmic, dental, and certain maxillofacial procedures and was commonly practiced by surgeons since many years. Blocks of the head and neck are usually performed by anaesthesiologists as an adjunct to provide perioperative pain relief. However, certain neurosurgical procedures require an awake patient for intraoperative neurological monitoring and hence are performed under scalp block or cervical plexus block as sole anaesthetic technique. The trigeminal nerve supplies majority of the scalp and face and branches out and emerges extracranially through various foramina. While the upper cervical nerves form a plexus and can be blocked easily with a single injection, the nerves of the face and scalp are widespread and need to be blocked individually at multiple sites. Besides blocking surgical areas certain regional blocks are exclusively performed as a part of establishing airway access in an awake patient. The unique submucosal course of nerves allows for transmucosal blocks in the upper airway. Apart from the sensory and motor blockade the contribution of autonomic nerves and their implication in chronic pain has increased the scope of head and neck blocks. Head and neck blocks present are not devoid of complications and respiratory compromise is a serious limitation in few blocks due to the blockade of nerves lying in close proximity. Additionally due to the proximity of the cervical nerves with the major vessels supplying the brain, intravascular injection can lead to catastrophic complications.

Keywords

Scalp · Airway block · Mandibular · Cervical plexus · Occipital nerve · Peribulbar

K. A. Theerth
Department of Neuronaesthesia and Critical Care, Medical Trust Hospital, Ernakulam, Kerala, India

M. K. Prasad (✉)
Department of Anaesthesiology, Teerthanker Mahaveer Medical College and Research Centre, Moradabad, India
e-mail: mukeshkumar2002@gmail.com

M. K. Prasad, S. J. S. Bajwa (eds.), *Steps to Successful Regional Anesthesia*,
https://doi.org/10.1007/978-981-97-4098-7_4

4.1 Scalp Block

4.1.1 Anatomy

The scalp is the soft tissue covering the roof of the skull. It is composed of five layers: skin, connective tissue, aponeurosis and muscle, loose areolar tissue, and periosteum. It has an extensive vascular and sensory nervous supply. The trigeminal nerve and spinal nerves from C2–4 forming the superficial cervical plexus innervate the scalp via 6 different nerves on each side (Table 4.1 and Fig. 4.1).

Table 4.1 Nerve supply of scalp

	Nerves	Origin	Course	Supply
1.	Supraorbital nerve/ supratrochlear nerve	Frontal branch of trigeminal nerve (V1)	This frontal branch enters the orbit through the superomedial aspect of the superior orbital fissure and divides into a larger lateral supraorbital nerve and a smaller medial supratrochlear nerve. The supraorbital nerve passes anteriorly over the levator palpebrae superioris and exits the orbit through the supraorbital notch lateral to the supratrochlear nerve. The supratrochlear nerve leaves the orbit between the supraorbital notch and the trochlea, passing in a superior direction over the forehead	Forehead and the anterior part of the scalp Supratrochlear additionally supply the medial part of the upper eyelid, and the root of the nose
2.	Zygomaticotemporal nerve	Maxillary branch of the trigeminal nerve	It passes through a small canal in the zygomatic bone and enters into the temporal fossa passing superiorly between the bone and the temporalis muscle subsequently piercing the muscle and the temporalis fascia	Small area of the forehead and the temporal region
3.	Auriculotemporal nerve	Posterior division of the mandibular branch of the trigeminal nerve	This nerve crosses over the root of the zygomatic process of the temporal bone and lies posterior to the superficial temporal artery	Temporal areas, lower lip, lower face, auricle and the scalp above the auricle
4.	Greater occipital nerve (GON)	Medial branch of dorsal ramus of the second cervical spinal nerve (C2) and some fibres from C3	The GON is a sensory nerve and after exiting the C2 spinal nerve posterior to the lateral part of atlanto-axial joint, it travels inferiorly and laterally reaching the inferior border of the obliquus capitis inferior muscle. It runs further between the obliqus capitis inferior and semispinalis capitis muscles before piercing the latter muscle. It then becomes subcutaneous by piercing the trapezius aponeurosis, slightly inferior to the superior nuchal line or passing through the tendinous arch between the trapezius muscle and the sternocleidomastoid muscle, where it lies medial to the occipital artery	Provides cutaneous innervation to the majority of the posterior scalp from the level of the external occipital protuberance to the vertex and skin over the auricle
5.	Lesser occipital nerve (LON)	Ventral rami of C2 and C3	The lesser occipital nerve runs superiorly towards the skull along the posterior aspect of the sternocleidomastoid muscle, then pierces the deep cervical fascia to emerge over the occipital bone and ascends along the posterior border of the sternocleidomastoid muscle	Lateral area of the scalp posterior to the auricle

(continued)

Table 4.1 (continued)

	Nerves	Origin	Course	Supply
6.	Greater auricular nerve (GAN)	Superficial branch of cervical plexus C2 and C3	This is the largest of the ascending branches of the cervical plexus. Minor contributions from the greater auricular nerve and third occipital nerve rarely encroach into each other Blockade of this nerve is included in scalp block especially in retromastoid surgical approaches	Skin overlying the parotid gland, external ear, mastoid process, and posterior auricular region

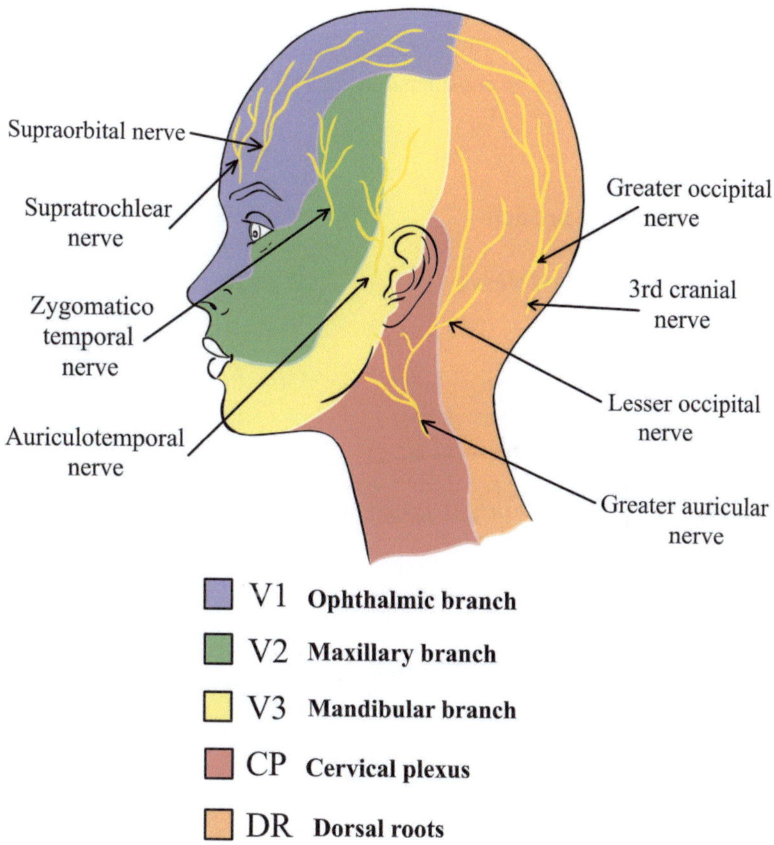

Fig. 4.1 Nerve Supply of scalp and face

4.1.2 Indications and Contraindications

Scalp block can be performed for various surgical procedures (Table 4.2). All the nerves can be blocked bilaterally or unilaterally and selective nerve blocks can be performed based on the indications.

4.1.3 Preparations

Refer to chapter on general considerations (Chap. 3).

4.1.4 Block Approach

4.1.4.1 Supraorbital Nerve

Landmark Technique

Position of patient—supine, sitting, and head in neutral position with the eyes closed.

Technique—The supraorbital nerve exits the superior surface of optic rim from supraorbital foramen and it can be blocked here. Under all aseptic precautions the supraorbital notch is located by palpation on superior orbit rim approximately 2–3 cm from midline in adults or on junction of medial one third and lateral two third of supraorbital margin. The 25–30-gauge needle is introduced perpendicularly 1 cm medial to the notch in medial and cephalad direction to avoid piercing the nerve with the needle. About 2 to 3 mL of LA (1% lidocaine, 0.25% bupivacaine or 0.5% ropivacaine) is injected 1 cm deep into the periosteum avoiding penetration of foramen itself (Fig. 4.2).

(**Tip**—Place a small roll of gauze firmly over the orbital rim to stop local anaesthetic from inflating at the superior aspect of the eyelid.)

Table 4.2 Indications and contraindications of scalp block

Indication	Contraindication
Scalp procedures—Repair of a laceration, skin grafting, rotational flaps, foreign body removal, wound exploration, abscess drainage, scalp tumour excision *Neurosurgical procedures*—Awake craniotomy, burr hole drainage of subdural haematomas, functional testing in deep brain stimulation for Parkinson's disease and stereotactic radiosurgeries, frontal ventroperitoneal shunt, analgesia for cranial surgeries and skull pin fixation *Chronic pain management*—Occipital neuralgia, migraine, cervicogenic headache, cluster headache, hemicrania continua, post-herpetic neuralgia involving ophthalmic division of trigeminal nerve	*Absolute* Patient refusal Absence of bone flap due to craniectomy Infection *Relative* Coagulation disorders Scars Allergy to the drugs

USG Technique

Position of patient—supine and head in neutral position.

Technique—Under all aseptic precautions a linear probe is placed in transverse direction over the orbital rim to locate the supraorbital notch, identified as small groove on bony surface (Fig. 4.3a). A 5 cm echogenic needle is used in either in-plane or out-of-plane approach and 2–3 mL drug is deposited after negative aspiration (Fig. 4.3b).

(**Tip**—Supraorbital artery can be identified in the groove by using colour Doppler and drug can be deposited besides it if supraorbital nerve is not visible.)

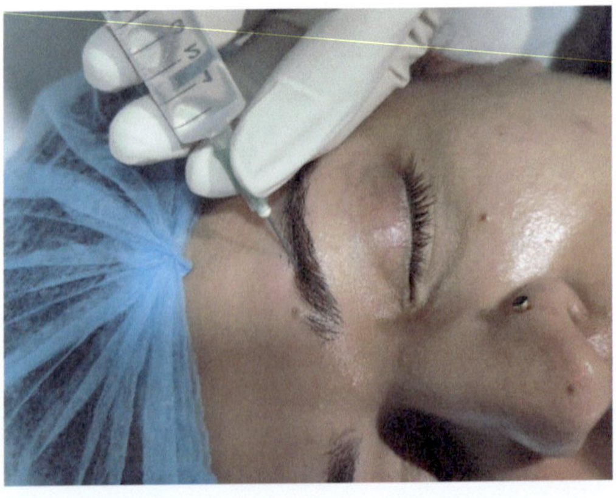

Fig. 4.2 Landmark-guided supraorbital and supratrochlear nerve block

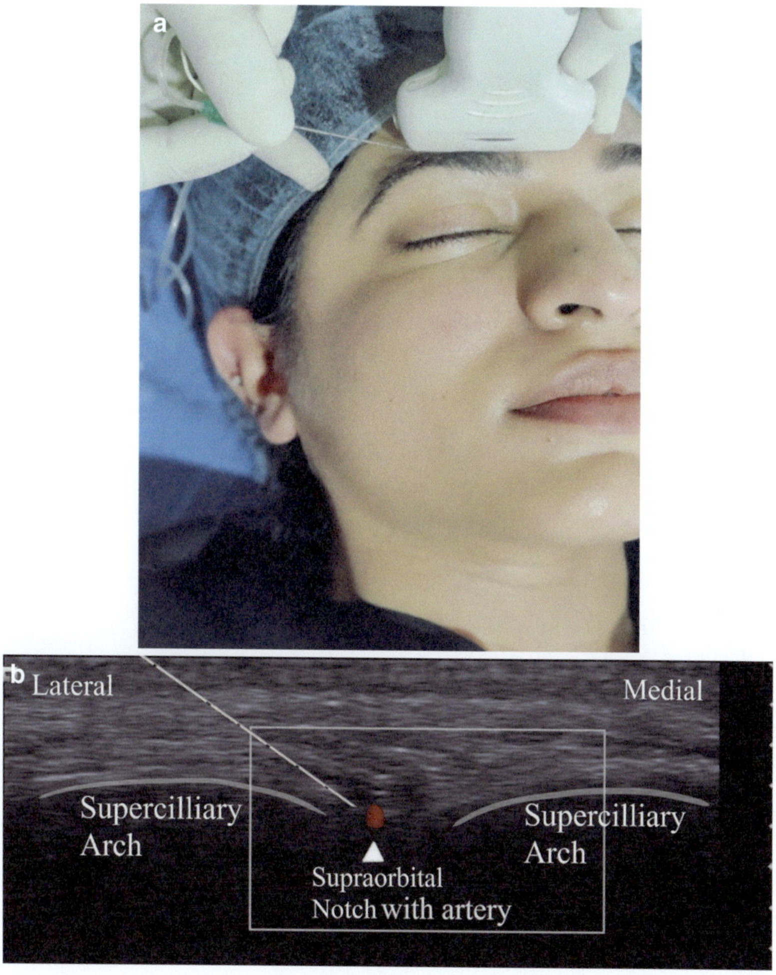

Fig. 4.3 (**a**) Probe position of supraorbital nerve block. (**b**) USG image of supraorbital nerve block

4.1.4.2 Supratrochlear Nerve

Position of patient—supine and head in neutral position.

Technique—The supratrochlear nerve runs about 1 fingerbreadth (3 mm medial to the vertical line) medial and parallel to the supraorbital nerve above the eyebrow. This nerve can be blocked from the same needle entry point as that of supraorbital nerve by directing the needle medially. A subcutaneous injection of 2 to 3 mL is injected directly into the subcutaneous space superior and medial to the supraorbital rim (Fig. 4.2).

After the needle is removed, mild pressure is applied to avoid bleeding and gentle massage helps in dispersing the drug.

4.1.4.3 Zygomaticotemporal Nerve

Position of patient—Head turned to one side so that the side to be blocked faces upward.

Technique—The zygomaticotemporal nerve branches as it pierces the temporalis fascia, hence both subcutaneous and deep injections are needed to block this nerve.

Under all aseptic precaution, groove is palpated along zygomatic arch lateral to lateral canthus of eye. The nerve is blocked by inserting the needle perpendicular to skin at the groove and when a 'pop' or loss of resistance is felt due to piercing of temporalis fascia, the needle is advanced further till it contacts with bone.

After negative aspiration, first 5 mL drug is infiltrated along lateral edge of supraorbital margin till distal aspect of zygomatic arch, then 1–2 mL is deposited when needle contacts the bone and another 3–4 mL is given by redirecting the needle laterally (Fig. 4.4).

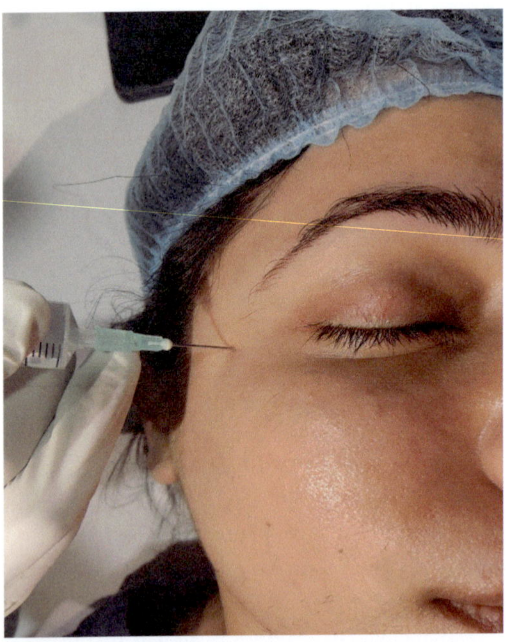

Fig. 4.4 Landmark-guided zygomaticotemporal nerve block

4.1.4.4 Auriculotemporal Nerve

Landmark Technique

Position of patient—Head turned to one side so that the side to be blocked faces upward.

Technique—Under all aseptic precaution the superior temporal artery is palpated about 1–1.5 cm cephalad to tragus of ear above the level of the temporomandibular joint. The needle is inserted perpendicular to skin and posterior to artery and as needle is advanced pop or loss of resistance is felt due to piercing of temporalis fascia at a distance of about 1–2 cm where 2–3 mL drug is deposited after negative aspiration (Fig. 4.5).

(Tip—Avoid deeper plane injections because they may result in a facial nerve block.)

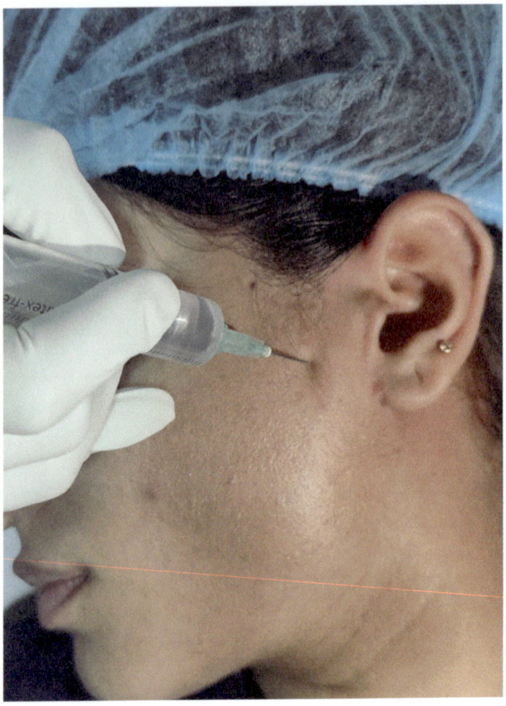

Fig. 4.5 Landmark-guided auriculotemporal nerve block posterior to superior temporal artery

Ultrasound-Guided Technique

Position of patient—Head turned to one side so that the side to be blocked faces upward.

Technique—Under all aseptic precaution the high frequency ultrasound probe is placed in horizontal direction parallel to and above the zygomatic arch. The superficial temporal artery is identified and 5 cm echogenic needle is inserted into deep surface of artery in out-of-plane technique and 2–3 mL local anaesthetic is deposited after negative aspiration (Fig. 4.6a, b).

4.1.4.5 Occipital Nerve Block

Indications

This nerve block is useful for postoperative analgesia after posterior craniotomies, shunt, as well as for diagnosis and pain treatment secondary to various headache syndromes described as chronic primary headaches (headaches more than 15 days per month) including occipital neuralgia, cervicogenic, migraines, tension and cluster headaches, and NSAID overuse. Patients can have

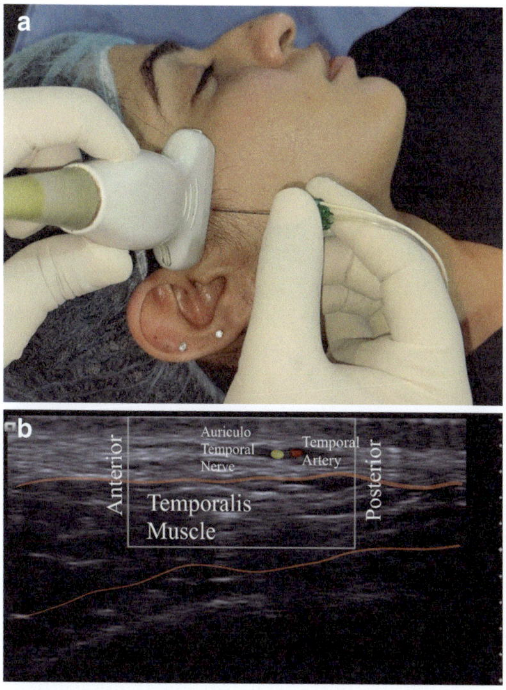

Fig. 4.6 (**a**) Probe position of patient for auriculotemporal nerve block. (**b**) USG image showing auriculotemporal artery and nerve

prolonged improvement in their pain up to 4 weeks after the procedure.

Block Approaches

Classical Landmark Technique

1. **For Greater Occipital Nerve (GON)**

Position of patient—Sitting with head flexed, lateral or prone.

Technique—A line is drawn between external occipital protuberance (EOP) and mastoid process on superior nuchal line. The occipital artery can be palpated on the medial one third of the line and GON is blocked medial to it (Fig. 4.7). Palpation in this area may elicit a paraesthesia or uncomfortable feeling in the distribution of the nerve. Under all aseptic precaution a 25- or 27-gauge needle can be used depending on the size of the patient. The needle is directed at 90° towards the occiput; after aspiration, 1–3 mL of local anaesthetic is injected. Numbness over the top of the head is a sign of a successful nerve block.

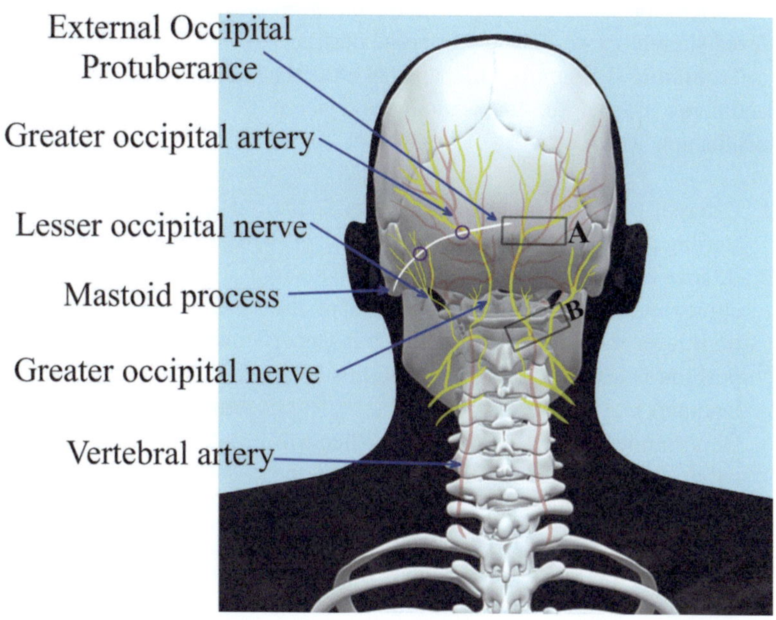

Fig. 4.7 Landmark and probe position (*A*—distal GON, *B*—proximal GON) for GON and LON blocks

There is considerable interpatient variability in the nerve location, with high variability (1.5–7.5 cm) of the distance of the GON to the midline at a horizontal level between the external occipital protuberance and the mastoid process. More recently, ultrasound guidance has been described to perform this nerve block.

2. **For Lesser Occipital Nerve (LON)**

Technique—The LON lies on lateral one third and medial two third along the superior nuchal line formed by joining EOP and mastoid process (Fig. 4.7). Anatomically, the LON can be located and blocked 5 cm lateral and 1 cm inferior to the EOP. At this point, under all aseptic precaution a 25- or 27-gauge needle is directed at 90° towards the occiput and after aspiration, 1–3 mL of local anaesthetic is injected. However, while performing GON block LA can spread to LON too.

Ultrasound-Guided Technique

1. For Greater Occipital Nerve (GON)

Patient position—Sitting up with the head flexed slightly forward, lateral or prone position.

Technique—A number of palpable external landmarks are helpful for scanning and nerve localization. They are:

1. External occipital protuberance: This is the starting point of a systematic scanning.
2. Inferior border of the mastoid process: This is approximately where the lateral end of the transducer should orient (the final transducer position is often slightly caudad to this bony landmark).
3. Bifid spinous process of axis (C2): When palpable, this is where the medial end of the transducer should orient.
4. The occipital artery can be found by palpating along the superior nuchal line until you locate the pulsating artery, normally about 3 cm lateral from the inion. The greater occipital nerve should be running medial to the artery. Colour flow Doppler can be utilized for confirmation.

- **Classical distal nerve block technique**

After skin and transducer preparation, place the linear high frequency 10–12 MHz transducer slightly lateral to external occipital protuberance at the level of superior nuchal line in transverse plane (position A in Fig. 4.7). In the transverse sonographic view, the hypoechoic GON is seen sandwiched between the semispinalis capitis muscle (SsCM) posteriorly and the obliquus capitis inferior muscle (OCIM) anteriorly (Fig. 4.8).

- Another more **proximal approach** at the level of the second cervical vertebra was developed by Greher et al. In this approach the linear probe is moved down over the atlas (C1) to the location of the spinous process of C2. The probe is then moved laterally to identify the obliquus capitis inferior muscle of the neck. The GON lies superficial to the obliquus capitis inferior muscle (OCIM); the relationship of the GON to this muscle appears constant and reliable (Fig. 4.9). Place the transducer in a slightly oblique plane to capture a transverse view of the OCIM slightly lateral to the spinous process of axis (position B in Fig. 4.7). The GON can be easily visualized at this level, crossing the obliquus capitis inferior muscle from caudal to rostral and lateral to medial.

Tip—Distinguish the GON from the second dorsal root ganglion which is deeper (anterior to OCIM).

Insert a 5 cm 22 G needle in-plane in the lateral to medial direction and aim to position the needle tip in the plane between OCIM and SsCM. Use hydro-dissection to confirm fluid distention in the correct plane before injecting 2–4 mL of LA.

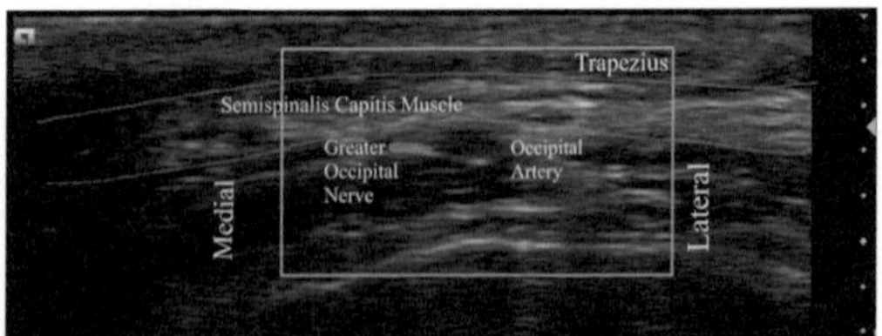

Fig. 4.8 USG approach to distal GON block

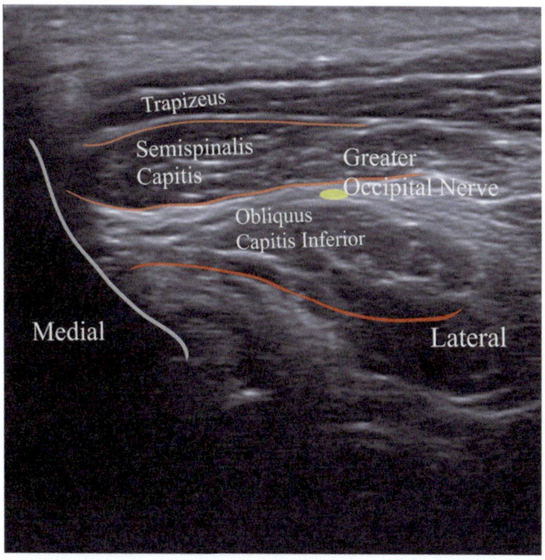

Fig. 4.9 USG approach for proximal GON block

2. **For Lesser Occipital Nerve (LON)**

Patient position—Sitting up with the head flexed slightly forward, lateral or prone position.

Technique—The linear probe is placed on the C2 spinous process in transverse plane (Fig. 4.10a). The attachment point of the SCM on the mastoid is identified while moving the probe laterally about 5 cm. The LON lies along the posterior border of the muscle (Fig. 4.10b). Insert a 2.5–5 cm 22 G needle using an out-of-plane technique and 1–2 mL of LA is injected after negative aspiration.

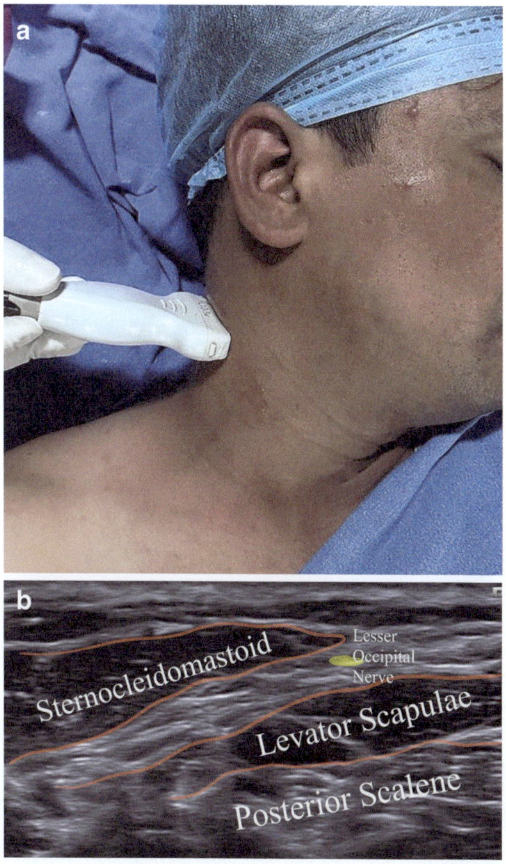

Fig. 4.10 (**a**) Probe position for LON block. (**b**) USG image of LON block

4.1.4.6 Greater Auricular Nerve

Classical Landmark-Guided Approach

Position of patient—Sitting up with the head flexed slightly forward, lateral or prone position.

Technique—Under all aseptic precaution identify the point below earlobe on posterior border of sternocleidomastoid 6–7 cm from external auditory meatus. Here greater auricular nerve (GAN) penetrates cervical fascia. Insert 3–5 cm long 25-25G needle subcutaneously (Fig. 4.11), The needle is directed towards mastoid process and at a depth of 2–4 cm 2 ml of LA is injected after negative aspiration.

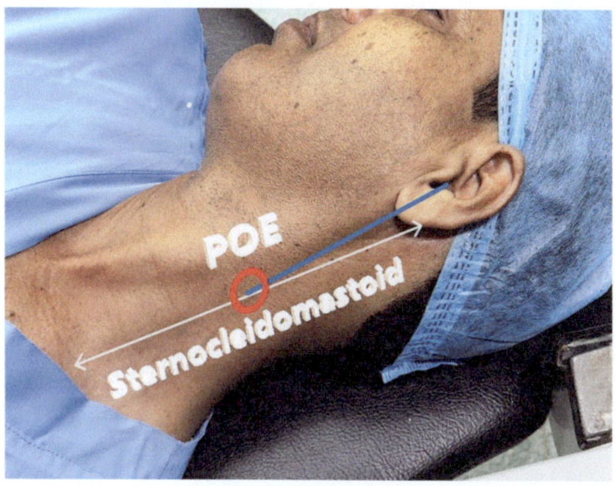

Fig. 4.11 Landmark-guided greater auricular nerve block

Ultrasound-Guided Approach

Position of patient—Sitting up with the head flexed slightly forward, lateral or prone position.

Technique—The linear probe is placed in transverse position at the middle of sternocleidomastoid muscle and traced slowly cranially towards the earlobe along posterior border of sternocleidomastoid. The GAN can be identified while moving the ultrasound probe cranially as it originates from the cervical plexus, courses in an anteromedial direction to lie on the anterior surface of the sternocleidomastoid (Fig. 4.12a, b). The needle is inserted in plane and 1–2 mL of drug is deposited after negative aspiration.

4.1.5 Complications

- Anaphylaxis.
- LA toxicity—Toxicity of LA. Addition of epinephrine can delay the systemic absorption of LA and prevent acute rise in the plasma levels. However, caution is advised to prevent intravascular injection as it can lead to arrhythmias and haemodynamic changes apart. Negative aspiration is a must in patients with cardiac disease.

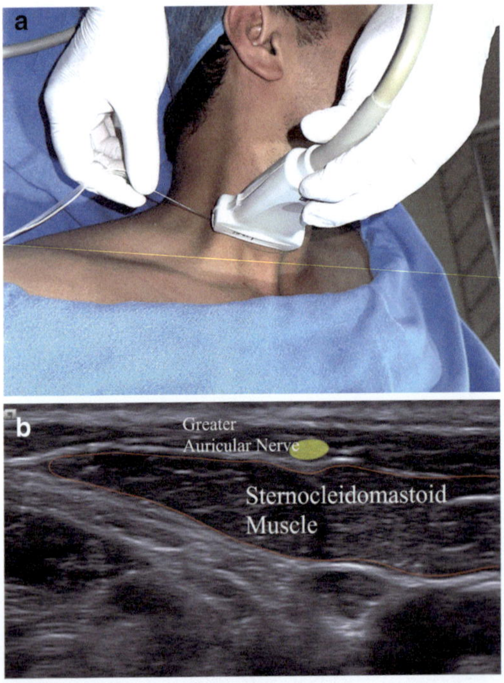

Fig. 4.12 (**a**) Probe position for greater auricular nerve block. (**b**) USG image of greater auricular nerve block

- Vascular puncture and haematoma formation especially during auriculotemporal and occipital blocks.
- Acute severe pain due to intraneural injection in supraorbital nerve block.
- Facial nerve palsy. This relatively rare complication (8.6%) can occur during the auriculotemporal block or zygomaticotemporal injections due to their proximity to the facial nerve. This is usually transient and caused by compression from haematoma, deep injection, oedema, or pressure due to local anaesthetic.
- Intracerebral or subarachnoid injection has been reported in patients with bony defects or previous craniectomies and occasionally with greater occipital nerve blocks. Caution needs to be taken because the vertebral artery and the spinal cord are close proximity to the GON. The vertebral artery is lateral to the GON deep to the obliquus capitis inferior muscle and the lamina of the atlas, while the spinal cord is medial and again deep to the muscle.
- Unilateral ptosis.
- Infection.
- A trigeminocardiac reflex can be activated during the scalp block and can cause severe bradycardia and hypotension. This occurs due to mechanical, electrical, or stretch stimuli over major or peripheral branches of the trigeminal nerve. Care should be taken to avoid rapid LA infiltration and direct infiltration into branches of the nerve.

4.1.6 Tips

- Care should be taken to protect the eyes during skin preparation with chlorhexidine.
- Sedation is recommended during administration of the block as multiple injections involving different point of entry are applied.
- When the needle is withdrawn, pressure should be maintained over the site of injection to promote soaking the nerve with local anaesthetic and to achieve haemostasis. Gentle massage helps in the spread of LA.

- As the dermatomal distribution exhibits enormous variability multiple nerves have to be blocked. Frequently, surgery on one side of the forehead requires a supplemental nerve block of the contralateral supratrochlear nerve because of overlapping distributions of the nerves.

4.2 Regional Anaesthesia for Ophthalmic Surgery

4.2.1 Anatomy

- **Orbit**

Each orbit is in the shape of an irregular pyramid with its base at the front of the skull and its axis pointing postero-medially. At the apex lies the optic foramen, transmitting the optic nerve and accompanying vessels. The superior and inferior orbital fissures transmitting the other nerves and vessels extend from the apex into the lateral walls of the pyramid. The angle between the lateral walls of the two orbits is approximately 90° and the angle between the lateral and medial walls of each orbit is nearly 45° (Fig. 4.13). Thus the medial walls of the orbit are almost parallel to the sagittal plane. The orbit measures 40–50 mm in depth with a volume of approximately 30 mL. The orbit contains the globe. Only 7 mL of this volume is occupied by the globe and its muscular cone with the rest mainly occupied by loose connective tissue containing orbital fat, extraocular muscles, nerves, blood vessels, and part of the lacrimal apparatus.

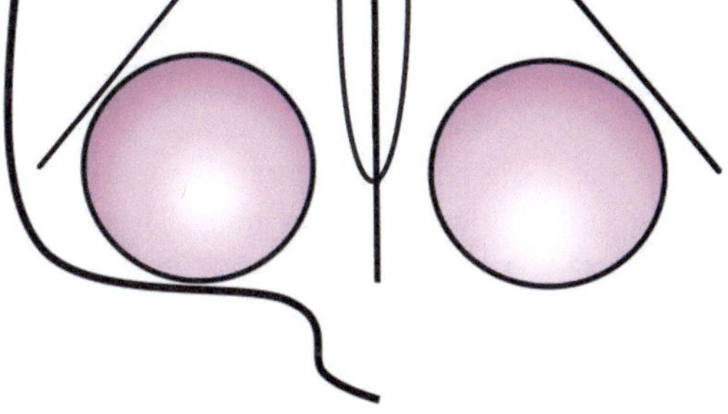

Fig. 4.13 Anatomy of orbit

- **The Globe** (Fig. 4.14) is situated in the anterior part of the orbital cavity closer to the roof than the floor and nearer the lateral than the medial wall. The sclera is the relatively tough fibrous layer of the eyeball completely surrounding the globe except in the anterior part, the cornea. The optic nerve penetrates the sclera posteriorly 1–2 mm medial to, and above, the posterior pole. The central retinal artery and vein accompany the optic nerve. Globe is covered by the Tenon's fascia. It arises from the corneo-scleral junction (the limbus) and fuses posteriorly with the dural sheath of the optic nerve. Tenon's fascia creates a potential space around the eye into which local anaesthetic can be placed, allowing diffusion of drugs to nerves that innervate the eye and its muscles as they pass through the fascia. The axial length of the globe measures around 25 mm in adults (range 12–35 mm). It is the distance from the corneal surface to the retina.
- **The Extraocular Muscles**
- There are four recti and two oblique muscles. The combined actions of these allow elevation, depression, adduction, and abduction of the eyeball. The cone refers to the cone-shaped structure formed by the extraocular muscles interconnected by a narrow circumferential band of intermuscular membrane. This small space extends from the annulus of Zinn at the orbital apex, to their penetration through Tenon's capsule before attaching to the globe. All the nerves supplying the extraocular muscles except the trochlear nerve transverse through the muscular cone of the orbit, thus injection of small volume of local anaesthetic (3-5 mL) via a retrobulbar injection in this area can reliably provide akinesia to the globe, thereby blocking both sensory and motor innervation. Under normal circumstances

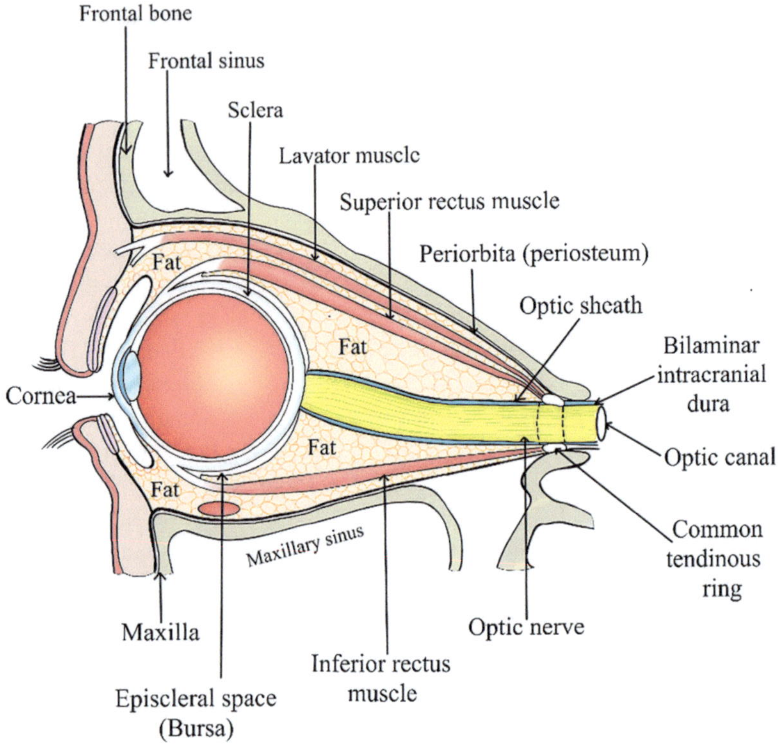

Fig. 4.14 Anatomy of eye globe, muscles, and fat

unmodified activity of one muscle is rare, but testing individual muscle function becomes necessary after local anaesthetic block to identify the unblocked nerve when some movement is still present.

- **The Orbital Fat** is divided into central (intraconal) and peripheral (periconal) compartments by the cone of the recti muscles. The central space contains the optic, oculomotor, abducens, and nasociliary nerves. The peripheral space contains the trochlear, lacrimal, frontal, and infraorbital nerves. All the motor and sensory nerves can be blocked by an extraconal injection via a peribulbar block into the orbital fat. However larger volumes (5–15 mL) are required for intraconal diffusion of the anaesthetic.

Intraocular pressure is described as the pressure the contents of the eyes produce on the surrounding wall. Increases in this pressure can have detrimental effects secondary to impairments in perfusion, resulting in a decrease in blood flow to ocular structures, including the retina, choroid, and optic nerve. Normal intraocular pressure is considered approximately to be 10 mm Hg to 21 mm Hg.

- **Nerve Supply**

The nerve supply to the orbital structures is by third to sixth cranial nerves entering the orbit via the superior orbital fissure. Lateral rectus is supplied by the sixth (abducens) cranial nerve and superior oblique is innervated by the fourth (trochlear) cranial nerve. Motor supply to the rest of the muscles is by branches of the third (oculomotor) nerve.

The sensory supply is mainly from the ophthalmic division of the fifth (trigeminal) cranial nerve. The lacrimal branch innervates the conjunctiva and the nasociliary branch supplies the cornea, sclera, iris, and ciliary body. The second cranial nerve (optic)provides vision.

Additionally, the iris muscles, ciliary muscle, smooth muscles of the eyelids, choroidal and conjunctival blood vessels, and the lacrimal gland have autonomic innervation. The parasympathetic supply is from the Edinger-Westphal nucleus. Fibres accompanying the third nerve synapse with the short ciliary nerves in the ciliary ganglion. The sympathetic fibres are from T1 and synapse in the superior cervical ganglion before joining the long and short ciliary nerves.

4.2.2 Indications and Contraindications

Almost all ophthalmic procedures can be done under regional anaesthesia except for extensive orbital exenteration surgeries (Table 4.3).

Table 4.3 Indications and contraindications

Indication	Contraindication
Cataract surgery Vitreoretinal surgery Trabeculectomy Strabismus correction	*Absolute* Local infection Allergy to the drugs *Relative* Severe coagulation abnormalities Ruptured globe Poor cooperation Movement disorders and altered mental state Postural problems

4.2.3 Troubleshoot

Most of the surgeries are performed in older patients with significant systemic illness which requires additional precautions while performing the procedure (Table 4.4).

4.2.4 Preparations

General preparations (Table 4.5).

Additional Care

- **Position**—Patient supine with eye in neutral gaze and clinician stand on side or head end
- Avoid fasting for low dose sedation and local anaesthetic techniques
- Prevent drapes from covering the mouth and face
- Provide squeaky ball for communication
- Topicalize the opposite eye to prevent the blink reflex
- Always inject with the bevel facing away from the sclera
- Explain the possibility of seeing unusual shapes shadows and kaleidoscopic colours

Equipment

Table 4.4 Troubleshoot

	Patient history	Anticipated problems	Optimization or alternative
1.	Previous surgery like scleral explant may encircle globe or lies in sub-Tenon space	Limit insertion of Tenon cannula; increased risk of perforation	Use of topical anaesthesia/peribulbar block
2.	**Cardiovascular comorbidities like** hypertension, angina, orthopnoea	Increased bleeding risk, intraoperative myocardial infarction, unable to lie flat	Use sedation Propped up position Continue antihypertensive and antianginal medications with adequate preoperative control Avoid adrenaline use
3.	**Respiratory comorbidities like** dyspnoea, asthma, COPD	Hypoxia Hypoxaemia CO_2 retention	Continue medical treatment Operation table adjustment Oxygen support Proper intraoperative draping to prevent CO_2 retention
4.	**Central nervous system involvement like** anxiety movement disorder, confusion, vertigo	Patient not able to lie flat/still	Sedation General anaesthesia may be considered

Table 4.5 General preparation of block

Pre-requisites	Equipment/materials required
Informed consent NPO status Optimal sedation if necessary Emergency, resuscitation drugs, and equipment Secure IV access Appropriate sedation, monitoring (HR, NIBP, Spo2, ECG, RR, etc.) and oxygen supply Site and side of block should be marked and confirmed	Sterile towels and 4 in. × 4-in. gauze packs 10–20 mL syringes with local anaesthetic Sterile gloves, marking pen, and surface electrode One 1.5 in., 25-gauge needle for skin infiltration

- 5% povidone iodine solution and paracaine solution for topical anaesthesia
- Sub-Tenon's cannula, short and long needles as per choice of technique
- Hyaluronic acid in the concentration of 5–70 IU/mL

4.2.5 Drugs

- Topical use—0.5% tetracaine, 0.5% proxymetacaine, 3.5% lignocaine, 0.4% oxybuprocaine.
- For infiltration—0.5% bupivacaine/levobupivacaine, 2% lignocaine, 0.75% ropivacaine.
- Adjuncts—Epinephrine 5 μ/ml or 1:20,0000.
  - Hyaluronidase (100 IU).

4.2.6 Block Approaches

4.2.6.1 Topical Anaesthesia

Local anaesthetic instillation is used predominantly especially in cataract surgery. Drugs are instilled 5–10 min before surgery and can be repeated as required.

Nerves blocked are trigeminal nerve terminals in the cornea and conjunctiva.

Limitation—Does not provide akinesia of globe and anaesthesia of intraocular structures, so patient can move eyeball intraoperatively.

4.2.6.2 Sub-Tenon's Block

Technique—Under all aseptic precaution a Barraquer speculum is inserted to keep the eye open. The inferonasal quadrant is exposed by asking the patient to look 'upwards and outwards' and hold that gaze. Inferonasal quadrant is preferred as it has no oblique muscles insertion (Fig. 4.15).

A non-toothed forceps is used to hold conjunctiva and Tenon's capsule 5–10 mm from the limbus in the exposed area and a small incision is made to expose the underlying white scleral area. A passage is created using round tipped scissor around the globe and sub-Tenons curved and blunt cannula is inserted following contour of the globe until the syringe is vertical. Local anaesthetic is then injected posterior to the equator of the globe. Three to five millilitre of LA (0.5% bupivacaine/levobupivacaine, 2% lignocaine, 0.75% ropivacaine) can be given. The use of gentle pressure to the closed eye encourages spread of the solution and reduces chemosis.

Limitations and Complications

- Need surgeon to administer
- Injection causes pain and may need sedation
- Conjunctival haemorrhage
- Retrobulbar haemorrhage
- Rectus muscle paresis
- Globe perforation
- Infection

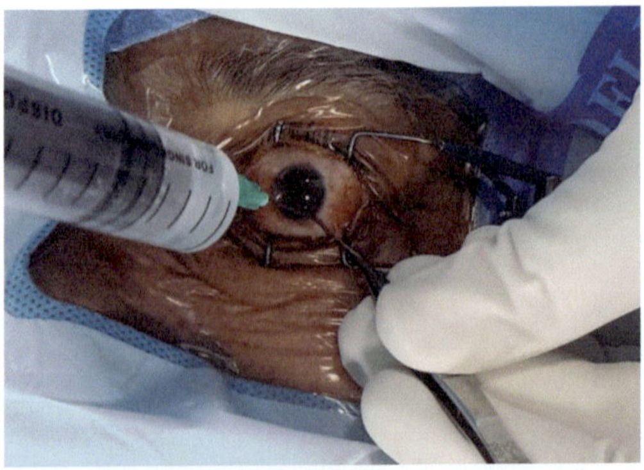

Fig. 4.15 Sub-Tenon's block

4.2.6.3 Peribulbar Block

Technique—The needle is inserted into extraconal space either via a trans-conjunctival or transcutaneous approach. This is an alternative to retrobulbar block.

Classically, two injections are performed. A 25-gauge, 2.5 cm needle is inserted at junction of medial 2/3rd and lateral 1/3rd of lower orbital rim perconjunctivally and the second injection between caruncle and medial canthus perconjunctivally or between the medial third and lateral two-thirds of the upper orbital rim and 6–12 mL LA is used.

Various approach followed for peribulbar block are inferotemporal, medial caruncular, and superonasal/nasal.

1. **Inferotemporal injection**

Technique—Under all aseptic precautions and after topical anaesthesia, the lower lid is retracted manually and the 3 cm needle is placed in inferolateral quadrant at the lower orbital rim. Alternatively, a transcutaneous injection is made when there is inadequate space for perconjunctival injection (Fig. 4.16).

The needle is advanced in along the orbital floor once needle is under the globe 5–8 mL of LA is slowly injected. The bevel of the needle should be oriented to face the globe so that any eye movement alert the anaesthetist of possible globe penetration.

Cross-section of eye showing needle directions as first peribulbar injection (Fig. 4.17).

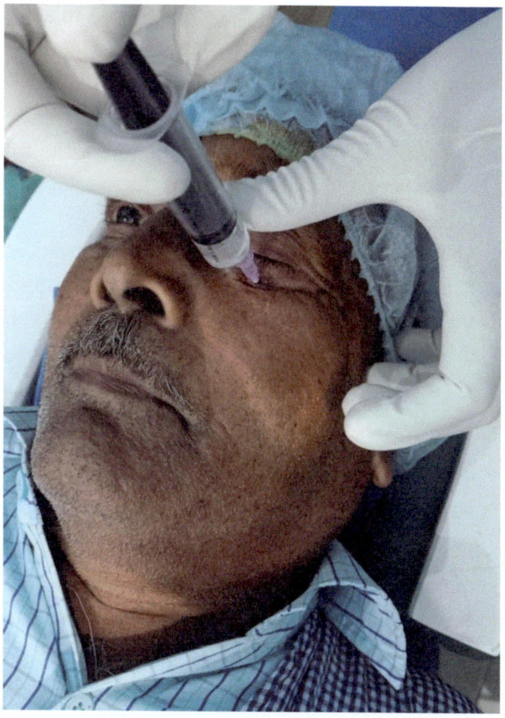

Fig. 4.16 Inferotemporal approach to peribulbar block

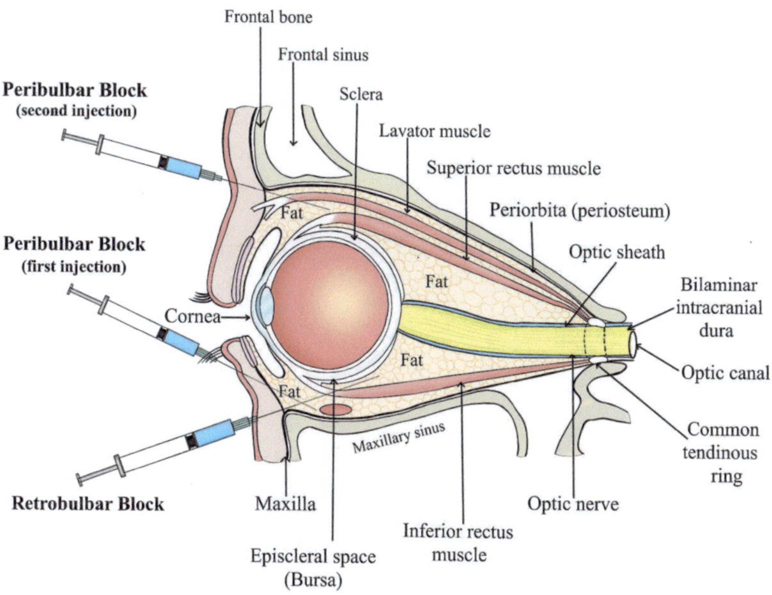

Fig. 4.17 Cross-section of eye showing needle directions as first peribulbar injection

Chemosis can occur due to LA filling the lower lid during the injection.

Tips

- A retrobulbar injection is suggestive of sudden ptosis, proptosis, and tense eyeball with lower volumes of LA. Stop injecting any further.
- There should not be any resistance while injecting. If resistance is encountered, the tip of the needle may be in one of the extraocular muscles and should be repositioned.
- Usually, adequate anaesthesia and akinesia is achieved within 5–10 min. In case of any sparing additional top-up of LA can be given either in same or different site.

2. **Nasal Injection**

Technique—Under all aseptic precautions and after topical anaesthesia the needle is placed medial to the caruncle on nasal side through the conjunctiva straight back parallel to the medial orbital wall and in slightly cephalad direction (Fig. 4.18).

Cross-section of eye showing needle directions as second peribulbar injection (Fig. 4.17).

After the needle crosses the medial canthal ligament 5 mL of LA is injected after negative aspiration. The entry into ligament may require gentle pressure.

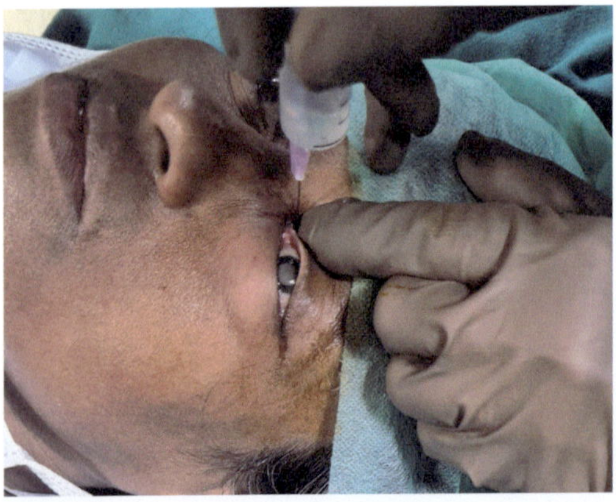

Fig. 4.18 Nasal approach to peribulbar block

Mild pressure is applied by putting gauze on closed eye to decrease the intraocular pressure. Assessment of the block is done after a period of 10 min. Ptosis, akinesia, and inability to fully close the eye mark the sign of successful block.

If after 10 min the block is inadequate a supplementary injection of 2–5 mL LA may be required.

Tips

- Prefer using fine 25 gauge short bevelled needle to avoid pain and better resistance appreciation.
- Prefer single injection technique and second injection for supplantation.
- Avoid going beyond 2.5 cm to prevent globe and optic nerve injury.
- Preferred needle insertion site is inferotemporal and nasal, superonasal site may injure superior oblique muscle and chances of globe injury are more as space between globe and orbit is very less here.

4.2.6.4 Retrobulbar Block

Technique—Under all aseptic precautions in classical Atkinson's method the 3.8 cm needle is inserted at the junction of medial 2/3rd and lateral 1/3rd of inferior orbital margin through the skin.

In modified retrobulbar approach, keeping eye in neutral gaze the needle is directed towards the apex within the muscle cone. Cross-section of eye showing needle direction as retrobulbar injection (Fig. 4.17).

The retrobulbar block can be administered after anaesthetizing the conjunctiva by topical anaesthesia. A 25 gauge, 2.5 cm needle is inserted in midpoint of line joining the lateral canthus and the lateral limbus in the lower conjunctiva. The needle is first pointed backwards behind the globe until it has reached the equator, at which point it is pointed upward at a 45° angle and inward to enter the space behind the globe between the inferior and lateral recti muscles. After confirming negative aspiration, 4–5 mL of LA is injected slowly.

The retrobulbar approach has largely been replaced by peribulbar block because of the higher incidence of complications.

4.2.7 Complications

Complications may result either due to the agents used or the block technique itself.

- Intravascular injection.
- Anaphylaxis.
- Haemorrhage—Retrobulbar haemorrhage (0.07–1.7%) is characterized by rapid orbital swelling and proptosis. There is sudden rise in IOP. Central retinal artery pulsations should be monitored, and the surgeon should be informed. If the IOP rises excessively, a lateral canthotomy may be necessary, and the operation must be delayed.
- Chemosis (subconjunctival oedema) occurs in 25–40% cases. Though resolves on its own but may interfere with suturing. Slowing the rate of injection and with gentle pressure, it disappears rapidly.
- Penetration or perforation of the globe (<0.1%)—More prevalent in myopic eyes, which are longer, thinner, and possibly developing staphyloma than normal. A weak red reflex, pain during the block, rapid loss of vision, or vitreous haemorrhage are all signs of perforation. Never direct the needle 'up and in' until the needle tip is clearly past the equator of the globe and patient should gaze straight ahead throughout block performance.
- Extraocular muscle injury especially inferior oblique and inferior rectus can lead to myonecrosis and contractions of muscle.
- Direct injection into dural cuff of the optic nerve may lead to drowsiness, vomiting, convulsions, respiratory depression, neurological deficits, contralateral blindness, and cardiac arrest.
- Oculocardiac reflex—The trigeminal nerve allows the afferent impulses to travel to the medulla, where they stimulate the efferent limb that travels through the vagus to the sinoatrial node leading to bradycardia. It can be triggered by pressure application on the globe or extraocular muscles traction.
- Partial or complete visual loss even immediately can occur if there is direct injury to optic nerve or central retinal artery injection.
- Sterile abscess formation can be seen with additive like hyaluronidase.
- Intramuscular LA injection may lead to postoperative strabismus.

4.2.8 Tips

- In high myopes elongation of eyeball causes thinning and weakness of the sclera leading to outpouching in the posterior and inferior areas (staphyloma) which increases the risk of globe perforation, especially during peribulbar or retrobulbar injections. Care should be taken for axial lengths >26 mm and other approaches like sub-Tenon's block or GA.
- Ophthalmic procedures can significantly raise intraocular pressure. Additionally, a 0.5-mL intravitreal injection can elevate intraocular pressure by more than 150%, and continued increases in intraocular pressure can impair blood flow to the retina and optic nerve, which can result in vision loss.
- Earlier practice of wiggling the needle to make sure that the globe is not engaged not recommended as it increases the chance of globe perforation.
- Anticoagulants and antiplatelet agents can be continued for patients undergoing cataract operations on day surgery.

4.3 Airway Block

4.3.1 Anatomy

The airway is divided into upper and lower airway as shown in Fig. 4.19.

The upper airways are innervated mainly by branches of the three cranial nerves, i.e. trigeminal, glossopharyngeal, and vagus nerves (Fig. 4.19).

The sensory distribution of nerve supply is shown in Table 4.6.

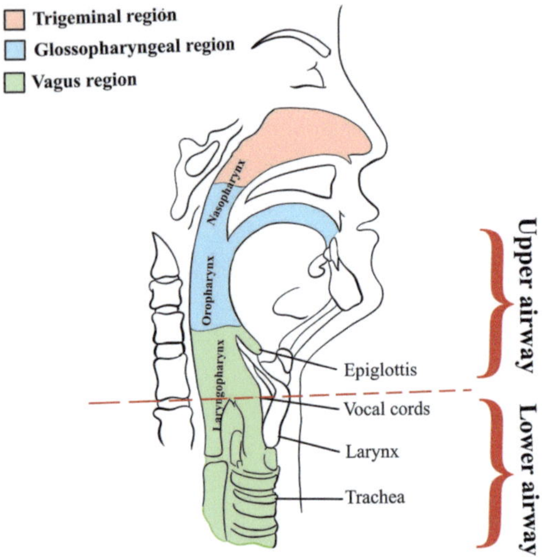

Fig. 4.19 Anatomy and nerve supply distribution of airway

Table 4.6 Sensory nerve supply of airway

Nasal cavity and septum	Anterior part—anterior ethmoidal nerve (branch of ophthalmic division of trigeminal, V1)
	Posterior part—greater and lesser sphenopalatine nerve (branch of maxillary division of trigeminal,V2)
Tongue	Anterior 2/3rd—lingual nerve (branch of mandibular division of trigeminal, V3)
	Posterior 1/3rd—glossopharyngeal nerve
Pharynx	Glossopharyngeal nerve
Larynx	Supply below epiglottis—vagus nerve Above vocal cord—internal laryngeal branch of superior laryngeal nerve from vagus Below vocal cord—recurrent laryngeal branch of vagus

The cricothyroid muscle is supplied by external branch of superior laryngeal nerve from vagus and posterior cricoarytenoid muscle is supplied by recurrent laryngeal nerve from vagus.

The glossopharyngeal and the vagal nerves are involved in brainstem-mediated reflex arcs which coordinate the processes involved in allowing breathing during feeding, providing protection against aspiration.

4.3.2 Indication

- Awake flexible fibreoptic bronchoscopy (FOB) for nasotracheal or orotracheal intubation with minimal discomfort and requires mild sedation. Fibreoptic laryngoscopy can be performed in an anaesthetized individual if the mask ventilation is not compromised by anaesthesia or in cases where FOB is done as a diagnostic procedure.
- Awake intubation using videolaryngoscopes and optical stylets especially when adequate mouth opening is present and bleeding and secretions obscure the visibility through a fibreoptic scope.
- Selective glossopharyngeal nerve block.
  - To prevent excessive gag in endoscopic procedures.
  - Glossopharyngeal neuralgia (trauma, Eagle's syndrome, elongated/ossified styloid process, cerebellopontine angle tumour, arachnoiditis, multiple sclerosis).

4.3.3 Preparation

- Patient counselling.
- Antisialogogues—It helps to dry the mucosa. Glycopyrrolate is 5 times more potent than atropine and atropine produces greater increase in heart rate.
  - Inj glycopyrrolate 5–10 μg/kg IV.
  - Inj Atropine 7–10 μg/kg IV.
- Sedative agents—Opioids such as fentanyl (1–2 μg/kg IV) or remifentanil (0.05–0.5 μg/kg IV).
  - Midazolam 0.15–0.3 mg/kg.
  - Dexmedetomidine IV infusion in the dose of 0.3–0.7 μg/kg per minute.
  - Dexmedetomidine also has potent antisialogogue action.
- Local anaesthetics.
  - Lignocaine 2%, 4% is used for infiltration and mucous membranes, respectively, and 10% is used as an atomized spray.
  - Mucosal anaesthesia can be achieved by using lignocaine gargles (2%), spray

(10%), and/or nebulization (2–4%). Nebulization can additionally anaesthetize the mucosa of the glottic and subglottic region. The nasal cavity can be anaesthetized by 2% lignocaine gel.
  - The maximum safe dosage is 3–4 mg/kg.
  - Benzocaine 20% for mucous membranes.
- Vasoconstrictors can be used along with LA to produce vasoconstriction and decrease the bleeding due to trauma during the insertion of the scope and especially the tube.
  - Cocaine nasal drops (0.5 mL in each nasal cavity of 4–10% concentration, maximum dose is 100–200 mg).
  - Lignocaine (4%) + Phenylephrine (1%) in a ratio 3:1.
  - Lignocaine spray (10%) + xylometazoline 0.1%/oxymetazoline 0.1%, 0.05% 1–2 sprays or 2–3 drops in each nostril.
  - Neosynephrine 0.25–0.5%, 2–3 sprays in each nostril.
- Oxygenation
- Oxygen can be administered in patients with compromised lung reserves and requiring moderate to severe sedation. Nasal cannula is usually used and a well-lubricated nasal airway can be inserted to maintain the airway patent as in case of deeper levels of sedation.
- Transnasal humidified rapid-insufflation ventilatory exchange (THRIVE) is the technique of providing relatively constant oxygen concentration (21–100%), temperature (31–37 °C), with high gas flows (up to 70 L min^{-1}). Optiflow™ (Fisher & Paykel Healthcare, Auckland, New Zealand) is a commercially available high-flow humidified transnasal oxygen-delivery system. The advantages of high flows are a washout of nasopharyngeal dead space, a reduction in the work of breathing, and the provision of a degree of positive airway pressure.

4.3.4 Block Approaches

Awake fiberoptic intubation needs blockade of nasal cavity (supplied by maxillary branch of the trigeminal nerve), oropharynx (supplied by glossopharyngeal nerve), larynx and trachea (supplied by vagus nerve). If the airway is not adequately prepared, it can cause autonomic reflexes leading to salivation, gagging, coughing, and haemodynamic changes. As airway anaesthesia involves blocking only the mucosal surface, these blocks can be performed by either topicalization or nerve block by infiltration.

4.3.4.1 Topical Anaesthesia

The structures needed to be anaesthetized depend on the route of insertion either via the nose or mouth. Various methods of topical anaesthesia which are also used in combination are given in Table 4.7.

Density of anaesthesia is variable and often requires supplementation to facilitate intubation.

4.3.4.2 Nerve Infiltration

Three main nerve blocks can be performed via infiltration.

Glossopharyngeal Nerve Block

This can be blocked via intraoral or extraoral approach based on the extent of mouth opening. Glossopharyngeal nerve block is commonly used to block gag reflex in endoscopic procedures.

1. **Intra-oral Approach**

In supine or semi-sitting position the mouth is opened widely. The posterior tonsillar pillar is identified.

The nerve is blocked by instilling 2–3 mL LA submucosally by a 22-gauge needle at the caudal aspect of the posterior tonsillar pillar. This approach is easier due to the consistent location of the nerve and easier identification of landmarks (Fig. 4.21).

There is chance of intravascular injection.

2. **Extraoral/Peristyloid Approach (Lateral Cervical Technique)**

Patient is placed supine with head in the neutral or head rotated 30° to contralateral side. A line is drawn between the angle of the mandible and the mastoid process.

Table 4.7 Various methods of topical anaesthesia for airway blocks

Topicalization	This is the simplest way of applying local anaesthetic to a mucosal area in order to block that area by local uptake of drug
Gargle	2–4 mL 2–4% lignocaine viscous solution is used for gargle for 30–40 s. However, anaesthesia to nasal cavity, the larynx or trachea is spared
Spray using pressurized canisters or atomizer syringes	They have long tubes and nozzles that produce a fine mist for the spray. In lignocaine 10% spray each dose (one spray) contains 10 mg of lidocaine. 2–3 puffs are optimum
McKenzie technique	This is an alternative to sprays where a 20 gauge cannula is attached to one end of three-way connector and a 5 mL syringe with local anaesthetic and oxygen source at the rate of 2–4 L/min are connected in a fashion as shown in figure (Fig. 4.20). A jet-like effect is seen and local anaesthetic is spread in the target area
Nebulization	Lidocaine 2–4% via face mask or oral nebulizer for 15–30 min can achieve highly effective anaesthesia of the oral cavity and trachea for intubation. This is simple and effective technique
Atomization	Used for airway topicalization by atomizing spray for endotracheal intubation
Anaesthetic-soaked cotton pledgets or swabs	Cotton pledgets or swabs soaked in either viscous or aqueous solutions of LA can be applied for 5–10 min on targeted mucosal surfaces. This technique is especially effective in sphenopalatine ganglion block but can also be applied to glossopharyngeal and superior laryngeal nerve blocks. Application of LA and vasoconstrictor-soaked cotton packing is commonly applied in the nasal cavity block before endoscopic nasal procedure. This can block the anterior ethmoidal, sphenopalatine branches
Spray-as-you-go (SAYGO)via epidural catheter	An epidural catheter cut 3 cm from the tip (to avoid dispersion of LA from the side ports) is inserted through working channel till it emerges out and the LA is injected with pressure onto vocal cord or desired part of airway under direct vision

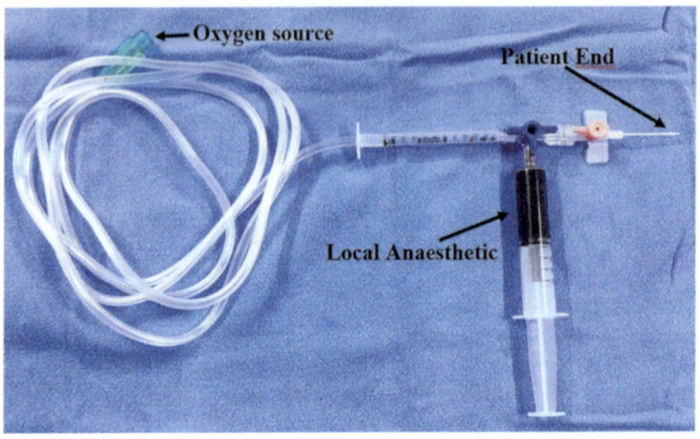

Fig. 4.20 McKenzie technique of topicalization

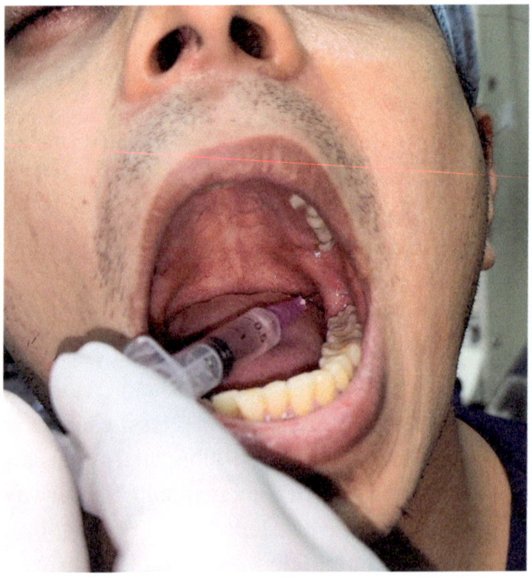

Fig. 4.21 Intraoral approach for glossopharyngeal nerve block

Under all aseptic precaution, the styloid process is palpated just posterior to the angle of the jaw approximately midway on the line drawn above using deep pressure, and a short, 25 gauge needle is inserted to contact the styloid process. The needle is then withdrawn slightly and directed posteriorly off the styloid process. As soon as bony contact is lost, 2–5 mL of LA solution is injected after careful aspiration for blood (Fig. 4.22).

Complications

- For both approaches, careful aspiration for blood must be carried out prior to injection as the glossopharyngeal nerve is closely associated with the internal carotid artery.

- Larger amount of LA can lead to blockade of vagus (collection of saliva in pyriformis fossa), spinal accessory nerve (weakness of trapezius), hypoglossal nerve (deviation of outstretched tongue towards blocked side), and superficial cervical ganglion.

Superior Laryngeal Block

The superior laryngeal nerve divides into a sensory (internal) and motor (external) branch lateral to the greater cornu of the hyoid bone. The nerve accompanies the superior laryngeal artery and pierces the thyrohyoid membrane approximately 2 mm inferior to the greater cornu of the hyoid bone. It passes submucosally in the pyriform recess and provides nerve supply to the base of the tongue, posterior surface of the epiglottis, aryepiglottic fold, and the arytenoids.

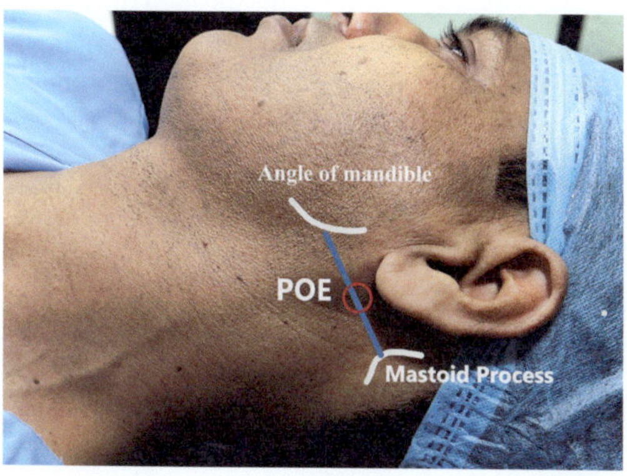

Fig. 4.22 Extra-oral approach for glossopharyngeal nerve block

The nerve can be blocked by intraoral or extraoral approach.

1. **Intraoral Approach**

Under all aseptic precaution Kraus or Jackson forceps or right-angled forceps can be used to hold a cotton pledget soaked in lidocaine 2–4% against the mucosa in the piriform fossa for about 1–2 min to block the superior laryngeal nerve.

2. **Extraoral Approach (Landmark-Guided)**

After skin preparation the hyoid bone can be displaced laterally towards the side of the block to make it more prominent. The greater cornu of the hyoid bone is then palpated and 25G needle is inserted perpendicular to the skin to contact the bone. The needle is then retracted and directed inferiorly to walk down the bone into the thyrohyoid ligament which can be identified by loss of resistance. The needle is placed between thyrohyoid ligament and laryngeal mucosa. At the depth of 1–2 cm 2 mL of LA is injected after negative aspiration to block both the branches of the superior laryngeal nerve. While withdrawing the needle another 1–2 mL drug is deposited in the tissues to reliably bathe the internal branch of the superior laryngeal nerve (Fig. 4.23a, b).

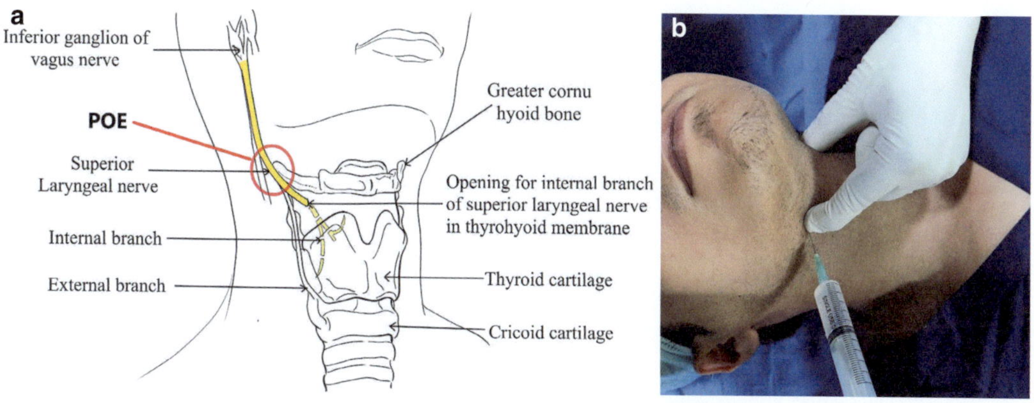

Fig. 4.23 (**a**) Anatomy of landmark-guided superior laryngeal nerve block. (**b**) Landmark-guided superior laryngeal nerve block

3. **Extraoral Approach (USG-guided)**

Under all aseptic precautions a high frequency probe is kept in parasagittal plane so that hyoid bone and thyroid cartilage are seen cranially and caudally, respectively. The thyrohyoid muscle is seen as hypoechoic band which passes over thyroid cartilage and inserted into hyoid bone and thyrohyoid membrane is seen as hyperechoic layer which delineates pre-epiglottic space below it. With slight tilting and rotating movement of probe superior laryngeal nerve can be seen below the thyrohyoid membrane. It can be sometimes visualized superficial to thyrohyoid membrane. The 23 gauge 5 cm needle is inserted in plane or out of plane and 2–3 mL of LA is deposited (Fig. 4.24a, b).

Alternatively, the probe is rotated over thyrohyoid membrane just below greater cornu of hyoid in transverse plane. In short-axis view thyroid muscle is seen anterior to the superior laryngeal nerve and artery, external carotid artery posterior and thyrohyoid membrane is deep to nerve. The 23 gauge 5 cm needle is inserted in plane and 2–3 mL of LA is deposited (Fig. 4.25a, b).

(Tip—If the nerve is not visible drug is deposited on surface of thyrohyoid membrane and anterior to external carotid artery. This area corresponds to internal branch of superior laryngeal nerve).

The hyoid bone can be easily fractured if excess pressure is applied. Blocking the external branch blockade may result in cricothyroid muscle weakness; however, the motor input of the recurrent laryngeal nerve is spared, and hence the laryngeal diameters are not significantly altered.

Recurrent Laryngeal Nerve Block/ Translaryngeal Block

Recurrent Laryngeal Nerve is a mixed nerve arising from the vagus and passes through the tracho-oesophageal groove. It provides sensory to the vocal cords and the trachea. As the motor and

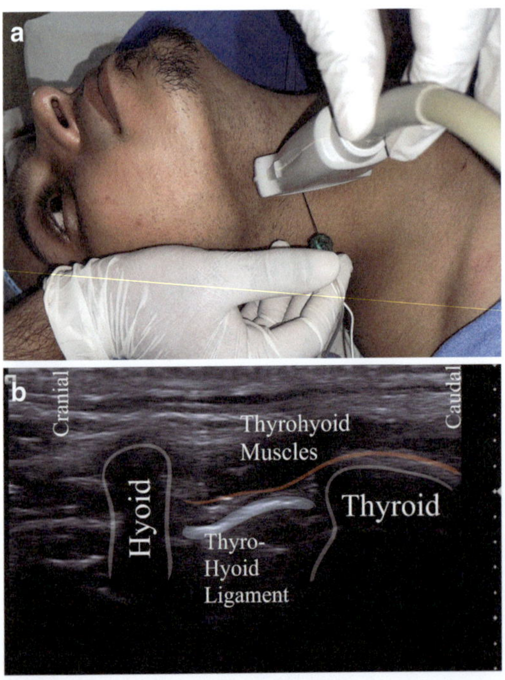

Fig. 4.24 (**a**) Parasagittal probe position for superior laryngeal nerve block. (**b**) USG image in parasagittal probe position for superior laryngeal nerve block

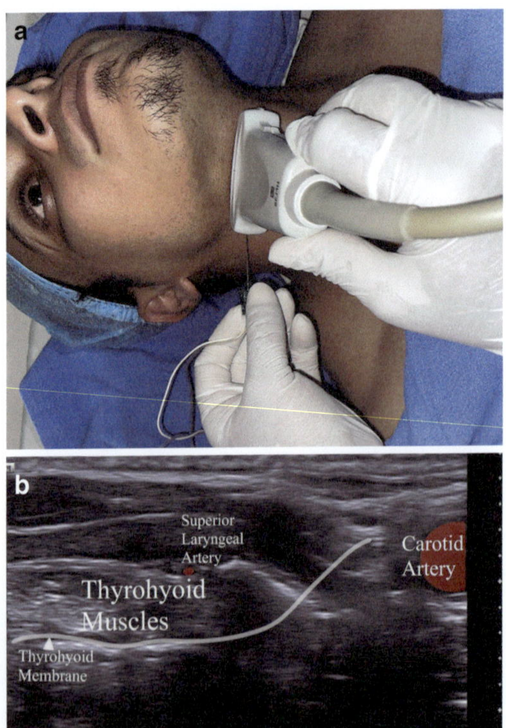

Fig. 4.25 (**a**) Transverse probe position for superior laryngeal nerve block. (**b**) USG image in transverse probe position for superior laryngeal nerve block

sensory fibres run together direct blockade of the nerve can cause motor weakness resulting in vocal cord palsy and airway obstruction. Hence, mucosal topicalization is performed via a percutaneous translaryngeal injection.

1. **Landmark-Guided Technique**

Position—The patient is placed in the supine position with maximum possible extension of neck.

Landmarks—Cricoid cartilage, thyroid cartilage, and median cricothyroid ligament.

Technique—The thyroid cartilage is palpated feeling for the thyroid notch in the midline and the finger is slid down caudally to feel the cricoid cartilage. The space between the thyroid and cricoid cartilage is felt and a 22 gauge 5 cm needle is inserted in the midline (poorly vascularized area) into cricothyroid membrane while the thyroid cartilage is stabilized by holding it between the thumb and the index finger of the other hand. The needle is advanced till a giveaway is felt and aspiration of air confirms the entry into the larynx. 2–5 mL of 2–4% lignocaine is injected rapidly and the needle should be withdrawn immediately as a cough will be stimulated which will help in the dispersion of the local anaesthetic in the larynx and the cords. The patient should be informed prior about the cough and should be reassured after the injection. Sedation may be needed to prevent excessive coughing (Fig. 4.26).

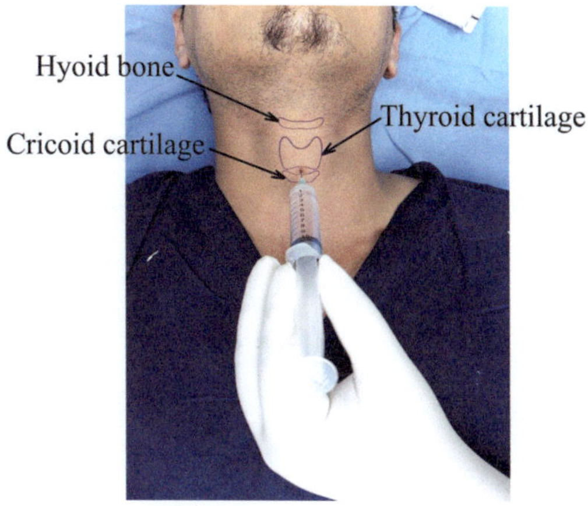

Fig. 4.26 Landmark-guided transtracheal injection

2. **Ultrasound-Guided Technique**

When the cartilages and the hyoid bone are difficult to palpate like in obese individuals, ultrasound can be used to identify these structures and increase the success rate of the block.

Position—The patient is placed in the supine position with maximum possible extension of neck.

Technique—Translaryngeal block can also be performed using the ultrasound by identifying the thyroid, cricoid cartilages, and the cricothyroid membrane in the sagittal plane. The probe is initially placed longitudinally in the midline above the suprasternal to identify the tracheal rings. By moving the probe cranially, the larger cricoid cartilage can be seen which is more superficial than the tracheal rings. The thyroid cartilage can be identified by further advancing the probe cranially. Once the cricothyroid space is identified the probe can be tilted parasagittally and the 22 gauge 5 cm needle can be inserted in an out-of-the plane technique and 2–5 mL of 2–4% lignocaine is injected rapidly after aspiration of air confirms the entry in to the larynx (Fig. 4.27a, b).

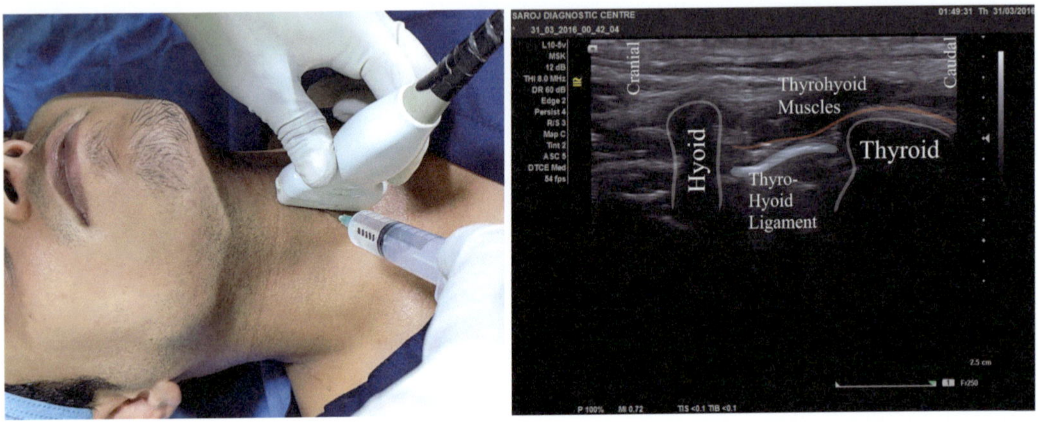

Fig. 4.27 (**a**) Probe position for transtracheal injection. (**b**) USG image showing transtracheal injection

4.4 Blocks of the Face

4.4.1 Infraorbital Nerve Block

4.4.1.1 Anatomy

Infraorbital nerve is the terminal branch of the maxillary division of the trigeminal nerve. As the maxillary division nerve exits the skull through the foramen rotundum it passes through the pterygopalatine fossa to enter into the infraorbital canal. It runs along the orbital floor to emerge through the infraorbital foramen. It divides into the anterior and middle maxillary alveolar nerves, inferior palpebral, lateral nasal, and superior labial branches giving sensory supply to the lower eyelid, lateral aspect of the nose, upper lip, upper incisor, canine, premolars, and mesiobuccal root of the first molar (Fig. 4.28).

4.4.1.2 Indications and Contraindications

Various indications and contraindications of infraorbital nerve block are tabulated (Table 4.8).

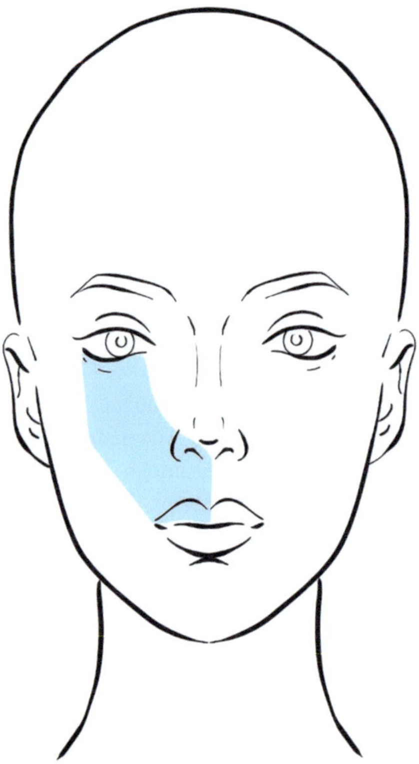

Fig. 4.28 Anatomical distribution of area supplied by inferior orbital nerve

Table 4.8 Indications and contraindications of infraorbital nerve block

Indications	Contraindications
Wound closure when local infiltration is not possible Dental procedures involving the maxillary teeth, apical abscess drainage Debridement Surgery and postoperative pain relief in endoscopic maxillary sinus surgeries, rhinoplasty, maxillary fixation, transsphenoidal hypophysectomy and cleft lip surgeries. A bilateral block is needed in case of surgeries involving the upper lip Any contraindication to general anaesthesia	Patient refusal Local infection Allergy to local anaesthetics Distorted anatomy (Lefort fracutres) Wound having multiple nerve innervation

4.4.1.3 Block Approaches

The nerve can be blocked by the extraoral and intaroral approaches in supine or sitting position.

1. **Intraoral Approach**

Landmark Technique

A line drawn down from the midpoint of the centred pupil passes through the infra orbital foramen, bicuspid teeth, and the mental foramen. The inferior border of the orbital ridge is palpated to locate the infraorbital foramen at the intersection of the vertical line along the centred pupil and horizontal line through alae nasi. While the infraorbital foramen is located with the finger of the other hand the needle is inserted into the ipsilateral superior buccal groove approximately at the upper second bicuspid tooth. The needle is inserted upward and outward in the direction of the finger palpating the inferior orbital foramen into the canine fossa (Fig. 4.29). After negative aspiration 1–3 mL LA is injected.

(Tip—The palpating finger should remain in place to prevent losing landmarks and stop the needle from entering the orbit.

- A firm pressure using the finger over the foramen can avoid injection of local anaesthetic into the canal and haematoma formation.)

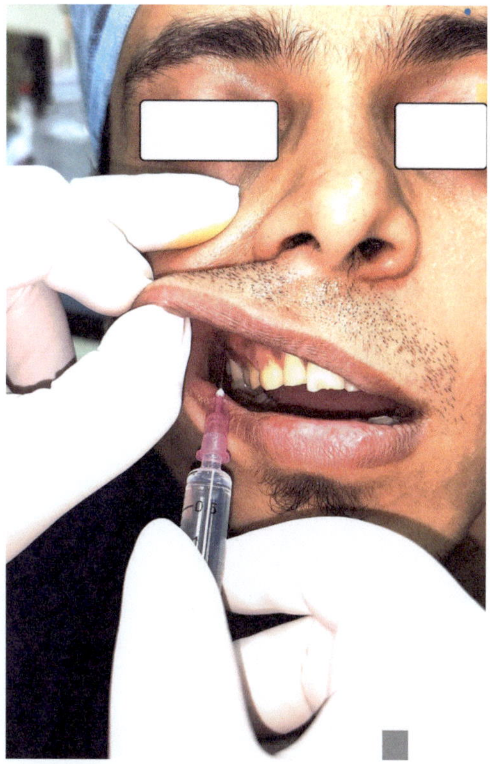

Fig. 4.29 Intraoral infraorbital nerve block

2. **Extraoral approach**

Landmark Technique

The infraorbital foramen is identified and palpated as mentioned above in intraoral approach. A 25–26G needle is inserted just below the foramen until contact is made with the bone and 2 to 3 mL of local anaesthetic is injected after withdrawing the needle slightly (Fig. 4.30).

(Tip—Care should be taken to avoid injecting the LA into the nerve or the canal. A lateral-to-medial approach lessens the chance of foramen penetration since the infraorbital foramen's axis is oriented caudally and medially.

- Mild pressure prevent any haematoma formation).

Ultrasound-Guided Approach

A high frequency linear probe is placed in transverse direction over the lower orbital rim to locate the infraorbital notch, identified as small groove

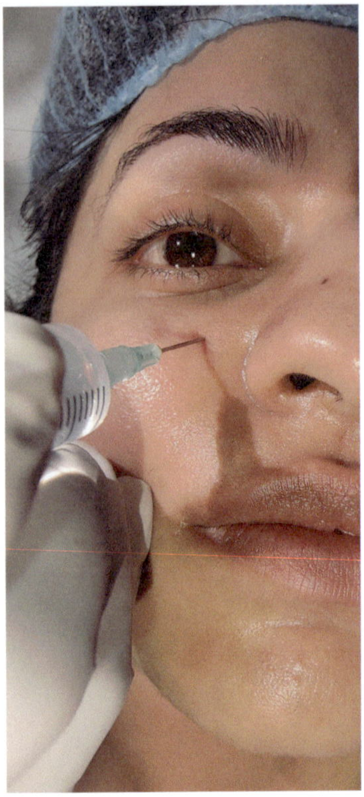

Fig. 4.30 Extraoral landmark-guided infraorbital nerve block

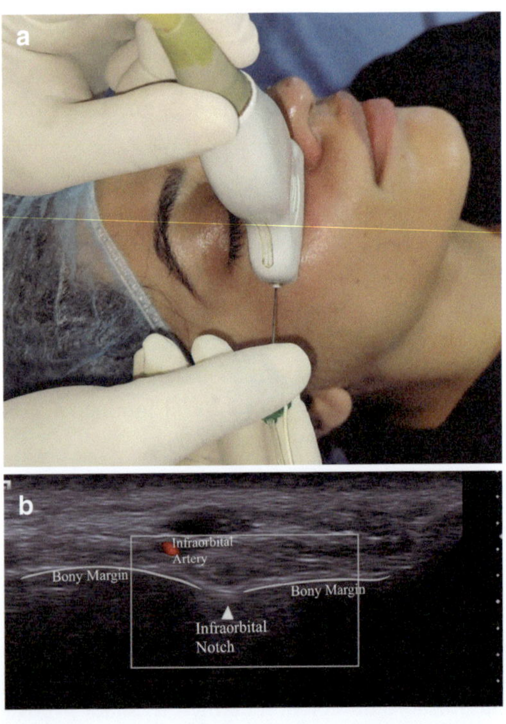

Fig. 4.31 (**a**) Probe position for infraorbital nerve block. (**b**) USG image showing for infraorbital nerve block

on bony surface. A 5 cm echogenic needle is used in either in-plane or out-of-plane approach and 2–3 mL drug is deposited after negative aspiration (Fig. 4.31a, b).

(Tip—Infraorbital artery can be identified in the groove by using colour Doppler and drug can be deposited besides it if nerve is not visible.

- If infraorbital groove is not visible slight downward movement of probe helps in identifying the groove).

4.4.1.4 Complications

Haematoma, bleeding, infection, intravascular injection, nerve damage and oedema. Injection of LA into the canal can rise the pressure within the canal and can cause damage to the nerve. Needle penetration into the orbit can damage orbital content.

4.4.2 Sphenopalatine Ganglion Block

The sphenopalatine ganglion (SPG) is an extracranial parasympathetic ganglion with multiple neural connections including sympathetic and sensory fibres. It is located in the pterygopalatine fossa (PPF) and is also called as the pterygopalatine ganglion (PPG). Though blockade of the ganglion using an intranasal approach had been described in the early 1900s due to its role in pain management. Sluder in 1908 described sphenopalatine neuralgia as a unilateral facial pain symptom complex with associated motor, sensory, and gustatory manifestations. The parasympathetic blockade also prevents vasodilation in the cerebral vessels and has established its role in the treatment of headaches.

4.4.2.1 Anatomy

The pterygopalatine fossa (PPF) is an inverted pyramid-shaped space bounded anteriorly by the posterior wall of the maxillary sinus and posteriorly by the medial pterygoid plate. The superior border is formed by the sphenoid sinus and the medial border is formed by the perpendicular plate of palatine bone. Laterally, the PPF communicates with the infratemporal fossa through the pterygomaxillary fissure. The parasympathetic preganglionic cell bodies originate in the superior salivatory nucleus in the pons, and the parasympathetic fibres run in the nervus intermedius (a branch from the facial nerve) through the geniculate ganglion, forming the greater petrosal nerve (GPN).

The postganglionic fibres from the PPG supply the lacrimal gland and the mucosa of the nasal cavity and nasopharynx and additionally supply branches to meningeal and cerebral blood vessels. The sympathetic fibres originate in the superior cervical ganglion around the internal carotid artery and give rise to the deep petrosal nerve, which joins the GPN to form the Vidian nerve, which enters the SPG. They pass without synapsing and supply the palate nasal cavity and the pharynx. The sphenopalatine, the lesser palatine, the greater palatine, the posterior superior lateral nasal, the posterior inferior lateral nasal, and pharyngeal nerves branch from the pterygopalatine ganglion (Fig. 4.32).

Apart from the ganglion the fossa contains fat, the maxillary division (V2) of the trigeminal nerve and its branches zygomatic nerve, posterior superior alveolar nerve(s), and the infraorbital nerve, the distal branches of the maxillary artery, and a few emissary veins.

4.4.2.2 Indications and Contraindications

Various indications and contraindications of sphenopalatine block are tabulated (Table 4.9).

4.4.2.3 Block Approaches

Various approaches have been used for SPG block.

Various local anaesthetics (4% cocaine, 2% to 4% lidocaine, or 0.5% bupivacaine, 0.5% Ropivacaine), depot steroids, or 6% phenol are used.

1. **Transnasal (Topical/injection)**

This is the simplest approach.

Patient position—supine position with extended cervical spine. A pillow or sheet can be placed under the shoulders to facilitate extension.

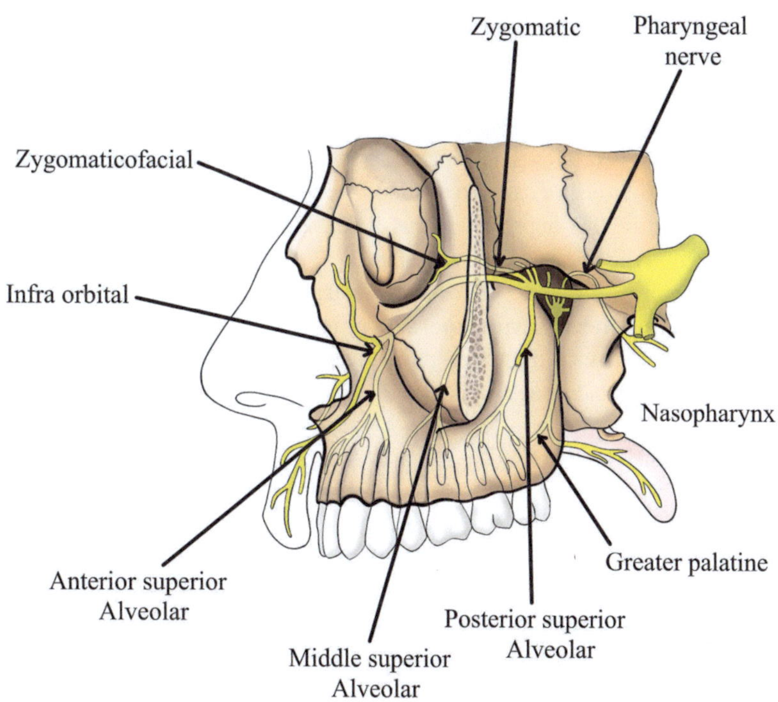

Fig. 4.32 Anatomy of sphenopalatine ganglion

Table 4.9 Indications and contraindications of sphenopalatine nerve block

Indications	Contraindications
Oral and maxillofacial surgeries Post-dural puncture headache Migraine and acute and chronic headaches Facial pain syndromes and neuralgias In reducing the need for analgesics after endoscopic sinus surgery	Patient refusal Local infection Allergy to local anaesthetics History of facial trauma

Technique—The nose should be inspected for obstruction and vasoconstrictor drops can be instilled to open up the passages. A long cotton tipped applicator soaked in the local anaesthetic solution (viscous lidocaine 4%) is inserted into the nose parallel to the floor above the middle turbinate till resistance is encountered. The applicator should be retained at this place for 30 min though initial effect is seen in 5 to 10 min (Fig. 4.33).

Alternatively a sphenocath device can be used (Fig. 4.34). This is a long flexible sheath with a curved tip and an inner catheter. Once the device is inserted as mentioned above and is in position, the inner catheter is advanced and 2 mL of local anaesthetic can be administered and the patient is advised to remain in the same position for 10 min. Needle tip position can be confirmed by injecting contrast under fluoroscopy before drug administration.

Other devices such as SPG Block Catheter and/or Tx360 Nasal Injector can also be used. The only disadvantage of this approach is that it requires transmucosal diffusion of local anaesthetic.

The more invasive **transoral, infrazygomatic, and lateral infratemporal** approaches are used exclusively by pain physicians and require training and image guidance.

2. **Transoral Approach**

A dental needle with a curved tip is inserted via the greater palatine foramen (GPF) in the posterior portion of the hard palate. To access the superior aspect of the pterygopalatine fossa, this should be placed just medial to the gum line opposite the third molar tooth and 2–3 mL LA is instilled. Though this technique provides direct access to the ganglion but is technically difficult and causes patient discomfort.

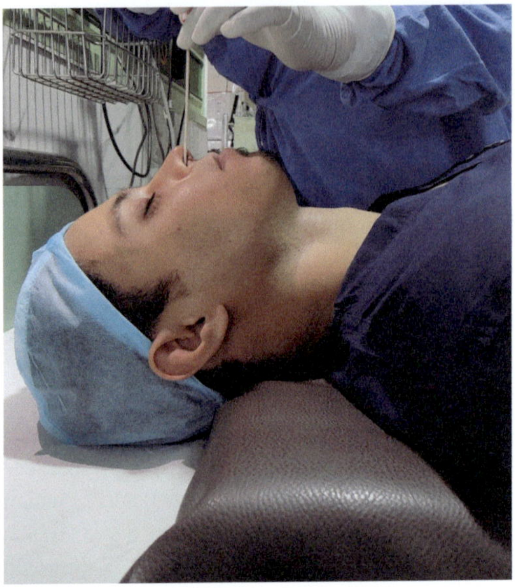

Fig. 4.33 Transnasal approach to SPG block

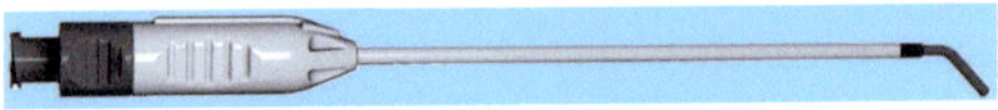

Fig. 4.34 Sphenocath for transnasal approach to SPG block

3. **Infrazygomatic Approach**

This approach is performed under computed tomography or fluoroscopy guidance. The patient position is supine. Under all aseptic precautions a 20–22 gauge 10 cm curved blunt needle is advanced in superior and medial direction towards pterygopalatine fossa when under lateral fluoroscopic view of face both the mandibular rami are superimposed.

Needle tip is advanced till ipsilateral nasal wall and position is confirmed by injecting contrast under fluoroscopy guidance and 1–2 mL LA is administered with or without adjuvants.

This technique is technically challenging though drug is directly deposited to SPG.

4.4.2.4 Complications

Epistaxis, haematoma, lacrimation of ipsilateral eye, infection, transient anaesthesia of pharynx, palate and root of nose.

4.4.3 Palatine Nerve Block

4.4.3.1 Greater and Lesser Palatine Nerve

Anatomy

The greater palatine nerve or the anterior palatine nerve is a branch of the maxillary division of the trigeminal nerve. It carries parasympathetic, taste, and the somatosensory fibres to supply the posterior aspect of the hard palate distal to the canines. As the nerve branches of from the maxillary division it enters the greater palatine canal to emerge from the greater palatine foramen in the hard palate and curves anteriorly under the hard palate.

The lesser palatine nerve or the posterior palatine nerves are a group of nerves carrying parasympathetic, taste, and the somatosensory fibres to supply the mucosa of the uvula, soft palate, and palatine tonsil. It arises from the pterygopalatine ganglion and travels through the lesser palatine canal which runs posterior to the greater palatine canal and emerges through the lesser palatine foramen behind the pyramidal process of the hard palate. Greater palatine block along with the lesser palatine nerve block can provide post-operative analgesia following cleft palate surgeries.

Block Approach

The nerve is blocked as it emerges through the foramen which is located opposite the anterior part of the third molar or posterior part of the second molar tooth.

Position—Supine or propped up and clinician standing on opposite side of side to be blocked.

Technique—The foramen can be located by pressing a small cotton swab opposite first molar tooth and proceeding posteriorly till it 'falls' into a depression created by the foramen near the posterior edge of the hard palate. Pain of needle insertion is minimized by application of 2% lignocaine in cotton tipped applicator. Around 0.6 to 1 mL of LA injected at an angle near the foramen is sufficient to block the nerve (Fig. 4.35). Greater palatine nerve block is commonly used in anaesthesia for dental procedures. Alternatively, a 25G spinal needle, bent 2–3 cm proximal to tip is inserted through foramen and 1–2 mL drug is deposited after negative aspiration. However, chances of sphenopalatine artery puncture are there with this approach.

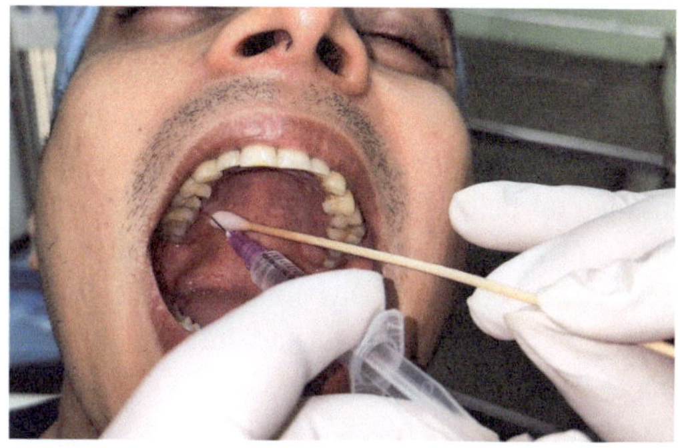

Fig. 4.35 Greater palatine nerve block

The greater and lesser palatine nerves as well as the nasociliary and nasopalatine nerves, which also contribute to the sensory innervation of the nasal cavity are anaesthetized.

Complications

Bleeding, infection, nerve injury, intravascular injection, and hypertension.

4.4.4 Mandibular Nerve Block

4.4.4.1 Anatomy

The mandibular nerve can be blocked as the nerve emerges extracranially through the foramen ovale. The more distal blockade of the inferior alveolar branches is usually performed by the dental surgeons.

The mandibular nerve is the largest branch of the trigeminal nerve.

As it exits through the foramen ovale it bifurcates into a smaller anterior trunk with motor branches supplying the primary muscles of mastication (temporalis, masseter, medial pterygoid, and lateral pterygoid muscles), the palatal muscles and the sensory branch, the buccal nerve. The larger posterior division divides into the auriculotemporal, lingual, and inferior alveolar nerve (IAN).

Complete nerve block results in anaesthesia of the ipsilateral mandibular bone, lower teeth up to the midline, buccal and lingual hard and soft tissue, anterior two-thirds of the tongue, floor of the mouth, the external acoustic meatus and auricle of the ear in its anterior zone, the skin over the jaw, the posterior part of the cheek, and the temporal area (except the area of the angle of the mandible, which is supplied by the superficial cervical plexus) (Fig. 4.1).

4.4.4.2 Indications

- Mandibular surgeries
- Dental procedure involving the lower teeth
- Neuralgias
- Chronic cancer pain

The mandibular nerve block has a success rate of 95–98%, whereas the IAN block is successful in only 65–85% of cases.

4.4.4.3 Block Approach

Position—supine with head slightly turned to opposite side.

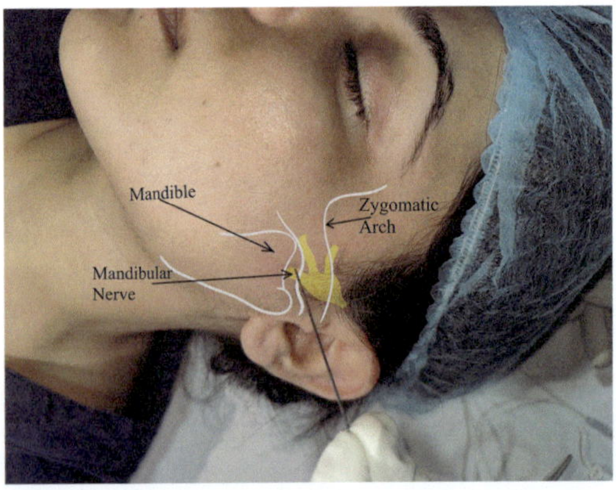

Fig. 4.36 Landmark/PNS-guided mandibular nerve block

Landmark—The tragus and the zygomatic processes are identified and the mandibular notch between the coronoid and the condylar process of the ramus of mandible is located inferior to the process.

Technique—The point of needle entry is the space between the mandibular notch and the zygomatic arch 5–10 cm (as high as possible) (Fig. 4.36). Under all aseptic precautions, a 22G, 5–10 cm nerve stimulator needle with an initial current strength of 1.5 mA is inserted perpendicular to the skin and advanced 2–4 cm towards the lateral pterygoid plate up to a maximal depth of 5–6 cm. The needle is withdrawn slightly after contacting the plate and is directed posteriorly and inferiorly until a motor response from temporalis and masseter muscles in the form of jaw jerk is achieved. After reducing the current to 0.5 mA with sustained motor response and confirming a negative aspiration up to 10 mL of local anaesthetic can be injected slowly.

4.4.4.4 Complications

- Internal maxillary artery injection
- Middle meningeal artery injection and seizures
- Transient facial nerve block

4.5 Cervical Plexus Block

Cervical plexus block was introduced in the early nineteenth century with the posterior and lateral approaches. Earlier techniques involved blockade at the level of the exit of the nerve roots from the vertebral column. It was simplified into a single injection technique by Winnie in the year 1975.

4.5.1 Anatomy

The plexus is formed by the anterior divisions of first to fourth cervical spinal nerves. Though the fifth cervical nerve is a part of brachial plexus, it contributes to the formation of phrenic nerve. These cervical nerves except the C1 divide into ascending and descending branches and unite with the adjacent nerves to form loops. They also receive contributions from the sympathetic trunk which descend from the superior cervical ganglion. The cervical plexus lies below the sternocleidomastoid muscle under the prevertebral fascia anterior to the middle scalene, levator anguli scapulae, and the cervical vertebrae. There are five main components of the cervical plexus. The cutaneous branches form the superficial cervical plexus while the deep branches supply the deeper structures and the muscles in the neck (Fig. 4.37).

1. The cutaneous branches are lesser occipital, greater auricular, transverse cervical and supraclavicular nerves
2. The ansa cervicalis, which innervates the infrahyoid and geniohyoid muscles
3. The phrenic nerve supplying the diaphragm
4. Contributions to the accessory nerve (CN XI), which innervates the sternocleidomastoid and trapezius muscles
5. Direct muscular branches, which supply prevertebral muscles of the neck

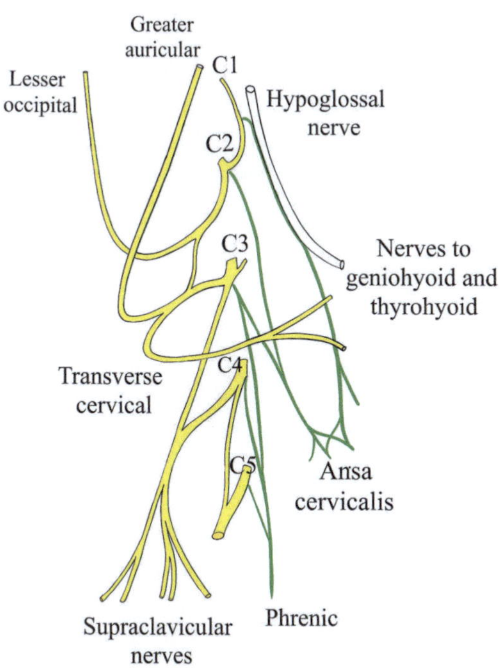

Fig. 4.37 Anatomy of cervical plexus

The four cutaneous branches are clustered around the middle of the sternocleidomastoid at the punctum nervosum and emerge from the posterior border branching out in different directions.

- The lesser occipital nerve arises from the C2 and supplies the lateral part of the scalp and the posterosuperior aspect of the pinna
- The greater auricular nerve arises from the C2 and C3 and provides sensory supply to the skin extending from the parotid gland till the angle of mandible, posteroinferior aspect of the auricle and the mastoid process
- The transverse cervical nerve is formed from the C2 and C3 and innervates the anterior triangle of the neck
- The supraclavicular nerves are a group of three nerves arising from the C3 and C4 spinal nerves and supply the skin over the clavicle and the shoulder.

4.5.2 Indications and Contraindications

Various indications and contraindications of cervical plexus block are mentioned in Table 4.10.

Table 4.10 Indications And Contraindications of cervical plexus block

Indication	Contraindication
Neck surgeries and lymph node dissection	Patient refusal
Thyroidectomy and parathyroid surgery	Local infection
Tympanomastoid and auricular surgeries	Allergy to local anaesthetics
Carotid endarterectomy for awake monitoring during cross clamping	Surgical or radiation-induced scarring
Excision of thyroglossal or branchial cleft cysts	Severe pulmonary compromise or contralateral phrenic nerve palsy (deep cervical plexus block)
Clavicle surgeries along with brachial plexus block	Coagulation disorders
	Scars
	Absence of bone flap due to craniectomy

4.5.3 Block Approaches

Superficial Cervical Plexus Block

1. **Landmark-guided technique**

Position—The patient is placed supine or in propped up position with the head turned to the opposite side.

Landmarks—The mastoid process, Chassaignac's tubercle, and the sternocleidomastoid muscle (SCM) are identified. In obese patients the sternocleidomastoid can be identified by asking the patient to lift the head.

Technique—A line is drawn along the posterior border of the SCM extending from the C6 tubercle to the mastoid process. A 25 gauge needle is inserted along the midpoint of this line and around 3 to 5 mL of local anaesthetic is deposited and the needle is fanned 2 to 3 cm above and below along the posterior border of SCM and around 2 to 3 mL is deposited in each direction. Avoid inserting the needle into deeper planes (Fig. 4.38).

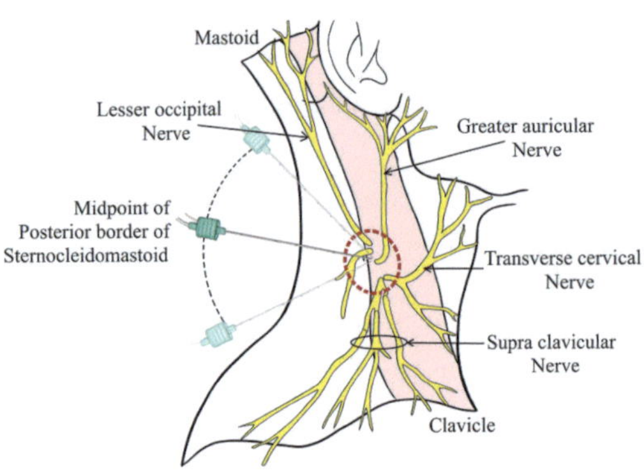

Fig. 4.38 Landmark-guided superficial cervical plexus block

2. **Ultrasound-guided technique**

Ultrasound can be used to identify the structures accurately and increase the success rate of the block.

Position—Supine, propped up position with the head turned to the opposite side. Patient can be placed in the lateral decubitus position when an ultrasound is used.

Technique—Under all aseptic condition a high frequency linear transducer is placed at the midpoint of posterior border of sternocleidomastoid transversely. The level approximates with the notch of thyroid and corresponds to the level of C4 (Fig. 4.39a).

The needle is inserted in in-plane approach from lateral to medial direction 1–2 cm below the posterior border of sternocleidomastoid or out-of-plane approach. 5 to 10 mL of local anaesthetic is deposited in the fascial layer deep to the posterolateral tapering sternocleidomastoid muscle and superior to the levator scapula (Fig. 4.39b).

Since superficial cervical plexus is a sensory plexus dilute concentration of local anaesthetic is sufficient to produce a blockade. However, higher concentrations can induce a dense blockade.

(Tips—The probe can be kept in longitudinal direction on posterior border of SCM and needle can be inserted in in-plane or out-of-plane direction

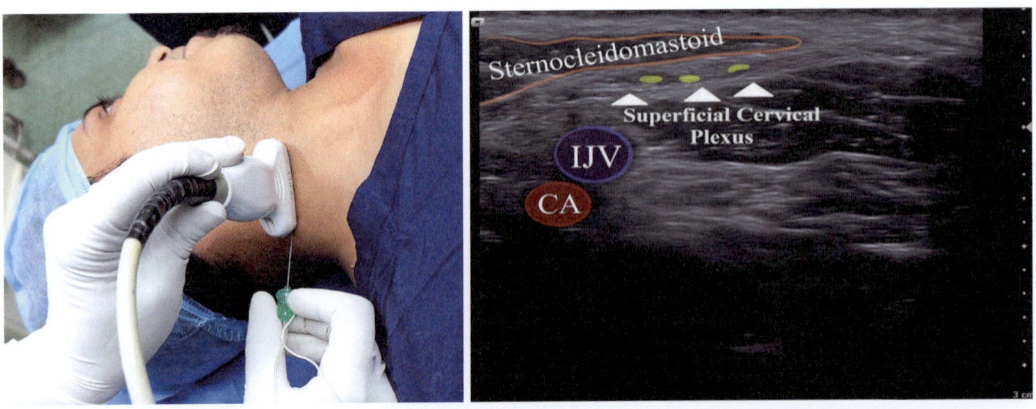

Fig. 4.39 (**a**) Probe position for superficial cervical plexus block. (**b**) USG image of superficial cervical plexus block

– If cervical plexus is not visible 10 ml of LA is deposited below SCM).

Intermediate Cervical Plexus Block

- Earlier the space between the investing layer of deep cervical fascia and the prevertebral fascia was targeted for cervical plexus block using landmarks and loss of resistance or pop technique. This technique was difficult and was later replaced by ultrasonography. Pandit et al. hypothesized that there is communication between the superficial and deep spaces through the prevertebral fascia, which may explain the similar efficacy of the superficial deep and combined blocks. Choquet et al. advocated the intermediate cervical plexus block targeting the posterior cervical space at the C4 level where the scalene disappears and the sternocleidomastoid lies against the prevertebral muscles. A linear array probe is placed on the lower neck to identify the C7 transverse process. Then, the probe is slid cranially till the C4 transverse process. The needle is inserted in a postero-anterior direction using an in-plane technique, and 10 mL of local anaesthetic is injected into the interfascial space between the investing fascia and the prevertebral fascia (Fig. 4.40). The local anaesthetic solution also spreads towards the carotid sheath and provides the glossopharyngeal blockade required in carotid surgeries.

Deep Cervical Plexus Block

- Landmark-guided approach

A line is drawn connecting the mastoid process and the Chassaignac's tubercle. The transverse process of C6 is located behind the clavicular head of the sternocleidomastoid. The transverse processes of C2, C3, and C4 are marked 2, 4, and 6 cm from the mastoid process along the line.

Under all aseptic technique the block can be achieved by a single injection at C3 or three separate injections. 3–5 mL of local anaesthetic per level is injected to ensure a reliable block. A 22G, 2.5–5 cm needle is inserted perpendicular to the skin in a slight caudal orientation to prevent inadvertent insertion of the needle towards the cervical spinal cord.

The needle should never be oriented cephalad. The needle is advanced slowly until the transverse process is contacted and is withdrawn 1–2 mm and LA is injected (Fig. 4.40). This procedure can be repeated at the consecutive levels.

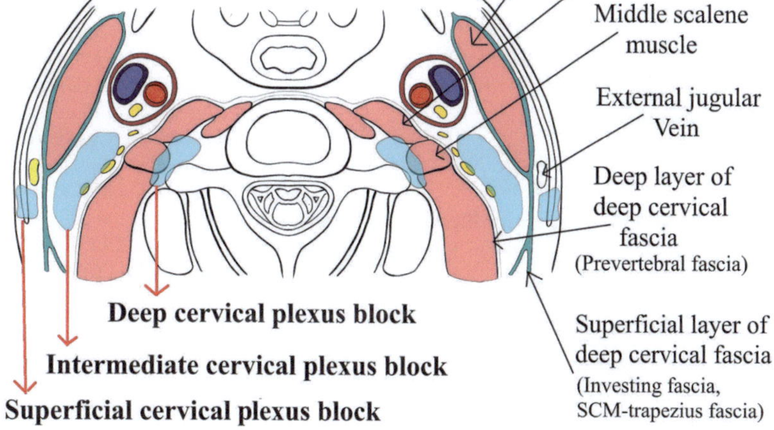

Fig. 4.40 Drug deposition of superficial, intermediate, and deep cervical plexus

(Tip—The transverse process is hit at a depth of 1–2 cm in majority of the patients. Hence the needle should never be inserted beyond the depth of 2.5 cm to avoid the risk of spinal cord injury)

- Ultrasound-guided approach

Under all aseptic condition, a high frequency linear probe is placed at the midpoint of posterior border of sternocleidomastoid in transverse orientation. The level approximates with the notch of thyroid and corresponds to the level of C4.

A 5–10 cm needle is inserted from lateral to medial direction under ultrasound guidance and LA is injected into the space between the prevertebral fascia and the cervical transverse process or it can be directed to touch the targeted transverse process and the LA can be deposited adjacent to it at multiple levels if needed.

Paresthesia is often elicited in proximity to the transverse process but has a nonspecific radiating pattern.

The deep cervical plexus block is associated with potentially devastating complications like intravascular (into vertebral artery) and intrathecal deposition of drug.

4.5.4 Complications

- Recurrent laryngeal nerve block causing hoarseness and stridor in bilateral blocks.
- Phrenic nerve blockade.
- Horner's syndrome.
- Injection into the internal jugular vein causing local anaesthetic systemic toxicity.
- Injection into the carotid or vertebral artery causing seizures.
- Dysphagia.
- Inadvertent deep injections can block the deep cervical and brachial plexus.
- Atheromatous plaques in the vessels could be dislodged with excessive head hyperextension. Care should be taken in patients with unstable plaques.
- Cerebral ischaemia can occur with extremes of rotation or extension due to compression of vertebral vessels. Strict monitoring and assessment of the patient should be done throughout the procedure.

Further Reading

Ahmad I. Regional and topical anesthesia for awake endotracheal intubation. Available from . Available from https://www.nysora.com/techniques/head-and-neck-blocks/airway/regional-topical-anesthesia-awake-endotracheal-intubation/.

Alexander CE, Dua A. Sphenopalatine ganglion block. [Updated 2022 Nov 16]. In: StatPearls [Internet]. Treasure Island: StatPearls Publishing; 2022 Jan. Available from: https://www.ncbi.nlm.nih.gov/books/NBK557751/

Anker R, Kaur N. Regional anaesthesia for ophthalmic surgery. BJA Educ. 2017;17:221–7.

Binfalah M, Alghawi E, Shosha E, Alhilly A, Bakhiet M. Sphenopalatine ganglion block for the treatment of acute migraine headache. Pain Res Treat. 2018;2018:2516953.

Candido KD, Massey ST, Sauer R, Darabad RR, Knezevic NN. A novel revision to the classical transnasal topical sphenopalatine ganglion block for the treatment of headache and facial pain. Pain Physician. 2013 Nov–Dec;16(6):E769–78.

Dsouza S, Sewell D. Cheen Ng S, editor. Scalp block: technique and applications. Available from https://resources.wfsahq.org/atotw/scalp-block-technique-and-applications/

Greher M, Moriggl B, Curatolo M, Kirchmair L, Eichenberger U. Sonographic visualization and ultrasound-guided block of the greater occipital nerve: a comparison of two selective techniques confirmed by anatomical dissection. Br J Anaesth. 2010;104:637–42.

Guise P. Sub-Tenon's anaesthesia: an update. Local Reg Anesth. 2012;5:35–46.

Guyer S, Shaw ES. Ocular ultrasound guided anaesthesia. In: Singh AD, editor. Ophthalmic ultrasonography. Amsterdam: Elsevier; 2012.

Jaichandran V. Ophthalmic regional anaesthesia: a review and update. Indian J Anaesth. 2013 Jan;57(1):7–13.

Johnson KD, Rai MR. Conscious sedation for awake fibreoptic intubation: a review of the literature. Can J Anaesth. 2013;60(6):584–99.

Kemp WJ 3rd, Tubbs RS, Cohen-Gadol AA. The innervation of the scalp: a comprehensive review includ-

ing anatomy, pathology, and neurosurgical correlates. Surg Neurol Int. 2011;2:178.
Kim JS, Ko JS, Bang S, Kim H, Lee SY. Cervical plexus block. Korean J Anesthesiol. 2018 Aug;71(4):274–88.
Mariappan R, Mehta J, Massicotte E, Nagappa M, Manninen P, Venkatraghavan L. Effect of superficial cervical plexus block on postoperative quality of recovery after anterior cervical discectomy and fusion: a randomized controlled trial. Can J Anaesth. 2015;62:883–90.
Nardi NM, Alvarado AC, Schaefer TJ. Infraorbital nerve block. [Updated 2022 Aug 8]. In: StatPearls [Internet]. Treasure Island: StatPearls Publishing; 2022 Jan. Available from: https://www.ncbi.nlm.nih.gov/books/NBK499881/
Osborn I. Sebeo "scalp block" during craniotomy: a classic technique revisited. J Neurosurg Anesthesiol. 2010;22(3):187–94.
Parate LH, Tejesh CA, Geetha CR, Mohan CV. Peripheral nerve stimulator-guided mandibular nerve block: a report of three cases. Saudi J Anaesth. 2016 Oct–Dec;10(4):491–49.
Perisanidis C, Saranteas T, Kostopanagiotou G. Ultrasound-guided combined intermediate and deep cervical plexus nerve block for regional anaesthesia in oral and maxillofacial surgery. Dentomaxillofac Radiol. 2013;42:29945724.
Preziosi BD, Hershkin AT, Seider PJ, Casey GM. Oral & maxillofacial regional anesthesia. Available from https://www.nysora.com/topics/regional-anesthesia-for-specific-surgical-procedures/head-and-neck/maxillofacial/oral-maxillofacial-regional-anesthesia/
Robbins MS, Robertson CE, Kaplan E, Ailani J, Charleston L, Kuruvilla D, et al. The sphenopalatine ganglion: anatomy, pathophysiology, and therapeutic targeting in headache. Headache. 2016;56:240–58.
Seidel R, Schulze M, Zukowski K, Wree A. Ultrasound-guided intermediate cervical plexus block. Anatomical study. Anaesthesist. 2015;64:446–50.
Standring S. Gray's anatomy. 41th ed. London: Churchill Livingstone Elsevier; 2016. p. 41.
Wang H, Liu G, Fu W, Li ST. The effect of infraorbital nerve block on emergence agitation in children undergoing cleft lip surgery under general anesthesia with sevoflurane. Paediatr Anaesth. 2015 Sept;25(9):906–10.

Approach and Troubleshooting to Upper Limb Blocks

5

Pulak Puneet, Ashish Ranjan Satapathy, and Santosh Kumar Sharma

Abstract

The tremendous progress in surgical techniques has its foundations in the even more prodigious growth in anesthetic techniques. Regional anesthesia is an important aspect of this evolution. Regional anesthesia involves least possible interference with the physiology of the patient for a given surgical procedure, which improves of the safety and comfort of the patient. The advent of ultrasonography (USG)-guided nerve and plexus blocks has revolutionized the practice of anesthesia. Regional anesthesia was used in the past for a variety of upper limb procedures and surgeries but gradually began falling out of favor due to possible complications. The emergence of USG and its widespread availability revived the interest in a wide variety of nerve and plexus blocks for a spectrum of indications, therapeutic as well as diagnostic. Some of the common blocks practiced are Phrenic nerve block, Suprascapular nerve (SSN) block, Clavipectoral fascia block, Stellate ganglion block, Brachial plexus blocks via different approaches (Interscalene, Supraclavicular, Infraclavicular, and Axillary) as well as individual nerve blocks in the arm such as Radial, Median, and Ulnar nerve blocks. Ongoing research is continuously widening the horizon in which these blocks are being employed.

Keywords

Ultrasound (USG)-guided blocks · Brachial plexus blocks · Phrenic block · Suprascapular nerve block · Stellate ganglion block · Clavipectoral fascia block

5.1 Introduction

It is a well-established fact that regional anesthesia has made significant inroads into the practice of Anesthesiology. A lot of potential complications can be avoided, and postoperative pain management better managed with its use.

There are four approaches to a nerve or plexus block:

1. The "blind" approach, based solely on anatomical landmarks.

The original version of the chapter has been revised. A correction to this chapter can be found at https://doi.org/10.1007/978-981-97-4098-7_21

P. Puneet (✉)
Department of Anaesthesia, Lifecare Hospital Musaffah, Abu Dhabi, United Arab Emirates

A. R. Satapathy
Department of Anaesthesia, Ng Teng Fong General Hospital (NUHS Jurong Campus), Singapore, Singapore

S. K. Sharma
Department Of Anaesthesia, AIIMS, Gorakhpur, Uttar Pradesh, India

M. K. Prasad, S. J. S. Bajwa (eds.), *Steps to Successful Regional Anesthesia*, https://doi.org/10.1007/978-981-97-4098-7_5

2. The use of Peripheral Nerve Locator/Stimulator (PNS) to locate the nerve and subsequently block.
3. Under real-time guidance of an Ultrasound (USG) machine with an "in-plane" or "out-of-plane" technique.
4. Using a combination of the USG as well as PNS.

It is worth noting that with the rapid evolution of imaging modalities and their ever-increasing availability, it might be safe to conclude that the "blind" approach should no longer be recommended and should be deemed an unsafe approach for all practical purposes.

Although imaging modalities such as CT scan are rapidly evolving, USG remains the more easily available, practical, and portable imaging technique. It is, however, to be noted that a combination of Peripheral Nerve Stimulator (PNS) guidance and USG guidance is considered to be superior to either of the techniques alone, as nerve injuries reported with USG guidance alone are also substantial enough to ignore.

Aside from central neuraxial blockade, upper limb blocks are perhaps the earliest to be put to productive use and among the most widely practiced ones today.

A simple way to classify them can be according to the site of injection of the local anesthetic:

(a) Injection site above the clavicle.
(b) Injection site below the clavicle.

5.2 Upper Limb Blocks with Injection Site Above the Clavicle

Some of the important upper limb blocks with injection site above the clavicle are:

1. Clavipectoral fascia block
2. Phrenic nerve block
3. Suprascapular nerve block
4. Interscalene brachial plexus block
5. Supraclavicular brachial plexus block
6. Stellate ganglion block

Going about any procedure, it helps to have an overview and a well laid out plan. There are various aspects to be considered.

5.2.1 Ergonomics and Positioning

The positioning of the patient and USG machine is the same for four of the above blocks viz.: **Phrenic nerve**, **Interscalene**, **Supraclavicular** and **Stellate ganglion block**.

The aim should be to have the injection site and the USG monitor in a single line of sight. The arrangement can be described as follows:

Patient—Supine, with head turned to the contralateral side. Some authors advocate the placement of a soft support beneath the shoulders midway between the two scapulae, to make structures in the supraclavicular area more prominent.

Operator and USG monitor

For **Right-sided block**:

Right-handed operator—Operator at the head-end and USG machine on the ipsilateral side of the patient at the level of the mid torso (Fig. 5.1).

Similar position is obtained by left-handed operator for performing a left-sided block on the left side.

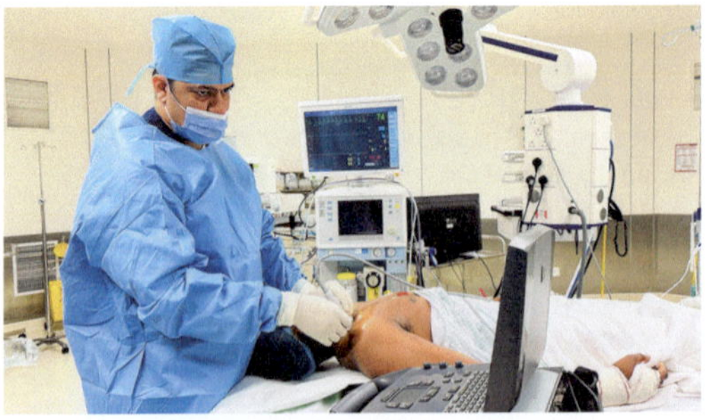

Fig. 5.1 Right-handed operator administering right-sided supraclavicular block. Note that the operator stands at the head-end and the machine by the side of the patient

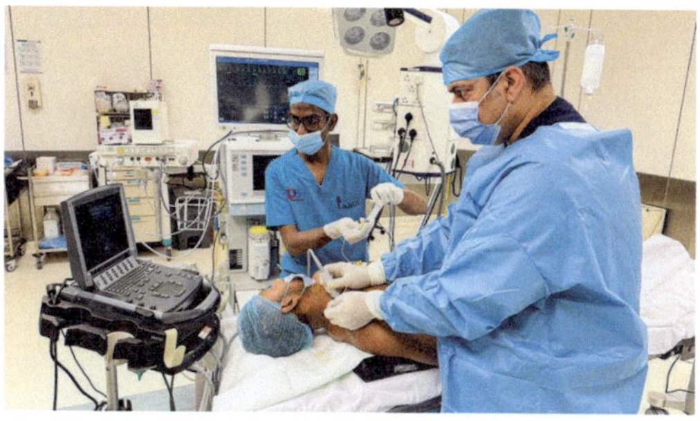

Fig. 5.2 Left-handed operator administering right-sided supraclavicular block, standing at the side of the patient at trunk level

Left-handed operator—USG machine at the head-end and operator on the ipsilateral side of the patient at the level of the mid torso (Fig. 5.2).

Similar position is obtained by a right-handed operator for performing a left-sided block on the right side.

5.2.2 Clavipectoral Fascia Block

It is universally accepted that the cutaneous innervation of the skin above the clavicle comes from the supraclavicular branch of the superficial cervical plexus, but the opinion on the nerve supply to the clavicle bone itself is not unanimous. It has been variously ascribed to nerves like suprascapular n., subclavian n., lateral pectoral n., and long thoracic n. and is not yet completely established due to a lack of validated cadaver studies.

Essentially, the clavicle and the anterior superior shoulder area derive its nerve supply from both the cervical and brachial plexus, making any single block insufficient to provide effective surgical or perioperative analgesia for surgical intervention. Multiple case reports suggest the efficacy of a combination of two blocks for clavicle surgeries (for instance, interscalene brachial plexus block and superficial cervical plexus or low volume brachial plexus block plus low volume selective supraclavicular nerve block), but it is time-consuming to perform two separate ultrasound-guided block and they have their own set of known possible complications.

In this backdrop, with its ease to perform with a single-injection and advanced safety profile, the Clavipectoral fascia block is fast becoming an attractive alternative. The CPB is likely safer due to its more lateral and superficial plane of injection and the clavicle serving as the natural backstop. Interestingly, the clavipectoral fascia block has proved effective in preventing pain despite not performing a separate supraclavicular nerve block.

It is increasingly being used in combination with sedation for clavicle fracture surgeries and is being considered as the sole anesthetic technique in some situations.

The primary advantage lies in the fact that it precludes the possible complications of prevalent techniques like phrenic nerve blockade, pneumothorax, Horner's syndrome, vertebral injections, etc.

5.2.2.1 Anatomy

The Clavipectoral fascia (costo-coracoid membrane/coraco-clavicular fascia) is a strong fascia situated under cover of the clavicular portion of the pectoralis major. It extends superiorly from the clavicle, medially from the costochondral joints and supero-laterally from the coracoid process.

The fascia converges in the axilla, where it forms a protective structure over the neurovascular structure of the axilla, essentially acting as a suspender for the floor of the axilla (Fig. 5.4). The primary relevance of the fascia here lies in the nerves that pierce it to constitute nerve supply of the clavicle.

5.2.2.2 Indications

For open surgery on the clavicle, including fracture fixation.

5.2.2.3 Contraindications (Table 5.1)

Table 5.1 Contraindications to Clavipectoral fascia block

Absolute	Relative
Patient refusal Local site infection Allergy to local anesthetics	Anticoagulation or bleeding disorders.

5.2.2.4 Preparation

Pre-requisite for block is tabulated in Table 5.2

5.2.2.5 Technique

Position—The aim should be to have the injection site and the USG monitor in a single line of sight.

Patient—Supine with head turned to the opposite side to create more working space.

Operator and USG monitor—(This suggestion is applicable for the block to be administered on either side).

Right-handed operator—By the right-hand side of patient at the chest level with the USG machine directly across, on the right side of patient, in direct line of sight (Fig. 5.3).

Similarly left-handed operator can perform by the left-hand side of patient at the chest level with the USG machine directly across, on the left side of patient, in direct line of sight.

The block can be administered for both sides, standing by the side of the patient.

5.2.2.6 Drug

15–20 ml of 0.5% ropivacaine, 0.5% bupivacaine/levobupivacaine.

Table 5.2 Pre-requisite for block

Pre-requisites	Equipment/Materials required
Informed consent. NPO status. Optimal sedation if necessary. Emergency, resuscitation drugs, and equipment. Secure IV access. Appropriate sedation, monitoring (HR, NIBP, Spo2, ECG, RR) and oxygen supply. Site and side of block should be marked and confirmed.	Ensure asepsis 10 ml syringes with local anesthetic Sterile gloves One 1.5 inch, 25-gauge needle for skin infiltration A 10 cm long, 21–22 gauge short-bevel, echogenic needle USG machine with linear transducer (8–18 MHz), sterile sleeve and gel. Peripheral nerve stimulator (as needed) Opening pressure injection monitoring device (if available)

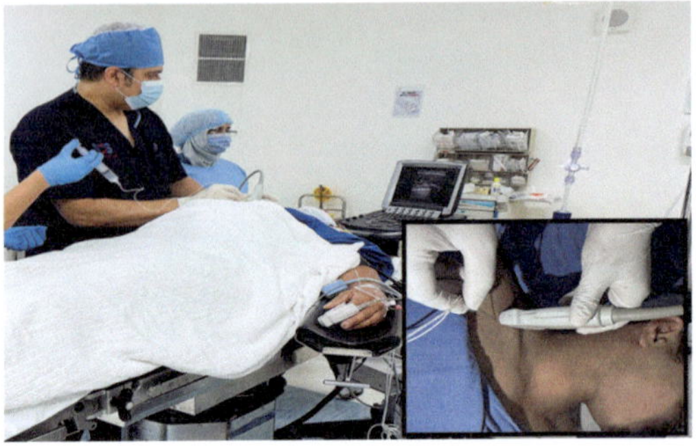

Fig. 5.3 Right-handed operator administering clavipectoral fascia block. Note the probe orientation and relative positions of the operator, patient, and the USG machine

5.2.2.7 Injection and Approach

PNS/Landmark-Guided

Given that the nerves blocked in this procedure are largely terminal, sensory branches, PNS stimulation-guided clavipectoral fascia block is not possible. Additionally, landmark-based technique consists of primarily being guided by the bony landmark of the clavicle. After palpating the clavicle on either side of the fracture, a 3–4 cm long needle is advanced in a paramedian plane from caudal to cephalad direction, entering the skin approximately 2–3 cm below the clavicle at an angle. Upon reaching the clavicle, the needle is withdrawn slightly and 10–15 of the LA is deposited there.

USG Guided

Under all aseptic precautions, 1–2 ml of local anesthetic is injected at the needle entry point. Under real-time USG guidance, with a high frequency (5–15 Hz) linear probe place in a paramedian plane, at the right angles to the long axis of the clavicle (Fig. 5.3), an 8–10 cm long, 22G short-bevel needle is advanced from the caudal to cephalic direction, to deposit the drug in between the clavipectoral fascia and the periosteum of the clavicle (Figs. 5.4 and 5.5).

5.2.2.8 Complications

The block has not been found to be associated with significant complications which highlights its promise.

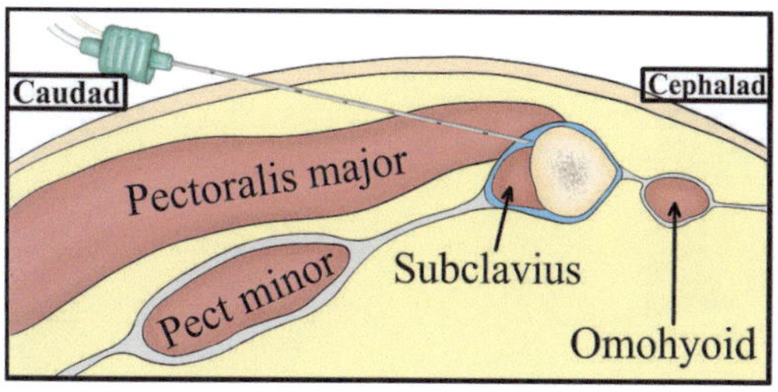

Fig. 5.4 Schematic representation of the area where local anesthetic needs to be deposited for clavipectoral fascia block

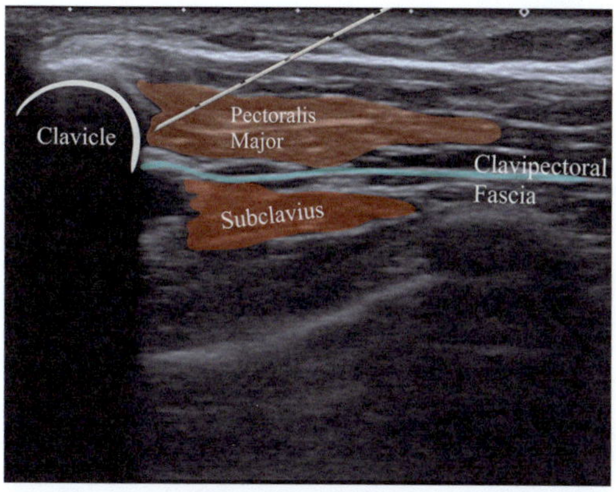

Fig. 5.5 Sonographic anatomy for clavipectoral fascia, also indicating the direction in which the needle is to be inserted

5.2.2.9 Tips

When there is clavicular fracture 10–12 ml of drug should be deposited on either side of the fracture.

5.2.3 Phrenic Nerve Block

The phrenic nerve arises from C3, C4 nerve roots and receives contributions from the third and fourth cranial nerves. It crosses the neck anterior to the scalenus anterior and enters the thorax to end by fanning out on the diaphragm to supply its musculature, the pleura, diaphragmatic peritoneum, and the peritoneal coat of upper abdominal organs. Along the way it also provides the sensory supply to the pericardium. A unilateral successful block paralyzes the hemidiaphragm and decreases the pulmonary capacity by 35–50%.

5.2.3.1 Indications

- Intractable treatment-resistant hiccoughs of various etiologies (after ruling out treatable causes). Some examples are psychogenic, CNS neoplasms, multiple sclerosis, vagal irritation, uremia, pericarditis, intravenous Pentazocine, malaria, tuberculosis, electrolyte imbalance, etc.
- Pain in innervation area (e.g., caused by tumors of lungs, mediastinum, etc.)

5.2.3.2 Contraindications

Apart from those described in Table 5.1, some specific contraindications are:

- Severe asthma/emphysema
- Paresis of the contralateral phrenic or recurrent laryngeal nerve.
- Contralateral pneumothorax

5.2.3.3 Preparation

Refer to Table 5.1 Pre-requisite for block

5.2.3.4 Position

Patient—Supine, with head turned to the contralateral side. Some advocate the placement of a soft support beneath the shoulders midway between the two scapulae, ostensibly to stretch and make structures in the supraclavicular area more prominent.

Operator and USG monitor

Refer to Sect. 5.2.1

5.2.3.5 Drug

As the space where the nerve is blocked is a confined space 3–5 ml local anesthetic is usually sufficient. 0.375% ropivacaine or 0.25–0.375% bupivacaine is generally used.

5.2.3.6 Injection and Approach

PNS/Landmark-Guided

It is recommended that this procedure is carried out only by an experienced anesthesiologist, or under their supervision.

The patient is positioned supine, with head turned to opposite side and landmarks identified.

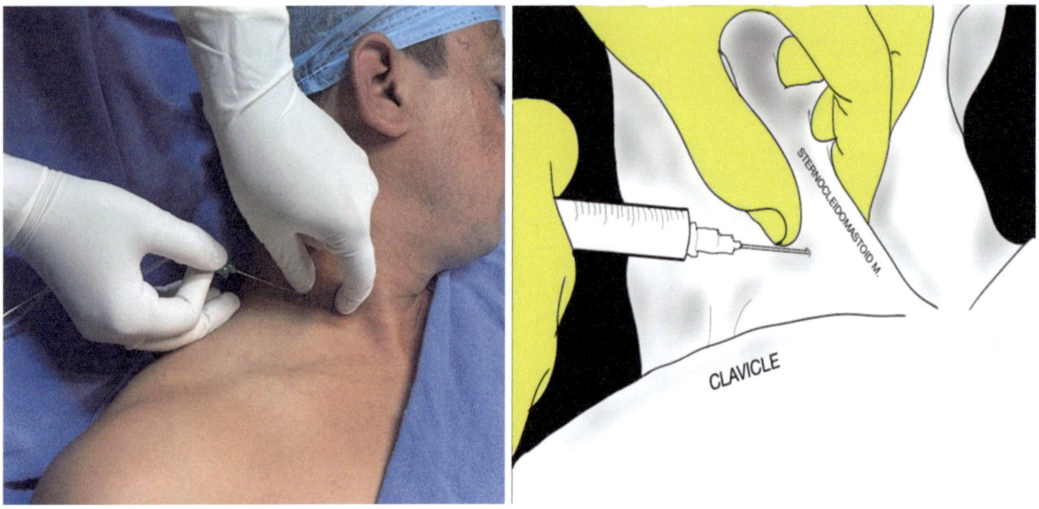

Fig. 5.6 Representation of landmark-based technique to block the phrenic nerve

Landmarks are lateral border of sternocleidomastoid (clavicular part); clavicle; scalenus anterior muscle.

Approximately 2–3 cm above the clavicle, at the lateral edge of the sternocleidomastoid muscle, at the right angle to the body and almost parallel to clavicle, the needle is inserted to an approximate depth of 2–3 cm directly medially (Fig. 5.6). The index finger is positioned in such a manner as to check the needle advancement. 3–5 ml of drug is then deposited after careful aspiration. The use of PNS is precluded due to the motor supply of the phrenic nerve, namely, the diaphragm. In any case, the idea is to bathe the nerve in local anesthetic solution, which is readily achieved by the method described.

USG Guided

With the positions arranged as described, a high frequency (5–15 Hz) linear probe is placed transversely at the level of C6, corresponding to the cricoid cartilage and the area is scanned to identify the sternocleidomastoid and scalenus anterior muscles. Between the two muscles a fascial expansion is looked for and that is the area to be aimed at (Fig. 5.7).

A 4–5 cm long 25G needle is advanced from the lateral to medial direction, constantly under vision to reach this space, cautious to avoid the cervical nerve roots which lie superficial and in close proximity.

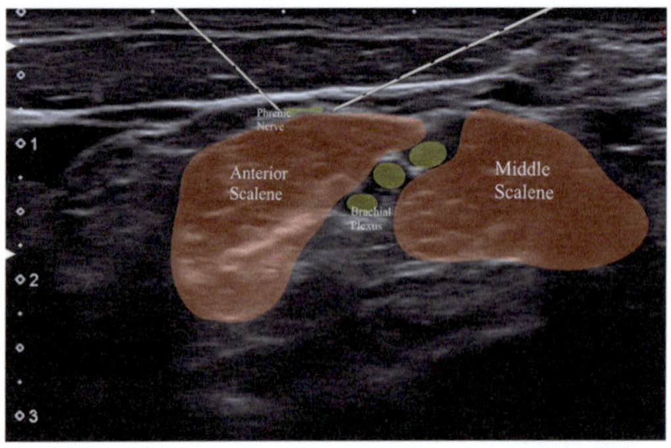

Fig. 5.7 USG appearance of phrenic nerve lying anterior to scalenus anterior as it crosses the neck. (*AS* Anterior Scalene muscle, *MS* Middle Scalene muscle)

After reaching the desired space, the drug is deposited after repeated negative aspirations, as described.

5.2.3.7 Complications

- Intravascular injection.
- Pneumothorax.
- Partial Stellate ganglion blockade (Horner's syndrome)

5.2.3.8 Tips

- The block should be carried out with an experienced anesthesiologist as it is deceptively risky.
- Simultaneous bilateral blockade should not be done. There should be a gap of at least 60–90 min.

5.2.4 Suprascapular Nerve Block

The suprascapular nerve (SSN) is the major sensory nerve supplying close to 70% of the shoulder, primarily to the posterior and superior aspects. The fact that it has a consistent course through the suprascapular notch the SSN is a suitable target for nerve blockade. Blockade of the SSN has been a diagnostic means for suprascapular neuropathy as well as therapeutic for the management of acute and chronic shoulder pain.

5.2.4.1 Anatomy

The SSN originates from C5, C6 ventral rami occasionally with a contribution from C4, carrying both sensory and motor fibers. Emerging from the upper trunk of the brachial plexus, it passes through the posterior triangle of neck deep to the trapezius and omohyoid, crosses the under the suprascapular ligament at the suprascapular notch, to enter the supraspinous fossa, running alongside the suprascapular artery in majority (78%) of the cases.

Immediately hereafter it gives a motor branch to supraspinatus and sensory to parts of the shoulder along its course before curving around the lateral border of the scapular spine to enter the infraspinous fossa and supply motor nerves to the infraspinatus (Fig. 5.8).

The consistency of its course in the suprascapular notch gives a reliable site of blockade particularly as the SSN hasn't divided into its branches as yet.

5.2.4.2 Indications

Acute postoperative shoulder pain (as an alternative to Interscalene blockade), chronic shoulder pain due to osteoarthritis, adhesive capsulitis, persistent rotator cuff tendinitis (pulsed radiofrequency).

5.2.4.3 Contraindications

As described in Table 5.1.

5.2.4.4 Preparation

Refer to Table 5.1 Pre-requisite for block

5.2.4.5 Technique

Patient position—The block can be performed with patient either sitting or lying prone. The prone position may offer the advantage of stability with patient less likely to move too much, but the sitting position is advantageous ergonomically in terms of reach.

Operator and USG monitor

The operator stands behind the sitting patient with the USG machine directly in front of both, as shown in Fig. 5.5.

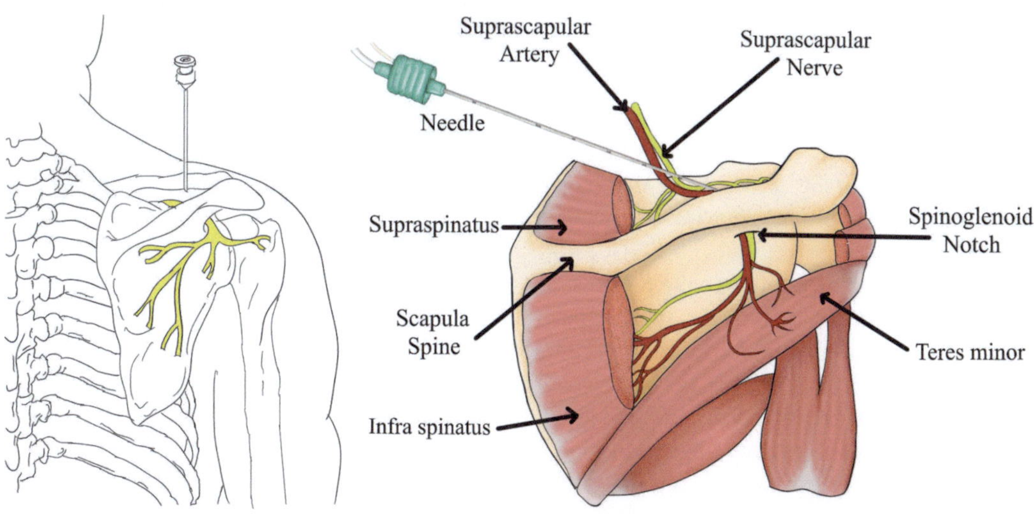

Fig. 5.8 Schematic representation of suprascapular nerve (right) in relation to bony and muscle landmarks

5.2.4.6 Drugs or Substances Used for Blockade

Various methods of blockade have been described, used alone or in combination, including local anesthetics, steroids, pulsed radiofrequency, and chemical neurolysis. The choice of agents depends on the indication with no established consensus. Bupivacaine (0.25–0.5%) with adrenaline (1:200,000) is a popular choice of local anesthetic. The volume of drug most widely accepted is 4–6 ml.

5.2.4.7 Injection and Approach

PNS/Landmark-Guided

Traditionally SSN blockade has been performed with a "blind" landmark-guided approach. Three landmark-based approaches have been described, namely, posterior, superior, and lateral approaches. The advent of PNS added to the accuracy in localization of the SSN, but the popularity of these approaches has declined with the introduction of radiological guidance.

USG-Guided

Both anterior and posterior approaches have been described, with the anterior approach aiming to block the SSN shortly after it branches off from the brachial plexus. The more widely practiced approach is the posterior approach where the nerve is approached far away from the brachial plexus. The most suitable site to perform the SSNB is at the floor of the suprascapular fossa.

With the patient in position, the high frequency (5–15 Hz) linear probe is placed in the coronal plane midway on an imaginary line joining the coracoid to the acromion. A slight anterior tilt to the probe may improve visualization (Fig. 5.9).

The operator should look for the SSN which frequently will be adjacent to the suprascapular artery (its pulsations can be looked for as a guide). These structures shall lie beneath the trapezius and supraspinatus muscle and just proximal to the scapular bony plate (Fig. 5.10).

1–2 ml of local anesthetic is injected at the needle entry point. An 8–10 cm long, 22G short-bevel needle is advanced with an in-plane technique, from medial to lateral and the drug deposited adjacent to the nerve.

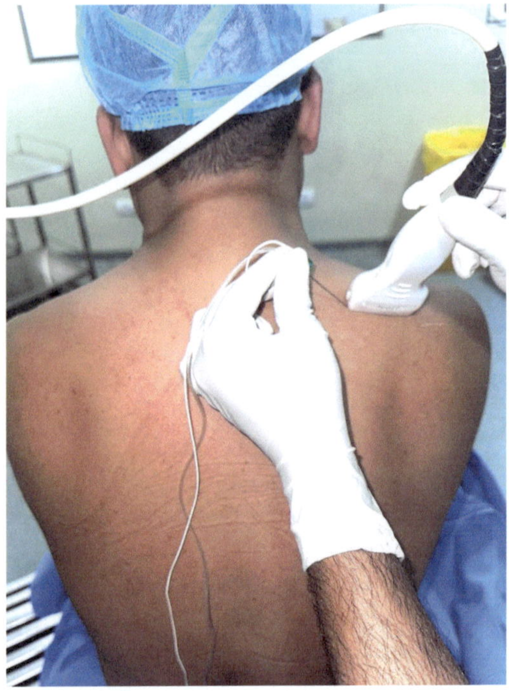

Fig. 5.9 Representation of the positioning for right-sided suprascapular nerve block by left-handed operator who stands behind the sitting patient, with the USG machine directly in front

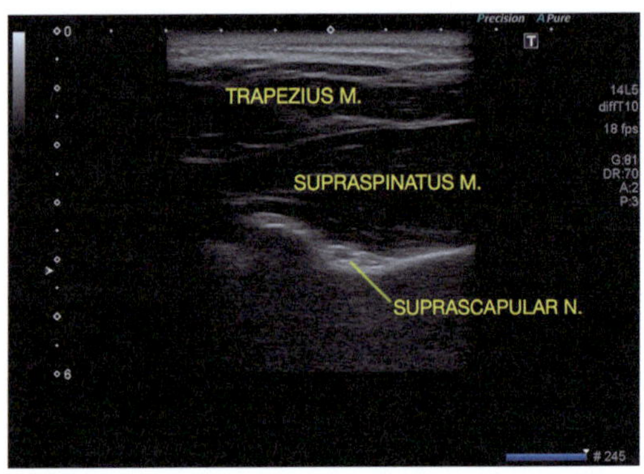

Fig. 5.10 USG appearance of the suprascapular nerve. Note that Doppler can be used to identify the suprascapular artery which frequently lies adjacent to the SSN

5.2.4.8 Complications

- SSNB is a relatively safe intervention with a generally low incidence of complications.

Though rare, pneumothorax (<1%), intravascular injection, vasovagal attack, and residual motor weakness are some of the known complications.

5.2.4.9 Tips

- The SSN runs along the floor of the supraspinous fossa, between the suprascapular notch and the spino-glenoid notch, contained in a compartment formed by the supraspinatus fascia, which thus limits the spread of the injectate. Consequently, even 5 ml of the injectate leads to adequate flooding of the nerve, thus making it the favored site of blockade.
- This approach renders the reliance on the suprascapular notch redundant, making the anatomical variations in the notch in some individuals irrelevant.
- The risk of pneumothorax is practically negligible due to the direction of the needle approach.
- Repeated aspirations (after every 1 ml of injections greatly reduce the risk of intravascular injection).

5.2.5 Brachial Plexus Blocks

The brachial plexus is a plexus formed by anterior rami of the nerves arising from spinal roots C5, C6, C7, C8, and T1 (Fig. 5.11). Occasionally, there is a contribution from the C4 root (referred to as "Pre-fixed" Brachial Plexus) and occasionally there is a contribution from the T2 root (referred to as "Post-fixed" Brachial Plexus).

Almost the entire superior extremity is innervated by nerves arising from this plexus (barring a small portion on the medial aspect of upper arm—supplied by intercostobrachial nerve [T2]; and upper part of the shoulder—supplied by supraclavicular nerve [C3–4]). It is therefore of extreme relevance to learn about the dermatomes, osteotomes, and neurotomes, as nerves arising from specific nerve roots supply specific portions of the upper limb (Figs. 5.12 and 5.13).

Consequently, depending on the area of proposed intervention, the brachial plexus can be blocked at an appropriate level to achieve desired surgical anesthesia and postoperative analgesia.

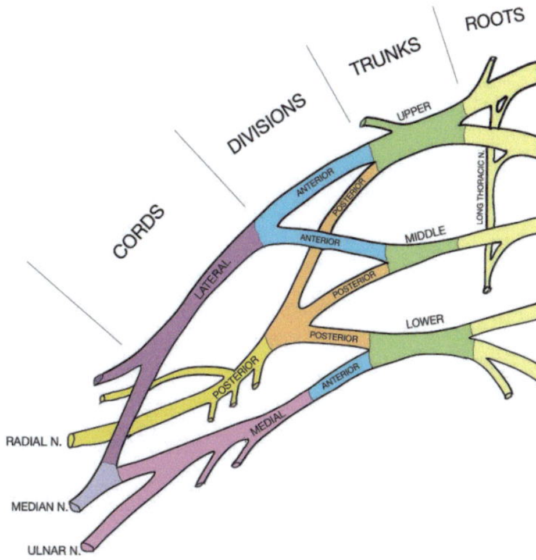

Fig. 5.11 A color-coded schematic representation of the brachial plexus. Yellow—Roots. Green—Trunks. Blue—Anterior divisions. Orange—Posterior divisions. Purple—Lateral cord. Pink—Medial cord. Mustard—Posterior cord

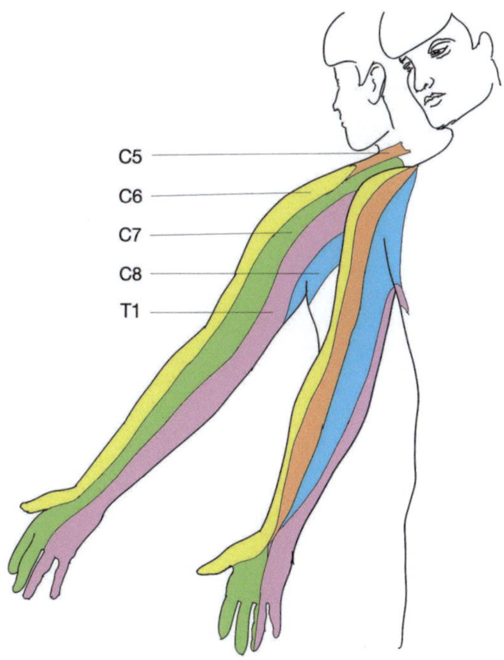

Fig. 5.12 Dermatomes supplied by brachial plexus. Orange—C5; Yellow—C6; Green—C7; Blue—C8; Purple—T1

Ultrasound (USG)-guided techniques of blockade are far more accurate and have proven predictable, superior success rate, and a reduced incidence of complications as well as require-

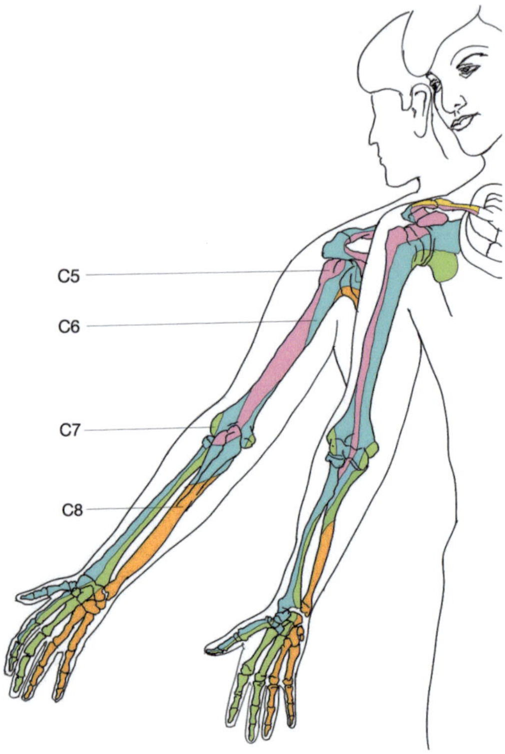

Fig. 5.13 Osteotomes supplied by the brachial plexus. Blue—C6; Purple—C5; Green—C7; Orange—C8

ment of local anesthetic volume as compared to traditional techniques. It seems reasonable to dwell more on this technique as it has rapidly become the most recommended one.

5.2.5.1 Anatomy

The brachial plexus lies deep to the prevertebral layer of the deep cervical fascia, which attaches to the C3–6 vertebrae on their anterior tubercles. The nerve roots from C5 through T1 exit their respective intervertebral foramina to traverse the interscalene groove between the scalenus anterior and scalenus medius muscles. It is here that the nerves form the upper, middle, and lower trunks. Subsequently each of these trunks divides into an anterior(ventral) and posterior(dorsal) division. The three posterior divisions come together to form the posterior cord (C5,6,7,8, T1). The upper trunk forms the lateral cord (C5,6,7) while the lower trunk continues as the medial cord (C8, T1) (Table 5.3, Figs 5.11, 5.12 and 5.13).

The posterior cord ends as the Radial nerve, the lateral cord receives a contribution from the medial cord to form the Median nerve and the medial cord continues as the Ulnar nerve.

Table 5.3 Motor supply by the terminal nerves of the brachial plexus

Nerve	Roots	Muscles	Motor Effect
Musculocutaneous (Lateral Cord)	C6	Biceps brachii, brachialis, and coracobrachialis	Flexion of the elbow and supination of the forearm
Axillary (Posterior Cord)	C5/6	Deltoid, teres minor	Abduction of shoulder and external rotation
Median (Lateral Cord and Medial Cord)	C5/6/7/8 & T1	Pronator teres, flexor carpi radialis, flexor digitorum superficialis, flexor digitorum profundus, palmaris longus, abductor pollicis brevis, opponens pollicis, flexor pollicis brevis and lumbricals	Flexion of the digits & wrist, pronation of the forearm, abduction of the wrist and abduction/flexion/opposition of the thumb
Radial (Posterior Cord)	C5/6/7/8 & T1	Triceps, extensor carpi radialis, extensor carpi ulnaris, extensor pollicis and supinator	Extension of elbow, wrist & fingers and supination of the forearm
Ulnar (Medial Cord)	C8/T1	Flexor carpi ulnaris, lumbricals, interossei, adductor pollicis, opponens digiti minimi, abductor digitorum minimi, flexor digiti minimi brevis and flexor digitorum profundus	Flexion & adduction of wrist, flexion/adduction & abduction of digits and opposition of little finger

Of the multiple approaches described for the Brachial plexus block, four are universally recognized. The most proximal Interscalene approach followed by the Supraclavicular, Infraclavicular, and Axillary approaches going progressively distal along the course of the plexus.

All of these approaches are based on the premise that a perivascular and perineural sheath contains the plexus along its entire course from the transverse processes to the axilla. The simplistic model of a single continuous sheath housing the entire plexus has since given way to a more intimate understanding of a multiseptated structure formed by a thin layer of fibrous surrounding the plexus creating individual fascial compartments for the nerves in the plexus.

The clinical significance of this understanding is yet to be unequivocally established but the "single injection for the whole plexus" stands challenged. In this light it seems reasonable to inject local anesthetic in divided doses at multiple sites within the sheath for optimal results.

5.2.5.2 Interscalene Block

Interscalene approach for the Brachial Plexus block involves injection of the local anesthetic at the interscalene level, between the anterior and middle scalene muscles, targeting the trunks of the plexus. This roughly corresponds with the level of the Cricoid cartilage.

The advent of USG-guided techniques has led to significant rise in safety and fall in the requirement of the volume of local anesthetic needed. The Interscalene block is suitable both for single-injection techniques and continuous techniques using a catheter.

Indications

Surgical—for open and arthroscopic shoulder surgeries (in combination with Superficial Cervical plexus block) and surgeries for fracture of proximal humerus.

Therapeutic—for chronic conditions of the shoulder including adhesive capsulitis where a continuous technique can provide analgesia and facilitate physiotherapy.

Contraindications

Apart from those described in Table 5.1, there are additional absolute contraindications.

- Contralateral interscalene block.
- Contralateral pneumonectomy or pneumothorax.
- Paresis of Phrenic or Recurrent laryngeal nerve on the contralateral side.

Preparation

Refer to Table 5.1 Pre-requisite for block

The importance of emergency airway management equipment cannot be overemphasized due to the very real risk of intrathecal injection, as well as diaphragmatic paralysis.

Position

Patient position—Supine, with head turned to the contralateral side. Some advocate the placement of a soft support beneath the shoulders midway between the two scapulae, ostensibly to stretch and make structures in the supraclavicular area more prominent. For the continuous injection technique, to insert a catheter, the patient lies in a lateral position with the intervention side placed nondependent.

Operator and USG monitor

The aim should be to have the injection site and the USG monitor in a single line of sight.

Refer to Sect. 5.2.1

Drug

When injecting at the accurate site, 10–15 ml of local anesthetic suffices to obtain surgical anesthesia of desired areas. 0.5–0.75% ropivacaine or 0.5% bupivacaine can be used.

Increasing the volume by 8–10 ml can often lead to blockade of Superficial Cervical Plexus too, but this outcome is rather inconsistent.

Injection and Approach

PNS/Landmark-Guided

With adequate sterile precautions and emergency preparedness, patient is positioned supine with head turned to contralateral side and arm drawn toward ipsilateral knee, the landmarks are identified.

Landmarks—Sternocleidomastoid muscle, interscalene groove between anterior and middle scalene muscles, C6 transverse process, and external jugular vein. The puncture site is located after identifying the landmarks.

Location of puncture site—The posterior edge of Sternocleidomastoid muscle is identified and posterior to this, the scalenus anterior muscle is palpated. The palpating finger is then "rolled" further posteriorly in the Interscalene groove between the scalenus anterior and scalenus medius muscle. The puncture site lies in this interscalene groove at the level of the cricoid cartilage, opposite to the C6 transverse process. The external jugular vein often crosses the interscalene groove at this level. In case it is difficult to identify structures, the patient can be asked to perform a Valsalva maneuver briefly, which makes the interscalene groove more prominent due to scalene muscles tensing up.

Technique—The block needle is inserted at an angle of 30° caudally and slight laterally directed approximately toward junction of middle and lateral third of the ipsilateral clavicle. A stimulation current of 1–2 mA and 2 Hz is selected with a duration of 0.1 ms. Once a motor response from the relevant musculature is elicited, the stimulation current is reduced to 0.2–0.3 mA. If slight twitching persists, it indicates the proper placement of the needle. A single injection of drug can be administered here, or a catheter can be inserted here in case of a continuous block.

USG-Guided

Among the various techniques prevalent, "forward tracing" from the vertebral transverse processes or "backward tracing" from the supraclavicular fossa is the more commonly used once. The authors recommend a variation of the "back tracing" from the supraclavicular area due to its uncomplicated nature and easily identifiable beginning targets.

After ensuring positioning as described above, the high frequency linear array transducer (10–13 MHz) is placed with a slight caudal tilt in the supraclavicular fossa, parallel and adjacent to the middle third of the clavicle (Fig. 5.14). The Subclavian artery is identified by scanning the area for a circular, hypoechoic pulsatile structure. Lateral to this is found a cluster of hypoechoic blobs contained in a sheath, classically described as a "bunch of grapes." This is the brachial plexus.

It is quite difficult to miss in spite of not infrequent variations in the relative positions of the two structures. The plexus can be found anywhere from immediately anterior to the Subclavian artery to anterolateral to far lateral in the fossa. One thing to remember is the plexus *is* there, regardless of variations and is never absent.

Once identified, the plexus is traced proximally, until it comes to lie between two muscles—the scalenus anterior and scalenus medius. Invariably, by the time you reach here, the plexus morphology changes to the aptly described "traffic light" pattern (Fig. 5.14), with three hypoechoic blobs appearing stacked in series between two muscle bellies. This generally is at C5–C6 level, with the blobs being the C5, C6, and C7 roots, C5 being the most superficial. At this level the neural structures have reduced connective tissue, making it easier to visualize the plexus.

1–2 ml of local anesthetic is injected at the needle entry point. With the "in-plane" technique, ensuring continuous visibility of the tip, an 8–10 cm long, 22G short-bevel needle is advanced in a lateral to medial direction to approach the plexus. It is recommended to scan for blood vessels in the planned needle trajectory using the color Doppler. As the needle pierces the prevertebral layer of the deep cervical fascia overlying the scalenus medius, a "pop" is felt, and a second "pop" is felt as the needle tip crosses the anterior border of the middle scalene muscle into the interscalene groove to enter the plexus sheath.

After ensuring adequate placement of needle tip, local anesthetic can be injected—superficial to C5 or between C5 and C6. Injection deep to C6

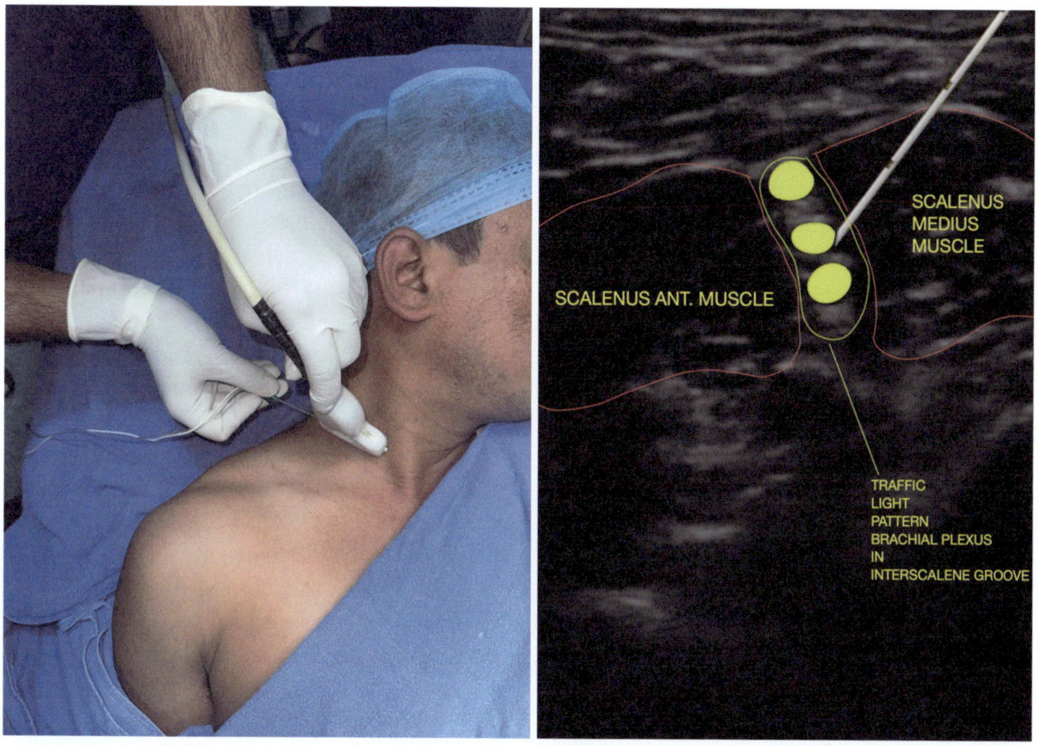

Fig. 5.14 Probe position and USG appearance of the brachial plexus for the interscalene approach. Note the linear arrangement of the nerve roots, which mimics the "traffic light" pattern

is better avoided for the fear of intraneural injection.

Pressure of injection should be carefully monitored as increased resistance or higher injection pressures suggest that the needle tip is intraneural. The needle should then be withdrawn and repositioned.

Complications

- Phrenic nerve block with ipsilateral diaphragm paralysis. Occurs commonly (Interscalene > Supraclavicular), due to cephalad spread of drug. Usually patient reassurance is sufficient management, but in patients with reduced pulmonary reserve it can cause significant respiratory compromise, even necessitating ventilatory support. The incidence is much less with USG-guided approach as opposed to traditional techniques.
- Horner's syndrome constituted by miosis, ptosis, and anhidrosis may result by the drug spreading to cause cervicothoracic sympathetic trunk block. It resolves as the action of the drugs wears off.
- Recurrent laryngeal nerve block may present as hoarseness or sensation of lump in throat.
- Pneumothorax is an increasingly rare complication with the use of USG guidance, but remains a significant threat, should it occur
- Epidural or intrathecal spread of drug or contralateral spread of drug is more likely to occur when higher dosages of local anesthetic are used, including bolus and infusion doses. It may lead to total spinal block which is life-threatening and may require management accordingly.
- Intravascular injection may result as the target area is a highly vascular zone including the vertebral artery and branches of the thyrocervical trunk. Accidental intravascular local anesthetic injection can rapidly lead to local anesthetic toxicity.
- Nerve injury occurring after intervention is of significant concern to both patients and health

care workers. The reported incidence is around 0.9 per 1000 blocks. There are various factors at play in such a situation, including surgical and patient related, and all possible causes should be considered before ascribing any neurologic injury to the regional anesthesia. Serious permanent neuropathy directly attributable the performance of plexus blocks is not very common.

- Catheter misplacement should be kept in mind with continuous technique.
- Cervical spinal cord injury has been reported due to local anesthetic being injected directly into the spinal cord while performing interscalene block under general anesthesia.

Tips

- Local anesthetic should be injected incrementally, with repeated aspiration every 2–3 ml to minimize risk of intravascular injection, given that it is a highly vascular area.
- Injection of local anesthetic inside the muscle belly of middle scalene muscle should be avoided.
- Stay alert for respiratory compromise, caused by diaphragmatic paralysis or accidental intrathecal injection following the block. Some patients may require assisted ventilation.
- Maintain high index of suspicion for pneumothorax and be prepared for needle thoracostomy if required.
- Use the color Doppler option while scanning before injecting the local anesthetic to identify blood vessels, which might appear similar to the hypoechoic shadows of the nerve roots or trunks.
- Injection of local anesthetic between C6 and C7 is better avoided for fear of intraneural injection.
- The nerves from C5 root such as the dorsal scapular nerve and the areas innervated by the lower trunk are likely to be spared with the Interscalene block.
- Going too close to the nerve roots should be avoided as nerve injury due to pressure effect is likely if the injection is too near the transverse foramen. Too deep injection tends to be intrafascicular or intraneural.
- For continuous technique, the needle entry point should be more cephalad and posterior. This allows space for tunneling of the catheter reducing chances of its displacement.

5.2.5.3 Supraclavicular Block

Brachial plexus block with the supraclavicular approach involves depositing the drug in the plexus sheath at the level where the trunks divide into anterior and posterior divisions.

Supraclavicular was one of the earliest approaches described for Brachial plexus block and was quite popular to begin with. However, as it became evident that this was associated with a high incidence of pneumothorax, its popularity waned. The emergence of USG-guided techniques has revived its popularity, albeit tempered with the understanding that it has similar or reduced efficacy as compared to other infraclavicular approaches. Delayed Ulnar nerve sensory blockade has also been demonstrated.

Indications

When performed well, the Supraclavicular Brachial plexus block can anesthetize the entire upper limb but is largely the block of choice for surgeries in the distal half of arm, elbow, and proximal forearm.

Due to the higher risk of catheter dislodgement, it is not an ideal technique for continuous catheter technique.

Contraindications

Apart from those described in Table 5.1, there are additional absolute contraindications.

- Contralateral Interscalene block.
- Contralateral pneumonectomy or pneumothorax.
- Paresis of Phrenic or Recurrent laryngeal nerve on the contralateral side.

Preparation

Refer to Table 5.1 Pre-requisite for block

Position

Patient Supine, with head turned to the contralateral side. Some advocate the placement of a soft support beneath the shoulders midway between the two scapulae, ostensibly to stretch and make structures in the supraclavicular area more prominent.

Operator and USG monitor

The aim should be to have the injection site and the USG monitor in a single line of sight.

Refer to Sect. 5.2.1

Drug

When injecting at the accurate site, 15–25 ml of local anesthetic suffices to obtain surgical anesthesia of desired areas. 0.5–0.75% ropivacaine or 0.5% bupivacaine can be suggested.

Injection and Approach

PNS/Landmark-Guided

With adequate sterile precautions and emergency preparedness, patient is positioned supine with head turned to contralateral side and arm drawn toward ipsilateral knee, the landmarks are identified.

Landmarks—The lateral border of the insertion of sternocleidomastoid on the clavicle, pulsation of the subclavian artery in the supraclavicular fossa. The puncture site is located after identifying the landmarks.

Location of puncture site—The subclavian artery pulsations are located in the supraclavicular fossa with the thumb of the non-dominant hand. This is approximately 2.5 cm lateral to the lateral end of the insertion of sternocleidomastoid on the clavicle and 1 cm proximal to the clavicle.

Technique—The block needle (typically 50 mm, 22G, short-bevel, insulated) is advanced in the parasagittal plain, parallel to the patient's midline. The nerve stimulator is initially set a current of 0.8 mA at 1 Hz with pulse width of 0.2–0.3 ms. The best results are obtained when a flexion or extension motor response is elicited in the fingers. In case the needle requires repositioning, it is redirected either anterior or posterior but in the same original parasagittal plane, always keeping the needle tip above the clavicle.

USG-Guided

The anatomy is approached as described above in the Interscalene block and the "bunch of grapes" is identified (Fig. 5.15). While performing the scan by a high frequency linear array transducer (10–13 MHz), it helps to identify and make a mental note of the "out of bound territories," namely the pleura, the subclavian artery, and the plethora of blood vessels as this is an even more vascular area. It is again recommended to scan for blood vessels in the planned needle trajectory using the color Doppler.

1–2 ml of local anesthetic is injected at the needle entry point. With the "in-plane" technique, ensuring continuous visibility of the tip, an 8–10 cm long, 22G short-bevel needle is advanced in a lateral to medial direction to approach the plexus. A slight caudal tilt of the transducer is maintained and positioned so as to have the 1st rib and pleura continuously visible to reduce the risk of pneumothorax. It is recommended to deposit around 5–7 ml of local anesthetic at the 6 o' clock position to begin with. Another 10–15 ml drug is deposited in the sheath containing the major cluster of nerves (the "bunch of grapes!")

Complications

- Phrenic nerve blockade
- Pneumothorax
- Intravascular injection
- Nerve injury—the incidence can be minimized by the use of needles with short-beveled tips. Intraneural positioning should be excluded and vasopressor additives should not be used.

Tips

- Local anesthetic should be injected incrementally, with repeated aspiration every 2–3 ml to minimize risk of intravascular injection, given that it is a highly vascular area.
- Maintain high index of suspicion for pneumothorax and be prepared for needle thoracostomy if required.
- Use the color Doppler option while scanning before injecting the local anesthetic to identify blood vessels, which might appear similar to

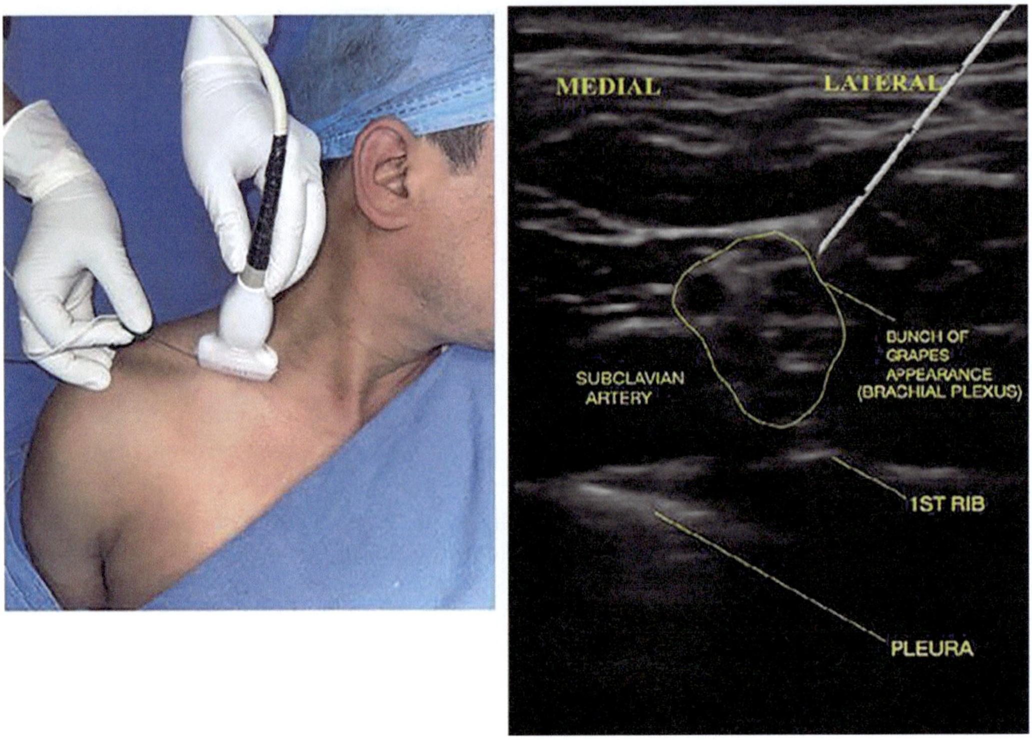

Fig. 5.15 Probe position and USG appearance of the brachial plexus for the supraclavicular approach. Note the appearance classically described as "bunch of grapes" lying anterolaterally to the subclavian artery

the hypoechoic shadows of the nerve roots or trunks.

- The nerves from C5 root such as the dorsal scapular nerve may be spared.
- High pressure of injection indicates intraneural position of the needle tip.
- The C8 and T1 distribution may have a delayed onset or incomplete blockade (medial border of forearm and hand)
- The block procedure is best avoided after general anesthesia.

5.2.6 Stellate Ganglion Block

Stellate ganglion is an oval structure and refers to the confluence of the first thoracic and inferior cervical sympathetic ganglia. It extends from the head of the first rib to the inferior border of the transverse process of the C7 vertebra and lies adjacent to the dome of the pleura, behind the Subclavian artery. This ganglion is absent in the classical description in 20% of the population, and a more appropriate name is Cervicothoracic sympathetic trunk. It is a conduit for all sympathetic outflow to the head and neck and the upper limb.

The traditional approach to the Stellate ganglion block is the anatomical landmark or fluoroscopy-guided paratracheal approach. It is rather unsafe and has significant potential of intravascular injection (can cause retropharyngeal and cervico-mediastinal hematoma—airway compromise) as well as puncture of the esophagus (more on left; can cause mediastinitis), pleura (pneumothorax), lateral lobe of the thyroid gland (hematoma) and cervical nerve roots.

The emergence of USG-guided techniques has significantly reduced potential complications (by affording identification of important soft tissue structures) (Fig. 5.16). Additionally, the accuracy and efficacy of block improves significantly, given that the drug spread in the appropriate subfascial plane can be ensured with real-time visualization. The drug goes in the subfascial plane as opposed to the pre-fascial plane as is the

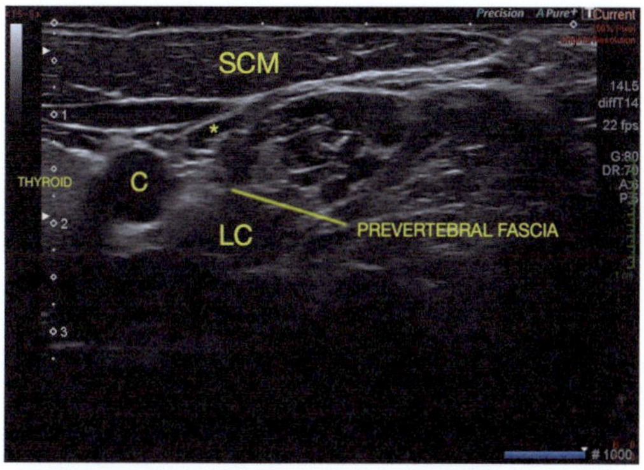

Fig. 5.16 USG appearance of the Stellate ganglion. It lies on the longus colli muscle. Note that the drug should be deposited superficial to the fascia investing the anterolateral surface of the longus colli muscle. SCM = Sternocleidomastoid muscle; C = Carotid artery; LC = Longus colli muscle; * = Internal jugular vein (collapsed)

case with landmark-based approach, where the needle is withdrawn after contact with the bony landmark.

5.2.6.1 Indications

Stellate ganglion block has been demonstrated to be of value in a variety of pain conditions such as:

- CRPS (complex regional pain syndrome)
- Refractory angina
- Phantom limb pain
- Pain in head, neck arm, or upper chest due to Herpes zoster
- Ischemic pain due to peripheral vascular disease.

It has been shown to be effective in managing refractory supraventricular tachycardia.

It has a role to play in post-traumatic stress disorder as it decreases dysfunctional sympathetic tone, hyperarousal state, and inability to relax.

5.2.6.2 Contraindications

As described in Table 5.1

5.2.6.3 Preparation

Refer to Table 5.1 Pre-requisite for block

5.2.6.4 Position

Patient position—In the lateral approach the most suitable position is with the patient in the lateral position with the proposed side of the block placed non-dominant, the neck extended, and head supported by a pillow.

Operator and USG monitor

Refer to Sect. 5.2.1

5.2.6.5 Drug

When injected in the subfascial plane 5 ml of 0.5% bupivacaine in 1:200,000 adrenaline has been demonstrated to be sufficient for spread from C4 to T1.

5.2.6.6 Injection and Approach

It is worth mentioning here that of the two USG-guided approaches in practice, the authors recommend the lateral approach with in-plane technique as it has significantly a lower risk of injury to vital soft tissues including the thyroid gland and inadvertent intravascular injection. The comfort of the patient also increases as the pressure on the trachea is avoided.

Landmark-Guided

In landmark or fluoroscopy-guided paratracheal approach, the needle is inserted toward the anterior tubercle of C6 (Chassaignac tubercle). The stellate ganglion is located opposite to the neck of the first rib, hence, this approach is more a blockade of the cervical sympathetic chain in proximity to the middle cervical ganglion.

USG-Guided

With the arrangement as described above, a high frequency linear array transducer (6–13 MHz) is placed transversely on the anterolateral aspect of the neck at the level of C6 such that the common carotid artery can be identified medially and the transverse process of C6 laterally.

A 4–5 cm long 25G needle is advanced in plane from lateral to medial to pierce the prevertebral fascia covering the longus colli muscle. The needle should be deep to the prevertebral fascia but superficial to the fascia investing the anterolateral surface of the longus colli because it is here that the cervical sympathetic chain is embedded.

1–2 ml of local anesthetic is injected at the needle entry point. 5–6 ml of local anesthetic is deposited as described above with frequent, careful negative aspiration.

5.2.6.7 Complications

- Retropharyngeal and cervico-mediastinal hematomas are reported despite repeated negative aspiration. This has the potential to cause airway compromise and become life-threatening.
- Esophageal puncture, leading to mediastinitis.
- Pleural puncture, leading to pneumothorax.
- Thyroid gland puncture, leading to hematoma in the substance of the gland.
- Cervical nerve root injury. Medial pressure on the probe can "push away" the cervical nerve roots during scanning.

5.2.6.8 Tips

- Real-time visualization of injectate with scanning is important as its absence may indicate intravascular injection.
- After the initial 0.1 ml signs of intravascular spread should be looked for (tinnitus, perioral tingling/numbness, lightheadedness, tachycardia, hypertension, etc.). Further injection should continue only after ensuring there is no intravascular spread.

5.3 Upper Limb Blocks with Injection Site Below the Clavicle

Some of the important upper limb blocks with injection site below the clavicle are:

- Infraclavicular brachial plexus block.
- Axillary brachial plexus block.
- Medial, lateral, and posterior cutaneous nerve of forearm.
- Median nerve block at the elbow.
- Radial nerve block at the elbow.
- Ulnar nerve block at the elbow.

5.3.1 Infraclavicular Brachial Plexus Block

The infraclavicular approach to the brachial plexus was first described by Bazy and Labat in the 1930s. The greater depth of the plexus under the clavicle and proximity to the pleura was a hindrance to its widespread adoption, and it was only after 1973 when Raj described his modified approach that it became popular. The discovery of lateral approaches to the plexus (under the coracoid process and outside the rib cage) and the emergence of USG have proven to be a game changer for infraclavicular brachial plexus block.

The infraclavicular fossa is an important anatomical area with brachial plexus blocks and central venous cannulation of the subclavian vein being routinely performed. The anterior border of the infraclavicular fossa is formed by the pectoralis minor and major muscles, the medial border by the ribs and intercostal muscles, the superior border by the clavicle and the coracoid process of the scapula, and the lateral border by the humerus (Fig. 5.17).

5.3.1.1 Anatomical Considerations

The trunks surround the **first part of the axillary artery** and pass over the first rib, deep to the clavicle, where they each divide into anterior and posterior divisions. The cords are therefore named according to their position relative to the **second part of the axillary artery** and are situated deep to the pectoralis major and minor muscles (Fig. 5.18). The terminal branches of the brachial plexus arise from the cords in the region of the **third part of the axillary artery**, inferior to the distal border of pectoralis minor, and supply skin and muscles of the upper limb (Fig. 5.19).

Surface Anatomy

Surface landmarks are relevant for nerve stimulator-based techniques.

Medial approach—Mid-point of the line joining the jugular notch and anterior process of acromion (corresponding to the mid-point of clavicle).

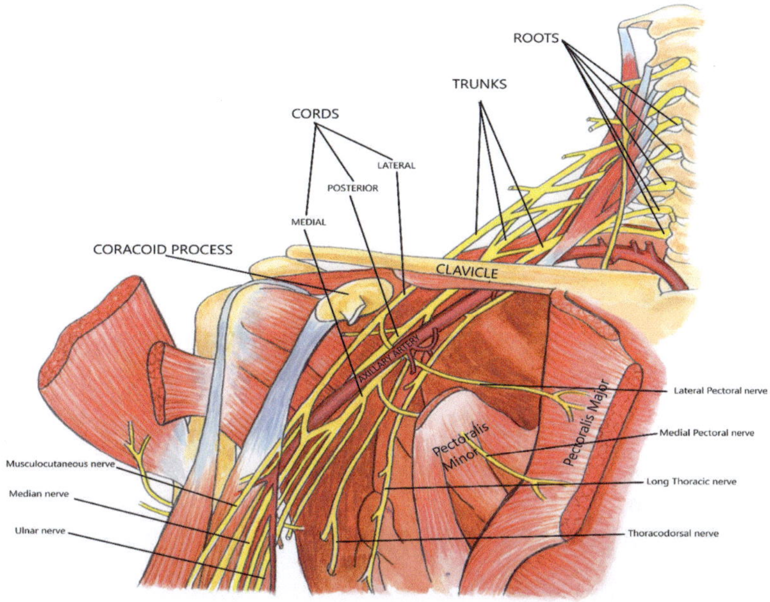

Fig. 5.17 Anatomy of the infraclavicular region and its contents. The pectoral muscles have been reflected out to show the position of the 3 cords around the axillary artery

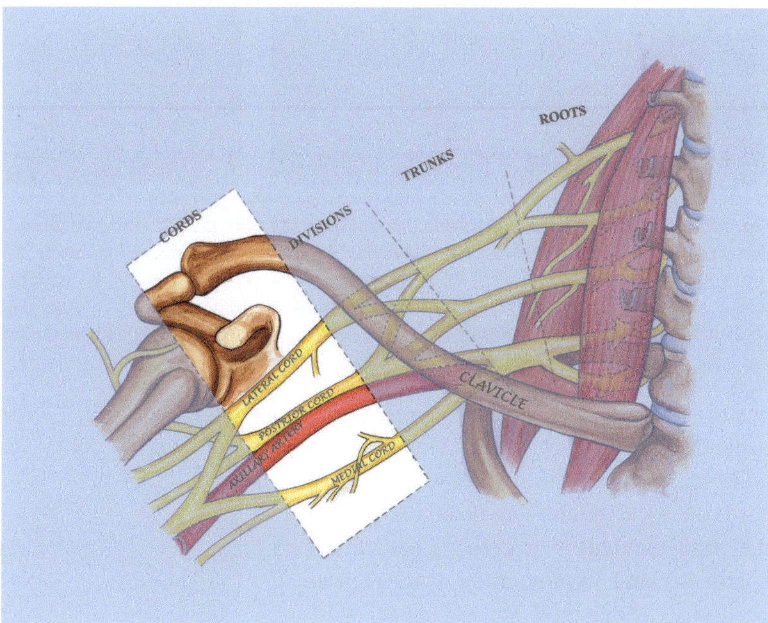

Fig. 5.18 Anatomical relationship of the 3 cords to the 2nd part of axillary artery. Note the position of the coracoid process at this point

Lateral approach—Most anterior prominence of the shoulder on shrugging (coracoid process).

The cords and their branches provide entire upper limb innervation below the shoulder except the medial upper arm (intercostobrachial nerve, which can be spared by the Infraclavicular Brachial Plexus Block and Axillary block).

Sonoanatomy for Infraclavicular Brachial Plexus Block

The pectoralis minor muscle divides the axillary artery into 3 divisions and the relative

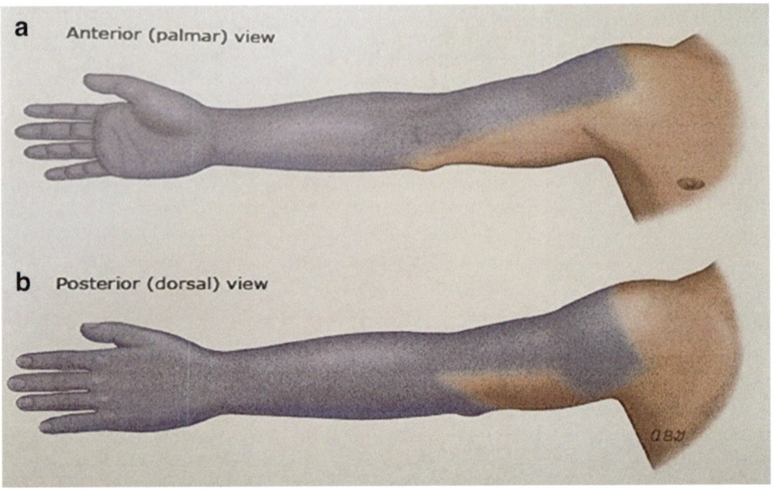

Fig. 5.19 Sensory innervation of the terminal branches of the infraclavicular portion of brachial plexus

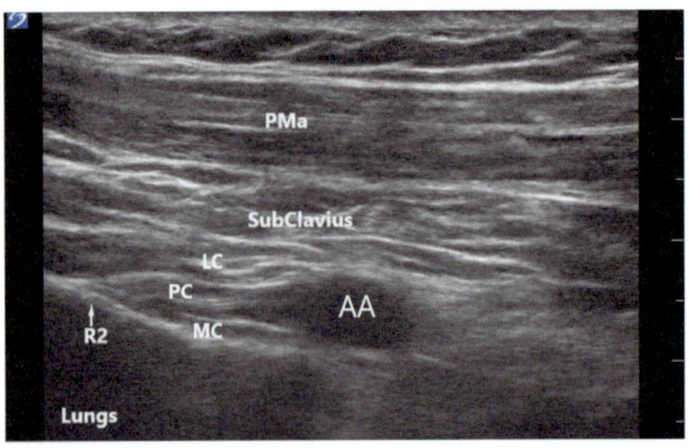

Fig. 5.20 Sonoanatomy of infraclavicular Space. *PMa* pectoralis major muscle, *Subclavius* subclavius muscle, *AA* axillary artery, *LC* lateral cord, *PC* posterior cord, *MC* medial cord, *R2* second rib. Note lateral position of all 3 cords in relation to the axillary artery

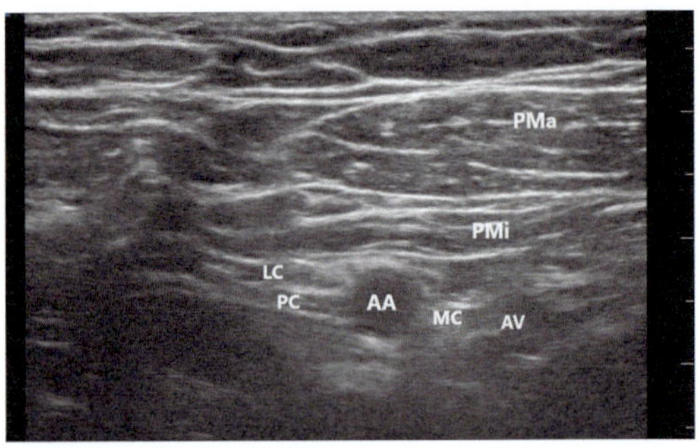

Fig. 5.21 Sonoanatomy of infraclavicular space. *PMa* pectoralis major muscle, *PMi* pectoralis minor muscle, *AA* axillary artery, *AV* axillary vein, *LC* lateral cord, *PC* posterior cord, *MC* medial cord. Note medial cord migrating to the medial side of the artery

position of the cords of the brachial plexus depends on the area scanned. Although there is wide variation in the anatomy, usually the 3 cords are located lateral to the axillary artery in the **mid-clavicular** region (Costoclavicular approach) and assume their true anatomical positions (as per their nomenclature) with the cords lying Lateral, Posterior, and Medial to the **second** part of the axillary artery in the **sub-coracoid** region (Figs. 5.20, 5.21, 5.22 and 5.23).

5.3.1.2 Indications

1. Surgical anesthesia for elbow, forearm, and hand procedures,

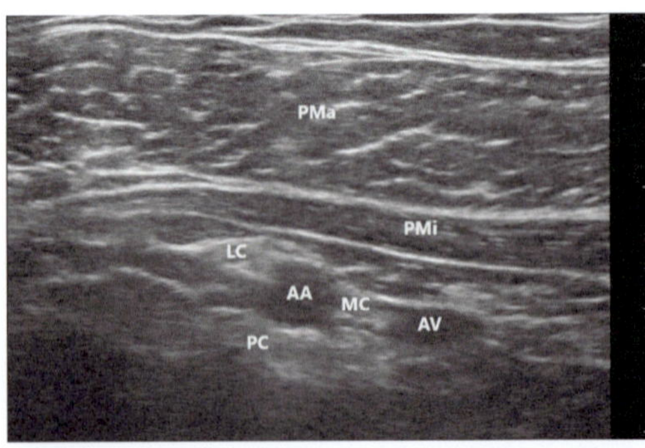

Fig. 5.22 Sonoanatomy in infraclavicular region. *PMa* pectoralis major muscle, *PMi* pectoralis minor muscle, *AA* axillary artery, *AV* axillary vein, *LC* lateral cord, *PC* posterior cord, *MC* medial cord. Note that the 3 cords are now in their true anatomical position

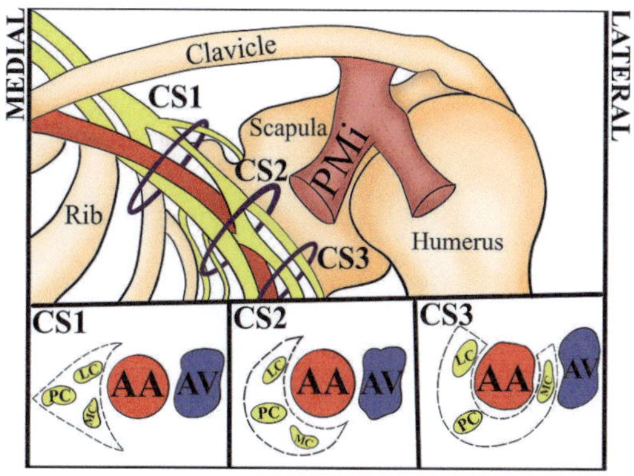

Fig. 5.23 Schematic representation of the rotation of cords around the axillary artery. The 3 rings represent the 3 Cross Sections (CS) at the 1st, 2nd, and 3rd part of the axillary artery with the relationship shown in the boxes below. *AA* axillary artery, *AV* axillary vein, *LC* lateral cord, *PC* posterior cord, *MC* medial cord

2. Cutaneous anesthesia for superficial procedures of the inner arm, for example, brachiobasilic fistula formation,
3. Chronic pain procedures.

5.3.1.3 Contraindications

Refer to Table 5.1

5.3.1.4 Preparation

Refer to Table 5.1 Pre-requisite for block

5.3.1.5 Position

Patient—The advantage of infraclavicular block over axillary block is that it can be performed with the arm adducted and in neutral position. This is very comfortable for the patient but can present significant challenges:

- The depth of the plexus from the skin can hinder visualization of the cords especially in obese and muscular patients.
- The angle of insertion needle insertion tends to be very steep which might make needle visualization very difficult.
- The options for needle insertion might be limited due to limited space under the clavicle (with medial approaches) and between the clavicle and shoulder (with lateral approaches).

Slight adjustments in the positioning can improve needle visualization as follows:

Arm Position—Abduct the arm to 90 degrees at shoulder and elbow and rotate the forearm externally—this elevates the clavicle and stretches the pectoral muscles, reducing the depth of the plexus from the skin and making visualization significantly easier.

Transducer Position—With the medial approach, the transducer is placed parallel to the clavicle with a slight cephalad tilt to view the costoclavicular space and with the lateral approaches, the probe should be placed in a parasagittal orientation with a slightly cephalad tilt. Both these positions and maneuvers help in visualization of the plexus and the reflected beam from the needle. Rocking the probe with a cephalad tilt also allows space for insertion of needle under the clavicle in a parasagittal approach.

Operator and USG monitor

The aim should be to have the clinician, the injection site, and the USG monitor in a single line of sight.

Refer to Sect. 5.2.1

5.3.1.6 Drug

20–25 ml of ropivacaine 0.75% or bupivacaine 0.5% may be suggested.

5.3.1.7 Ultrasound Probe

A high frequency linear transducer (8–14 MHz) is most appropriate for this block. A low frequency curved array probe may sometimes offer better figure quality in a patient with thick chest wall.

5.3.1.8 Injection and Approach

There are two approaches commonly practiced for the Infraclavicular approach to brachial plexus block with the lateral approach gaining favor for obvious reasons of less potential for complications (Fig. 5.24).

A. Medial Approach:
   1. Nerve stimulator-guided—Vertical Infraclavicular Block (VIB)
   2. USG-guided—Costoclavicular approach.

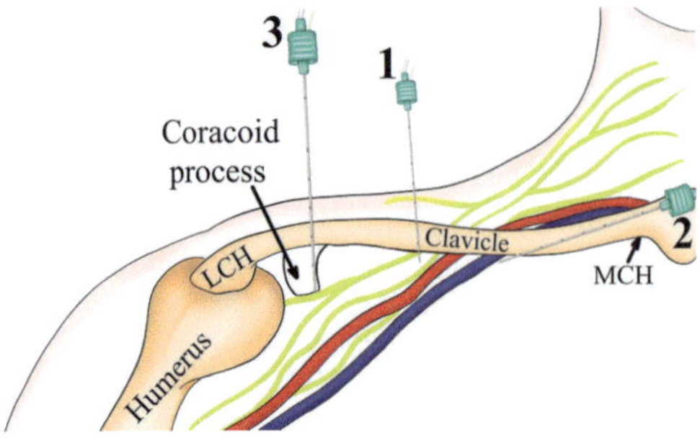

Fig. 5.24 Medial and lateral approaches to infraclavicular brachial plexus block. 1 = vertical infraclavicular block (nerve stimulation), 2 = costoclavicular block (ultrasound) and 3 = sub-coracoid (both ultrasound and nerve stimulation). *MCH* medial clavicular head, *LCH* lateral clavicular head

Table 5.4 Response to nerve stimulation at the plexus below the clavicle level

Motor response	Cord	Acceptability
Wrist or Finger Extension	Posterior Cord	Yes
Pectoral muscle twitch	None: Direct stimulation of muscle or pectoral nerves	Not acceptable, too superficial or too close to lateral cord
Elbow Flexion	Lateral Cord, too cephalad or superficial	Not acceptable, too superficial or close to lateral cord
Post-scapular movement	None: Stimulation of long thoracic nerve	Do not accept, too deep
Wrist flexion/ thumb adduction	Medial Cord	Only acceptable for surgery along ulnar distribution

B. Lateral Approach:
   1. Nerve stimulator-guided—Peri-coracoid & Parasagittal.
   2. USG-guided—Sub-coracoid approach.

Medial Approach

PNS-Guided (Vertical Infraclavicular Block)

This is a popular approach, where the needle is inserted perpendicular to all planes below the mid-point of the clavicle (between the jugular notch and the medial acromion process). In smaller patients the needle insertion point is moved laterally by 0.2 cm for every cm the clavicle measures <22 cm. The plexus is usually encountered at an average depth of 2–3 cm. If the plexus is not encountered by 4 cm, check your landmarks again and move the needle medially or laterally along the inferior surface of the clavicle. Various responses to nerve stimulation at plexus below the clavicle are tabulated in Table 5.4.

Clinical Tips

- Keep needle absolutely vertical and close to clavicle and move it in horizontal plane only (medial or lateral)
- Do not advance the needle beyond 4 cm even in obese patients.
- Care should be taken during advancement in small patients since the plexus maybe very superficial and easily damaged.

A variation to this approach was proposed by Raj and Borgeat where the needle insertion point is still at the mid-point below the clavicle, but the direction of angulation is along the sheath, i.e., laterally toward the axilla.

USG-Guided (*Costoclavicular Approach*) This is a proximal/medial approach described recently. The brachial plexus is scanned for in the costoclavicular space under the mid-point of the clavicle. The two perceived advantages of this technique are (a) clear separation of the artery from the 3 cords and (b) organization of the divisions seen in supraclavicular fossa into 3 distinct cords. This also makes it an ideal location for insertion of catheters.

A high frequency linear probe is placed at the mid-point of the clavicle in a transverse orientation on the clavicle. The probe is then gently rolled off the inferior border of the clavicle and the subclavian artery and vein visualized (Fig. 5.25). A gentle cephalad tilt reveals the costoclavicular space (between the posterior surface of the clavicle and the second rib) with the 3 cords arranged beside the artery.

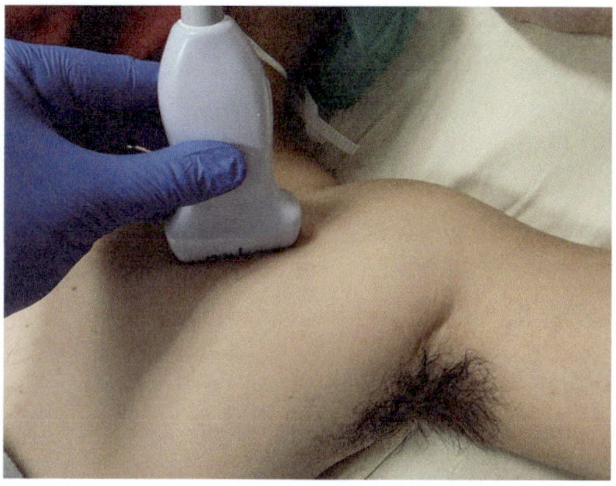

Fig. 5.25 Patient and probe position for costoclavicular approach. Note the position of linear probe parallel to the clavicle and just under it.

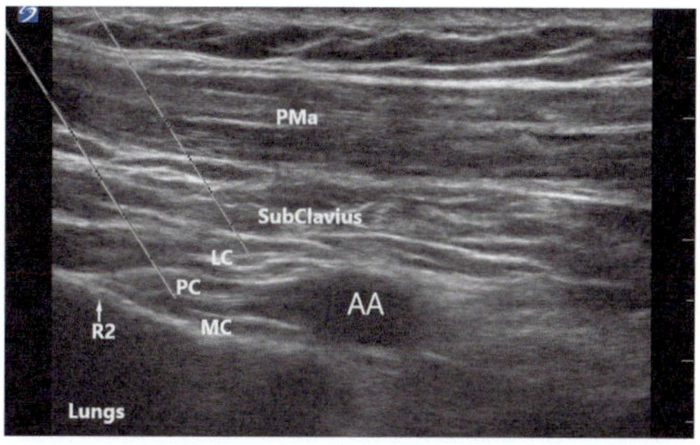

Fig. 5.26 Double injection technique for costoclavicular block under ultrasound. Note the septa separating lateral cord (LC) from posterior cord (PC) and medial cord (MC). *PMa* pectoralis major muscle, *Subclavius* subclavius muscle, *AA* axillary artery, *R2* 2nd rib

The skin is infiltrated with 1–2 2% lidocaine and a 22G short-bevel echogenic needle is advanced in-plane with a lateral to medial approach and positioned in the center of the "cord-cluster." After ruling out intra-epineural position with a 1 ml test dose of 5% dextrose (no cord swelling seen and the 3 cords are pushed apart), a further 10–15 ml of LA is then deposited in 5 ml aliquots with repeated negative aspiration for blood. Monitor the patient throughout for discomfort/pain along the arm and if using a pressure gauge keep the pressure less than 15 psi during injection of LA.

Single vs Double injection—The fascial layers surrounding the plexus may compartmentalize it by forming complete/incomplete septae hindering the spread of LA with single-injection techniques. A. Hadzic and colleagues demonstrated that there exists a linear septum separating the brachial plexus into 2 compartments—a superficial compartment containing the lateral cord and a medial compartment containing the medial and posterior cords. They have advocated using a double injection technique for successful block at this level (Fig. 5.26). This is in keeping with the observation by Morimoto and colleagues who reported the existence of setae posterolateral to the subclavian artery hindering LA spread during infraclavicular brachial plexus block. The initial identification of the septum is a challenge, but it becomes more apparent after the hypoechoic LA starts to fill in the space and the septum prevents its spread to medial and posterior cords. Further advancement of the needle also gives tactile feedback of a "give" sensation and complete LA spread into all quadrants.

Clinical Tips

Tilt the probe (cephalad/caudad) and rotate it gently (clockwise/anti-clockwise) to get the artery in a true cross-section, like a "circle" (beam at right angle to artery).

- Identify the cephalic vein (and its insertion into the subclavian vein) by sliding the probe laterally and avoid injection at this point.
- Keep the subclavius muscle in view during the block (true costoclavicular block) especially for catheter insertions since it helps to anchor the catheter.

Lateral Approach

PNS-Guided (*Peri-Coracoid Approach*) Palpate the coracoid process (after asking patient to shrug his/her shoulder) and mark a point 2 cm inferior and medial to it. Insert a stimulating needle perpendicular to all planes (with no medial angulation) and only in sagittal plane.

USG-Guided (Sub-Coracoid Approach)

The goal of this technique is to avoid pleura, avoid the 2 vessels and achieve a U-shaped spread of local anesthetic under the axillary artery. A high frequency linear array probe is placed under the coracoid process (Figs. 5.27 and 5.28) and the axillary artery identified under the pectoral muscle (usually at a depth of 3–5 cm). Scanning medially and laterally allows the chest wall and pleura to be identified and avoided.

Once the axillary vessels are identified, an attempt is made to reduce the depth and identify the 3 cords around the axillary artery which appear as hyperechoic structures at 10–11 o'clock (lateral cord), 1–2 o'clock (medial cord) and 5–7 o'clock (posterior cord), respectively.

1–2 ml of 2% lidocaine is infiltrated in the skin at the point of injection. A 5 cm 22G short-bevel needle is advanced in-plane from the cephalad end of the probe to pass the pectoral muscles toward the lateral cord. Negative aspiration and injection of 1 ml of local anesthetic under low pressure makes the cord more apparent and pushes it away from the needle tip.

The needle is then gently advanced to 6 o'clock position and placed just under the artery (avoid going too deep). After negative aspiration, injection of 1 ml of local anesthetic should produce a double-bubble appearance from the "artery" and the "local anesthetic" under it. Further injection of local anesthetic results in flattening of the artery from below and spread of local toward the medial cord (located in the groove between the artery and the vein). Toward the end a U-shaped hypoechoic shadow appears *under* the axillary artery from the deposition of local anesthetic.

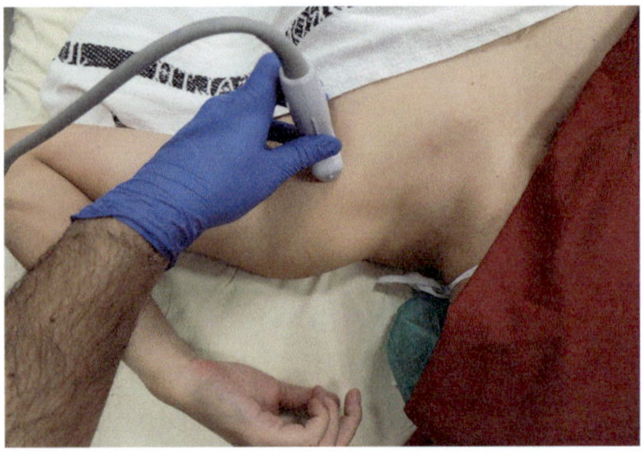

Fig. 5.27 Patient and probe position for sub-coracoid infraclavicular brachial plexus block. Note the parasagittal position of the probe under the coracoid process

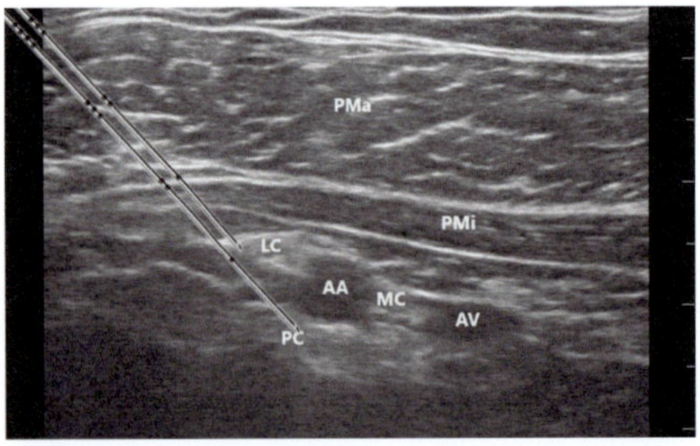

Fig. 5.28 Sub-coracoid block technique. The lateral cord (LC) nearest to the clavicle is targeted first followed by the posterior cord (PC) and the medial cord (MC) is blocked by the spread of local anesthetic from these two. AA = axillary artery and AV = axillary vein

Clinical Tips

- Always locate the ribs and pleura first by scanning medial and lateral.
- Locate the axillary vein by reducing the pressure on the probe since the vein is easily obliterated under pressure. It is vital to locate the vein since it allows identification of the medial cord. Additionally, it can easily be punctured leading to unrecognized/accidental intravascular injection of local anesthetic.
- A "heel-up" maneuver (rocking the probe toward the patients head in a parasagittal plane, depressing the tissues caudad to the probe) makes it easier to visualize the vessels and manipulate the probe.
- Avoid targeting the medial cord unless the spread toward the medial cord is inadequate while depositing local anesthetic under the artery. This can be avoided by not going too deep under the artery while looking for the "double-bubble" sign.

5.3.1.9 Complications

- Most commonly reported is vascular puncture. Axillary vein puncture is more likely in the PNS-guided approach. No significant long-term effects have been reported with accidental vascular puncture here.
- Pneumothorax, though reported, can largely be avoided with an appropriate technique.

- Phrenic nerve palsy has been reported with vertical infraclavicular block.

5.3.1.10 Tips

- The anatomy of the brachial plexus changes along the axillary artery as one moves proximal to lateral.
- Use of ultrasound has made identification of the anatomy and subtle variations easier. This does not necessarily translate into increased success and reduction in complications since ultrasound is user dependent.
- Choosing the best approach to infraclavicular block should depend on right patient selection, thorough anatomical and sono-anatomical knowledge.

5.3.2 Axillary Brachial Plexus Block

The axillary approach to brachial plexus was first demonstrated by William Halsted in 1884 where he injected cocaine under direct vision. Though the first percutaneous approach was performed by **G Hirschel in 1911 it was not until 1959 (after Burnham's publication**) that this approach gained popularity. It has since, become the most used peripheral nerve block for forearm and hand surgery especially due to a lower incidence of complications compared to the more proximal approaches to the brachial plexus. With the advent of USG the more proximal approaches are fast gaining popularity due to increased safety.

5.3.2.1 Anatomical Considerations

The axilla is a pyramid-shaped space inferior to the glenohumeral joint and superior to the axillary fascia with the base of the pyramid on the surface. The apex of the axilla is the cervico-medullary canal bounded by the clavicle, first rib, and upper part of the scapula. The pectoralis major and minor muscles and pectoral and clavipectoral fascia form the anterior wall. The scapular and subscapularis muscle in the upper part and latissimus dorsi and teres major muscles in the inferior part make up the posterior wall. The first four ribs and associated intercostal and serratus anterior muscles comprise the medial wall. The humeral head and neck comprise the lateral wall of the axilla (Fig. 5.29).

Contents of the Axilla The contents of the axilla region include muscles, nerves, vessels, and lymphatics (Fig. 5.30):

- Axillary artery (and branches).
- Axillary vein (and tributaries).
- Brachial plexus (and branches).
- Axillary lymph nodes.
- Biceps brachii (short head) and coracobrachialis.

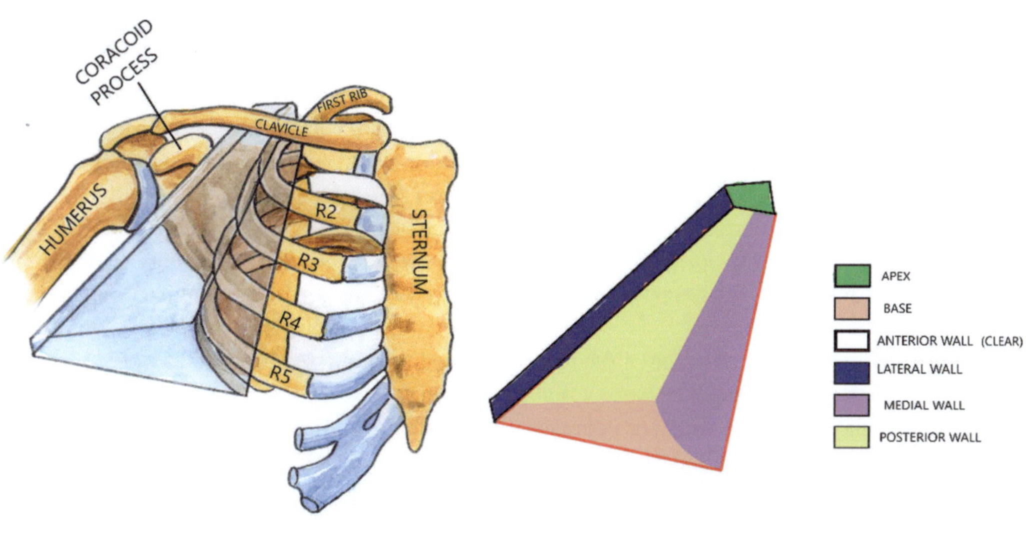

Fig. 5.29 Boundaries of the axilla—Note the pyramidal structure and the walls encompassing the axilla

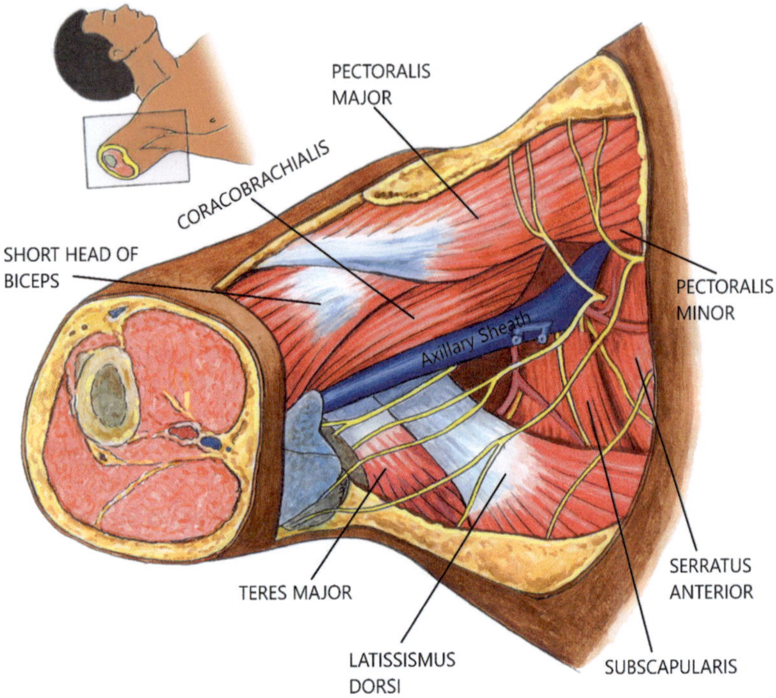

Fig. 5.30 Contents of the axilla. Note the various muscles surrounding the "axillary sheath" containing the neurovascular bundle-brachial plexus, axillary artery, and the axillary vein.

The neurovascular bundle of the axilla is enclosed in a fibrous layer called the **axillary sheath** which encloses the axillary artery and the three cords of the brachial plexus. It is surrounded by the axillary fat. It is an extension of the prevertebral fascia of the deep cervical fascia and is continuous with the carotid sheath at the venous angle.

Brachial Plexus in the Axilla

The brachial plexus supplies the nerve supply to the upper limb and is formed by the ventral rami of the lower four cervical nerves and the first thoracic nerve. It consists of roots, trunks, divisions, and cords. The roots are arranged between the scalenus anterior and medius muscles, and they combine in the posterior triangle to form three trunks: upper, middle, and lower.

On approaching the clavicle, each of the three trunks divides into an anterior and posterior division to supply the flexor and extensor compartments of the arm, respectively. Anterior divisions of the upper and middle trunk unite to form the lateral cord, anterior division of the lower trunk continues as the medial cord, and posterior divisions of all the three trunks assemble to form the posterior cord.

The three cords enter the axilla at the apex and are arranged, according to the names, around the second and third parts of the axillary artery. In relation to the first part of the artery, however, the lateral and posterior cords are lateral, and the medial cord lies posterior to the artery (Fig. 5.31).

At the lateral border of the pectoralis minor muscle, the cords divide into terminal nerves of the brachial plexus: musculocutaneous, median, ulnar, radial, axillary, medial cutaneous nerve of arm (MCNA), and medial cutaneous nerve of forearm (MCNF), which along with the intercostobrachial nerve (ICB) provide the sensory and motor supply to the whole upper extremity (Fig. 5.30). The cords, the terminal branches, and the vessels lie within an incomplete fascial sheath derived from the scalene fascia, which is in turn derived from the prevertebral fascial layer.

At the level of axilla, the median, radial, and ulnar nerves lie within the neurovascular bundle, whereas the median cutaneous nerve of the arm and forearm may lie either inside or outside the sheath. The musculocutaneous nerve always lies

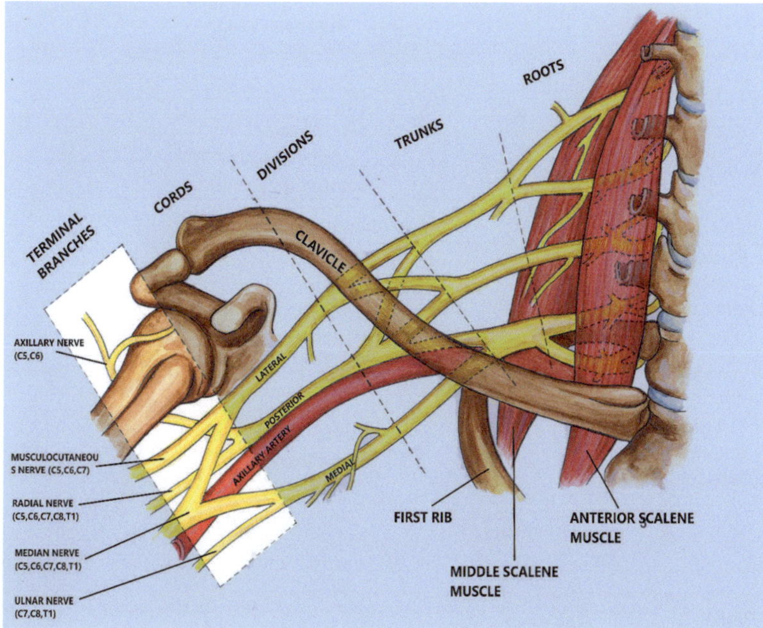

Fig. 5.31 Brachial plexus in the axilla. Note the 3 cords, its terminal branches and their relationship to the axillary artery.

outside the sheath (in the plane between the biceps and coracobrachialis muscle or in the body of coracobrachialis), because it leaves the lateral cord before the cords enter the axilla. Within the fascia, in relation to the axillary artery, the nerves are arranged as follows: (1) median-lateral and anterior, (2) ulnar-medial and anterior, and (3) radial-medial and posterior. The musculocutaneous nerve appears lateral and posterior to the artery.

Surface Anatomy for Axillary Brachial Plexus Block

Pertinent surface anatomy landmark for nerve stimulator-based techniques is the pulse of the axillary artery just distal to the pectoralis major near the anterior axillary wall. Superior to this point, one can identify the coracobrachialis muscle for the associated musculocutaneous nerve block. Cutaneous innervation of the upper extremity is depicted in Fig. 5.32.

Sonoanatomy for Axillary Brachial Plexus Block

Sonoanatomy of the brachial plexus in the axilla readily reveals the axillary artery and the surrounding hypoechoic nerves inside the fascia. With the ultrasound probe placed transversely at the mid to distal axilla: the median nerve may be identified lateral and superficial to the axillary artery, the ulnar nerve is typically medial and superficial to the artery, and the radial nerve location is posterior to the artery (Fig. 5.33). There is, however, variation to the exact nerve location around the artery. The musculocutaneous nerve is usually found within the fascial plane between the biceps and coracobrachialis muscles or piercing the coracobrachialis muscle belly.

5.3.2.2 Indications

1. Surgical anesthesia/analgesia for elbow, forearm, and hand procedures.
2. Cutaneous anesthesia for superficial procedures of the inner arm, for example, brachiobasilic fistula formation.
3. Chronic pain procedures.

5.3.2.3 Contraindications

Refer to Table 5.1

5.3.2.4 Preparation

Refer to Table 5.1 Pre-requisite for block

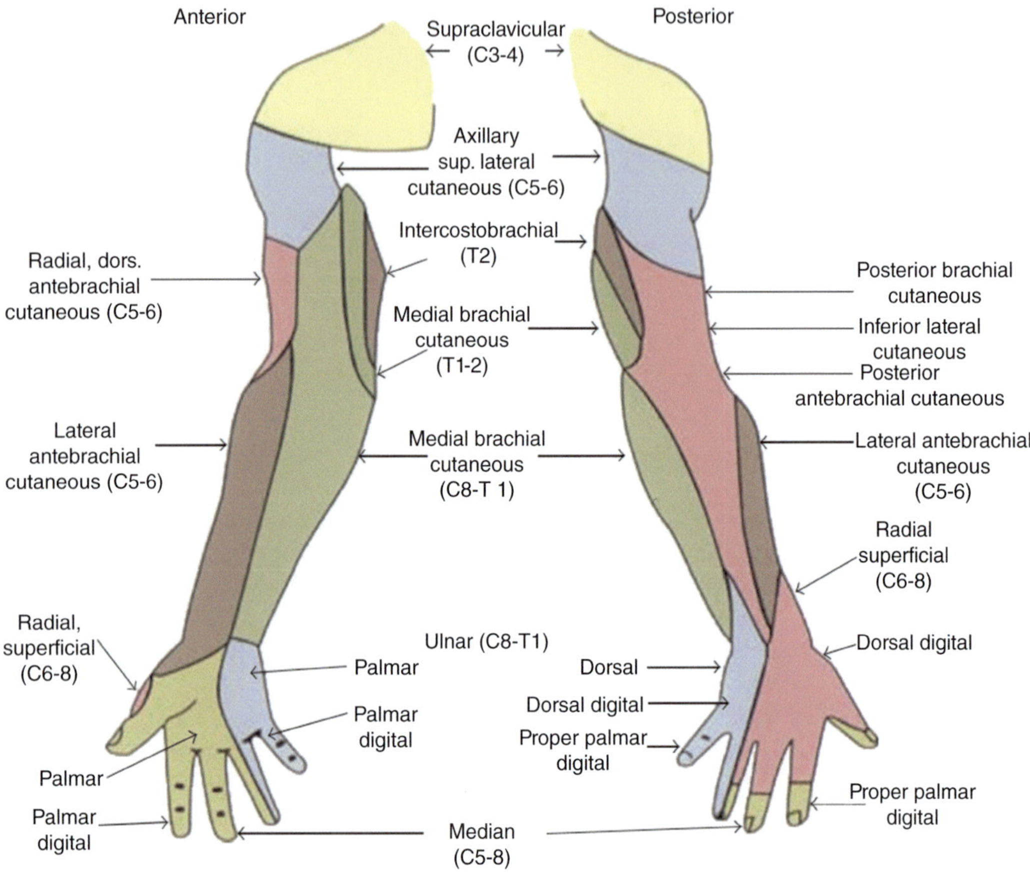

Fig. 5.32 Cutaneous innervation of the upper extremity. Note the significant contributions of the cutaneous branches of the plexus. (Courtesy from Wikimedia Commons, file: Gray's Anatomy 812 and 814.PNG)

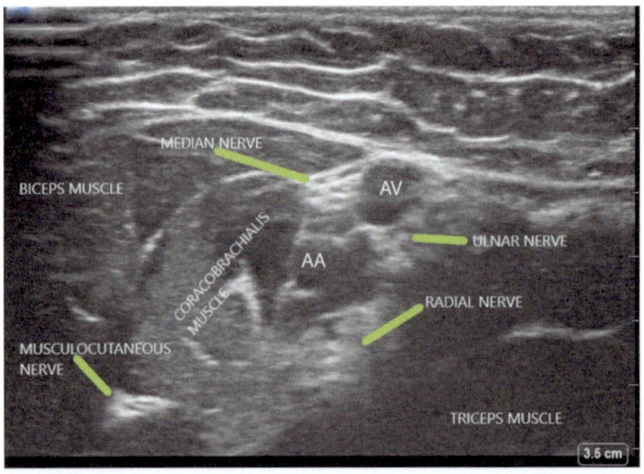

Fig. 5.33 Ultrasound scan of axilla. AA: axillary artery, AV = axillary vein. Note the position of the 4 nerves around the vessels

5.3.2.5 Position

The aim should be to have the injection site and the USG monitor in a single line of sight.

Patient position—For the ease of palpation of the landmarks, needle insertion/manipulation and probe position optimal positioning require arm abduction (at least 90 degrees) to access the axilla. The forearm may be propped comfortably, whether supported horizontally at 90 degrees or above or behind the head.

Operator and USG monitor

The aim should be to have the clinician, the injection site, and the USG monitor in a single line of sight.

Refer to Sect. 5.2.1

5.3.2.6 Drug

20-25 ml of ropivacaine 0.75% or bupivacaine 0.5% can be used.

5.3.2.7 Injection and Approach

There are two approaches commonly practiced:

1. PNS (Peripheral Nerve Stimulator)-guided.
2. USG (Ultrasonography)-guided.

1. **PNS-guided**—A multi-injection technique using a PNS was found to be associated with a higher success rate, as traditional single-injection approaches demonstrated lack of circumferential spread of local anesthetic due to the septate axillary sheath. Knowledge of the arrangement of the nerves around the axillary artery is integral to performing this block. With the arm out in the "anatomical position" the median nerve usually lies superior to the artery, the ulnar nerve inferiorly and the radial nerve posterior to the artery. The musculocutaneous nerve lies outside the sheath and is usually superior and lateral to the artery (Fig. 5.34).

The patient is positioned with the arm abducted to 90 degrees and elbow flexed. The axillary artery is palpated under the anterior axillary fold (pectoralis major muscle) and stabilized with index and middle fingers. With all aseptic precautions, after infiltrating the skin with 1–2 ml of 2% lidocaine the insulated stimulating needle is inserted above the artery for **median** nerve; above and deep for **musculocutaneous** nerve; below the artery for **ulnar** nerve, and behind the artery for **radial** nerve.

Start with an initial current (1–2 mA), pulse duration (0.1 ms), and frequency (2 Hz). The needle is advanced until the desired motor twitch is obtained. Various responses to stimulation are tabulated in Table 5.5. The current is then reduced until motor response disappears. The displayed current on the nerve stimulator is noted. A current between 0.2–0.5 mA is accepted as an ideal threshold current. Below 0.5 has been shown to give a high success rate. Below 0.2 mA may mean that the needle tip is in the nerve and should be withdrawn. Once the nerve has been located satisfactorily, the syringe is aspirated to ensure against intravascular placement. The local anesthetic is then injected in 5 ml increments without moving the needle tip. The motor twitch should disappear as soon as 0.5 ml to 1 ml of local anesthetic is injected. This is thought to be either due to mechanical displacement of the nerve from the needle (Raj test) or due to change in the electrical conductivity around the nerve. Failure of the twitch to disappear, pain on injection or high injection pressures suggests intraneural placement of the needle tip and warrants withdrawing it by 0.5–1 mm.

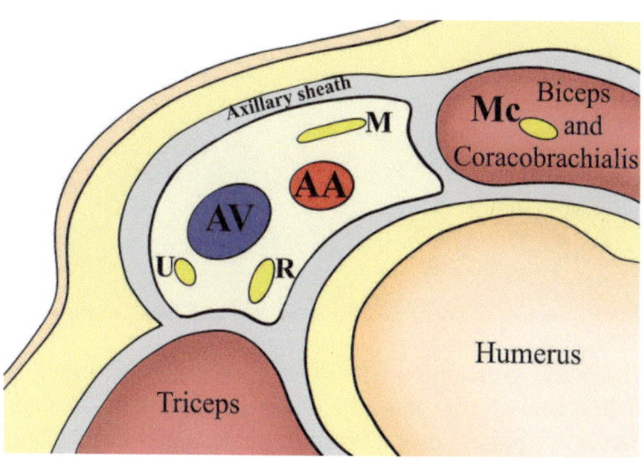

Fig. 5.34 Cross-section anatomy at axilla. Note the position of the 4 terminal nerves, especially the musculocutaneous nerve which is outside the "axillary sheath."

2. **USG-guided**—In 1981, Abramowitz and Cohen first described the use of Doppler USG to identify the axillary artery, thereby aiding the performance of axillary plexus block for upper limb surgery. However, it was the use of

Table 5.5 Response to nerve stimulation at the level of axilla

Motor response	Nerve	Acceptable
Index/middle finger flexion	Median Nerve	Yes
Flexion of the little finger or Adduction of thumb	Ulnar Nerve	Yes
Extension of thumb	Radial Nerve	Yes
Flexion of Elbow	Musculocutaneous Nerve	Yes

B-mode ultrasound in 1989 for axillary block performance that heralded the era of USG-guided peripheral nerve block. Ultrasonographic visualization of target nerve, needle, and local anesthetic injectate spread has been associated with improved block success rates, decreased block onset times, and a decrease in the local anesthetic dose needed for successful nerve block.

The patient is positioned with the arm abducted to 90 degrees and elbow flexed. A high frequency linear transducer (8–14 MHz) is placed in a transverse plane at the lateral border of pectoralis major muscle (Fig. 5.35). The pulsating axillary artery is visualized, and the transducer moved to locate the individual nerves around the artery. Easing the pressure off the transducer usually reveals the position of the axillary vein. The nerves at this level have a honeycomb appearance, but their locations relative to the artery are variable. The **median** nerve usually lies around 9–12 o'clock position, the **ulnar** nerve often in the corresponding 2 o'clock position, and the **radial** nerve at the 5 o'clock position in relation to the artery (Fig. 5.36).

The musculocutaneous nerve usually lies in the plane between the biceps and coracobrachialis muscles or in the body of coracobrachialis and has a flattened appearance with a bright border and hypoechoic core. As we scan up and down the arm, the musculocutaneous nerve appears to glide in the fascial plane, either moving toward the artery as we scan proximally or away from he artery as we scan distally down the arm.

The radial nerve, which lies deeper, below, and medial to the artery is one of the most difficult to visualize with ultrasound. It is important to exclude "post-cystic ultrasonographic enhancement" beneath the artery, with which the radial nerve is most often confused. Various measures have been tried to obviate this clinical problem including the use of a PNS. Injection of local anesthetic in a "horseshoe" pattern underneath the artery, with the needle tip at 5 o'clock position, in our experience, effectively blocks the radial nerve in most cases. A similar "donut" technique has been described by Imasogie et al., where the authors achieved successful block of the median, ulnar, and radial nerves by circumferential deposition of local anesthetic around the axillary artery, instead of targeting them individually.

After positioning of the probe, it is recommended to infiltrate local anesthetic distal to the probe, subcutaneously, to cover the injection site and to block the intercostobrachial nerve.

A short-beveled 5 cm needle can then be inserted either in-plane or out-of-plane relative to the probe, toward the four nerves and each blocked individually. The "in-plane" approach to

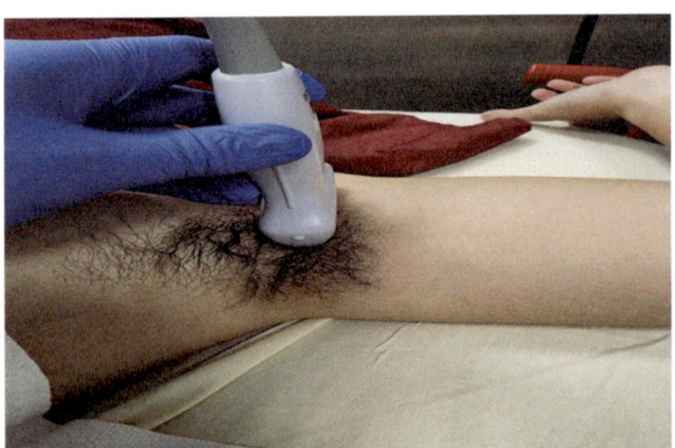

Fig. 5.35 Patient, arm, and probe position for ultrasound-guided in-plane approach for axillary brachial plexus block. An out-of-plane approach has also been described in this probe position

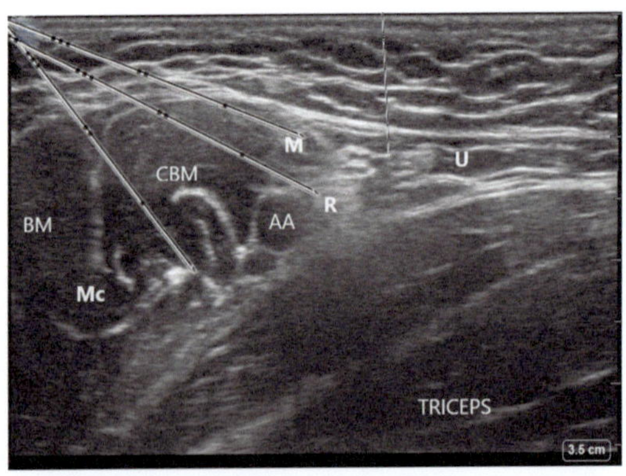

Fig. 5.36 Ultrasound scan of axilla. *AA* axillary artery, *R* radial nerve, *Mc* musculocutaneous nerve, *M* median nerve, *U* ulnar nerve. Both in-plane and out-of-plane approaches can be seen above. This is the same patient as in Fig. 5.33 above but with additional pressure on the probe which has obliterated the axillary vein (AV). *BM* biceps muscle, *CBM* coracobrachialis muscle

axillary block involves the insertion of the needle keeping its entire length in view during the procedure. The "out-of-plane approach," in contrast, involves insertion of the needle along the short axis of the probe, and hydro-location of the needle tip may be necessary to confirm the position of the tip of the needle. In terms of safety, the in-plane approach offers better visualization of the needle tip but the out-of-plane approach has been shown to be more comfortable of the two, for the patient, in some studies. After careful positioning of needle tip, gentle negative aspiration, and an asymptomatic initial 0.5–1 mL perineural injection, further local anesthetic is injected in 2 mL aliquots to surround each nerve.

5.3.2.8 Complications

- The most common complication encountered is accidental intravascular injection of the local anesthetic.
- Intraneural injection of local anesthetic.

5.3.2.9 Tips

- After identification of the AA and the 4 nerves around it, release pressure on the probe and identify the AV [figure above] to prevent accidental intravascular injection of local anesthetic.
- There are usually multiple veins as a normal variation of anatomy and it is important to locate them first before beginning injection. Frequent aspiration of local anesthetic and visible small aliquot injection is the key to avoid injection of local anesthetic into the veins.
- Gentle sliding of the probe proximal and distal to the axilla helps identify the hyperechoic musculocutaneous outside the brachial plexus sheath.
- Identifying the nerves in the mid-humeral region and tracing the nerves up to the axilla might help identify the terminal nerves faster. This is especially true for the radial nerve which stays "hidden" behind the AA under ultrasound.
- Choice of local anesthetic: The choice of local anesthetic is determined by the duration of sensory analgesia desired. Lidocaine 1.5–2% with adrenaline 5 mcg·mL−1 and mepivacaine 1% provide effective nerve blockade for 2.5–3 h and are ideal for shorter duration procedures. For longer-duration procedures, it is possible to achieve sensory blockade for 9 h with ropivacaine 0.5% and 11 h with levobupivacaine 0.33%. When used for surgical anesthesia decreasing the concentration of both local anesthetics further would lengthen the onset of block and increase the risk of inadequate blocks.
- Volume of Local Anesthetic: In the past, it was necessary to use large volumes of local anesthetic to achieve acceptable success rates for peripheral regional anesthetic techniques. Recent studies have shown that volume of local anesthetic can be significantly reduced when axillary blocks are performed under ultrasound guidance.
- The anatomy of the axillary brachial plexus involves three additional cutaneous nerves (ICB, MCNA, and MCNF) with extensive distribution in the arm and forearm, and the use of such low volumes may risk inadequate block in the distribution of these nerves.

5.3.2.10 Cutaneous Nerves in the Axilla

The **medial brachial cutaneous nerve** (MBCN—also known as the medial cutaneous nerve of the arm) arises from the medial cord of the brachial plexus. Originally posterior to the axillary vein, it comes to lie medial to it in the axilla and upper arm. It then passes medial to the brachial artery in the middle arm to pierce the deep fascia to supply sensation of the medial and posterior aspect of the lower arm, reaching the medial epicondyle and the olecranon area. The nerve is also known as the **nerve of Wrisberg** (after Heinrich Wrisberg, who described the anatomy of the nerve).

The **medial antebrachial cutaneous nerve** (also known as the medial/lesser internal cutaneous nerve of the forearm) also arises from the medial cord of the brachial plexus and lies medial to the axillary artery in the axilla. At the lower axilla the nerve gives a small branch which pierces the fascia to supply the skin over the biceps muscle. The main trunk of the nerve then descents medial to the brachial artery to pierce the fascia in the middle part of the arm. The nerve then terminates in a volar branch (supplying the skin of ulnar side of the forearm) and an ulnar branch (supplying the skin on the posterior-ulnar aspect of the forearm).

The **intercostobrachial nerve (ICBN)** is a lateral cutaneous branch of the second intercostal nerve that supplies sensation to the skin of the axilla. It leaves the second intercostal space at the midaxillary line and subsequently pierces the serratus anterior muscle to enter the subcutaneous tissues of the axilla. At times the lateral cutaneous branch of the third intercostal nerve may give rise to a second intercostobrachial nerve. Along with the medial brachial cutaneous nerve, it supplies the skin of the medial arm.

Of the three nerves mentioned above, the MBCN and the ICBN lie together and outside the brachial sheath in the axilla and tend to be spared in Axillary Brachial Plexus Block. As mentioned above, these two nerves together provide sensory innervation to the whole of the medial side of the arm from axilla to the elbow and it is very important to block them for surgery involving this region (e.g. proximal fistuloplasty) and to obtund tourniquet pain. In contrast to these two, the medial antebrachial cutaneous nerve lies between the median and ulnar nerves in the axilla and is usually blocked during an axillary brachial plexus block. This can be specifically targeted beside the basilic vein, at the elbow, under ultrasound guidance.

Ultrasound-guided techniques tend to have a higher success rate than landmark techniques for the two cutaneous nerves. MBCN and ICBN can be located under high-resolution ultrasound guidance above the conjoint tendon, 2–3 cm distal to the axillary vessels in axillary sheath. Even without visualization, infiltration of local anesthetic in this fascial plane above the latissimus dorsi muscle results in good sensory analgesia in the distribution of the nerves.

Axillary nerve block is a safe and effective regional anesthetic technique suitable for a wide variety of procedures, for both inpatient and outpatient care. The axillary approach to the brachial plexus is considered the safest of the four approaches because of reduced risk to surrounding structures such as the risk of phrenic nerve blockade and/or pneumothorax, but the general risks of accidental intravascular and intraneural injection still exist.

5.4 Selective Distal Nerve Blocks of Upper Limb

5.4.1 Introduction

The introduction of ultrasound has transformed the field of regional anesthesia, has improved the efficacy of the nerve blocks of upper limb, making performance of these blocks easier. While the proximal blocks of upper limb like interscalene, supraclavicular, infraclavicular, and axillary approaches to brachial plexus block continue to be preferred for surgeries of the upper limb, ultrasound has made the distal nerve blocks of the upper limb a technically feasible, safer, and efficacious option. With the introduction of complex hand and wrist surgeries there has been need for motor sparing distal nerve blocks. This chapter is dedicated to review the relevant anatomy of the selective nerves of upper limb and the technical pre-requisites while performing the distal blocks of the upper limb.

The upper limb is innervated by eight nerves out of which seven arise directly from the brachial plexus while the eight (the intercostobrachial) is a branch of the second thoracic intercostal nerve (T2). Out of the seven nerves, the four major nerves are median, ulnar, radial and musculocutaneous nerves. Rest three nerves are the medial brachial cutaneous nerve or medial cutaneous nerve of arm, the medial antebrachial cutaneous nerve or medial cutaneous nerve of forearm and the axillary nerve which also arise directly from the brachial plexus. While median, ulnar, and radial nerves provide sensory-motor supply to the forearm and hand, the lateral cutaneous nerve of forearm (a continuation of musculocutaneous nerve), posterior cutaneous nerve of forearm (a branch of radial nerve) along with medial cutaneous nerve of forearm provide sensory supply to the skin of the forearm up to the wrist.

The musculocutaneous nerve and median cutaneous nerve of arm are blocked in the axillary approach to the brachial plexus block and will not be discussed here. The axillary nerve which supplies shoulder joint and upper lateral aspect of arm will also not be discussed here.

The median, ulnar, and radial nerves are the primary targets for selective nerve blocks in the forearm. While landmark and peripheral nerve (PNS) stimulation-based techniques are used widely to block these three main nerves, ultrasound (US) imaging provides reliability in blocking these individual nerves in the distal upper limb. The lateral, medial, and posterior cutaneous nerves of forearm which are purely sensory can also be blocked around the elbow using landmark-based infiltration techniques as well as under ultrasound guidance. There are four different sites in the upper limb where the nerves can be easily blocked under guidance. They are the mid-humeral/above elbow, antecubital, mid forearm and at the level of the wrist. Of these the mid forearm and mid-humeral/above elbow are most common sites for blockade, while blockade at wrist is rarely done.

5.4.2 Indications

- SURGICAL ANESTHESIA/ANALGESIA
  - Hand and wrist surgery (*motor sparing*).
  - Supplementation or rescue of failed/patchy proximal brachial plexus block.
  - Regional anesthesia for minor procedures, dressing and attending to wounds and lacerations of upper limb below elbow in the Emergency unit.
- NON-SURGICAL
  - Forearm fractures
  - Neuralgia
  - Cancer pain
  - Complex regional pain syndrome

5.4.3 Contraindications

- Patient refusal
- Severe coagulopathy
- Local infection
- Allergy to local anesthetics (rare, usually allergy is to the preservative)
- Untreated sepsis
- Compartment syndrome
- Paresthesias, tingling, or weakness of the limb

5.4.4 Advantages

- Lower amount of LA needed when done under US guidance.
- The puncture site is away from critical structures, hence the inadvertent risk of intravascular or pleural puncture, phrenic nerve injury are avoided.
- Proximal muscle functions are well preserved allowing early discharge of patients and greater patient satisfaction. Preservation of motor function is vital while performing complex hand surgeries.
- Suitable for patients where local infiltration is contraindicated like trauma or wound of surgical site.
- Allow better operating conditions without anatomical distortion at the site of surgery.
- Onset time of distal nerve being blocked is shortened, especially when combined with proximal blocks.

5.4.5 Disadvantages

- With sole distal nerve blocks tourniquet pain cannot be prevented in an awake patient.
- May not cover all surgical procedures involving wider surgical areas.
- Patient discomfort is more as there blocks need multiple punctures.
- Anisotropy of distal nerves makes ultrasound scanning of these nerves more challenging.

5.4.6 Relevant Anatomy

5.4.6.1 Median Nerve (C5, C6, C7, C8, and T1)

The median nerve is a mixed sensory-motor nerve which originates from medial and lateral cord of the brachial plexus. It traverses along the anteromedial side of humerus in the upper arm lying lateral to brachial artery and then enters the forearm compartment crossing the artery just above the elbow to lie medial to the brachial artery in the cubital fossa. It initially lies between the biceps brachii and brachialis. It passes between the two heads of pronator teres in the forearm and then it traverses further between flexor digitorum superficialis and flexor digitorum profundus before entering the carpel tunnel deep to flexor retinaculum at the wrist. The anterior interosseous nerve branches from the median nerve distal to the elbow. Figure 5.37 is a schematic illustration of the course and branches of the median nerve.

5.4.6.2 Ulnar Nerve (C8, T1)

The ulnar nerve is a mixed sensory-motor nerve which originates from medial cord having C8 T1 roots of brachial plexus. It traverses the posteromedial side of humerus and enters the forearm compartment through the cubital tunnel formed by medial epicondyle of humerus and olecranon. It emerges in forearm between two heads of flexor carpi ulnaris and lies medial to ulnar artery, initially separated away from the artery in upper third of forearm, then in the distal forearm the nerve traverses along with the artery deep to the flexor carpi ulnaris tendon to enter the palm superficial to flexor retinaculum through the ulnar tunnel. This relationship with ulnar artery is useful for identifying the nerve. The ulnar nerve gives dorsal and palmar cutaneous branches before entering the palm. Figure 5.38 is a schematic illustration of the course and branches of the ulnar nerve.

5.4.6.3 Radial Nerve (C5, C6, C7, C8, and T1)

The radial nerve is a mixed sensory-motor nerve which originates from posterior cord of the brachial plexus (along with axillary nerve). It traverses posteriorly in the spiral groove of humerus deep to the triceps in the upper arm and enters the forearm compartment anterior to lateral epicondyle. It lies in the fascia between brachialis and brachioradialis laterally above the elbow. It then divides into superficial sensory and deep motor branch at the elbow. The deep branch continues as the posterior interosseous nerve. Figure 5.39 is a schematic illustration of the course and branches of the radial nerve.

5.4.6.4 The Lateral Antebrachial Cutaneous Nerve (LACN) or Lateral Cutaneous Nerve of Forearm (C5, C6, C7)

The lateral cutaneous nerve of forearm is a continuation of the musculocutaneous nerve in the forearm and originates between the coraco-

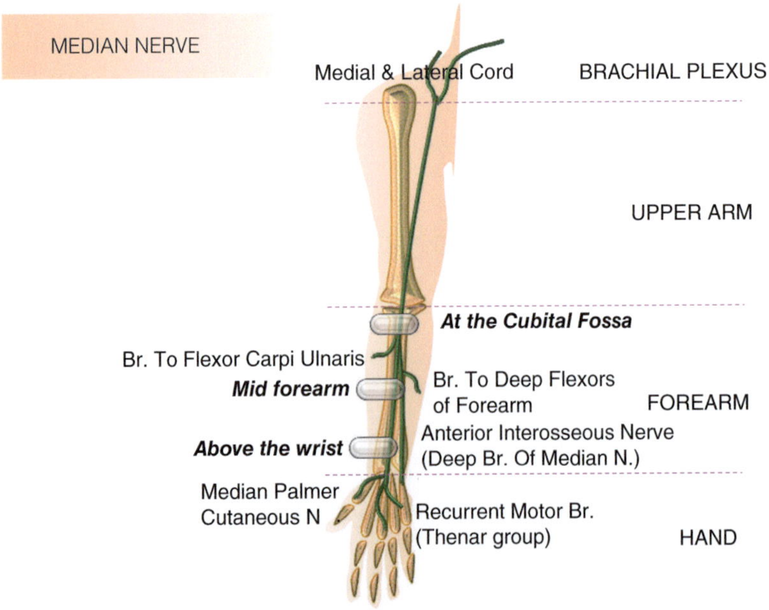

Fig. 5.37 Schematic illustration of the course and branches of median nerve. Also shown in the diagram are the levels for US-guided median nerve blockade

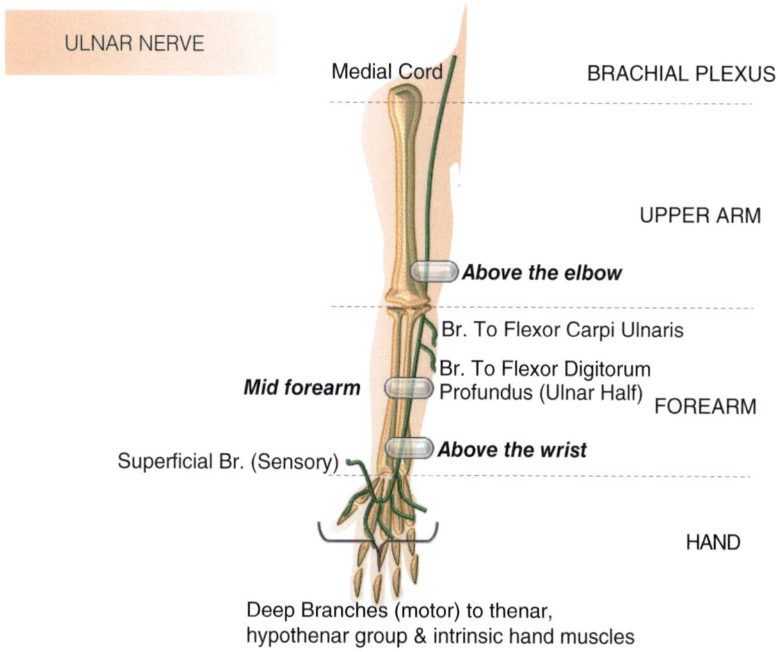

Fig. 5.38 Schematic illustration of the course and branches of ulnar nerve. Also shown in the diagram are the levels for US-guided ulnar nerve blockade

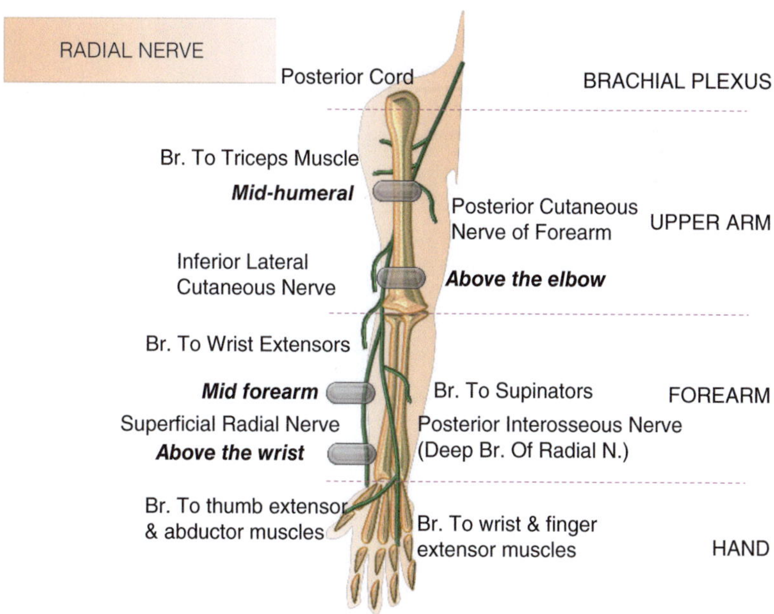

Fig. 5.39 Schematic illustration of the course and branches of radial nerve. Also shown in the diagram are the levels for US-guided radial nerve blockade

brachialis, biceps, and brachialis muscles. It then ascends to lie subcutaneously along the lateral border of biceps brachii tendon and continues on the lateral aspect of the forearm running parallel and volar to the cephalic vein (Fig. 5.40).

5.4.6.5 The Medial Antebrachial Cutaneous Nerve (MACN) or Medial Cutaneous Nerve of Forearm (C8, T1)

The medial cutaneous nerve of forearm is a direct branch from the medial cord of brachial plexus. It lies medial to axillary artery at its origin, and it then runs along the medial aspect of upper arm. It lies medial to the brachial artery at mid-humeral level deep within the brachial fascia (Fig. 5.41). At mid arm level (Fig. 5.42) it pierces the fascia along with the basilic vein and divides into anterior and posterior branches which run along the anteromedial and posteromedial aspect in the forearm, respectively.

5.4.6.6 The Posterior Antebrachial Cutaneous Nerve (PACN) or Posterior Cutaneous Nerve of Forearm (C5, C6, C7, C8)

The posterior cutaneous nerve of forearm is a branch of radial nerve arising just at the level of spiral groove of humerus proximal to elbow joint (Fig. 5.43). The nerve ascends up in the fascial plane to reach the subcutaneous plane between triceps and brachioradialis and gives an upper branch which runs in the lateral aspect of lower arm while the lower branch continues in the posterior aspect of forearm.

5.4.7 Area of Distribution

Median nerve supplies the anterolateral aspect of hand and includes thumb, index. and middle finger.

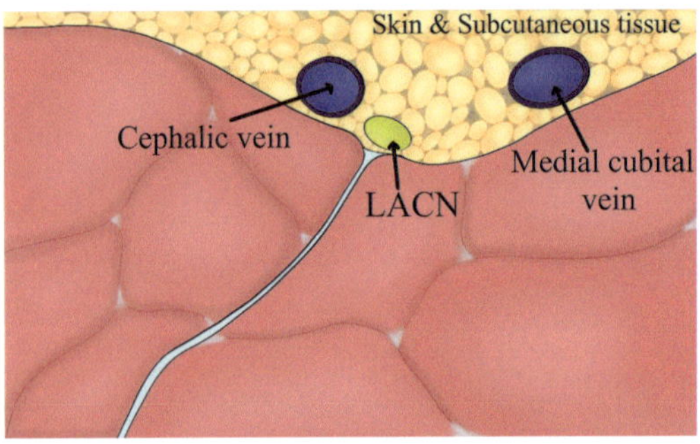

Fig. 5.40 Schematic illustration of transverse section of the arm at the mid forearm level. LACN runs subcutaneously parallel to the cephalic vein

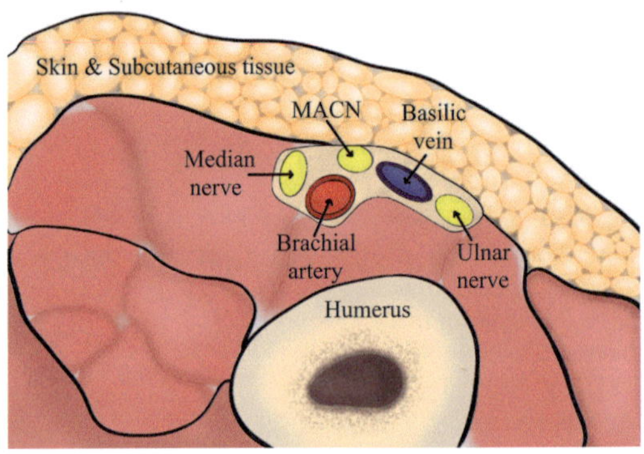

Fig. 5.41 Schematic illustration of transverse section of the arm at the mid-humeral level. MACN is in close proximity to the brachial artery and basilic vein.

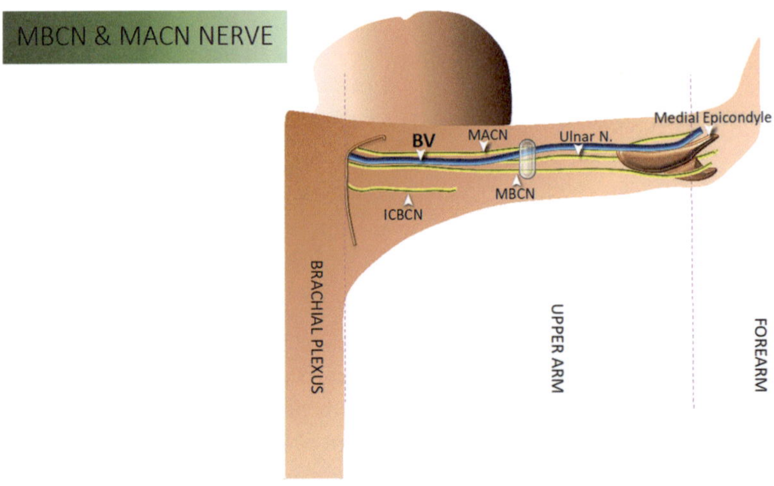

Fig. 5.42 Schematic illustration of the course of MBCN & MACN. Also shown in the diagram is the level for US-guided MACN blockade

Ulnar nerve provides sensory supply to the medial aspect of hand and includes the fifth digit and the medial half of the fourth digit.

Radial nerve supplies sensation to dorsolateral side of hand including thumb, index, middle, and lateral half of ring finger up to distal interphalangeal joint.

The lateral cutaneous nerve of forearm provides sensory innervation to the lateral aspect of the forearm up to the wrist and occasionally up to the base of the thumb. The medial cutaneous nerve of forearm provides innervation to the skin over the biceps brachii muscle in upper arm up to elbow and the skin over the medial side of forearm (both anteromedial and posteromedial aspect) up to the wrist.

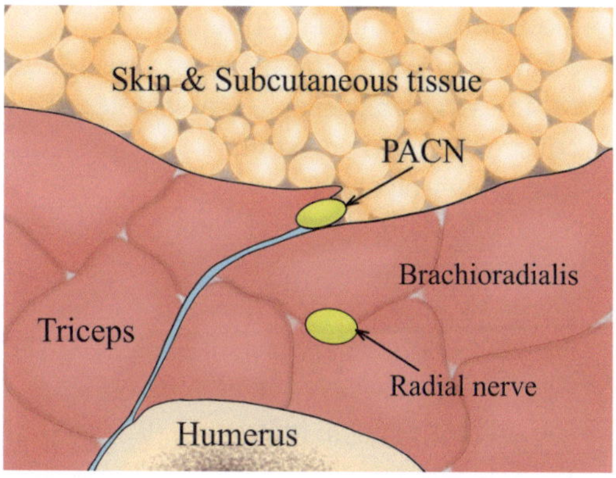

Fig. 5.43 Schematic illustration of the transverse section of arm below spiral groove of humerus, PACN.

The posterior cutaneous nerve of forearm supplies the skin on the posterior aspect of forearm up to the wrist. An upper branch supplies skin on the lateral aspect of lower arm. Figure 5.44 is a schematic illustration of the area of distribution of the individual nerves innervating the upper limb.

5.4.8 Peripheral Nerve Stimulation-Guided Nerve Block

5.4.8.1 Preparation and Technique

The landmark and PNS-guided techniques for median, ulnar, and radial nerves are described below. The blocks for medial, lateral, and posterior cutaneous nerves of forearm are described separately in the ultrasound section later in the chapter.

5.4.8.2 Patient Position

The patient lies supine with arm abducted to 90° and elbow extended for median and radial n., while it is flexed to 90° for ulnar n.

5.4.8.3 Anatomical Landmarks

The important landmarks to note are the elbow crease, biceps brachii, and brachioradialis for

Fig. 5.44 Schematic illustration of the area of distribution of the individual nerves innervating the upper limb. (B Cut—Brachial cutaneous, AB cut—Antebrachial cutaneous)

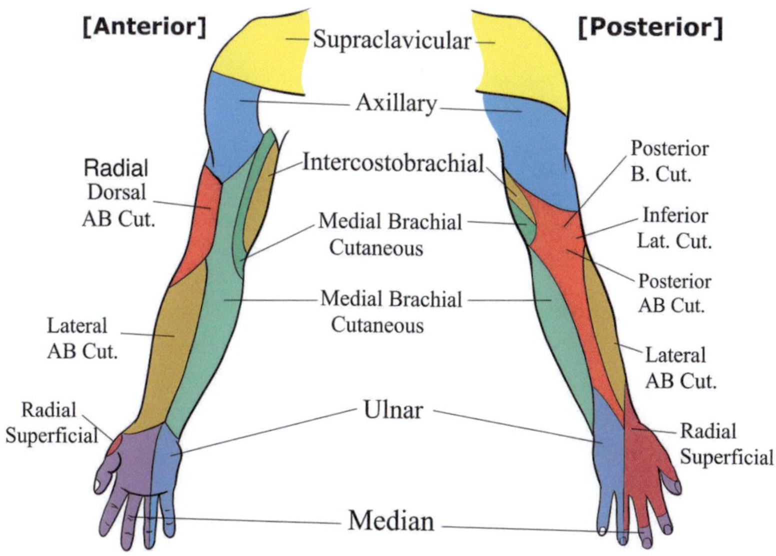

radial n., pulsation of brachial artery for median n., and medial epicondyle and ulnar styloid process for ulnar n.

5.4.8.4 Point of Entry (POE)

Median Nerve—below the elbow crease, medial to brachial artery.

Ulnar Nerve—junction of proximal 1/3rd and distal 2/3rd of line joining medial epicondyle of humerus and ulnar styloid process. Alternatively ulnar nerve may be blocked 1–2 cm proximal to the ulnar sulcus (between medial epicondyle of humerus & olecranon process).

Radial Nerve—below the elbow crease, between brachioradialis and biceps. Alternatively radial nerve may be blocked 2 cm proximal to elbow crease, between brachioradialis & biceps.

5.4.8.5 Needle Entry

The needle is always kept perpendicular to the skin in PNS technique, and the depth of injection varies from 0.5–2 cm for below elbow motor nerve blocks.

5.4.8.6 Evoked Motor Response (EMR)

Median Nerve—Flexion of fingers and wrist.

Ulnar Nerve—Thumb adduction, flexion of 5th finger, ulnar deviation of wrist.

Radial Nerve—Wrist and finger extension.

5.4.8.7 Dosages

It is suggested that 5–8 ml of local anesthetic (LA) drug is appropriate for each nerve. The concentration varies from 1–2% for lignocaine, 0.25–0.5% for bupivacaine, and 0.2–0.5% for ropivacaine.

5.4.9 Ultrasound-Guided Selective Distal Nerve Block

5.4.9.1 Salient Features

- These block techniques result in individual nerve specific block
- They are easy to learn and safer than proximal blocks above the clavicle (less risk of neural injury and intravascular injection)
- Ultrasound guidance aids in blocking the nerves at any level proximal to wrist and not limiting to wrist only
- They can be performed either as single nerve or multiple nerve injection
- The duration of anesthesia is 3–4 h, while analgesia lasts for 8–18 h when using 0.25–0.5% bupivacaine
- Lower doses required in these blocks permit feasibility for multiple blocks at different sites, peripheral nerves blocks of both limbs or doing repeat blocks without exceeding safe dose of LA

5.4.9.2 Equipment

- A high-resolution ultrasound machine with availability of color flow Doppler.
- High frequency linear array transducer (8–15 MHz frequency) with sterile probe cover or Tegaderm dressing.
- Sterile ultrasound gel.
- 5 cm 22G short-bevel and blunt nerve blocking echogenic needles.
- Sterile skin preparation (povidone iodine or 2% chlorhexidine) for cleaning injection site thoroughly.
- LA solution for skin infiltration (0.5–1 ml of 1–2% lignocaine)
- LA solution for nerve block (bupivacaine 0.25–0.5% or ropivacaine 0.2–0.5%) to partially surround the nerve (3–5 ml per nerve).
- IV sedation (midazolam 1–2 mg) & opioid analgesia (fentanyl 25–50 μg) for awake patient.

5.4.9.3 Preparation and Ergonomics

- Patient position: supine (sitting is also an alternative way) with arm of side to be blocked being abducted, supinated, and elbow extended on an OT table. For radial block above elbow the arm of the side to be blocked is adducted, pronated, and hand rested on the abdomen.
- Examiner standing/sitting on same side of limb to be blocked, while ultrasound screen placed straight in front of him on the other side of the patient; thus, maintaining an in-line orientation between performer, puncture site, and ultrasound screen.

- Depth of screen set at 2–5 cm.
- Probe placed transversely at elbow or forearm to visualize cross-section of nerve (short axis of nerve).

5.4.9.4 Sonoanatomy, Scanning, Probe Position, and Needling Techniques

Each individual nerve can be scanned just distal to the elbow and traced downwards or alternately by placing probe proximal to the wrist and then traced back proximally up to mid forearm or above. Fanning or tilting the probe can help visualize the nerve better. This technique counteracts anisotropy and thus helps differentiate the nerve from tendons and ligaments.

Median Nerve

(i) At the mid forearm level (Fig. 5.45): The median nerve is best blocked at the mid forearm where it lies consistently between the flexor digitorum superficialis and the flexor digitorum profundus. The patient lies supine with forearm supinated and elbow extended, and the probe is placed transversely directly over the ventral aspect of forearm. The probe may need to be tilted back and forth to overcome anisotropy and obtain the best sono-Figure of the median nerve. The needle is inserted in-plane from radial side of the probe or out of plane directing the needle tip tangentially to the nerve till the needle tip lies within the fascial sheath containing the nerve and then 5–8 ml of LA is injected to encircle the nerve.

(ii) Distal one third of forearm proximal to the wrist (Fig. 5.46): We can also block the nerve further distally by placing probe transversely at the carpel tunnel proximal to the wrist. The nerve is viewed in axial section and appears hyperechoic and round or elliptical similar to tendons. The nerve is then traced a little proximally where the tendons just change to muscle belly while the median nerve continues looking hyperechoic. This position is particularly preferred for motor sparing blockade for hand surgery.

(iii) At the elbow (Fig. 5.47): Alternatively, we can block the nerve higher up at the elbow by placing the probe transversely at the elbow crease where the nerve lies just medial to the brachial artery. Care must be taken not to puncture the artery while needling.

Ulnar Nerve

(i) At the mid forearm level (Fig. 5.48): After blocking the median nerve, ulnar nerve may be blocked at mid forearm closer to the wrist without any repositioning of the forearm in supination. We begin by palpating the ulnar artery proximal to wrist. Then we place the probe transversely over the artery. Ulnar nerve lies medial to the artery. The probe is now traced back proximally and the nerve can be seen distancing away from the artery as the probe is moved proximally. The nerve appearing as oval hyperechoic structure

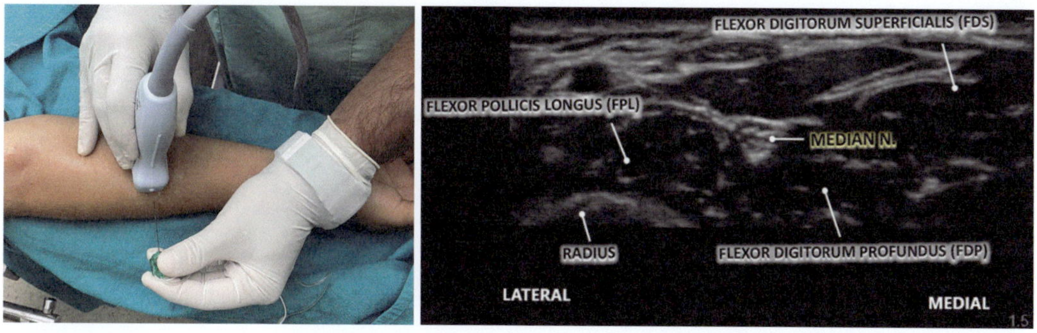

Fig. 5.45 Probe position and USG image of median nerve block at mid forearm level

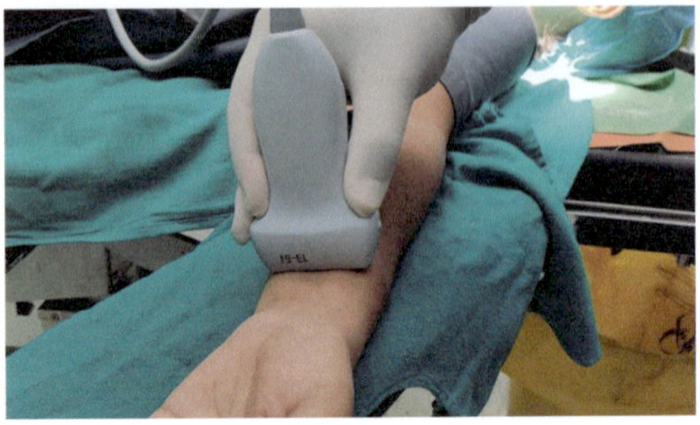

Fig. 5.46 Median nerve block at wrist

(sandwiched between the flexor carpi ulnaris above and flexor digitorum profundus below) can now be safely blocked away from the artery using in-plane or out-of-plane technique with needle tip placed tangentially to the nerve within the fascial sheath with a 5–8 ml of LA injected to circumscribe the nerve. Blocking the nerve at forearm is especially suited for hand surgeries.

(ii) At the mid-humeral level: Alternatively, ulnar nerve can also be blocked at mid-

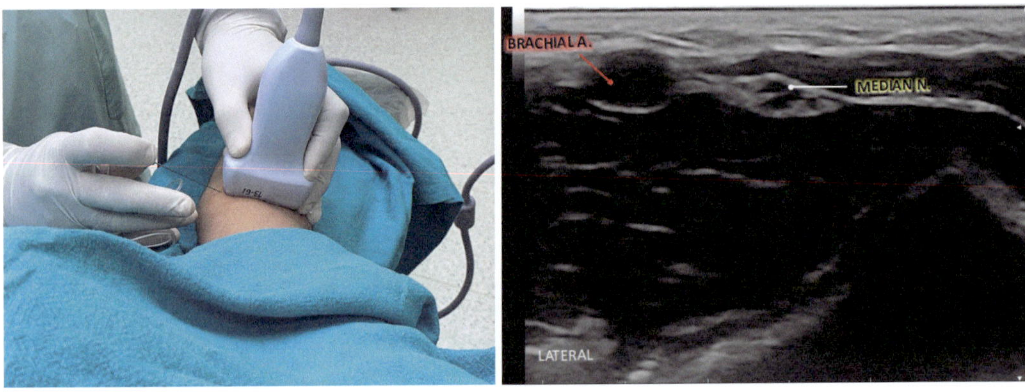

Fig. 5.47 Probe position and USG image of median nerve block at the elbow level

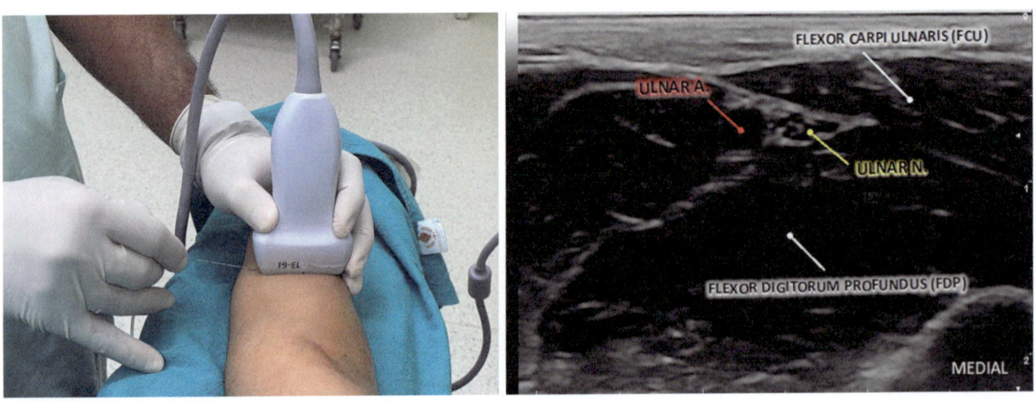

Fig. 5.48 Probe position and USG image of ulnar nerve block at the mid forearm level

humeral level superficial and medial to brachial artery. This is preferred technique in procedures of forearm as it blocks forearm muscles as well.

A note of caution is that ulnar nerve should never be blocked in the elbow where the nerve lies between olecranon and medial epicondyle as it may lead to ischemia and nerve damage.

Radial Nerve

Radial nerve is the most challenging nerve to block among the three. Two techniques have been described for radial nerve blockade.

(i) Above the elbow just distal to spiral groove (Fig. 5.49): The first technique which is preferred involves scanning the nerve 3–4 cm above the elbow. The patient lies supine, his arm adducted and internally rotated with the hand placed over the chest. The probe is placed transversely and postero-laterally at mid-humeral level above the elbow and slid proximal to distal so as to identify the nerve emerging from the spiral groove of the humerus. The nerve is visible as a triangular hyperechoic structure with a characteristic honey combing. The probe is slid distally and anteromedially to identify the radial nerve lying between brachialis and brachioradialis. The advantage of this technique is that the nerve is undivided and appears larger and is easily visible. The needle can now be inserted in-plane (from lateral or medial side) or out-of-plane and LA injected in the fascial sheath to encircle the nerve.

(ii) Below the elbow: In the second technique the radial artery is first palpated proximal to wrist and probe placed over the artery to find the radial nerve lateral to artery. Here patient lies supine, arm kept straight in supination with extension at the elbow. Then the nerve is traced proximally and blocked below the elbow (Fig. 5.50). This technique blocks

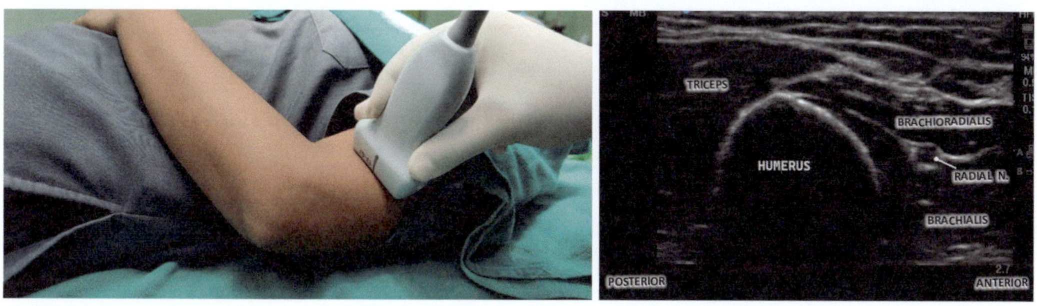

Fig. 5.49 Probe position and USG of radial nerve block above the elbow

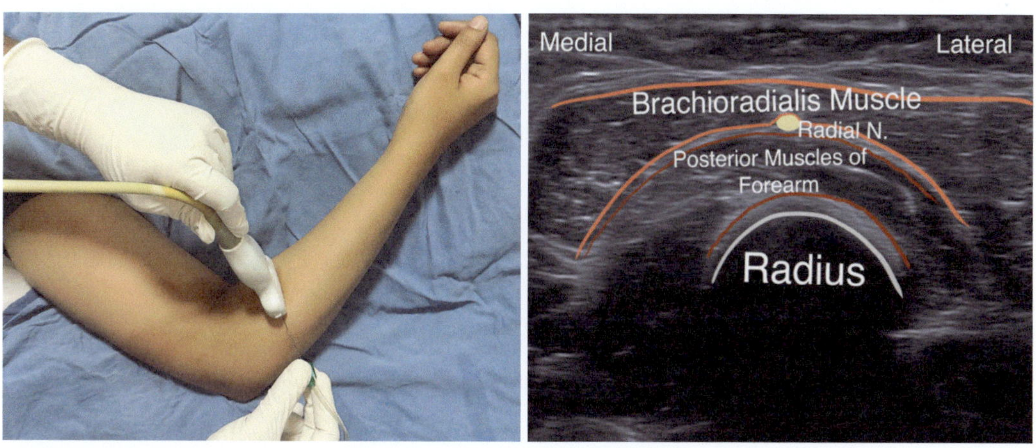

Fig. 5.50 Probe position and USG of radial nerve block below the elbow (upper third of forearm)

only the superficial radial nerve while sparing the deep branch as well as posterior interosseous nerve. This technique is difficult and less popular. It is done only when sparing of the extensor group of forearm muscles is needed.

Medial, Lateral, and Posterior Cutaneous Nerves of Forearm

These nerves are very superficial and can be blocked by landmark-based infiltration technique. Ultrasound guidance may be utilized for identifying relevant anatomical structures in their vicinity. It may be noted that ulnar or median nerves do not supply any structures proximal to the wrist in the forearm and hence blockade of these cutaneous nerves is important for any incisions proximal to the wrist crease.

(i) The medial antebrachial cutaneous nerve or the medial cutaneous nerve of forearm
  - Landmark technique: MACN is blocked by subcutaneous LA infiltration between head of pronator teres and biceps tendon above the elbow.
  - US-guided: MACN can be blocked with ultrasound guidance using a linear probe placed transversely at mid-humeral level. The patient lies supine, arm abducted 90° and externally rotated, elbow flexed while the hand is placed beside the head. The nerve can be visualized as a hyperechoic oval structure lying superficially lateral to the basilic vein. The other structures visualized are the brachial artery, median and ulnar nerves. A 23–25 G hypodermic needle introduced in-plane in lateral to medial direction and 2–3 ml of LA is deposited in the fascial plane next to basilic vein after negative aspiration.

(ii) The lateral antebrachial cutaneous nerve or the lateral cutaneous nerve of forearm
  - Landmark technique: LACN is blocked by subcutaneous LA infiltration between brachioradialis and biceps tendon above the elbow.
  - US-guided: LACN can be blocked with ultrasound guidance using a linear probe placed transversely proximal to the elbow to identify the biceps tendon. The nerve can be visualized as a hyperechoic structure lying lateral to the tendon which becomes subcutaneous upon sliding the probe distally to lie medial to the cephalic vein. A 23–25 G hypodermic needle introduced in-plane in lateral to medial direction and 2–3 ml of LA is deposited in the fascial plane next to cephalic vein after negative aspiration.

(iii) The posterior antebrachial cutaneous nerve or the posterior cutaneous nerve of forearm
  - Landmark technique: PACN can be blocked by SC infiltration of LA drug deposited between lateral epicondyle of humerus and olecranon.
  - US-guided (Fig. 5.51): PACN can be blocked with ultrasound guidance at mid-humeral level along with the radial nerve as it emerges from the spiral groove. The patient lies supine, arm adducted and internally rotated, elbow flexed while the hand is placed on the chest. A linear probe is placed transversely over the spiral groove to identify the triceps, brachioradialis muscles, and the radial nerve. Upon sliding the probe distally, the PACN can be visualized as a small hyperechoic structure lying subcu-

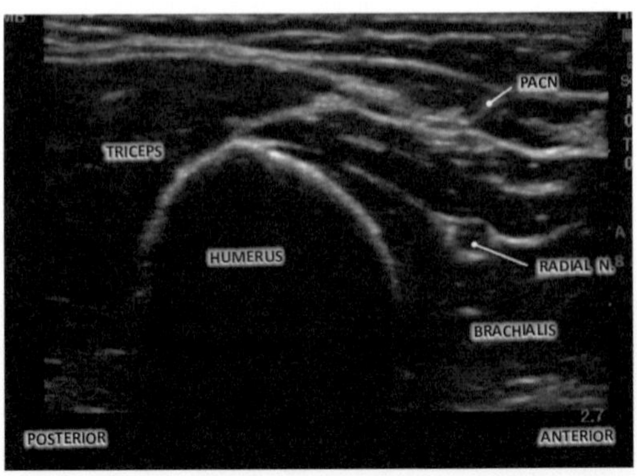

Fig. 5.51 PACN block above the elbow (just below spiral groove)

taneously between the two muscles. A 23–25 G hypodermic needle is introduced in-plane in anterior to posterior direction and 2–3 ml of LA is deposited in the subcutaneous plane next to the PACN.

5.4.9.5 Complications

Ultrasound guidance provides utmost safety while performing these blocks. But block failure and vascular puncture are possible in rare occasions.

5.4.9.6 Summary

- **Position of patient**: supine
- **Mode of anesthesia**: can be performed in awake or anesthetized patients
- **Type of probe and orientation:** linear (8–15 MHz) and in transverse orientation
- **Needle:** 22G, 5 cm echogenic needle with blunt tip
- **Direction of needle:** in-plane technique is recommended; out-of-plane may be used
- **Progression of the needle**: monitored using continuous direct visualization of needle tip (double echo), tissue traction, jiggling, see-saw movement and hydro-localization
- **Nerve stimulation**: usually not needed
- **Drug & dose:** LA (lignocaine 1.5–2%, bupivacaine 0.25–0.5% or ropivacaine 0.2–0.5%), 5–8 ml per nerve (partially surround the nerve)

5.4.9.7 Clinical Tips

- Use blunt, echogenic needles with depth markings.
- Injected LA slowly in small aliquots (avoid forceful injection at high pressure).
- Aspirate for blood before injection of LA solution.
- Knowing your needle tip location at all times is essential.
- Hydro-location with non-active fluid should be used for confirming needle tip position.
- Ulnar nerve should never be blocked at the elbow.
- Radial nerve is best blocked just above the elbow where it is undivided.

Further Reading

Abell DJ, Barrington MJ. Pneumothorax after ultrasound-guided supraclavicular block: presenting features, risk, and related training. Reg Anesth Pain Med. 2014;39(2):164–7.

Blanco R, Gómez BM, González JM. Ultrasound appearance of the cutaneous nerves of the upper limb: a novel description in pain management. J Pain Relief. 2012;1:e109.

Chiavaras MM, Jacobson JA, Billone L, Lawton JM, Lawton J. Sonography of the lateral antebrachial cutaneous nerve with magnetic resonance imaging and anatomic correlation. J Ultrasound Med. 2014;33:1475–83.

Dufeu N, Marchand-Maillet F, Atchabahian A, et al. Efficacy and safety of ultrasound-guided distal blocks for analgesia without motor block after ambulatory hand surgery. J Hand Surg Am. 2014;39:737–43.

Fredrickson MJ, Ting FS, Chinchanwala S, Boland MR. Concomitant infraclavicular plus distal median, radial, and ulnar nerve blockade accelerates upper extremity anaesthesia and improves block consistency compared with infraclavicular block alone. Br J Anaesth. 2011;107:236–42.

Fritsch G, Hudelmaier M, Danninger T, Brummett C, Bock M, McCoy M. Bilateral loss of neural function after interscalene plexus blockade may be caused by epidural spread of local anesthetics: a cadaveric study. Reg Anesth Pain Med. 2013;38(1):64–8.

Fugelli CG, Westlye ET, Ersdal H, Strand K, Bjørshol C. Combined interscalene brachial plexus and superficial cervical plexus nerve block for midshaft clavicle surgery: a case series. AANA J. 2019;87:374–8.

Gadsden JC, Choi JJ, Lin E, Robinson A. Opening injection pressure consistently detects needle-nerve contact during ultrasound-guided interscalene brachial plexus block. Anesthesiology. 2014;120(5):1246–53.

Hansen JT, Netter FH. Netter's Atlas of human anatomy. 6th ed. Philadelphia: Sanders Elsevier; 2014.

Jankovic D, Peng P. Regional nerve blocks in anesthesia and pain therapy: traditional and ultrasound techniques. 4th ed. Cham: Springer; 2015.

Johnson RL, Kopp SL, Kessler J, Gray AT. Miller's Anesthesia, 2-Volume Set, 9th Edition. Philadelphia, PA: Elsevier; 2020. Peripheral nerve blocks and ultrasound guidance for regional anesthesia;1460–61.

Kessler J, Marhofer P, Hopkins PM, Hollmann MW. Peripheral regional anaesthesia and outcome: lessons learned from the last 10 years. Br J Anaesth. 2015;114(5):728–45.

Li JW, Songthamwat B, Samy W, et al. Ultrasound-guided costoclavicular brachial plexus block: sonoanatomy, technique and block dynamics. Reg Anaesth Pain Med. 2017;42:233.

Lin E, Choi J, Hadzic A. Peripheral nerve blocks for outpatient surgery: evidence-based indications. Curr Opin Anaesthesiol. 2013;26:467–74.

Magazzeni P, Jochum D, Iohom G, Mekler G, Albuisson E, Bouaziz H. Reg Anaesth Pain Med. 2018;43:832–7.

Moritz T, Prosch H, Pivec CH, et al. High-resolution ultrasound visualization of the subcutaneous nerves of the forearm: a feasibility study in anatomic specimens. Muscle Nerve. 2014a;49:676–9.

Moritz T, Prosch H, Pivec CH, Sachs A, Pretterklieber ML, Kriechbaumer L, et al. High-resolution ultrasound visualization of the subcutaneous nerves of the forearm: a feasibility study in anatomic specimens. Muscle Nerve. 2014b;49:676–9.

Munirama S, McLeod G. A systematic review and meta-analysis of ultrasound versus electrical stimulation for peripheral nerve location and blockade. Anaesthesia. 2015 Sep;70(9):1084–91.

Olofsson M, Taffé P, Kirkham KR, Vauclair F, Morin B, Albrecht E. Interscalene brachial plexus block for surgical repair of clavicle fracture: a matched case-controlled study. BMC Anesthesiol. 2020;20:91.

Sala-Blanch X, Reina MA, Pangthipampai P, Karmakar MK. Anatomic basis for brachial plexus block at the costoclavicular space: a cadaver anatomic study. Reg Anaesth Pain Med. 2016;41:387.

Salviz EA, Xu D, Frulla A, Kwofi e K, Shastri U, Chen J, et al. Continuous interscalene block in patients having outpatient rotator cuff repair surgery: a prospective randomized trial. Anesth Analg. 2013;117(6):1485–92.

Satapathy AR, Coventry DM. Axillary brachial plexus block. Anaesthesiol Res Pract. 2011:173796.

Siegenthaler A, Mlekusch S, Schliessbach J, Curatolo M, Eichenberger U. Ultrasound imaging to estimate risk of esophageal and vascular puncture after conventional stellate ganglion block. Reg Anesth Pain Med. 2012;37:224–7.

Standring S, editor. 41st ed. London: Elsevier; 2016. Shoulder girdle and arm. Gray's anatomy: the anatomical basis of clinical practice; pp. 832–33.

Takayuki Y, Yoshiko W, Kenta F. Proximal approach for ultrasound-guided infraclavicular brachial plexus block. Acta Anaesthesiol Taiwan. 2016;54:31–2.

Thallaj A, Marhofer P, Kettner SC, Al-Majed M, Al-Ahaideb A, Moriggl B. High-resolution ultrasound accurately identifies the medial antebrachial cutaneous nerve at the midarm level: a clinical anatomic study. Reg Anesth Pain Med. 2011;36:499–501.

Tsui BC, Lou L. Learning the 'traceback' approach for interscalene block. Anaesthesia. 2014;69(1):83–5.

Varela V, et al. Reg Anesth Pain Med. 2019;44:929–33.

Wongkerdsook W, Agthong S, Amarase C, Yotnuengnit P, Huanmanop T, Chentanez V. Anatomy of the lateral antebrachial cutaneous nerve in relation to the lateral epicondyle and cephalic vein. Clin Anat. 2011;24:56–61.

Approach and Troubleshooting to Thoracic Blocks

6

Payal Jain, Rajnish Kumar,
and Mukesh Kumar Prasad

Abstract

Peripheral nerve blocks for thoracic region are used for operative anaesthesia and/or postoperative analgesia for a variety of surgeries of the chest. Introduction and acceptance of these blocks has helped in lowering the opioid consumption to a large extent. This chapter will discuss the relevant anatomy, clinical applications, techniques and drugs used for these blocks and complications common to all nerve blocks. The blocks covered in this chapter include Pectoral Nerve Block, Serratus Anterior Plane Nerve Block and Transversus Thoracic Muscle Plane block. These blocks have stolen the limelight due to their less invasive nature in comparison with paravertebral blocks. These techniques are simple for the clinician to perform and require little or no sedation in the pre-operative holding area. Thoracic Blocks have found their way into a lot of clinically relevant applications like cessation of postoperative pain following pacemaker insertion, fractured ribs, superficial mastectomy, breast reconstruction, ICD insertion.

Keywords

Thoracic nerves · Serratus plane block · Peripheral nerves · Pectoral nerve · Intercostal nerve

6.1 Pec(pectoral) Blocks

6.1.1 Introduction

Pectoral nerve blocks (Pecs) are superficial thoracic wall blocks which through blockade of the pectoral intercostobrachial, the long thoracic nerve and intercostal nerves provide analgesia for breast surgery and other procedures/surgery involving the anterior chest wall. This ultrasound-guided technique was first described by Blanco et al in 2011 as Pec I block. This was an interfascial plane block where local anaesthetic is deposited between pectoralis major and pectoralis minor. Blanco et al in 2012 came up with modified Pec block or Pec II block where drug was deposited in interfacial plane formed between pectoralis minor and serratus anterior muscles. A combination of Pec I and Pec II provides excellent analgesia for thoracic especially breast surgeries. A combination of bilateral Pecs and

P. Jain (✉) · M. K. Prasad
Department of Anaesthesiology, Teerthanker Mahaveer Medical College and Research Centre, Moradabad, India
e-mail: mukeshkumar2002@gmail.com

R. Kumar
Department of Anaesthesiology, AIIMS, Patna, India

M. K. Prasad, S. J. S. Bajwa (eds.), *Steps to Successful Regional Anesthesia*,
https://doi.org/10.1007/978-981-97-4098-7_6

Transversus Thoracic Muscle Plane Block (TTMPB) provides analgesia in various thoracic procedures. Pecs block are simple to perform, reduce postoperative analgesic requirements and avoid the use of more invasive techniques such as paravertebral blockade.

6.1.2 Anatomy

PEC block involves Lateral pectoral, Medial pectoral, Long thoracic nerve, Thoracodorsal nerve, Intercostal nerves and Intercostobrachial nerve (Table 6.1, Figs. 6.1 and 6.2).

Table 6.1 Pectoral and intercostal nerves anatomy

Nerve	Lateral Pectoral Nerve (LPN)	Medial Pectoral Nerve (MPN)	Intercostal Nerve (IN)	Long Thoracic Nerve (LTN)	Thoracodorsal nerve
Roots	Lateral cord of brachial plexus (C5, C6, C7)	Medial cord of brachial plexus (C8, T1)	Anterior rami of thoracic spinal nerves (T2–T6))	Lateral branch of brachial plexus. (C5, C6, C7)	Posterior cord of brachial plexus (C6, C7, C8)
Course/ Innervations	LPN pierces the clavipectoral fascia to reach and provides motor supply to the pectoralis major muscle. Also provides minor communications to pectoralis minor muscle. There is no cutaneous branch.	MPN receives communicating branches from LPN forming loop around pectoralis minor and pierces the deep surface of the pectoralis minor to give motor innervation to this muscle and penetrate it to supply the pectoralis major muscle.	Intercostal nerves course in intercostal space along with vessels providing lateral, anterior, and posterior cutaneous branches.	LTN descends posteriorly to the brachial plexus along with axillary vessels anterior to the scalenus posterior muscle and then courses distally and laterally, deep to the clavicle and superficial to the first and second ribs. LTN continues along the anterior thoracic wall in the mid-axillary line, and supplying the serratus anterior muscle. (SAM) motor nerve that provides innervation to the serratus anterior	TDN originates from apex of axilla runs between superior and inferior subscapular nerves (hence also called middle subscapular or long subscapular nerve), then to posterior axillary wall thoracodorsal vessels and supplies latissimus dorsi muscle (LDM)
Actions	On Shoulder joint—Arm adduction, internal rotation, flexion (clavicular head) and arm extension (sternocostal head)On Scapulothoracic joint— Draws scapula anteroinferiorly		Supply segmental somatic sensory innervation to skin of pectoral and axillary region.	SAM helps in breathing by lifting the ribs and anterolateral movement of scapula anteriorly to allow forearm anteversion. Also helps in upward lifting by upward rotation of the scapula along with the trapezius muscle.	LDM along with teres major and pectoralis major adducts, medially rotate and extend arm at glenohumeral joint.

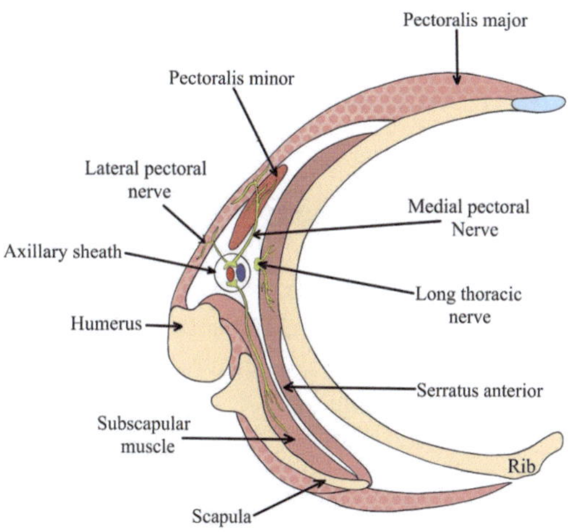

Fig. 6.1 Cross-sectional image of pectoral region

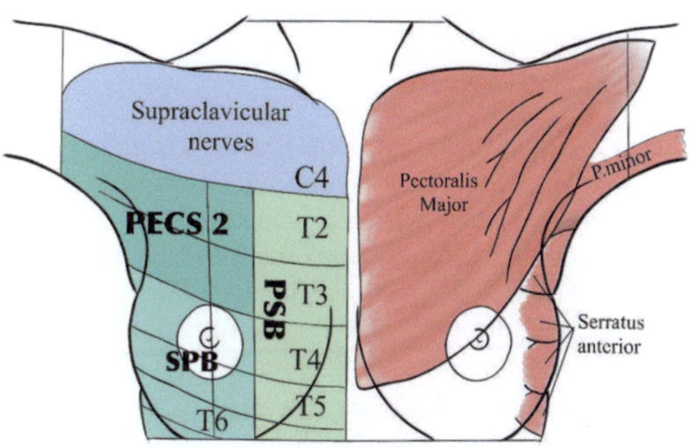

Fig. 6.2 Dermatomes of pectoral and axillary region

A PEC II block can also provide additional analgesia via exposing the long thoracic nerve (C5–7) to the local anaesthetic (arises from and innervates the serratus anterior muscle), and the thoracodorsal nerve (C6–8), which innervates the latissimus dorsi muscle.

6.1.3 Indications

Pecs I and II blocks are widely used for analgesia after various surgeries involving the anterior thorax like mastectomies, sentinel node biopsy, axillary dissection, anterior thoracotomies, breast surgeries (insertion of breast expanders and submuscular prostheses), pacemakers/implantable cardiac defibrillators, anterior shoulder surgery, tumour resection, rib fracture, minimally invasive cardiothoracic surgery.

6.1.4 Contraindications (Table 6.2)

6.1.5 Preparations (Table 6.3)

6.1.6 Drugs

Drugs used for PEC block (Table 6.4)

Table 6.2 Contraindication of PEC block

Absolute	Relative
Patient refusal. Known allergy to local anaesthetics Infection at the proposed injection site.	Patient receiving ongoing anticoagulation therapy or suffering from bleeding diathesis. Neuromuscular disease Lack of expertise. Inadequate assessment of sonoanatomy (e.g. obese patient)

Table 6.3 Preparation of block

Pre-requisites	Equipment/Materials required
Informed consent. NPO status. Optimal sedation if necessary. Emergency, resuscitation drugs and equipment. Secure IV access. Appropriate sedation, monitoring (HR, NIBP, Spo2, ECG, RR, etc.) and oxygen supply. Site and side of block should be marked and confirmed.	Sterile towels and 4 in. × 4-in. gauze packs 10–20 ml syringes with local anaesthetic Sterile gloves, marking pen, and surface electrode One 1.5 in., 25-gauge needle for skin infiltration A 10-cm long, 21–22 gauge short-bevel, insulated stimulating needle Peripheral nerve stimulator Injection pressure monitor USG machine with curvilinear transducer (2–5 MHz), sterile sleeve and gel.

Table 6.4 Drugs used for PEC block

Drug	Onset (min)	Anaesthesia (h)	Analgesia (h)
2% Lignocaine	10–20	2–5	3–8
0.5% Ropivacaine	15–30	4–8	5–12
0.75% Ropivacaine	10–15	5–10	6–24
0.5% Bupivacaine	15–30	5–15	8–30

6.1.7 Block Approaches

6.1.7.1 Ultrasound-Guided (Table 6.5)

6.1.8 Complications

Complications are rare as Pecs block is performed under ultrasound guidance and the pleura and major blood vessels are visible throughout the procedure (Table 6.6).

Table 6.5 Ultrasound approach to PECS block

Position	Patient is placed in the supine position with the arm abducted 90° or kept by his/her side	
Landmark (Fig. 6.3a)	Under all aseptic precautions a high-frequency ultrasound probe is placed under the clavicle at the midclavicular line and angled inferolateral to locate the axillary artery and vein and 2nd rib under the pectoralis major and minor muscles. (Tip—Usually, the rib that is identified while moving inferolateral after clavicular shadow is 2nd rib). or The coracoid process is identified in paramedian sagittal plane then transducer is rotated slightly in inferolateral direction in such a way that proximal margin of transducer is fixed and caudal margin is rotated. This rotation aids in visualizing the thoracoacromial artery's pectoral branch. For Pec I probe is then moved inferolateral towards the axilla as you visualize and count the ribs till you reach the 3rd rib where pectoralis major is identified above and pectoralis minor below. For Pec II block, three muscle layers: pectoral major, pectoralis minor and serratus anterior muscles are identified while moving inferolateral from above downwards at the level of the 3rd and 4th ribs.	
POE (Fig. 6.3b)	For the PECS I block, after image optimization, the needle is inserted medial to lateral in an oblique manner in an in-plane technique until the tip enters the plane between the pectoralis major and minor muscles between the 3rd and 4th ribs.	For the PECS II block, the needle is then advanced into the plane between the pectoralis minor and serratus muscles between the 3rd and 4th ribs.
Needle	A 5–10 cm long, 21–22 gauge short-bevel, echogenic insulated stimulating needle	
End point	10 ml of local anaesthetic is injected in Pec I block and 20 ml of local anaesthetic is injected in Pec II block watching for spread between the muscle layers under ultrasound guidance.	
Drug dosage	10 ml in Pec I and 20 ml in Pec II or 0.2 ml/kg of 0.25% bupivacaine/levobupivacaine or 0.5% ropivacaine not to exceed maximum permissible dose for the patient	
Highlights/Tips	Always identify the pleura prior to needling The depth is usually 1–3 cm for the first injection and 3–6 cm for the second injection. The proper fascial plane is confirmed by hydro dissection to open the space between the pectoralis muscles. Small blood vessels are present in fascial planes which can be identified by using colour Doppler If ribs not visible try to locate ribs by tilting probe more medially Needle approach of in-plane technique is from medial side as lateral approach is more painful. Perform Pec II block first followed by Pec I to avoid distortion in anatomy of interfacial plane between pectoralis major and pectoralis minor In obese patients out-of-plane approach hitting the 4th rib and injecting drug below serratus anterior muscle can be performed.	

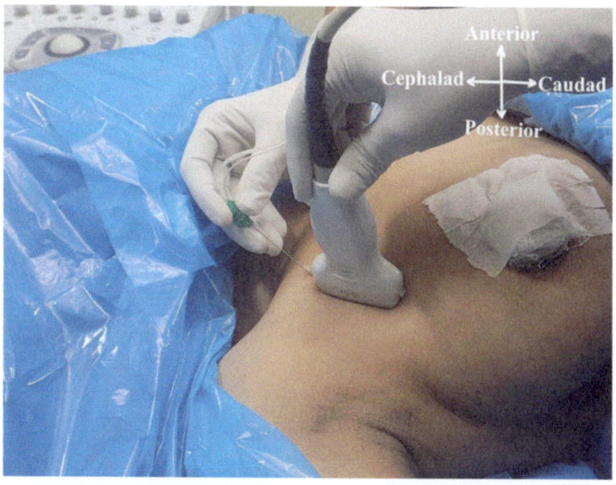

Fig. 6.3a Probe position and POE of PEC block

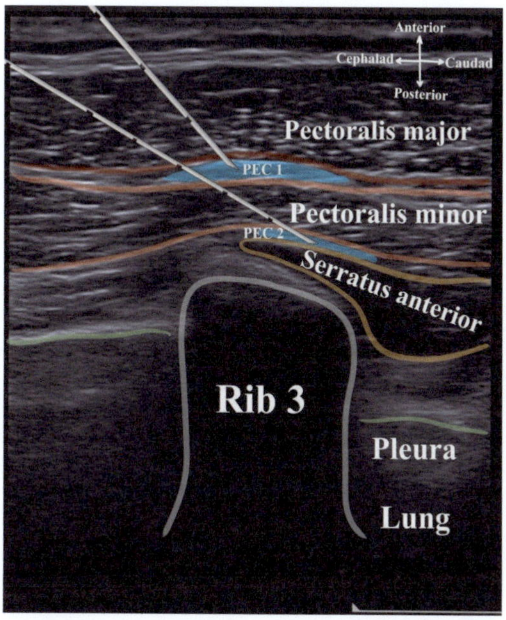

Fig. 6.3b USG image of PEC 1 and PEC 2 block

Table 6.6 Complications of PEC block

Due to needle puncture	Due to local anaesthetic	Due to catheter
Pleura puncture causing pneumothorax Vascular puncture (use colour Doppler to prevent it) Infection (Tip—Strict adherence to aseptic measure)	Local anaesthetic systemic toxicity (LAST) Allergy	Infection (Tip—Remove the catheter within 72 h)

6.2 Serratus Anterior Plane Block

6.2.1 Introduction

Serratus Anterior plane blocks (SAP) is a newer ultrasound-guided regional anaesthesia techniques of the thorax. It was first introduced by Blanco in 2013. It is an interfascial plane block in which local anaesthetic is deposited between latissimus dorsi and serratus anterior muscle. It is a relatively simple and safe technique with minimal complications and can be used for providing analgesia to anterolateral chest wall.

6.2.2 Anatomy

The surgeries involving anterolateral chest wall which extends from the posterior axillary line to mid clavicular line are covered in SAP block used either alone or in combination with PEC block. The main muscles of interest are Serratus anterior and Latissimus dorsi muscle. The serratus anterior overlies the lateral aspect of first to eighth ribs and intercostal muscles and originates as multiple slips of muscle attached to the approximate mid-point of the first 10 ribs (corresponding roughly to the anterior axillary line). These slips expand and merge as they run posteriorly to insert on the anterior surface of the scapula. Posteriorly, the Serratus Anterior muscle is covered by the latissimus dorsi and anteriorly by the pectoralis major and minor muscles. Primary nerve targets are the lateral cutaneous and muscular branches of T3–T10 intercostal nerves. These arise from the main nerve trunk close to the mid-axillary line and ascend through intercostal and serratus anterior muscles before dividing further into anterior and posterior branches that innervate the anterolateral and posterolateral torso. The other nerves covered in SAP block are lateral cutaneous branch of T2, i.e. the intercostobrachial nerve, long thoracic nerve, and thoracodorsal nerve. The nerves are described above in PEC block section.

6.2.3 Indications

Lateral rib fractures, Breast Surgery, Chronic pain after mastectomy, Thoracotomy, minimally invasive cardiac surgeries

6.2.4 Contraindications

Refer to Table 6.2

6.2.5 Preparations

Refer to Table 6.3

6.2.6 Drugs (Table 6.7)

6.2.7 Block Approach

6.2.7.1 Landmark and PNS-Guided SAP Block

Landmark and PNS-guided SAP Block (Table 6.8)

6.2.7.2 Ultrasound-Guided approach

USG approach to Serratus Anterior Plane block (Table 6.9)

6.2.8 Continuous Sap Block

After identifying the correct plane, needle is inserted in plane, after confirming the needle placement 20 G catheter can be introduced to a distance of 5–6 cm in the SAP, i.e. between the serratus anterior muscle and the rib. Needle is

Table 6.7 Drugs to be used in SAP Block

Drug	Onset (min)	Analgesia (h)
2% Lignocaine	10–20	3–8
0.5% Ropivacaine	15–30	5–12
0.2% Ropivacaine	10–15	6–24
0.5% Bupivacaine	15–30	8–30

Table 6.8 Landmark and PNS-guided SAP Block

Position	Supine or lateral position with ipsilateral arm abducted
Landmark (Fig. 6.4)	Under all aseptic precautions palpate and identify the 5th rib in mid-axillary line (Tips—Ribs can be counted from sternal angle which corresponds to the 2nd rib Drug can be deposited on lower ribs like 6th to 8th as per area of analgesia required)
POE	POE is perpendicular to surface of fifth rib in mid-axillary line
Needle	A 5–10 cm long, 21–22 gauge short-bevel stimulating needle
PNS stimulation	Nerve stimulator set at a current intensity of 1.5 mA (2 Hz, 0.1–0.3 msec)
End point	Motor stimulation twitches of chest wall (Serratus Anterior) at current intensity of 0.5 mA when decreased from initial set of 1.5 mA. After negative aspiration, LA is injected in 3–5 ml aliquots along with reduction in muscle twitches. Tip— Rib should be hit as target before deposition of drug.
Drug dosage	10–20 ml of 0.25–0.5% bupivacaine or levobupivacaine, 0.2–0.5% ropivacaine, 1–2% lignocaine with epinephrine 1:2,00,000–1:4,00,000
Highlights	Long thoracic is the target nerve for PNS stimulation

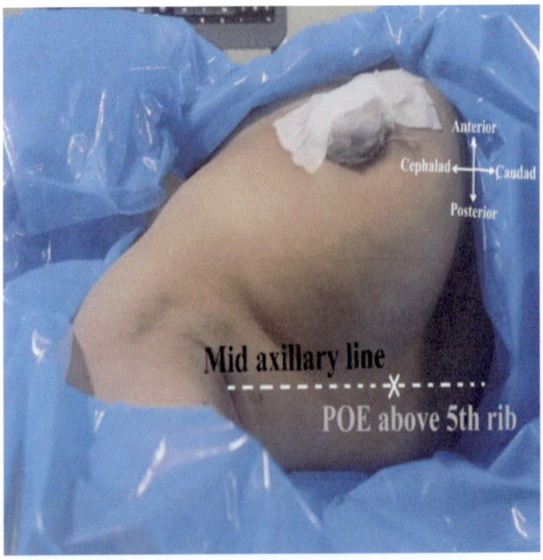

Fig. 6.4 Landmark-guided SAP showing POE

Table 6.9 USG approach to Serratus Anterior Plane block

Position	Supine with arm abducted to 90 degrees or lateral position with arm away from the lateral chest wall
Landmark and Sonoanatomy	Under all aseptic conditions place high frequency transducer in parasagittal plane below midclavicular region angled inferolaterally to locate the axillary artery and vein and 2nd rib under the pectoralis major and minor muscles. Move the transducer inferolaterally towards mid/posterior axillary line till fourth rib is identified by counting down from above. At this level thick latissimus dorsi muscle is identified superficially by tilting the transducer posteriorly in coronal plane. Deep to the latissimus dorsi, a thick hypoechoic muscle, i.e. serratus anterior is imaged over the ribs. Moving the transducer more posteriorly helps in the identification of the plane between the serratus anterior and latissimus dorsi muscles. Another method is to place the transducer across the axilla, where the latissimus dorsi will appear more prominent. The superficial l plane lies in between the latissimus dorsi and serratus anterior muscles, whereas the deep plane extends between the serratus anterior and underlying ribs (Tip—Usually, the 1st rib that is identified while moving inferolaterally after clavicular shadow is 2nd rib)
POE (Figs. 6.5a and 6.5b)	Both in-plane and out-of-plane approaches can be adopted. After identification of sonographic landmarks, a skin wheal of LA is made 1–1.5 cm away from the lateral edge of the transducer. The needle is inserted in plane in the mid-axillary line. The needle is coursed through latissimus dorsi, the outer sheath of serratus anterior muscle (superficial SAP), the serratus anterior muscle and intercostal muscles and ribs (deep SAP)
Needle	A 50–100 mm long, 21–22 gauge short-bevel, echogenic and insulated stimulating needle
Drug dosage	0.2–0.4 ml/kg or 20–40 ml of 0.25% bupivacaine/levobupivacaine or 0.5% ropivacaine can be used not to exceed maximum permissible dose for the patient.
End point	10–20 ml of LA is injected in superficial SAP block and 10–20 ml of LA is injected in deep SAP block watching for spread between latissimus dorsi and serratus anterior and between serratus anterior and ribs, respectively (Fig. 6.5b). Alternatively, drug can be deposited only between serratus anterior and between serratus anterior and ribs.
Highlights/Tips	Always identify the pleura below the ribs prior to needling Imaging should be such that the pleural line and lung are in the bottom third of your image at all times during the procedure Identification of **thoracodorsal artery** is of utmost importance, it lies in the plane between the LD and SA muscles and should be identified using colour Doppler before performing the block The depth is usually 1–4 cm for the injection. Consider needle repositioning if separation of the plane is not seen, or if there is resistance to injection The proper fascial plane is confirmed by hydrodissection to open the space between the muscles Use the ribs as a backstop whilst injecting to prevent pneumothorax/pleural puncture. If ribs not visible try to locate ribs by tilting probe more medially In obese patients out-of-plane approach hitting the 4th rib and injecting drug below serratus anterior muscle can be performed.

removed and catheter secured with adhesive. A continuous infusion of local anaesthetic can be started at the rate of 5–8 ml/h.

Tips

1. In-plane approach is always preferred for catheter insertion.
2. If any resistance is encountered during catheter placement, then it should be withdrawn and plane of insertion should be confirmed again.

6.2.9 Complications

Complications are rare as SAP block is performed under ultrasound guidance and the pleura and major blood vessels are visible throughout the procedure (Table 6.10).

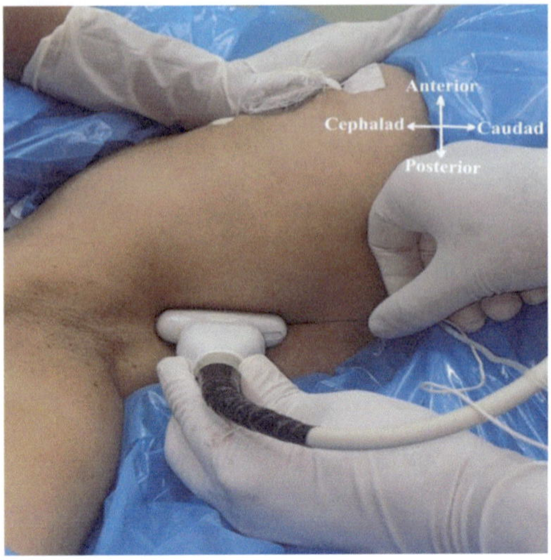

Fig. 6.5a USG probe position for SAP

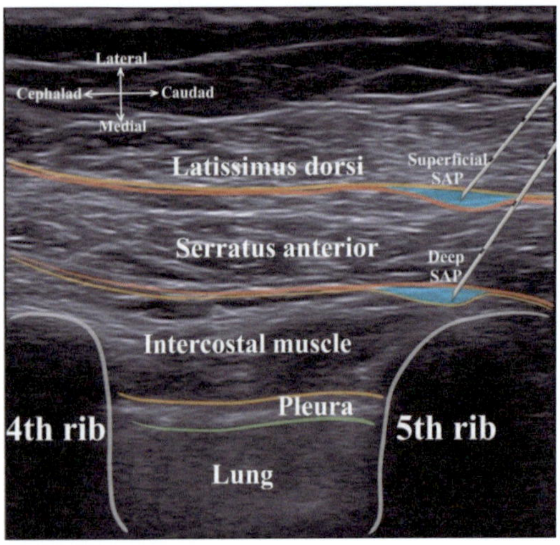

Fig. 6.5b USG image of SAP block showing drug deposition

Table 6.10 Complications of SAP

Due to needle puncture	Due to local anaesthetic	Due to catheter
Pleura puncture causing pneumothorax, vascular puncture (use colour Doppler to prevent it) Infection (Tip— Strict adherence to aseptic measure)	Local anaesthetic systemic toxicity (LAST) Allergy	Infection (Tip— Remove the catheter within 72 h)

6.3 Transversus Thoracic Muscle Plane Block (TTMPB)

6.3.1 Introduction

TTMPB is a newer ultrasound-guided fascial plane block first defined by Ueshima in 2015. In TTMPB drug is deposited in between transversus thoracic muscle and the internal intercostal muscles which provides analgesia to the medial side of anterior chest wall. The TTMP block is targeted to anaesthetize the anterior cutaneous terminal branches of the intercostal nerves that supply the medial coverage to breast and parasternal areas of the chest wall (T2–T6). The TTMP block is performed in combination with Pecs and serratus anterior block for complete chest wall coverage. Recently the block has been added into the enhanced recovery after surgery (ERAS) protocol for cardiothoracic surgeries with positive outcomes as the block helps facilitate early and pain-free extubations in patients undergoing median sternotomy. TTMPB is a great alternative in patients that cannot be given conventional neuraxial or epidural analgesia owing to coagulopathies or risk of epidural hematomas.

6.3.2 Anatomy

Intercostal nerve anatomy (Table 6.11 and Fig. 6.6)

6.3.3 Indications

Acute Pain
Conventional cardiac surgery (bilateral TPVB) thoracotomy, Chest wound exploration, Thoracoabdominal esophageal surgery, Video-assisted thoracoscopic surgery, Cholecystectomy, Renal surgery, Breast surgery, Herniorrhaphy, Liver resection, Appendicectomy, Minimally invasive cardiac surgery.

Chronic Pain
Postherpetic neuralgia, Benign and malignant neuralgia

Table 6.11 Intercostal nerve anatomy

Roots	Originate from the anterior rami of the T1–T11 spinal nerves T1–T2 and T7–T11 are atypical spinal nerves (Also supply/branches to other region besides thoracic wall) T3–T6 are typical intercostal nerve (travel solely in their own intercostal spaces)	
Course	As thoracic spinal nerves T1–T12 emerge from their respective intervertebral foramina, they divide into paired grey and white ventral rami communicantes, which passes anteriorly to the sympathetic ganglion chain and dorsal cutaneous ramus, supplying skin and muscle in the paravertebral region. ICN after coming out from intervertebral foramen penetrates the posterior intercostal membrane after about 3 cm (in adults) to enter the subcostal groove found in lower margin of ribs. Within the thorax it is sandwiched between the parietal pleura and innermost intercostal (intercostal lisintimus) muscles and the external and internal intercostal muscle, it gives off the lateral cutaneous branch arises just anterior to the mid-axillary line. T2–T11 lateral cutaneous branches penetrate the internal and external intercostal muscles and divide into the anterior and posterior branches except T12. T12 ventral ramus joins that of L1 to form the iliohypogastric, ilioinguinal and genitofemoral nerves; the rest penetrates and travels between transverse abdominal muscle and the internal oblique muscle. Near midline it turns anteriorly and pierces the overlying muscles giving anterior cutaneous branch and terminate in skin. ICN carry both sensory and motor fibres.	
Innervations/Actions	**Lateral Cutaneous Branch** Supply the muscles and skin of the lateral thorax. The anterior branches of T7–T11 innervate the skin till the lateral edge of the rectus abdominis. The posterior branches of T7–T11 supply the skin overlying the latissimus dorsi.	**Anterior Cutaneous Branch** T1–T6 supply the skin of the anterior part of the thorax near the midline, the intercostal muscles and parietal pleura, and these branches may cross to adjoining intercostal spaces. T7–T12 pierces the posterior rectus sheath and gives motor supply to the rectus muscle and sensory supply to the skin of the anterior abdominal wall. Terminal branches of T7–T12 along with L1, innervate the parietal peritoneum of the abdominal wall and cutaneous innervation near the linea alba.

Liver capsule pain after blunt abdominal trauma, Chronic sternal pain syndrome, Miscellaneous

Relief of pleuritic chest pain, Multiple fractured ribs, Treatment of hyperhidrosis

6.3.4 Contraindications

Refer to Table 6.2

6.3.5 Preparations

Refer to Table 6.3

6.3.6 Drugs (Table 6.12)

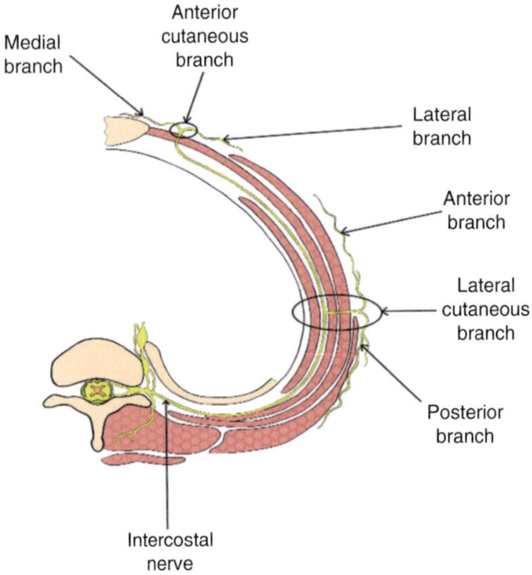

Fig. 6.6 Cross-section of intercostal nerve anatomy

6.3.7 Block Approaches

6.3.7.1 Ultrasound-Guided TTMPB (Table 6.13)

6.3.8 Complications

Due to Needle Puncture Pneumothorax, Hemothorax, Pericardial puncture, resulting in potential hemopericardium or pericardial injection, Intravascular injection, Damage to the internal thoracic artery, Hematoma, Neural injury, Infection (Tip—Strict adherence to aseptic measure).

Table 6.12 Doses of LAs

Drug	Onset (min)	Anaesthesia (h)	Analgesia (h)
2% Lignocaine	10–20	2–5	3–8
0.5% Ropivacaine	15–30	4–8	5–12
0.75% Ropivacaine	10–15	5–10	6–24
0.5% Bupivacaine	15–30	5–15	8–30

Table 6.13 Ultrasound-guided TTMPB

Position	Supine/Lateral
Landmark (Fig. 6.7a)	Under all aseptic precautions, high frequency linear (10–15 MHz) transducer placed in a parasagittal plane in the midsternal area at the level of third and fourth ribs. ↓ Visualize the ribs, intercostal muscles, pleura, and identify lung sliding. ↓ The intercostal muscle lies in between the ribs. If the transducer is moved medially to contact the sternum, all muscles and pleural structures will disappear and will be replaced with this hyperechoic structure. ↓ From the sternum, slowly slide the transducer laterally until structures reappear and keep scanning laterally until a dark, black, hypoechoic, and linear structure appears below and deep to the intercostal muscle. This thin band is the TTM
POE (Fig. 6.7b)	Once identified, a skin wheal of LA is made 1–1.5 cm away from the lateral edge of the transducer. ↓ Needle inserted in a cephalad to caudad direction (caudad to cephalad is also acceptable) and place the tip of needle between the intercostal muscle and the TTM between the ribs and above the pleura. (Before needle placement, the surrounding area should be scanned carefully to identify the internal thoracic artery (previously known as the internal mammary). Doppler can be used to identify arterial flow. This artery must be avoided during injections.)
Needle	A 5-cm long, 21–22 gauge short-bevel needle
End point	After negative aspiration, inject 10 mL of LA in 5-mL increments, aspirating between injections
Drug dosage	1–2 ml of drug injected to identify the correct position of the needle; 15–20 ml of drug deposited.
Highlights	Hydro dissection should be used to avoid deeper penetration to the pleura

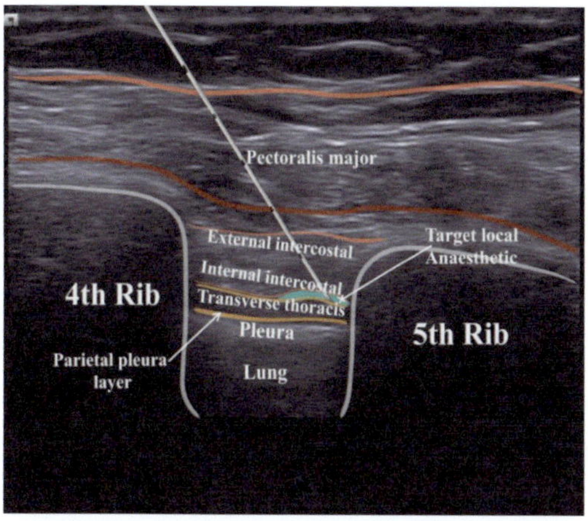

Fig. 6.7a USG probe position for TTMPB

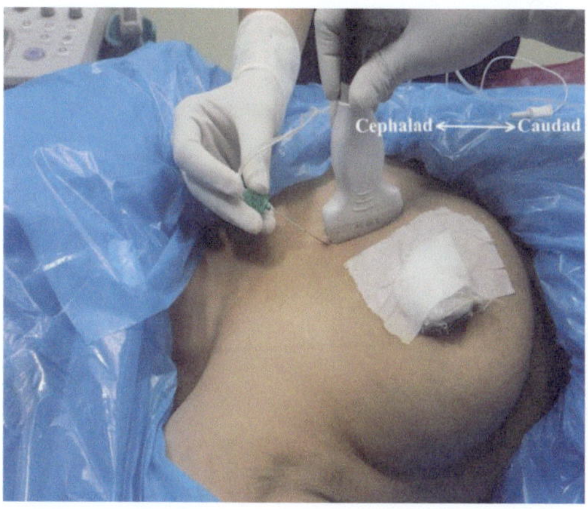

Fig. 6.7b USG Image showing TTMPB

Due to Local Anaesthetic Local anaesthetic Systemic toxicity (LAST)

Further Reading

Aydin ME, Ahiskalioglu A, Ates I, Tor IH, Borulu F, Erguney OD, Celik M, Dogan N. Efficacy of ultrasound-guided transversus thoracic muscle plane block on postoperative opioid consumption after cardiac surgery: a prospective, randomized, double-blind study. J Cardiothorac Vasc Anesth. 2020;34(11):2996–3003.

Bhatt HV, Hernandez N, Shariat A. Successful use of serratus and transversus thoracic plane blocks for subcutaneous implantable cardioverter-defibrillator placement. J Cardiothorac Vasc Anesth. 2018;32(1):e22–3.

Blanco R. The "pecs nerve block": a novel technique for providing analgesia after breast surgery. Anaesthesia. 2011;66:847–8.

Blanco R, Parras T, McDonnell JG, Prats-Galino A. Serratus plane block: a novel ultrasound-guided thoracic wall nerve block. Anaesthesia. 2013;68:1107–13.

Camacho FCO, Segura-Grau E. O bloqueio contínuo do plano serrátil anterior fornece analgesia em fraturas múltiplas de costelas: relato de caso [Continuous serratus anterior plane block provides analgesia in multiple rib fractures: a case report]. Braz J Anesthesiol. 2019;69(1):87–90.

Fujii T, Shibata Y, Akane A, Aoki W, Sekiguchi A, Takahashi K, et al. A randomised controlled trial of pectoral nerve-2 (PECS 2) block vs. serratus plane block for chronic pain after mastectomy. Anaesthesia. 2019;74:1558–62.

Fujiwara S, Komasawa N, Minami T. Pectoral nerve blocks and serratus intercostal plane nerve block for intractable post thoracotomy syndrome. J Clin Anesth. 2015;27:275–6.

May L, Hillermann C, Patil S. Rib fracture management. BJA Edu. 2016;16(1):26–32.

Okmen K, Okmen BM, Uysal S. Serratus anterior plane (SAP) block used for thoracotomy analgesia: a case report. Korean J Pain. 2016;29(3):189–92.

Sun Q, Liu S, Wu H, Kang W, Dong S, Cui Y, et al. Clinical analgesic efficacy of pectoral nerve block in patients undergoing breast cancer surgery: a systematic review and meta-analysis. Medicine. 2020;99:e19614.

Szamborski M, Janc J, Rosińczuk J, Janc J, Leśnik P, Lysenko L. Use of ultrasound-guided interfascial plane blocks in anterior and lateral thoracic wall region as safe method for patient anesthesia and analgesia: review of techniques and approaches during COVID-19 pandemic. Int J Environ Res Public Health. 2022;19:8696.

Varghese L, Johnson M, Barbeau M, Rakesh SV, Magsaysay P, Ganapathy S. The Serratus anterior plane (SAP) block: an anatomical investigation of the regional spread of anesthetic using ultrasound-guided injection. FASEB J. 2016;30:560.

Zhang Y, Li X, Chen S. Bilateral transversus thoracis muscle plane block provides effective analgesia and enhances recovery after open cardiac surgery. J Card Surg. 2021;36(8):2818–23.

Approach and Troubleshooting to Anterior Truncal Blocks

7

Ritesh Roy and Gaurav Agarwal

Abstract

Anterior trunk or the anterior abdominal wall blocks are one of the common blocks for the surgery of the abdomen. The blocks, namely transversus abdominis plane (TAP) block, rectus sheath block (RSB), the lower abdomen nerves ilioinguinal and iliohypogastric nerve block are blocked in the interfascial compartments of the anterior abdominal wall muscles. The fascial plane blocks are performed as a part of multimodal analgesia technique for postoperative pain management for open and laparoscopic abdominal surgeries. This chapter describes the functional anatomy, approaches, indications, and contraindications of the anterior truncal blocks with a stepwise approach and their troubleshooting.

Keywords

Transversus abdominis plane (TAP) block · Rectus sheath block · Ilioinguinal and iliohypogastric

R. Roy · G. Agarwal (✉)
Department of Anaesthesiology & Pain management, CARE Hospitals, Bhubaneswar, India

7.1 Transversus Abdominis Plane (Tap) Block

7.1.1 Introduction

Transversus abdominis plane (TAP) block is the common ultrasound (US)-guided block used for analgesia of the trunk. TAP is the interfascial plane between the transversus abdominis (TA) and internal oblique (IO) muscles of the abdominal wall. The TAP contains the thoracolumbar, the subcostal, ilioinguinal, and iliohypogastric nerves. The US-guided TAP block can provide somatic analgesia for the anterior abdominal wall.

TAP block was first described by Rafi in 2001, who described the Petit triangle, landmark approach. In 2006, O'Donnell coined the term transverse abdominis plane (TAP) block and the double pop technique to the block. Hebbard et al. in 2007 described the US-guided lateral/mid-axillary approach to the TAP block. The subcostal approach to TAP block was described by Lee et al. in 2010 to be a higher sensory block for upper abdominal surgery.

TAP blocks are performed as a multimodal analgesia technique for postoperative pain management for open and laparoscopic abdominal surgeries, reducing the opioid requirements. This chapter describes the functional anatomy, approaches, indications and contraindications of the US-guided TAP block.

M. K. Prasad, S. J. S. Bajwa (eds.), *Steps to Successful Regional Anesthesia*,
https://doi.org/10.1007/978-981-97-4098-7_7

7.1.2 Functional Anatomy

The anterolateral abdominal wall is formed of the four muscles, namely, transversus abdominis (TA), internal oblique (IO), external oblique (EO), and rectus abdominis muscle (RAM). The TAP is an interfascial plane between the TA and IO. The TAP compartment consists of the cutaneous branches of the thoracolumbar nerves from the sixth thoracic to first lumbar levels (T6-L1), which are responsible for the somatic sensation of the anterolateral abdominal wall. The thoracolumbar nerves exit the intervertebral foramen to form the ventral and dorsal primary ramus, the ventral primary ramus divides to give cutaneous branches, the anterior and the lateral cutaneous branches, which lie in the TAP compartment, a fascial compartment between the transversus abdominis and the internal oblique muscles (Fig. 7.1).

The segmental nerves T6-T9 emerge from the costal margin to enter the TAP compartment, between the anterior axillary line and midline. The segmental nerves T10-T11, subcostal nerve T12, and L1 emerge in TAP compartment posterior to mid-axillary line. The nerves form an intercommunicating longitudinal plexus of nerves in the TAP compartment, at the anterior axillary line, lateral to the ascending branch of deep circumflex artery (Fig. 7.2). The segmental nerves re-emerge from the plexus to traverse through the linea semilunaris and posterior surface of the rectus abdominis muscle (RAM) to reform a plexus of nerves lateral to the deep inferior epigastric artery (Fig. 7.2). The nerves traverse through the RAM to form the superficial anterior cutaneous nerves supplying the skin at the midline (Fig. 7.3). The segmental nerves give off the muscular branches innervating the obliques and the RAM.

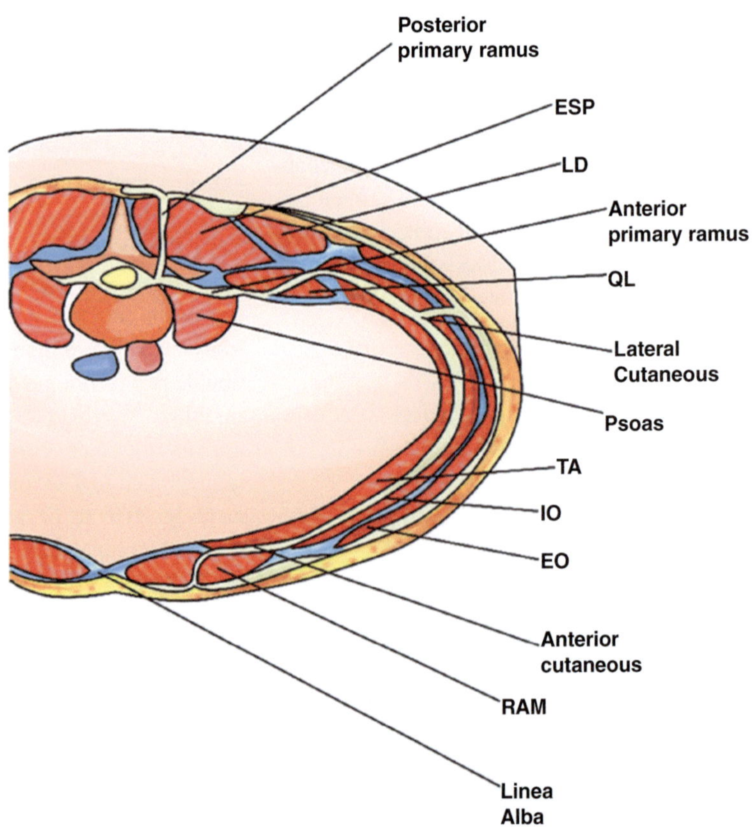

Fig. 7.1 Schematic diagram of the course of thoracolumbar nerves in the transversus abdominis plane. *ESP* erector spinae muscle, *LD* latissimus dorsi muscle, *QL* quadratus lumborum muscle, *TA* transversus abdominis muscle, *IO* internal oblique muscle, *EO* external oblique muscle, *RAM* rectus abdominis muscle

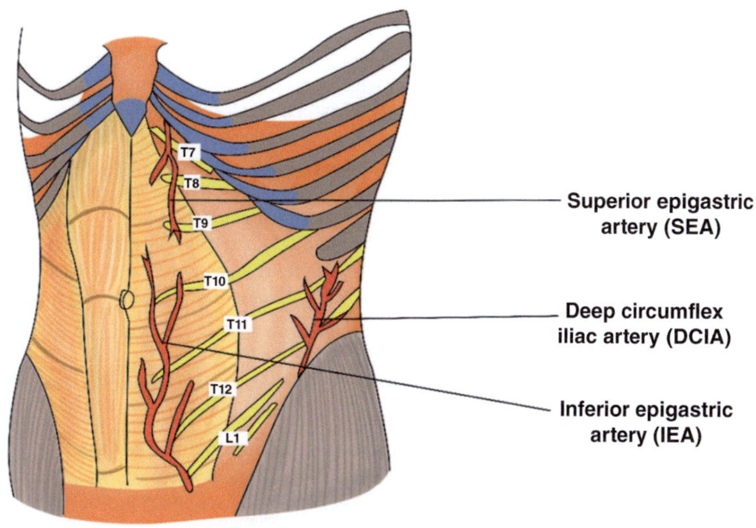

Fig. 7.2 Schematic diagram of the arteries in transversus abdominis plane

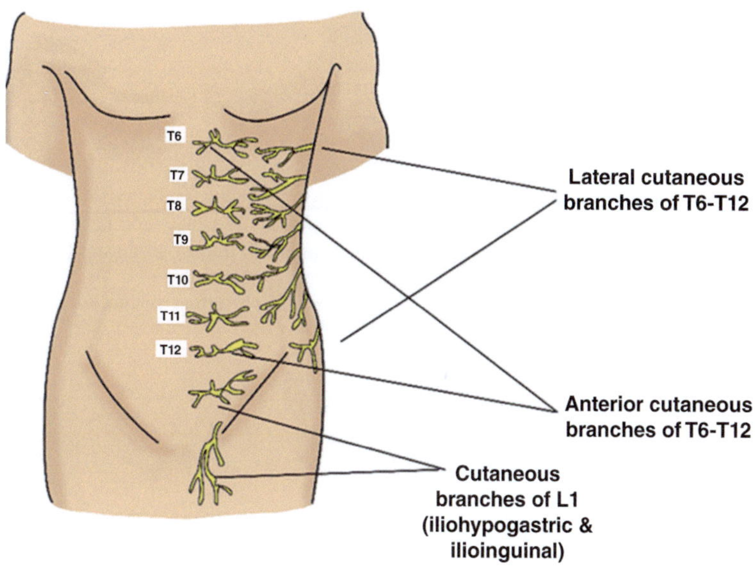

Fig. 7.3 Schematic diagram showing the lateral cutaneous and the anterior cutaneous branches along the dermatomal distribution

7.1.3 Indications

TAP block in different approaches is performed for analgesia of the anterior abdominal wall procedures.

Indications for TAP block (Table 7.1)

The transverse abdominal incision and midline incisions require a bilateral block or a combination of the various approaches of the TAP block.

7.1.4 Contraindications

Contraindications for TAP block (Table 7.2)

7.1.5 Pre-requisite

Pre-requisite for TAP block (Table 7.3)

Table 7.1 Indications for TAP block

Subcostal TAP	Lateral or posterior TAP
Analgesia for subcostal surgery Analgesia for laparoscopic cholecystectomy Analgesia for open cholecystectomy Analgesia for roof top incision or subcostal incision	Analgesia for obstetrics & gynecology surgery (cesarean section, open hysterectomy, laparoscopic hysterectomy, diagnostic hysteroscopy-laparoscopy) Analgesia for open laparotomy surgery (exploratory laparotomy, appendicectomy, colon resection, renal transplant, nephrectomy, prostatectomy, inguinal hernia) Analgesia for laparoscopy surgery (diagnostic laparoscopy, cholecystectomy, appendicectomy, colectomy, nephrectomy, renal transplant prostatectomy, inguinal hernia)

Table 7.2 Contraindications for TAP block

Absolute	Relative
Patient refusal Local site infection Allergy to local anesthetics	Anticoagulation or bleeding disorders. Peritoneal infection Difficult anatomical situations (scars, fibrosis, very thin, or elderly) Restriction to the volume of drug required

Table 7.3 Pre-requisite for TAP block

Pre-requisites	Equipment/Materials required
Informed consent. NPO status. Optimal sedation if necessary. Emergency, resuscitation drugs and equipment. Secure IV access. Appropriate sedation, monitoring (HR, NIBP, Spo2, ECG, RR) and oxygen supply. Site and side of block should be marked and confirmed.	Ensure asepsis 10 ml syringes with local anesthetic Sterile gloves One 1.5 inch, 25-gauge needle for skin infiltration A 10 cm long, 21–22 gauge short bevel, echogenic needle USG machine with linear transducer (8-18 MHz), sterile sleeve and gel. Peripheral nerve stimulator Opening pressure injection monitoring device (if available)

7.1.6 Block Approaches

7.1.6.1 Landmark Approach

Landmark approach for TAP block (Table 7.4)

7.1.6.2 PNS Approach

PNS approach for TAP block (Table 7.5)

7.1.6.3 USG Approach

Ultrasound approach is the gold standard for the TAP block, as it is safer, easier to identify, perform, and get the best desired block. TAP block can be achieved by the three approaches, the subcostal, lateral, or classical and the posterior approach.

Subcostal TAP Block

Subcostal TAP block approach (Table 7.6)

Lateral/Classical Approach

Lateral/classical approach for TAP block (Table 7.7)

Posterior Approach

Posterior approach for TAP block (Table 7.8)

7.1.7 Tips and Tricks

Tips and tricks for TAP block (Table 7.9)

Table 7.4 Landmark approach for TAP block

Position	Supine, anterolateral abdominal wall draped after asepsis
Landmark	The lumbar triangle of Petit is marked with borders of external oblique muscle anteriorly, the border of latissimus dorsi posteriorly and the base of the triangle by the Iliac crest (Fig. 7.4).
Point of needle insertion	The needle is used to feel the pops of the EO fascia and IO fascia to reach the TAP compartment between TA & IO in the lumbar triangle of Petit. After creating a skin wheal with local anesthetic Needle is inserted perpendicular to skin to feel the 2 pops (Fig. 7.5)
Needle	10 cm 22G short bevel, blunt tip needle
End point	Drug is deposited in the plane in between TA & IO after feeling of 2 pops
Drug	25–30 ml of local anesthetic (0.2% ropivacaine or 0.25% bupivacaine/levobupivacaine) with or without adjuvant each side
Highlights	The drug after a generous volume will backflow from the needle to assure the right plane of placement This approach blocks the anterior cutaneous branches of the T9-T12 thoracolumbar nerves (Fig. 7.3)

Table 7.5 PNS approach for TAP block

Position	Supine, anterolateral abdominal wall draped after asepsis
Landmark	The Lumbar triangle of Petit is marked with borders of external oblique muscle anteriorly, the border of latissimus dorsi posteriorly and the base of the triangle by the Iliac crest (Fig. 7.4).
Point of needle insertion	The stimulating needle is used to stimulate the contraction of the anterior abdominal wall muscles as the end point After creating a skin wheal with local anesthetic Needle is inserted perpendicular to skin (Fig. 7.5) After the needle crossing the skin the PNS is set at 1 Hz, 1.0 mA, 2 ms setting After getting the anterior abdominal wall muscle contractions the current is reduced to 0.5–0.3 mA
Needle	10 cm 22G short bevel, blunt tip, stimulating, insulated needle
End point	Drug is deposited in the plane in between TA & IO after getting the abdominal wall muscle contraction at 0.3–0.5 mA current.
Drug	15–20 ml of local anesthetic (0.2% ropivacaine or 0.25% bupivacaine/levobupivacaine) with or without adjuvant each side) after ensuring the stimulation at 0.5–0.3 mA current
Highlights	This approach blocks the anterior cutaneous branches of the T9-T12 thoracolumbar nerves (Fig. 7.3)

Table 7.6 Subcostal TAP block approach

Position	Supine, anterior abdominal wall draped after asepsis
Landmark	Under all aseptic technique high frequency linear probe (10–15 Hz) is placed on midline parallel to subcostal margin (Fig. 7.6) Identify the linea alba and RAM (Fig. 7.7) Slide laterally from midline to identify the lateral margin of RAM at the linea semilunaris and EO, IO & TA (Figs. 7.8 and 7.9)
Point of needle insertion	The point of needle tip placement is between the TA & PRS at the level of linea semilunaris/mid-clavicular line (Fig. 7.10) After creating a skin wheal with local anesthetic Needle is inserted in-plane (Fig. 7.10)
Needle	10 cm 22G short bevel, blunt tip, echogenic needle
End point	Drug is deposited in the plane in between PRS and TA (Fig. 7.10)
Drug	15–20 ml of local anesthetic (0.2% ropivacaine or 0.25% bupivacaine/levobupivacaine) with or without adjuvant each side
Highlights	Compiled ultrasound image (Fig. 7.11) This approach blocks the anterior cutaneous branches of the T6-T9 thoracolumbar nerves (Fig. 7.12)

Table 7.7 Lateral/classical approach for TAP block

Position	Supine, anterior, and lateral abdominal wall draped after asepsis
Landmark	Under all aseptic technique high frequency linear probe (10–15 Hz) is placed transversely above the umbilicus on midline, to slide laterally toward the mid-axillary line, to reach midpoint between subcostal margin and iliac crest (Fig. 7.13) Identify the three abdominal muscles, counting from below upwards, identify peritoneal cavity, peritoneum, TA, IO, EO, subcutaneous tissue, and skin (Fig. 7.14)
Point of needle insertion	The point of needle tip placement is between the TA & IO at the level of mid-axillary line After creating a skin wheal with local anesthetic Needle is inserted in-plane (Fig. 7.15)
Needle	10 cm 22G short bevel, blunt tip, echogenic needle
End point	Drug is deposited in the plane in between TA & IO
Drug	15–20 ml of local anesthetic (0.2% ropivacaine or 0.25% bupivacaine/levobupivacaine) with or without adjuvant each side
Highlights	The injection of drug opens the plane in a zip-like fashion This approach blocks the anterior cutaneous branches of the T10-T12 thoracolumbar nerves (Fig. 7.16)

Table 7.8 Posterior approach for TAP block

Position	Supine, anterior, and lateral abdominal wall draped after asepsis
Landmark	Under all aseptic technique high frequency linear probe (10–15 Hz) is placed transversely above the umbilicus on midline, to slide laterally similar to lateral, but posterior to mid-axillary line (Fig. 7.17). Identify the three abdominal muscles at the lateral most margin of the muscles, counting from below upwards, identify peritoneal cavity, peritoneum, TA, TA aponeurosis, IO, EO, subcutaneous tissue, and skin (Fig. 7.18)
Point of needle insertion	The point of needle tip placement is between the TA aponeurosis & IO at the level posterior to mid-axillary line, at the lateral margin of the abdominal muscles. After creating a skin wheal with local anesthetic Needle is inserted in-plane from mid-axillary line to posterior direction till it reaches the posterior end of TAP (Fig. 7.19)
Needle	10 cm 22G short bevel, blunt tip, echogenic needle
End point	Drug is deposited in the plane in between TA aponeurosis & IO
Drug	15–20 ml of local anesthetic (0.2% ropivacaine or 0.25% bupivacaine/levobupivacaine) with or without adjuvant each side
Highlights	The injection of drug opens the plane in a zip-like fashion This approach blocks the anterior and lateral cutaneous branches of the T9-T12 thoracolumbar nerves (Fig. 7.20)

Table 7.9 Tips and tricks

1. TAP compartment confirmation	Count the layers in the US-guided blocks from below up, as it is easier to identify the peritoneal compartment and count above from below the peritoneum, TA, IO, EO, subcutaneous layer, and skin
2. Subcostal TAP	Keep the probe parallel to the subcostal margin while scanning and performing the block Identify the layer with small aliquot injection and visualize the drug getting spread toward the lateral side of the layer for successful block
3. Lateral TAP	Inject the drug in small aliquots to confirm the fascial compartment for a successful block
4. Posterior TAP	The lateral most limit of the three muscles is identified before performing this approach A low frequency curvilinear probe might be required in an obese individual to visualize the structures

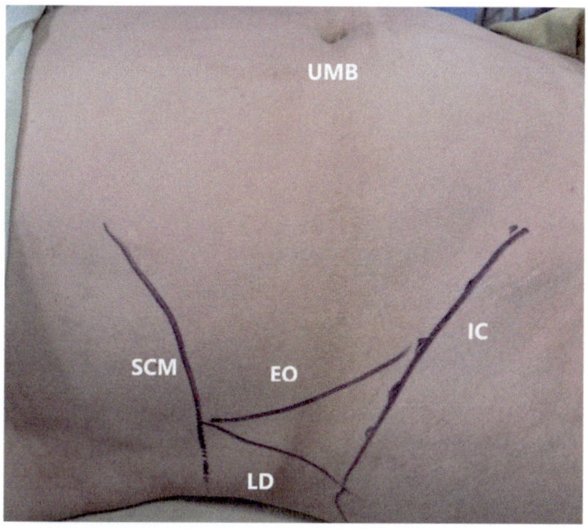

Fig. 7.4 Identification of the triangle of Petit for landmark approach to TAP block. *EO* External oblique lateral margin, *LD* border of latissimus dorsi, *SCM* subcostal margin, *IC* iliac crest, *UMB* umbilicus

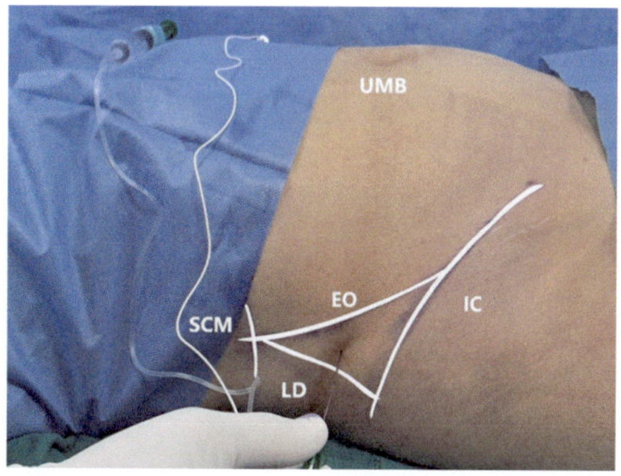

Fig. 7.5 Needling at the triangle of Petit for landmark approach to TAP block. *EO* External oblique lateral margin, *LD* border of latissimus dorsi, *SCM* subcostal margin, *IC* iliac crest, *UMB* umbilicus

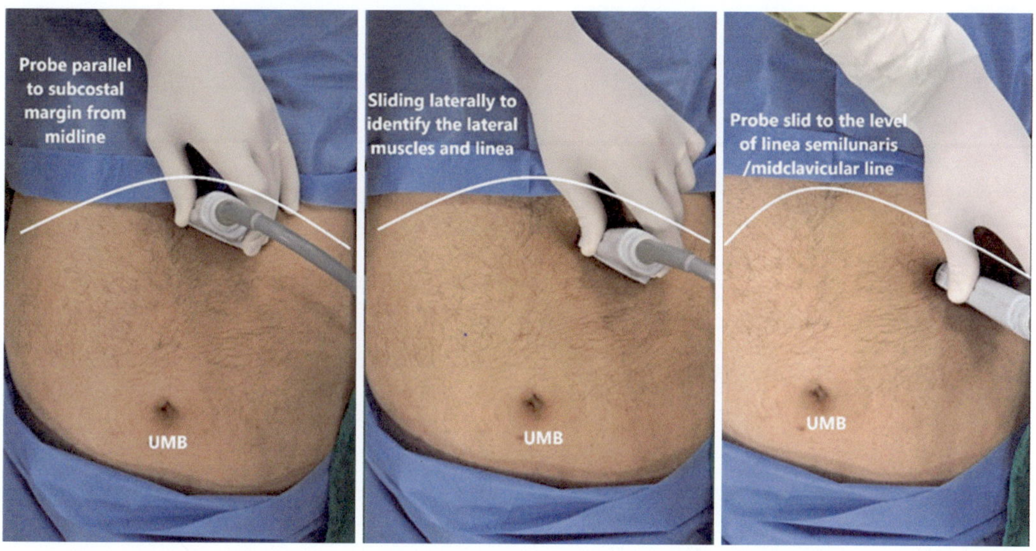

Fig. 7.6 Probe position and sliding for the subcostal TAP starting from midline. *UMB* umbilicus

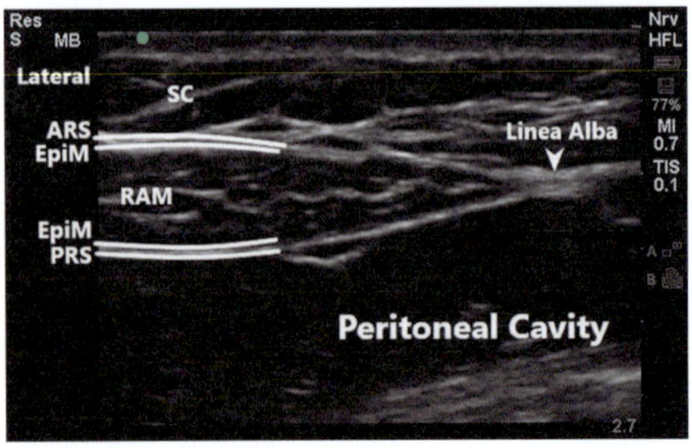

Fig. 7.7 Sonoanatomy approach of the subcostal approach to TAP block starting from midline. *SC* subcutaneous tissue, *ARS* anterior rectus sheath, *RAM* rectus abdominis muscle, *PRS* posterior rectus sheath, *EpiM* epimysium of RAM

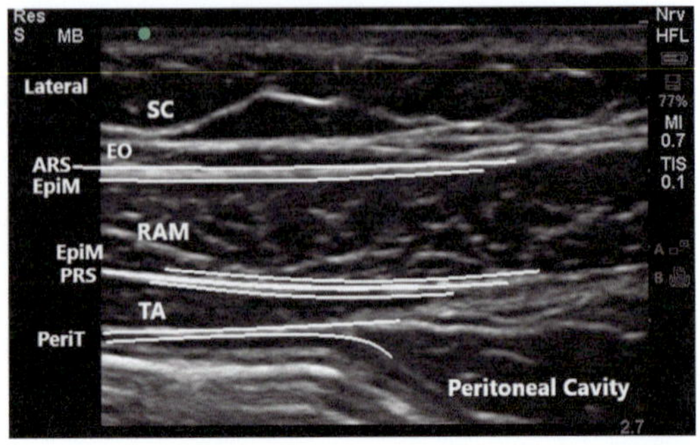

Fig. 7.8 Sonoanatomy approach of the subcostal approach to TAP block sliding laterally from midline. *SC* subcutaneous tissue, *EO* external oblique, *ARS* anterior rectus sheath, *RAM* rectus abdominis muscle, *PRS*: posterior rectus sheath *EpiM* epimysium of RAM, *PeriT* peritoneum

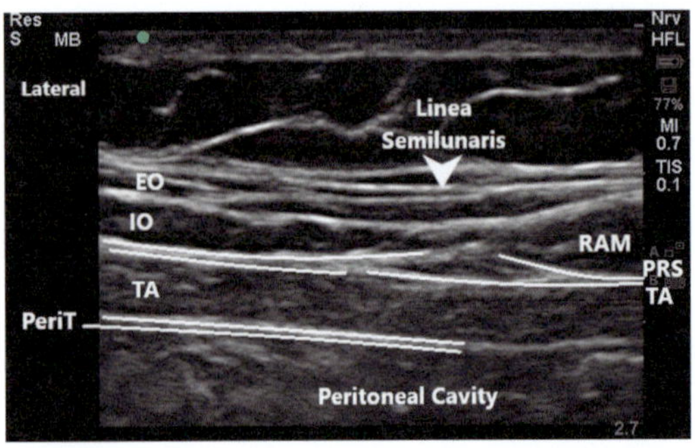

Fig. 7.9 Sonoanatomy of landmark for the subcostal approach to TAP block. *SC* subcutaneous tissue, *EO* external oblique, *IO* internal oblique, *TA* transversus abdominis, *RAM* rectus abdominis muscle, *PRS* posterior rectus sheath, *EpiM* epimysium of RAM, *PeriT* peritoneum

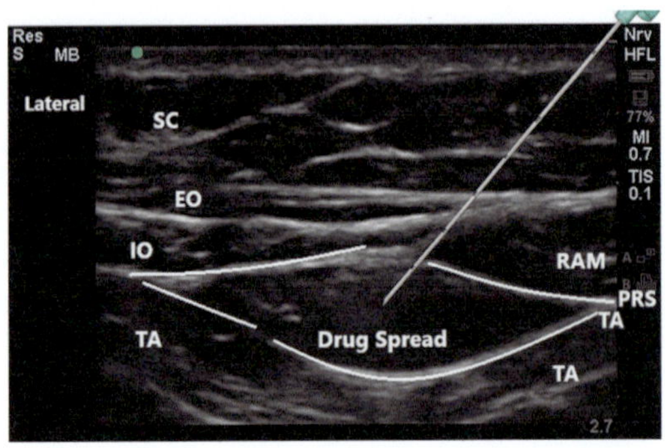

Fig. 7.10 Needle trajectory and the drug spread of the subcostal approach to TAP block. *SC* subcutaneous tissue, *EO* external oblique, *IO* internal oblique, *TA* transversus abdominis, *RAM* rectus abdominis muscle, *PRS* posterior rectus sheath

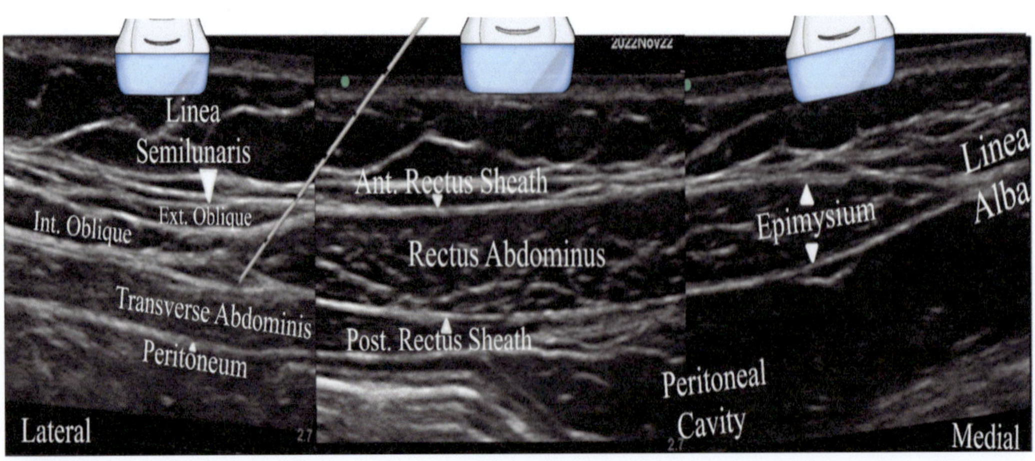

Fig. 7.11 Compiled image of Figs. 7.7, 7.8, 7.9, 7.10

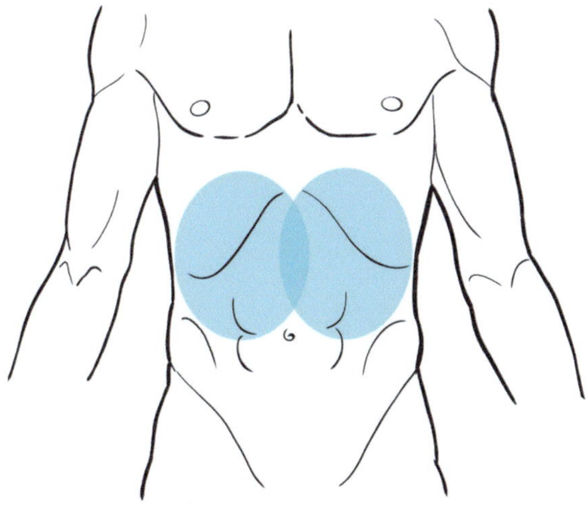

Fig. 7.12 Schematic somatic analgesia distribution of the subcostal approach to TAP block

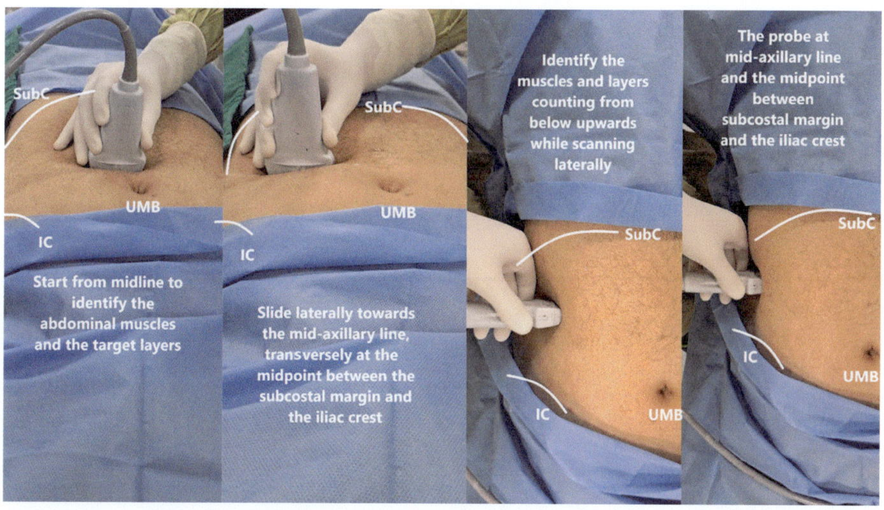

Fig. 7.13 Probe position and sliding for the lateral TAP starting from midline. *UMB* umbilicus, *SubC* subcostal margin, *IC* iliac crest

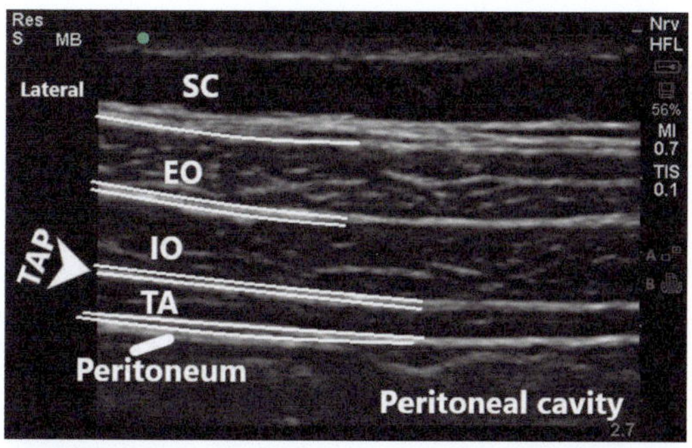

Fig. 7.14 Sonoanatomy of the lateral approach to TAP block. *TA* transversus abdominis muscle, *IO* internal oblique, *EO* external oblique, *SC* subcutaneous tissue, *TAP* transversus abdominis plane

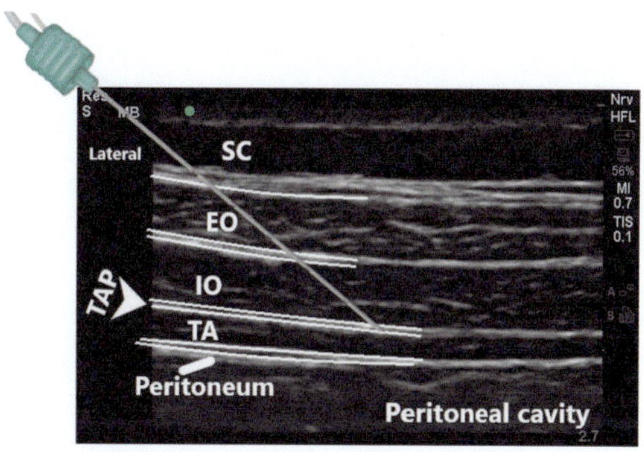

Fig. 7.15 Needle trajectory of the lateral approach to TAP block. *TA* transversus abdominis muscle, *IO* internal oblique, *EO* external oblique, *SC* subcutaneous tissue, *TAP* transversus abdominis plane, straight line denotes the needle trajectory

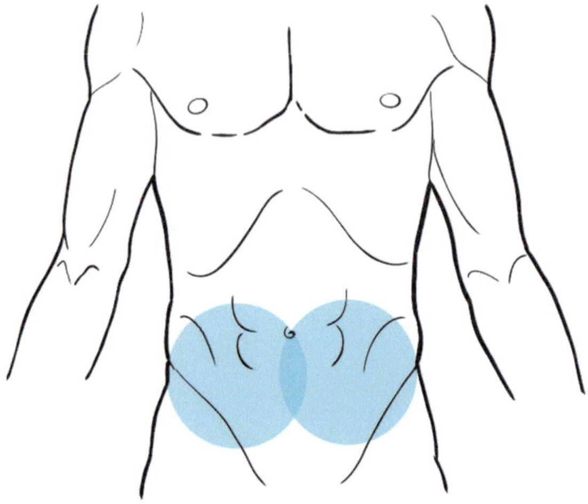

Fig. 7.16 Schematic somatic analgesia distribution of the lateral approach to TAP block

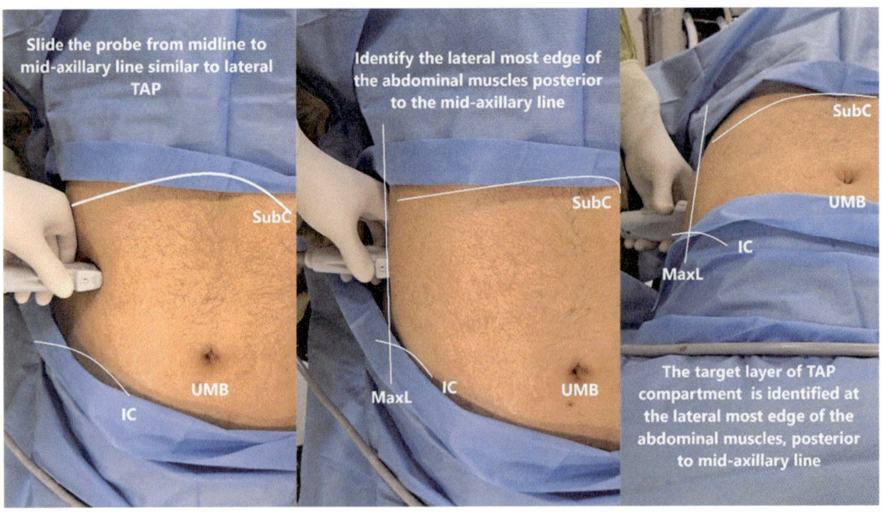

Fig. 7.17 Probe position and sliding for the lateral TAP starting from midline. *UMB* umbilicus, *SubC* subcostal margin, *IC* iliac crest, *MaxL* mid-axillary line

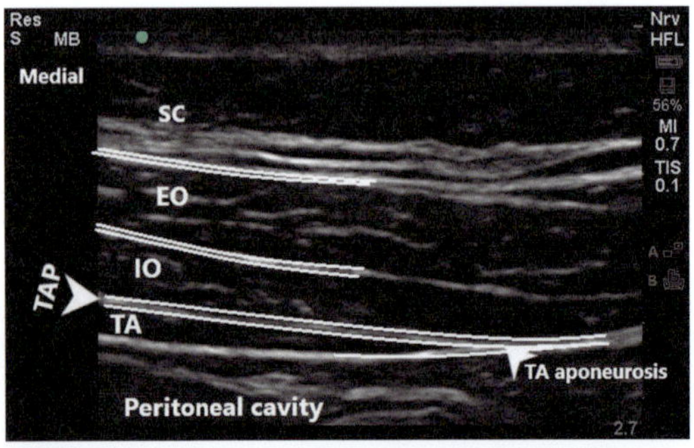

Fig. 7.18 Sonoanatomy of the posterior approach to TAP block at the lateral limits of the muscles. *TA* transversus abdominis muscle *IO* internal oblique, *EO* external oblique, *SC* subcutaneous tissue, *TAP* transversus abdominis plane

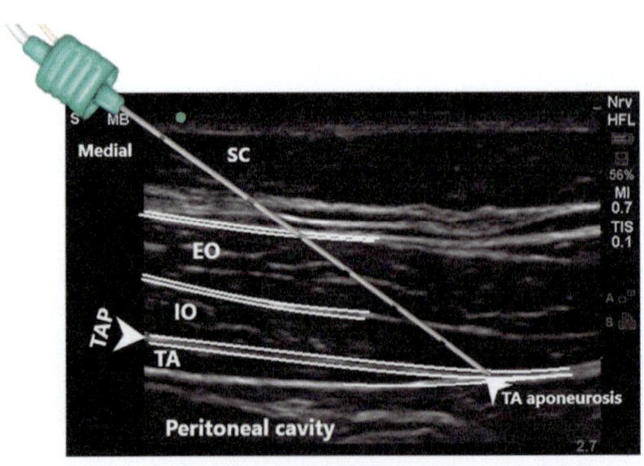

Fig. 7.19 Needle trajectory into the TAP compartment of the posterior approach to TAP block at the lateral limits of the muscles. *TA* transversus abdominis muscle, *IO* internal oblique, *EO* external oblique, *SC* subcutaneous tissue, *TAP* transversus abdominis plane

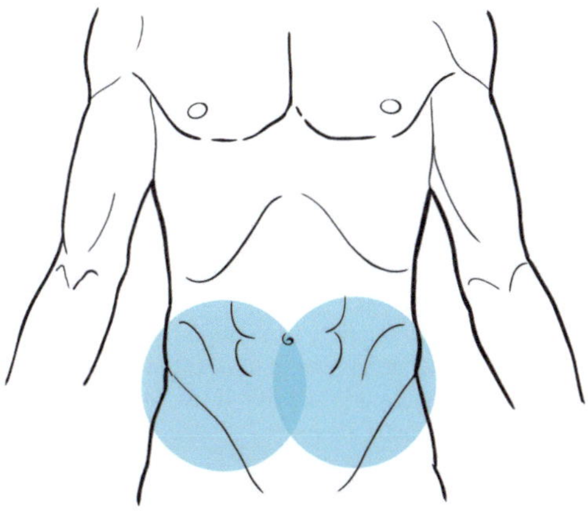

Fig. 7.20 Schematic somatic analgesia distribution of the posterior approach to TAP block

7.2 Ultrasound-Guided Rectus Sheath Block (RSB)

7.2.1 Introduction

Rectus sheath block (RSB) is a common ultrasound (US)-guided blocks used for analgesia of the abdominal midline surgery. The rectus abdominis muscles (RAM) are paired vertical muscle of abdominal wall separated in midline by the linea alba covered on by the thin sheath of fascia formed of the lateral abdominal muscle aponeuroses. RSB is the injection of required drug in the interfascial plane between the RAM and the posterior rectus sheath (PRS). The RSB can block the anterior cutaneous branches of the T7-T11 thoracolumbar nerves supplying the anterior abdominal wall at midline. The RSB gives a denser somatic analgesia for the midline surgery as compared to TAP block, though of a shorter duration.

Schleich described the RSB, way back in 1899, to provide relaxation of the anterior abdominal wall for midline surgery. Fergusson and colleagues, in 1996, described the RSB as an analgesia technique or umbilical hernia repair in children. US guidance for RSB has made the technique popular as a part of multimodal analgesia for midline surgery of the abdominal wall. The block needs to be performed bilaterally for midline surgery.

7.2.2 Functional Anatomy

The anterolateral abdominal wall is formed of the four muscles, namely, transversus abdominis (TA), internal oblique (IO), external oblique (EO), and rectus abdominis muscle (RAM). RAM is the vertical midline muscle separated by the linea alba in midline and covered by the fascial sheath formed by the aponeurosis of the lateral muscles, forming the anterior rectus sheath (ARS) and the posterior rectus sheath (PRS). Below arcuate line, the one-third distance from umbilicus to pubic symphysis, the aponeurosis of the TA & IO traverses anterior to RAM, leaving the fascial sheath formed by a thin fascia transversalis. The TAP is an interfascial plane between the TA and IO. The cutaneous branches of the thoracolumbar nerves traverse in the TAP compartment (Fig. 7.1) and through the linea semilunaris enter the posterior surface of the rectus abdominis muscle (RAM) to reform a plexus of nerves lateral to the deep inferior epigastric artery (Fig. 7.2). The nerves traverse through the RAM to form the superficial anterior cutaneous nerves supplying the skin at the midline (Fig. 7.3). RSB can block the anterior cutaneous nerves of the T9-T11 thoracolumbar nerves, but a higher injection can also block the cutaneous branches of the T6-T9 thoracolumbar nerves. The tendinous intersections don't tend to fuse at the PRS, the single injection in RSB can block multiple dermatomal levels.

RSB has proven to provide dense somatic analgesia in midline. The RSB with continuous catheter technique has also been compared to thoracic epidural analgesia (TEA) for postoperative analgesia for midline incisions.

7.2.3 Indications

Indications for rectus sheath block (Table 7.10)

7.2.4 Contraindications

Contraindications for rectus sheath block (Table 7.11)

Table 7.10 Indications for rectus sheath block (RSB)

Analgesia of midline for umbilical hernia surgery
Analgesia of midline incisions for laparotomy surgery
Analgesia of midline ports for laparoscopy surgery
Analgesia for abdominal wall surgery of midline

Table 7.11 Contraindications for rectus sheath block

Absolute	Relative
Patient refusal Local site infection Allergy to local anesthetics	Anticoagulation or bleeding disorders. Peritoneal infection Difficult anatomical situations (scars, fibrosis, very thin, or elderly) Restriction to the volume of drug required

7.2.5 Pre-requisites

Same as Table 7.3

7.2.6 Approach to Rectus Sheath Block

USG Approach to rectus sheath block (Table 7.12)

7.2.7 Tips and Tricks

Tips and tricks for rectus sheath block (Table 7.13)

Table 7.12 USG approach to rectus sheath block

Position	Supine, anterior abdominal wall draped after asepsis
Landmark	Under all aseptic technique high frequency linear probe (10–15 Hz) is placed transversely 2 cm above the umbilicus on midline (Fig. 7.21) Identify the linea alba and RAM (Fig. 7.22) Slide laterally from midline to identify the lateral margin of RAM at the linea semilunaris and EO, IO & TA aponeurosis (Figs 7.23 and 7.24)
Point of needle insertion	After creating a skin wheal with local anesthetic At the lateral margin of RAM, needle is inserted in-plane (Fig. 7.25)
Needle	10 cm 22G short bevel, blunt tip, echogenic needle
End point	Drug is deposited in the plane in between PRS and epimysium of the RAM (Fig. 7.26)
Drug	10–15 ml of local anesthetic (0.2% ropivacaine or 0.25% bupivacaine/ levobupivacaine) with or without adjuvant each side
Highlights	Compiled ultrasound images of RSB (Fig. 7.27) EO: external oblique muscle, IOA/TAA: internal oblique and transversus abdominis aponeurosis; RSB at higher level closer to the subcostal margin can ensure the blockade of cutaneous branches from T6-T8, making a four-injection technique a complete analgesia for somatic blockade of T6-T11 (Fig. 7.28)

Table 7.13 Tips and tricks for rectus sheath block

1. RSB confirmation	Scan the layers from midline identifying the linea alba, RAM, lateral margin of RAM, lateral abdominal muscles, PRS
2. Successful block	Inject in the layer between RAM & PRS in small aliquots to open the space in a zip-like fashion, free of any fibrous bands
3. Complete Analgesia	The midline analgesia will be complete after bilateral block The block at T6-T8 needs additional injection(s) at higher level (four-point injection)

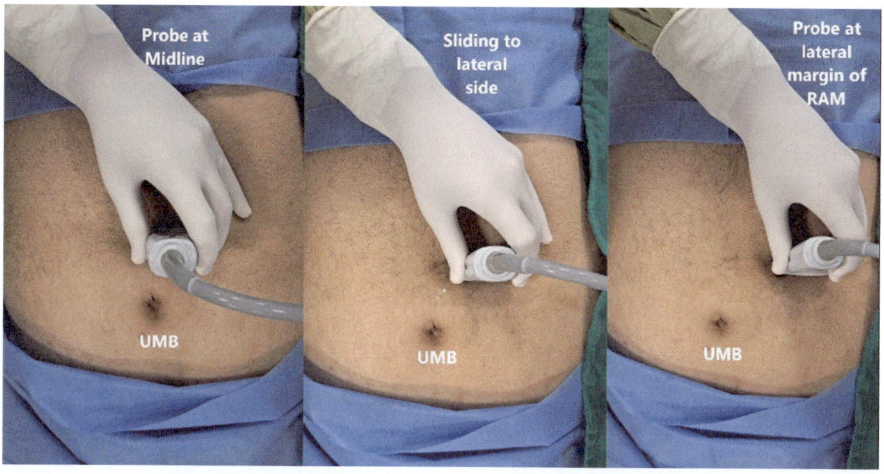

Fig. 7.21 Probe position and sliding for the RSB starting from midline. *UMB: umbilicus*

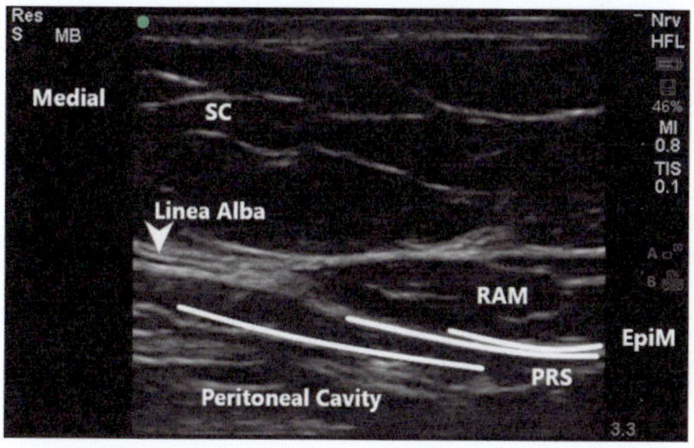

Fig. 7.22 Sonoanatomy approach of the RSB starting from midline. *SC* subcutaneous tissue, *RAM* rectus abdominis muscle, *PRS* posterior rectus sheath, *EpiM* epimysium of RAM, *PeriT* peritoneum

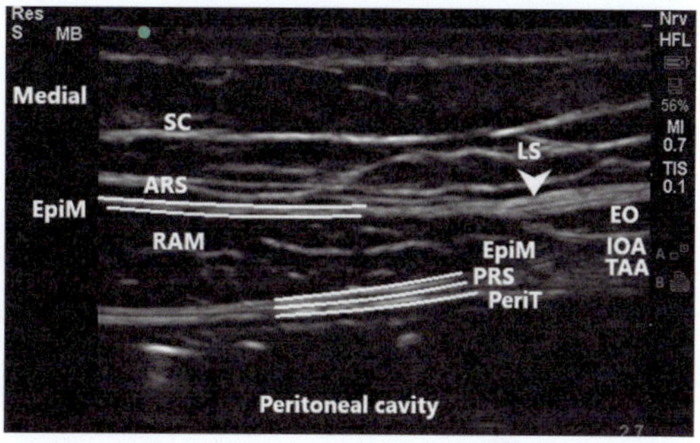

Fig. 7.24 Sonoanatomy approach of the RSB sliding laterally from midline to lateral margin of RAM. *SC* subcutaneous tissue, *RAM* rectus abdominis muscle, *ARS* anterior rectus sheath, *PRS* posterior rectus sheath, *EpiM* epimysium of RAM, *PeriT* peritoneum, *LS* linea semilunaris, *EO* external oblique muscle, *IOA/TAA* internal oblique and transversus abdominis aponeurosis

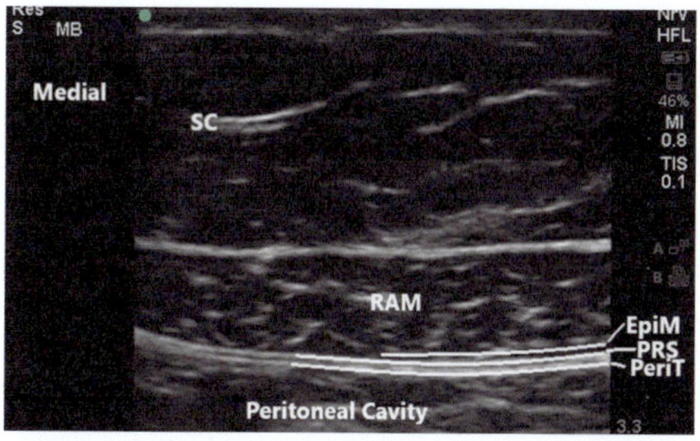

Fig. 7.23 Sonoanatomy approach of the RSB sliding laterally from midline to midpoint of RAM. *SC* subcutaneous tissue, *RAM* rectus abdominis muscle, *PRS* posterior rectus sheath, *EpiM* epimysium of RAM, *PeriT* peritoneum

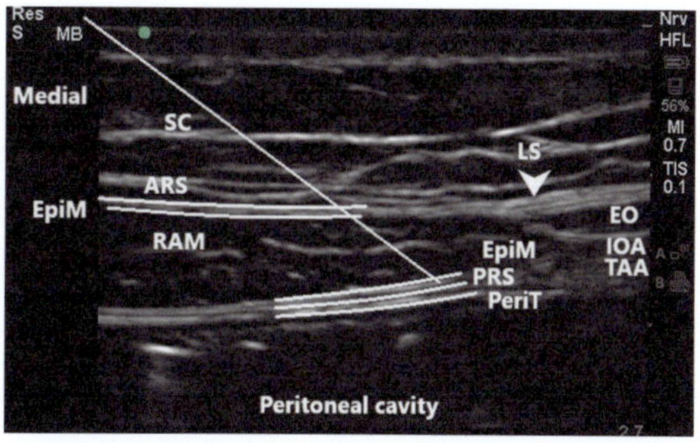

Fig. 7.25 Needle trajectory of RSB. *SC* subcutaneous tissue, *RAM* rectus abdominis muscle, *ARS* anterior rectus sheath, *PRS* posterior rectus sheath, *EpiM* epimysium of RAM, *PeriT* peritoneum, *LS* linea semilunaris, *EO* external oblique muscle, *IOA/TAA* internal oblique and transversus abdominis aponeurosis

Fig. 7.26 Drug spread of RSB. *SC* subcutaneous tissue, *RAM* rectus abdominis muscle, *ARS* anterior rectus sheath, *PRS* posterior rectus sheath, *EpiM* epimysium of RAM, *PeriT* peritoneum, *LS* linea semilunaris, *EO* external oblique muscle, *IOA/TAA* internal oblique and transversus abdominis aponeurosis

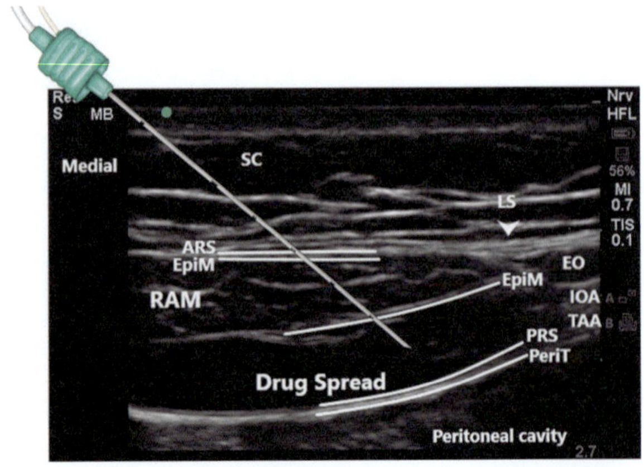

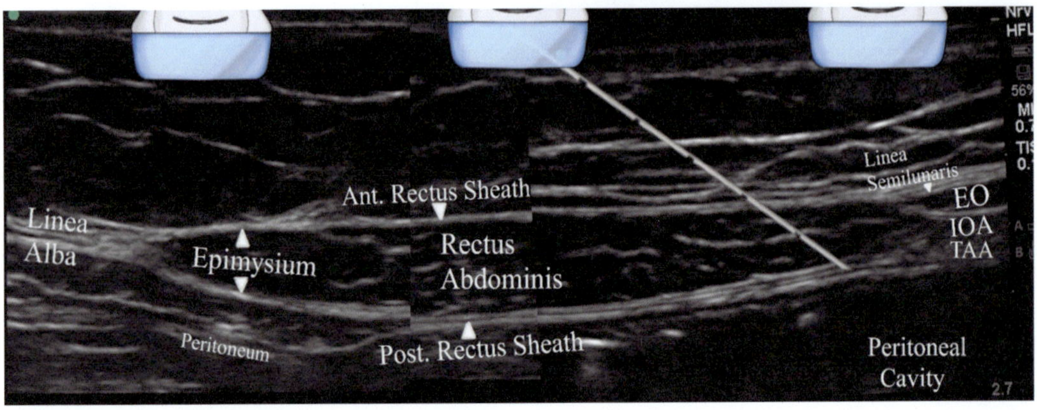

Fig. 7.27 Compiled ultrasound images of RSB (Figs. 7.21, 7.22, 7.23 and 7.24). *EO* external oblique muscle, *IOA/TAA* internal oblique and transversus abdominis aponeurosis

Fig. 7.28 Schematic somatic analgesia distribution of the RSB (four-point injection)

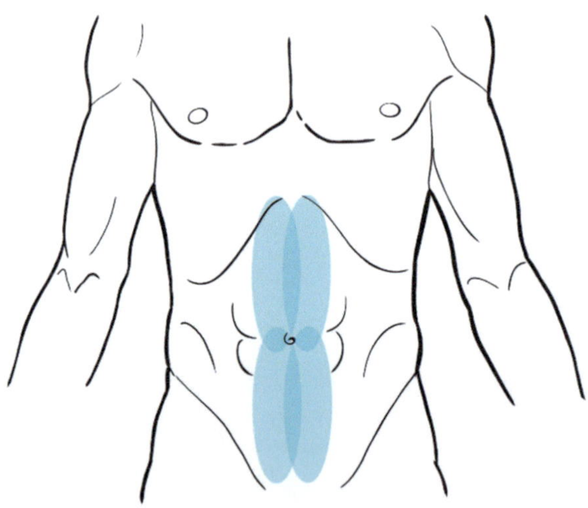

7.3 Ilioinguinal and Iliohypogastric Nerve Block

7.3.1 Functional Anatomy of Ilioinguinal and Iliohypogastric Nerve

Ilioinguinal (IIN) and iliohypogastric (IIH) nerve arises from the lumbar plexus (ventral ramus of L1 spinal nerve). The nerves start their course in the posterior abdominal wall and emerge from the upper border of psoas major muscle. The nerves pass anterior to quadratus lumborum muscle and initially lie between the transversus abdominis muscle and transversalis fascia (Fig. 7.29). The nerves pierce the transversus abdominis muscle posterior and cranial to anterior superior iliac spine and run in the TAP plane between the transversus abdominis muscle and internal oblique muscle. The nerves pierce the internal oblique and external oblique muscle medial and caudal to anterior superior iliac spine to provide cutaneous innervation (Fig. 7.30).

Iliohypogastric nerve divides into medial and lateral branch (Fig. 7.31). The medial branch provides sensory innervation to abdominal wall above symphysis pubis and lateral branch provides sensory innervation to skin over lateral gluteal area. It also provides motor innervation to internal oblique and transversus abdominis muscle.

Ilioinguinal nerve provides sensory innervation to skin over anteromedial thigh, anterior region of scrotum in males and mons pubis and labia majora in females (Fig. 7.31).

7.3.2 Indications

Indications for anterior to ASIS approach/PNS-guided block (Table 7.14)

7.3.3 Contraindications

Contraindications for ilioinguinal and iliohypogastric nerve (Table 7.15)

7.3.4 Pre-requisites

Same as Table 7.3

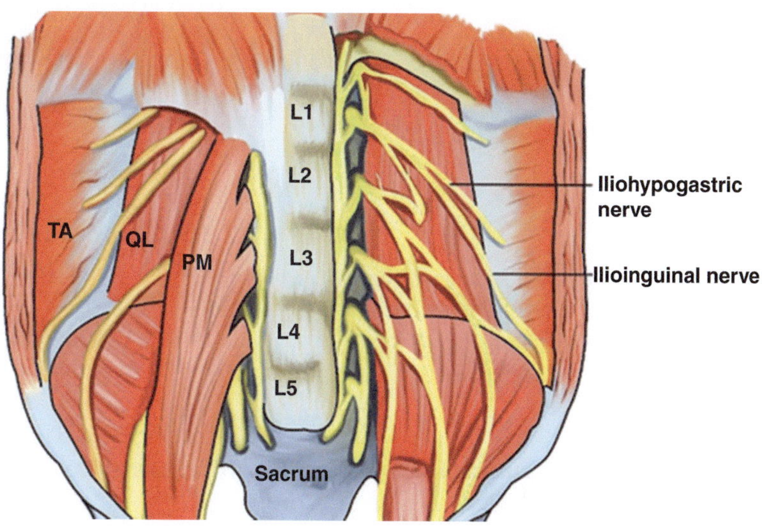

Fig. 7.29 Schematic image showing the origin and initial course of iliohypogastric and ilioinguinal nerve. *PM* psoas major muscle, *QL* quadratus lumborum muscle, *TA* transversus abdominis muscle

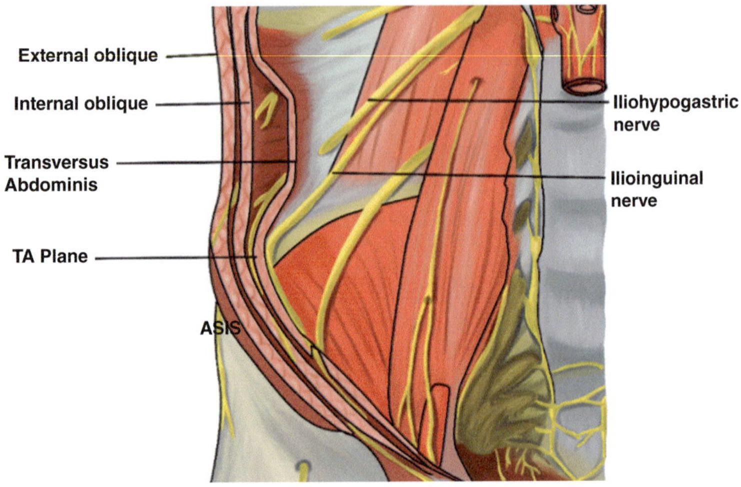

Fig. 7.30 Schematic image showing the anterior course of ilioinguinal and iliohypogastric nerve. *TA plane* transversus abdominis plane, *ASIS* anterior superior iliac spine

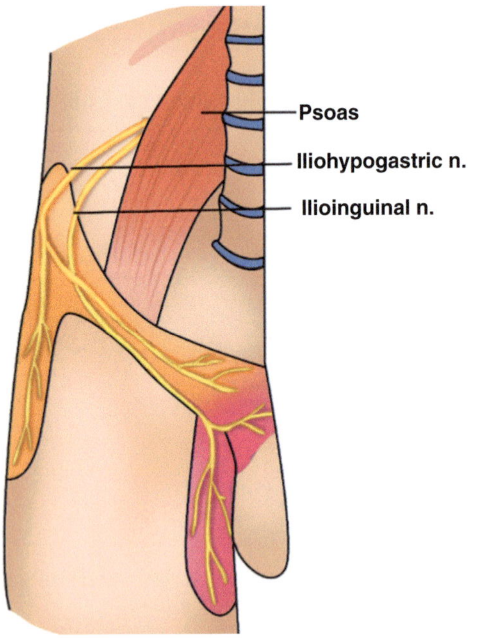

Fig. 7.31 Schematic image showing the innervation of ilioinguinal and iliohypogastric nerve

7.3.5 Approaches

At the level of anterior superior iliac spine (ASIS) between the transversus abdominis and internal oblique muscle

7.3.5.1 PNS-Guided Approach

PNS-guided approach for ilioinguinal and iliohypogastric nerve (Table 7.16)

Table 7.14 Indications for anterior to ASIS approach/PNS-guided block

Any surgery in L1 dermatome medial to ASIS
Inguinal hernia repairs
Pfannenstiel incision
Scrotoplasty

Table 7.15 Contraindications for ilioinguinal and iliohypogastric nerve

Absolute	Relative
Patient refusal Local site infection Allergy to local anesthetics	Anticoagulation or bleeding disorders Peritoneal infection Difficult anatomical situations (scars, fibrosis, very thin, or elderly) Restriction to the volume of drug required

7.3.5.2 Ultrasound-Guided Approach

Approach at the level of anterior superior iliac spine (Table 7.17)

ASIS: anterior superior iliac spine, EO: external oblique muscle, IO: internal oblique muscle, TA: transversus abdominis muscle, DCIA: ascending branch of deep circumflex iliac artery, IIIH: ilioinguinal and iliohypogastric nerve

7.3.6 Tips and Tricks

Tips and tricks for ilioinguinal and iliohypogastric nerve (Table 7.18)

Table 7.16 PNS-guided approach for ilioinguinal and iliohypogastric nerve

Position	Supine, anterolateral abdominal wall draped after asepsis
Landmark	Anterior superior iliac spine (ASIS) is the most important landmark which is marked Adult: A line is drawn 5 cm cephalad from the highest point of ASIS Second line is drawn 5 cm posterior from the first line (end of this line is the point of needle entry) (Fig. 7.32). Children: A line is drawn 2 cm cephalad from the highest point of ASIS Second line is drawn 2 cm posterior from the first line (end of this line is the point of needle entry)
Point of needle insertion	Adult: Point of needle insertion is 5 cm cephalad and 5 cm posterior from the highest point of ASIS (Fig. 7.33). Children: Point of needle insertion is 2 cm cephalad and 2 cm posterior from the highest point of ASIS.
Needle	5 cm 22G short bevel, blunt tip, insulated needle
Procedure	5 cm insulated needle is inserted perpendicular to the skin Feel for the pop of external oblique and internal oblique muscle fascia (2 pops) Switch on the PNS machine at initial setting of Current—1-1.5 mA, Frequency—1-2 Hz or SENSe and pulse duration— 0.1 msec Expected motor response— The twitches in the lower abdominal wall and the inguinal region (T10-L1 territory)
Acceptable motor response	The twitches in the lower abdominal wall and the inguinal region (T10-L1 territory) at a current of 0.4–0.5 mA.
Local anesthesia volume and concentration:	Adult: Anesthesia: 10–15 ml of local anesthetic (0.5% ropivacaine or 0.5% bupivacaine) with or without adjuvant Analgesia: 10–15 ml of local anesthetic (0.2% ropivacaine or 0.25% bupivacaine) with or without adjuvant per side Children: A volume of 0.15 mL/kg per side (0.2% ropivacaine or 0.25% bupivacaine) with or without adjuvant is adequate for effective analgesia

Table 7.17 Approach at the level of anterior superior iliac spine (ASIS)

Position	Supine, anterolateral abdominal wall draped after asepsis
Landmark	Under all aseptic technique high frequency (10-15 Hz) linear probe is placed just superior and medial to the ASIS parallel to the line joining the ASIS and umbilicus (Fig. 7.34) Three abdominal muscle, separated by hyperechoic fascia: counting from below up, the innermost TA, IO and the outermost EO are identified The iliohypogastric and ilioinguinal nerves appear as a hypoechoic oval structure and lie in the plane between the transversus abdominis muscle and the internal oblique muscle (TA Plane) either side by side or up to 1 cm apart (Fig. 7.35).
Point of needle insertion	After creating a skin wheal with local anesthetic A needle is inserted in-plane medial to lateral to reach the TA plane to block both the nerves (Fig. 7.36)
Needle	10 cm 22G short bevel, blunt tip, echogenic needle
End point	Drug is deposited in the plane in between TA & IO in TA plane to wash both nerves, opening the layer in a zip-like fashion.

(continued)

Table 7.17 (continued)

Local anesthesia volume and concentration:	Adult: Anesthesia: 10–15 ml of local anesthetic (0.5% ropivacaine or 0.5% bupivacaine) with or without adjuvant Analgesia: 10–15 ml of local anesthetic (0.2% ropivacaine or 0.25% bupivacaine) with or without adjuvant per side Children: A volume of 0.15 mL/kg each side (0.2% ropivacaine or 0.25% bupivacaine) with or without adjuvant is adequate for effective analgesia.
Highlights	The hyperechoic osseous prominence of the anterior superior iliac spine (ASIS) and the hypoechoic acoustic shadow below is a useful landmark which can be used as a reference and is seen on the lateral side of the US image. Color Doppler can be used to identify the ascending branch of deep circumflex iliac artery, which lies adjacent to the nerves in the same plane (TA plane) as an additional landmark useful in identifying the nerves (Fig. 7.37).

Table 7.18 Tips and tricks for ilioinguinal and iliohypogastric nerve

1. Plane Confirmation	(a) Start with linear transducer placed just superior and medial to ASIS on line joining ASIS and umbilicus (b) Always identify the three muscle layers counting from below up on ultrasound screen. (c) Ilioinguinal iliohypogastric nerves appear hypoechoic oval structure in TA plane close to ASIS
2. Safety	(a) Watch for pulsation of ascending branch of deep circumflex iliac artery and confirm by color Doppler
3. Plan B	(a) If nerves not identified deposit drug in the TA plane close to ASIS

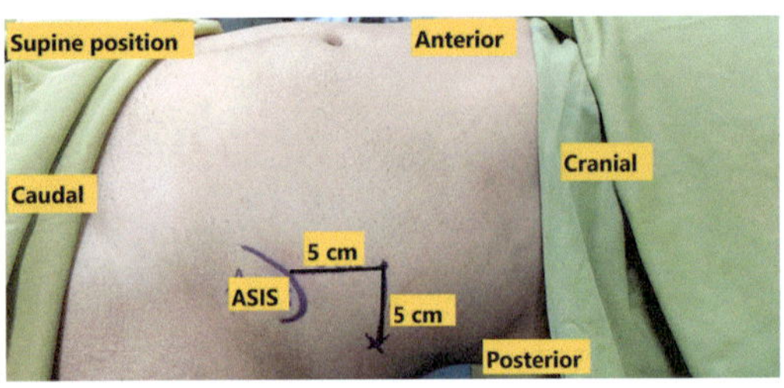

Fig. 7.32 Landmark for PNS-guided approach. *ASIS* Anterior superior iliac spine

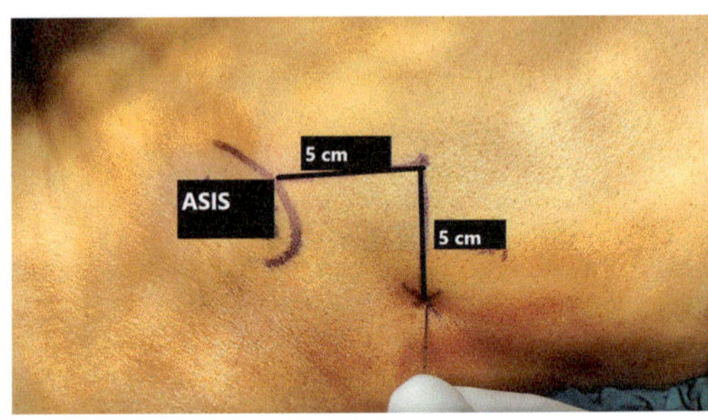

Fig. 7.33 Point of needle insertion in PNS-guided approach

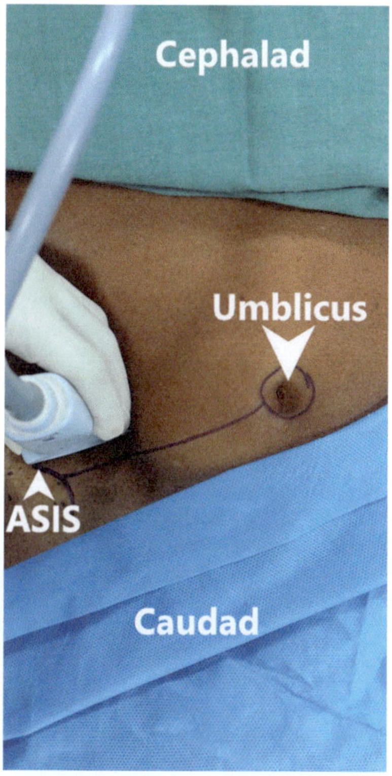

Fig. 7.34 Transducer position to image the ilioinguinal and iliohypogastric nerves at the level of anterior superior iliac spine (ASIS). The transducer is positioned in a transverse orientation superior and medial to the anterior superior iliac spine parallel to the line joining ASIS and umbilicus

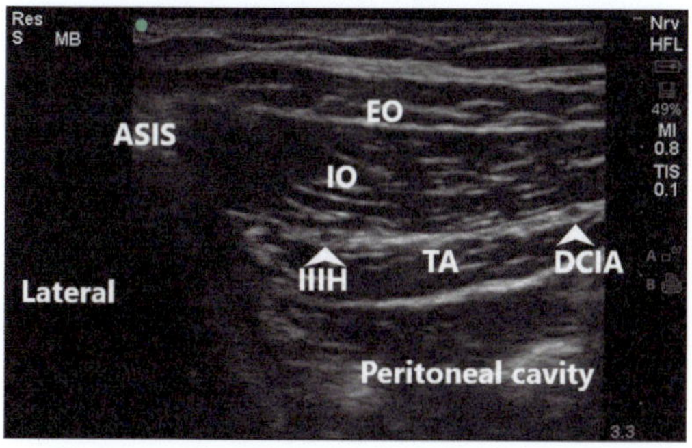

Fig. 7.35 Ultrasound anatomy of ilioinguinal and iliohypogastric nerve at the level of anterior superior iliac spine

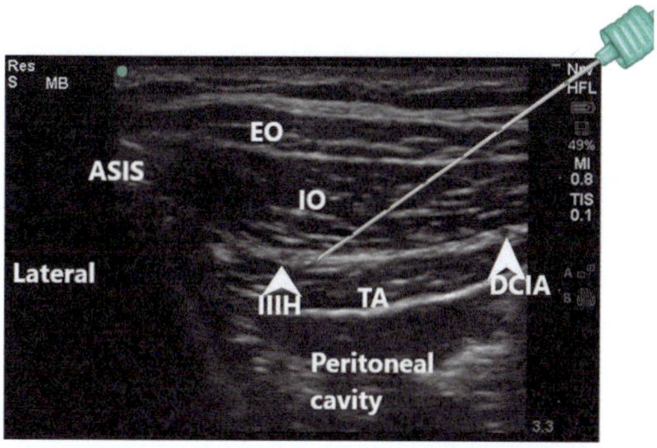

Fig. 7.36 Ultrasound image showing the in-plane needling from medial to lateral to block the ilioinguinal and iliohypogastric nerve (IIIH). *ASIS* anterior superior iliac spine, *EO* external oblique muscle, *IO* internal oblique muscle, *TA* transversus abdominis muscle, *DCIA* ascending branch of deep circumflex iliac artery

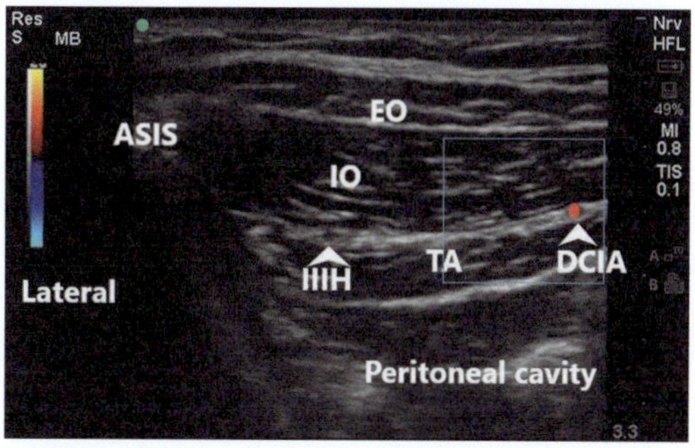

Fig. 7.37 Ultrasound anatomy of ilioinguinal and iliohypogastric nerve at the level of anterior superior iliac spine with color Doppler enhancing ascending branch of deep circumflex iliac artery. *ASIS* anterior superior iliac spine, *EO* external oblique muscle, *IO* internal oblique muscle, *TA* transversus abdominis muscle, *DCIA* ascending branch of deep circumflex iliac artery, *IIIH* ilioinguinal and iliohypogastric nerve

7.4 Transversalis Fascia Plane Block or TFP Block

The transversalis fascia plane block, or TFP block, is a truncal block that targets anterior and lateral branches of the subcostal nerve (T12), the ilioinguinal (L1) and iliohypogastric nerves (L1) between transversus abdominis muscle and its deep investing transversalis fascia posterior to the anterior superior iliac spine (ASIS). It was first described by Hebbard in 2009.

7.4.1 Indications

Indications for transversalis fascia block (Table 7.19)

7.4.2 Contraindications

Same as ilioinguinal and iliohypogastric nerve block

7.4.3 Pre-requisites

Same as ilioinguinal and iliohypogastric nerve block

7.4.4 Approaches

USG approach to TFP block (Table 7.20)

7.4.5 Tips and Tricks

Tips and tricks for TFP block (Table 7.21)

Table 7.19 Indications transversalis fascia block (TFP block)

Inguinal hernia repairs
Open appendectomy
Any surgery on L1 dermatomes
Anterior iliac crest bone graft harvesting
Pfannenstiel incision

Table 7.20 USG approach to TFP block

Position	Lateral, side to be blocked up, draped after asepsis
Landmark	Under all aseptic technique low frequency (3–5 Hz) curvilinear probe is placed above and posterior to ASIS (Fig. 7.38). Three abdominal muscle, separated by hyperechoic fascia: counting from below up, the innermost TA, IO, and the outermost EO are identified Transversus abdominis muscle tapers off into an aponeurosis (TA aponeurosis) which joins with the aponeurosis of internal oblique muscle to form the thoracolumbar fascia The tapering of transversus abdominis muscle into aponeurosis also called transversus abdominis aponeurosis (TAA) which is an important guide for needle placement is identified (Fig. 7.39) Lying below the transversus abdominis muscle and thoracolumbar fascia is hyperechoic transversalis fascia and extraperitoneal fascia which are difficult to identify separately
Point of needle insertion	After creating a skin wheal with local anesthetic The needle is inserted in plane to reach the plane between the TA and transversalis fascia near the TAA (Fig. 7.40)
Needle	10 cm 22G short bevel, blunt tip, echogenic needle
End point	Drug is deposited in the plane in between TA & transversalis fascia opening the layer in a zip-like fashion. (Fig. 7.40)
Local anesthesia volume and concentration:	Adult: Anesthesia: 10–15 ml of local anesthetic (0.5% ropivacaine or 0.5% bupivacaine) with or without adjuvant Analgesia: 10–15 ml of local anesthetic (0.2% ropivacaine or 0.25% bupivacaine) with or without adjuvant per side Children: A volume of 0.15 mL/kg per side (0.2% ropivacaine or 0.25% bupivacaine) with or without adjuvant is adequate for effective analgesia

Table 7.20 (continued)

Highlights	Correct needle tip location will open the space between transversus abdominis fascia and fascia transversalis and push the retroperitoneal fat down on injection of local anesthetic (Fig. 7.41).

Table 7.21 Tips and tricks for TFP block

1. Plane Confirmation	(a) Position the patient in lateral position with block side up for better block performance and ergonomics (b) Always identify the three muscle layers counting from below up on ultrasound screen (c) Transversus abdominis aponeurosis (TAA) is the most important guide for needle tip placement (d) Target of needle tip placement is below the transversus abdominis muscle fascia and transversalis fascia near the TAA Correct needle tip location will open the space between transversus abdominis fascia and fascia transversalis and push the retroperitoneal fat pad down on injection of local anesthetic.
2. Safety	If injection of local anesthetic causes swelling of transversus abdominis muscle advance the needle If injection of local anesthetic causes swelling of retroperitoneal fat pad withdraw the needle Always perform the block closure to iliac crest for extra safety as retroperitoneal fat pad is prominent and thickest and peritoneum is more posterior

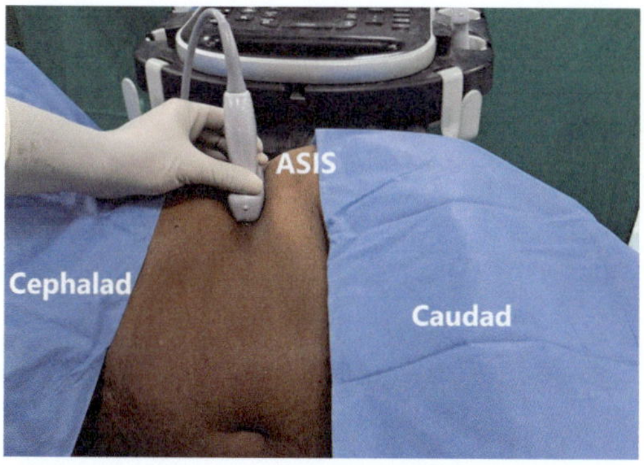

Fig. 7.38 Patient position and curvilinear probe placement for TFP block. *ASIS* anterior superior iliac spine

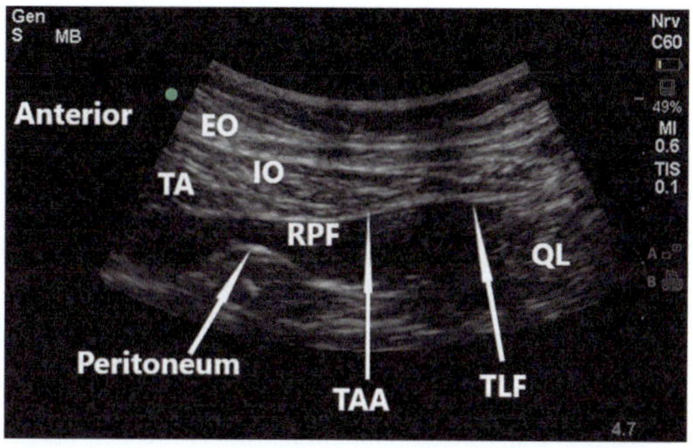

Fig. 7.39 Sonoanatomy of transversalis fascia plane block. *QL* quadratus lumborum muscle, *TA* transversus abdominis muscle, *IO* internal oblique muscle, *EO* external oblique muscle, *TAA* transversus abdominis aponeurosis, *TLF* thoracolumbar fascia, *RPF* retroperitoneal fat

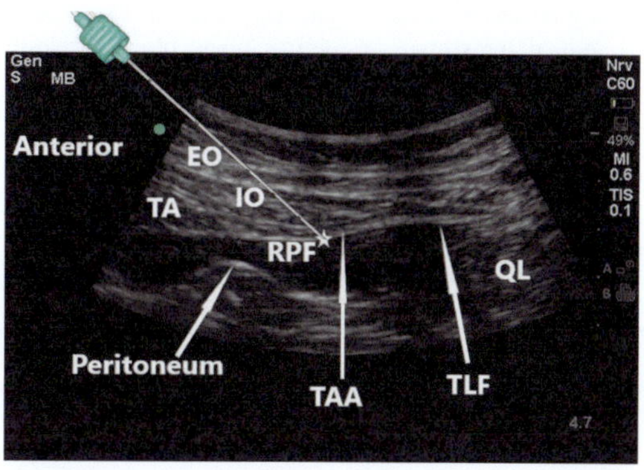

Fig. 7.40 In-plane needling and needle tip location of transversalis fascia plane block. *QL* quadratus lumborum muscle, *TA* transversus abdominis muscle, *IO* internal oblique muscle, *EO* external oblique muscle, *TAA* transversus abdominis aponeurosis, *TLF* thoracolumbar fascia, *RPF* retroperitoneal fat. White star—Needle tip location

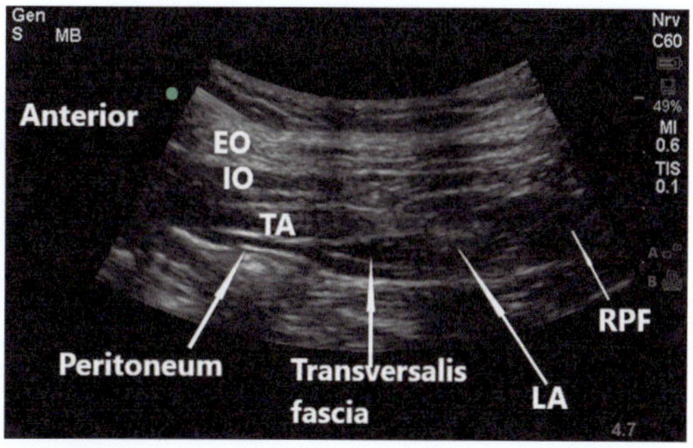

Fig. 7.41 Post injection sonoanatomy of transversalis fascia plane block. *TA* transversus abdominis muscle, *IO* internal oblique muscle, *EO* external oblique muscle, *TAA* transversus abdominis aponeurosis, *RPF* retroperitoneal fat

Further Reading

Clebone A, Finkle JH, Ruskin KJ, Burian BK. Ultrasound guided procedures and radiologic imaging for pediatric anesthesiologists. Oxford University Press; 2021 225 p.

Editor DT. Section 1, Chapter 3: Anatomy of the lumbar nerves [Internet]. Wheeless' textbook of orthopaedics. 2018 [cited 2023 Feb 16]. Available from: https://www.wheelessonline.com/issls/lumbar-nerves-anatomy/

Hebbard P, Fujiwara Y, Shibata Y, Royse C. Ultrasound-guided transversus abdominis plane (TAP) block. Anaesth Intensive Care. 2007;35(4):616–7.

Kaye AD, Green JB, Davidson KS, Gennuso SA, Brown ML, Pinner AM, et al. Newer nerve blocks in pediatric surgery. Best Pract Res Clin Anaesthesiol. 2019;33(4):447–63.

Lee THW, Barrington MJ, Tran TMN, Wong D, Hebbard PD. Comparison of extent of sensory block following posterior and subcostal approaches to ultrasound-guided transversus abdominis plane block. Anaesth Intensive Care. 2010 May;38(3):452–60.

Mavarez AC, Ahmed AA. Transabdominal Plane Block [Internet]. StatPearls [Internet]. StatPearls Publishing; 2022 [cited 2023 Jan 7]. Available from: https://www.ncbi.nlm.nih.gov/books/NBK560527/

O'Donnell BD, McDonnell JG, McShane AJ. The transversus abdominis plane (TAP) block in open retropubic prostatectomy. Reg Anesth Pain Med. 2006;31(1):91.

Quek KHY, Phua DSK. Bilateral rectus sheath block as the single anaesthetic technique for an open infraumbilical hernia repair. Singapore Med J. 2014;55(3):e39–41.

Rafi AN. Abdominal field block: a new approach via the lumbar triangle. Anaesthesia. 2001;56(10):1024–6.

Rozen WM, Tran TMN, Ashton MW, Barrington MJ, Ivanusic JJ, Taylor GI. Refining the course of the thoracolumbar nerves: a new understanding of the innervation of the anterior abdominal wall. Clin Anat. 2008;21(4):325–33.

Tsai HC, Yoshida T, Chuang TY, Yang SF, Chang CC, Yao HY, et al. Transversus abdominis plane block: an updated review of anatomy and techniques. BioMed Res Int. 2017;2017:8284363.

Uppal V, Sancheti S, Kalagara H. Transversus abdominis plane (TAP) and rectus sheath blocks: a technical description and evidence review. Curr Anesthesiol Rep. 2019;9(4):479–87.

Willschke H, Marhofer P, Bösenberg A, Johnston S, Wanzel O, Cox SG, et al. Ultrasonography for ilioinguinal/iliohypogastric nerve blocks in children†. BJA Br J Anaesth. 2005;95(2):226–30.

Willschke H, Bösenberg A, Marhofer P, Johnston S, Kettner SC, Wanzel O, et al. Ultrasonography-guided rectus sheath block in paediatric anaesthesia—a new approach to an old technique. Br J Anaesth. 2006;97(2):244–9.

Willschke H, Marhofer P, Machata AM, Lönnqvist PA. Current trends in paediatric regional anaesthesia. Anaesthesia. 2010;65(s1):97–104.

Approach and Troubleshooting to Posterior Truncal Blocks

8

Vanita Ahuja and Mukesh Kumar Prasad

Abstract

The regional anaesthesia practice using landmark technique has observed a change to peripheral nerve stimulator technique and now has been steered to ultrasound-guided regional nerve blocks. With the advent of fascial plane blocks the role of landmark and peripheral nerve stimulator is no longer considered precise. The modern-day anaesthesiologist has to master the regional anaesthesia techniques for nerve and fascial plane blocks. For this, a detailed knowledge of anatomy and stereoscopic skills are required. The regional anaesthesia performed on trunk is called truncal blocks. The present chapter will cover the relevant anatomy, sonoanatomy, commonly performed techniques of different posterior truncal blocks and any required troubleshooting. The posterior truncal blocks which are included in this chapter are Paravertebral block (PVB), Erector spinae plane block (ESPB), Retrolaminar block (RLB), Intercostal nerve block, Quadratus lumborum (QL) block, and thoracolumbar interfacial plane (TLIP) block. The growing importance of posterior truncal blocks can be understood with the fact that it cover both somatic and visceral pain as it is close to the spinal cord and also do not have the risk associated as reported in neuraxial procedures.

Keywords

Analgesia · Erector spinae plane block · Intercostal nerve · Local anaesthetic · Nerve blocks · Pain · Paravertebral block · Postoperative · Quadratus lumborum · Truncal blocks, Pain · Regional anaesthesia · Retrolaminar block · TLIP block · Ultrasonography

8.1 Introduction

Currently, majority of the surgical procedures are being done under laparoscopic or minimally invasive approach which allows early discharge from hospital. Perioperative pain management is now undergoing a shift from neuraxial procedures like epidural analgesia to regional analgesia. The pragmatic shift from landmark technique to peripheral nerve stimulator technique to ultrasound-guided blocks is well appreciated in the multimodal perioperative pain management. The most commonly practiced posterior truncal

V. Ahuja
Department of Anaesthesia and Intensive Care, Government Medical College, Chandigarh, India

M. K. Prasad (✉)
Department of Anaesthesiology, Teerthanker Mahaveer Medical College and Research Centre, Moradabad, India
e-mail: mukeshkumar2002@gmail.com

M. K. Prasad, S. J. S. Bajwa (eds.), *Steps to Successful Regional Anesthesia*,
https://doi.org/10.1007/978-981-97-4098-7_8

blocks are paravertebral block, intercostal nerve block, erector spinae plane block, quadratus lumborum block, and many more. The objectives for each block described are relevant anatomy, indications, contraindications, procedural details, and troubleshooting. The most commonly used methods have been described here and no claim is made to include all approaches whilst performing a block. However, the readers should note that with evolving techniques variations in approaches are possible.

8.2 Anatomy

The human body has an outer skin, followed by subcutaneous tissue, fibrous connective tissues, muscles, nerves, vessels, bones, and organs. Anatomically, there are three main layers of fasciae encountered in human body. The outermost is superficial fascia, then deep fascia, and then fascia surrounding muscles. The fascia surrounding muscles are namely; epimysium, perimysium, and endomysium. The deep fascial layer is an identifiable structure during ultrasound-guided interfascial plane blocks and anatomically maintains basal tension of the torso. The deep fascial layer has several attachments, envelopes muscles, nerves, vessels, organs, and is devoid of adipose tissue.

8.2.1 Fascia of Abdomen

The thoracolumbar fascia (TLF), which functions almost like a tendon in the abdomen, is movable and connects medially to the tip of the transverse process and laterally to the muscles of the anterior abdominal wall. The anterior, intermediate, and posterior layers make up the TLF. The quadrates lumborum muscle's anterior surface is covered by the anterior layer. The anterior surface of the erector spinae muscle and the posterior surface of the quadratus lumborum are both covered by the intermediate layer. The erector spinae muscle's posterior surface is covered by the TLF's posterior layer. The varied techniques for performing a quadrates lumborum block and an erector spinae block correspond to the therapeutic consequences of TLF. From L4 to subcostal level, the quadratus lumborum and psoas major muscles share a continuous fascial plane. The details of the extent of TLF are shown in Fig. 8.1.

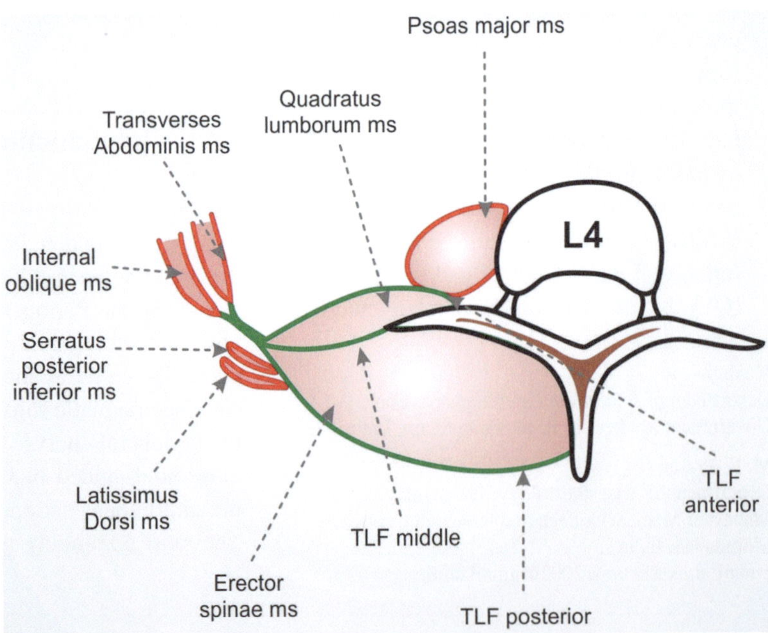

Fig. 8.1 Thoracolumbar fascia (TLF) and muscles of posterior lower trunk

8.2.2 Muscles of the Posterior Trunk

The muscles of the posterior trunk (Fig. 8.2) can be classified as:

- Extrinsic muscles (superficial): Trapezius, Latissimus dorsi, levator scapula, Rhomboid major, Rhomboid minor.
- Extrinsic muscle (deep): Serratus posterior superior, Serratus posterior inferior.
- Intrinsic muscles (superficial): Erector spinae muscles (Spinalis, Longissimus, Iliocostalis).
- Intrinsic muscle (intermediate): Spinotransverse group (semispinalis, multifidus, rotatores).
- Intrinsic muscle (deep): Interspinales, Intertransversarii.

8.2.3 Nerves of the Posterior Trunk

There are 12 intercostal nerves in the thoracic spine, 6 on each side of the chest. The chest wall, abdominal wall, pleura, peritoneum, groin, and intercostal nerves are all sensory organs. The ventral rami of the corresponding thoracic spinal nerve from T1 to T12 is where the intercostal nerve starts. The posterior intercostal membrane is punctured by the intercostal nerve as it travels along the lower edge of the rib and then dips into the thoracic pleura, about 3 cm distal to the intervertebral foramen, to enter the subcostal grove. Intercostal nerves give a lateral cutaneous branch at the midaxillary line. Then moving anteriorly, intercostal nerve gives branches and pierces the overlying muscles, fascia and finally terminates into anterior cutaneous branches (Fig. 8.3).

- Before splitting into anterior and posterior branches, T2–T11's lateral cutaneous branches pierce the internal and external intercostal muscles. T7–T11 anterior branches provide skin up to the rectus abdominis. The skin above the latissimus dorsi is supplied by posterior branches T7–T11.

8.2.4 Anatomical Landmarks

- The T12 lateral cutaneous branch does not split.
- The L1 and T12 ventral rami combine to form the genitofemoral, iliohypogastric, and ilioinguinal nerves.
- The anterior cutaneous branch T2–T6 pierces the pectoralis major and external intercostals; more information on this branch is provided in the section on chest wall blocks.
- The lumbar and sacral plexus are formed by the ventral nerves in the lumbar spine. Medial, intermediate, and lateral branches are created when the dorsal ramus divides.
- The T1 intercostal nerve joins C8 after exiting the intercostal space; it lacks an anterior cuta-

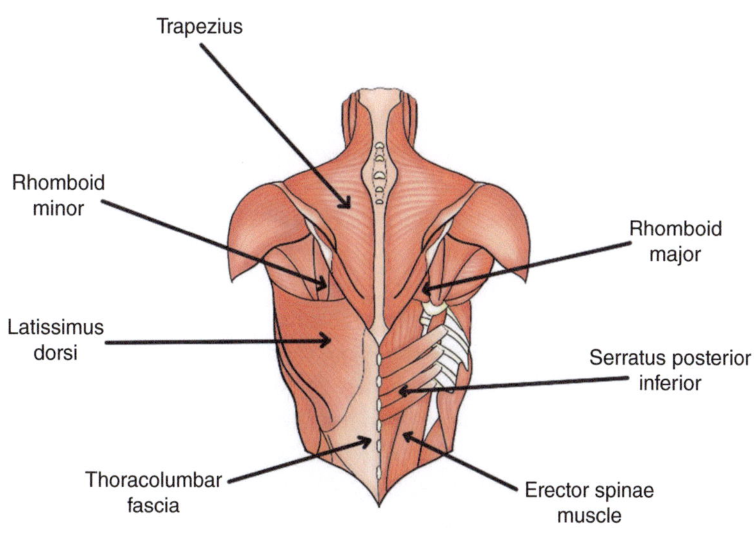

Fig. 8.2 Muscles of the posterior trunk

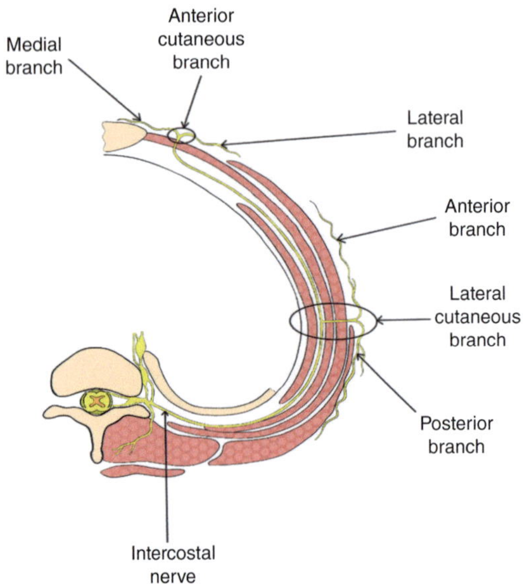

Fig. 8.3 Intercostal nerves and their branches

neous nerve and, in most cases, no lateral cutaneous nerve.

- Fibres of T2 and T3 form intercostobrachial nerve.
- T12 is known as subcostal nerve.

8.3 Mechanism of Spread of Drug

1. Injecting the local anaesthetic solution in the correct anatomic plane has a passive spread of the drug via path of least resistance.
2. Local anaesthetic solution is disseminated in plane by pumping action when a muscle contracts because it transfers 30% of the muscular force to the connective tissue around the muscle.
3. The autonomous contractile elements of deep connective fascia result in the spread of solution via force generation.
4. The fascial layers can act as biomechanical elastic spring which can absorb, store, and release energy. The deep fascial planes do not only have A and C fibres but are predominated by "wide dynamic range" neurons, which can detect and propagate multiple sensory signals. This mechanism may be present in combination or only a few may be present depending on the fascia of which region of the body is being subjected to fascial plane block.
5. A few questions still remain unanswered about whether the presence of solid organs like liver on the right side impedes the spread of local anaesthetic solution cranially. Does spontaneous versus controlled ventilation affect the spread of injectate solution effect in thoracic fascial blocks?
6. More research is needed to determine the best location to provide local anaesthetic, how and where the solution spreads in the interfascial planes, and whether open or laparoscopic thoracic or abdominal surgery may have an impact on the solution's spread. Cassette studies might not be able to provide the answers to these queries; instead, a living animal model or human subjects would be needed.

8.4 Equipment Required and Preparations for Performing Block

Preparation of block (Table 8.1).

Table 8.1 Preparation of block

Pre-requisites	Equipment/Materials required
Informed consent NPO status Optimal sedation if necessary Emergency, resuscitation drugs, and equipment Secure IV access Appropriate sedation, monitoring (HR, NIBP, Spo2, ECG, RR etc.) and oxygen supply Site and side of block should be marked and confirmed	Sterile towels and 4 inches × 4-inch gauze packs 10–20 ml syringes with local anaesthetic Sterile gloves, marking pen, and surface electrode One 1.5 in., 25-gauge needle for skin infiltration A 10-cm long, 21–22 gauge short-bevel, insulated stimulating needle Peripheral nerve stimulator Injection pressure monitor USG machine with curvilinear transducer (2–5 MHz), sterile sleeve, and gel

8.5 Paravertebral Block

The paravertebral block (PVB) induces unilateral somatosensory and sympathetic block at any level in thoracic and lumbar areas. The block is indicated in acute pain and in chronic pain conditions. PVB was found to be superior to intercostal nerve block, intrapleural neuralgia, intrathecal opioids, and non-inferior to thoracic epidural analgesia.

8.5.1 Anatomy

The thoracic PVB is a wedge-shaped space that communicates through the intercostal space, medial epidural space, and adjacent paravertebral space on both the superior and inferior sides. The paravertebral space's boundaries in the thoracic region are:

- Base-Posterolateral portion of the vertebral body, intervertebral disc, the articular processes, and the intervertebral foramen.
- Posterior boundary—the transverse process, superior costotransverse ligament, and heads of ribs collectively.
- Anterolateral border—The parietal pleura.

Contents—Spinal nerves, the sympathetic chain, the ramus communicans, blood arteries, and adipose tissue make up the PVBs (Fig. 8.4).

In lumbar PVB, the boundaries are anterolaterally psoas muscle, medially are vertebral bodies, intervertebral disc, intervertebral foramen with its contents, and the posterior boundary is a transverse process with the intertransverse ligaments.

The lumbar PVB space is occupied by psoas major muscle. Psoas major muscle has two

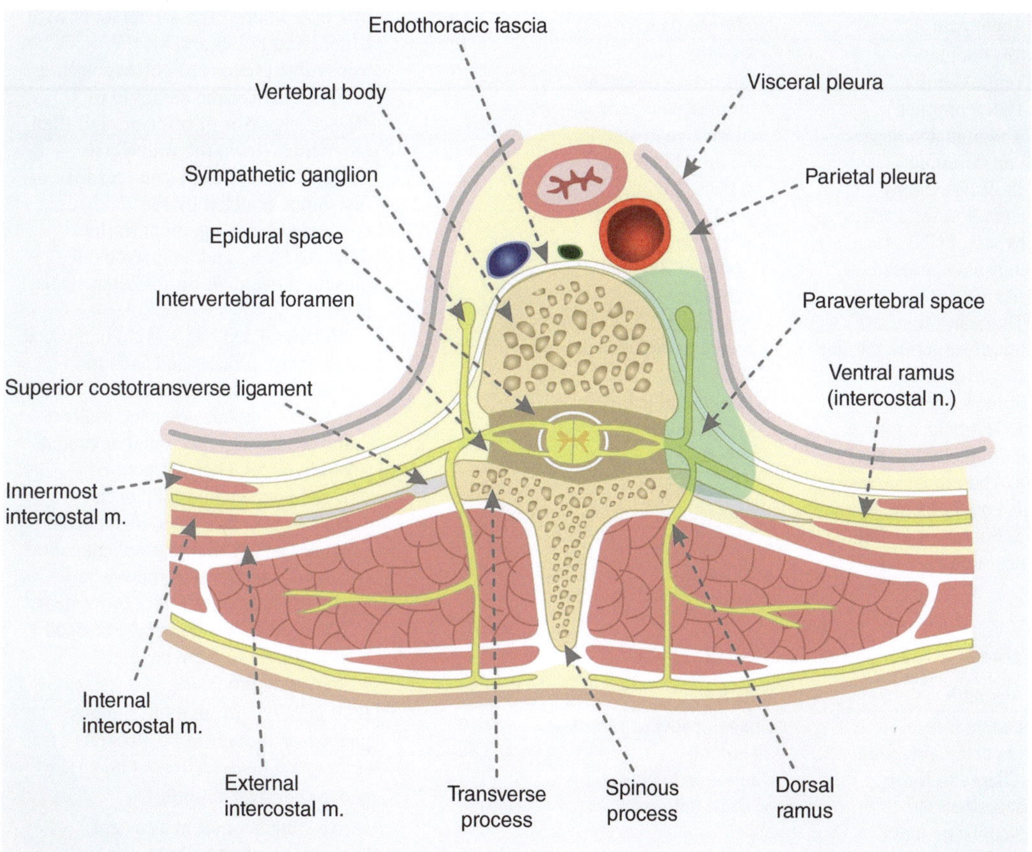

Fig. 8.4 Boundaries of thoracic paravertebral space

parts; the anterior part originates from the anterolateral part of vertebral bodies and the accessory psoas muscle originates from a transverse process. The lumbar spinal nerve roots are located in the triangle-shaped area between the two psoas muscle sections. The epidural space and the lumbar paravertebral space communicate.

8.5.2 Indications

(Table 8.2 Indications of PVB).

8.5.3 Contraindications

Contraindications of PVB (Table 8.3).

Table 8.2 Indications of PVB

Acute pain	Chronic pain
Rib fractures Ventral hernia Thoracotomies Abdominal surgeries: Laparoscopic cholecystectomy, laparotomies, gastric bypass, PCNL, renal transplant, caesarean section Thoracic surgeries: VATS, breast surgeries, cardiac surgeries Spine surgeries 1. Thoracic surgeries 2. Flail chest trauma 3. Abdominal surgeries 4. Post-herpetic neuralgias 5. Benign or malignant neuralgia	Shoulder pain Refractory headache Lumbar pain as an alternative to anterior epidural block for patients having radiculopathy pain, facet joint pain etc. Complex Regional Pain Syndrome Neuralgias-postherpetic, benign/malignant Myofascial pain Treatment of hyperhidrosis

Table 8.3 Contraindications of PVB

Absolute	Relative
Patient refusal Local site infection Allergy to local anaesthetics Neoplastic mass occupying paravertebral space	Coagulopathy or bleeding disorder Caution in kyphoscoliosis or spine deformity

8.5.4 Approaches to Block

8.5.4.1 Landmark Technique of Paravertebral Block

Landmark/PNS-guided PV Block (Table 8.4).

Table 8.4 Landmark/PNS-guided PV Block

Position	Sitting, lateral, or prone position
Landmark (Fig. 8.5)	Under all aseptic precautions palpate and identify the spinous process and draw a vertical line joining the vertebral spinous processes (Line 1) Draw a line parallel to line 1 at a distance of 2–2.5 cm (Line 2) Required vertebral level can be identified by counting above from tuffier line (L4 level) or counting below from C7 (the most prominent cervical vertebra) Then at required level transverse line is drawn transecting the 2 lines (Line 3) Insert the needle perpendicularly at junction where Line 4 intersects with Line 2 and line 3 and hit the transverse process of corresponding vertebra then make an angle of 10–15° superior or inferior, and then move away from the transverse process' border until you feel loss of resistance (caused by the costotransverse ligament in the thoracic PVB) and/or intercostal muscle movement on ipsilateral side (Tips Maximum depth is 3–4 cm in thoracic transverse process and 5–6 cm in lumbar transverse process If there is no bony contact, redirect the needle slightly cranial or caudal until you hit a bony structure If adequate intercostal muscle response is not elicited then needle should be slightly adjusted cranial or caudal at the level of transverse process to achieve motor movement The needle should not be advanced more than 1–1.5 cm beyond transverse process)
POE	POE is 2–2.5 cm lateral to spinous process on the side to be blocked
Needle	A 22 G Touhy or 8–10 cm long, 21–22 gauge short-bevel needle
PNS stimulation	Nerve stimulator set at a current intensity of 1.5 mA (2 Hz, 0.1–0.3 msec)

(continued)

Table 8.4 (continued)

End point	Feeling of loss of resistance in landmark-guided block and initiation of motor response in chest wall (intercostal muscle movement) is elicited at a current of <0.5 mA and > 0.3 mA. The local anaesthetic drug is injected and after 1–2 ml there is reduction in motor movement
Drug dosage	After negative aspiration, in a single shot block 2.5 ml for one level or 10 ml for 2–3 thoracic levels is administered. Drugs used are 0.25–0.5% bupivacaine or levobupivacaine, 0.2–0.5% ropivacaine, 1–2% lignocaine with epinephrine 1:2,00,000–1:4,00,000 It is estimated that 4–6 dermatomes will be blocked with injection of 20 ml local anaesthetic
Highlights	A continuous technique may be used by putting an epidural catheter or commercial perineural catheter. For catheter technique an initial priming of the paravertebral space is required with 5–10 ml of normal saline or 5% dextrose

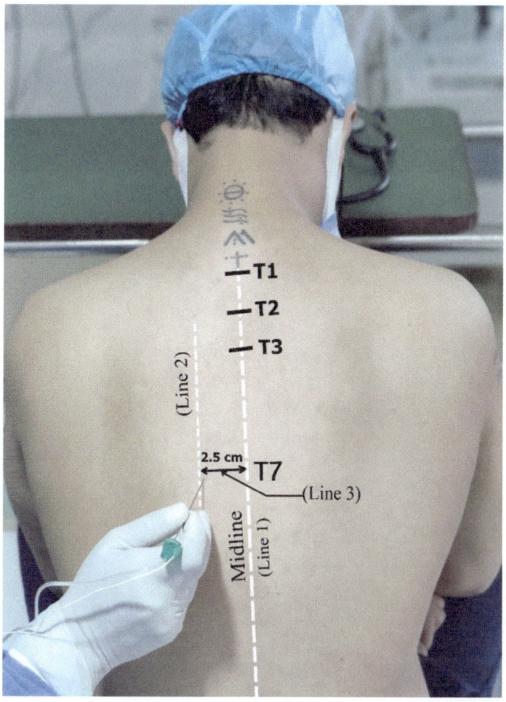

Fig. 8.5 Landmark/PNS-guided paravertebral block

8.5.4.2 Troubleshooting

The performer should be informed that the catheter was placed intrapleurally rather than in the paravertebral space if there was an unexpected smooth insertion of >6 cm and respiratory difficulties. To prevent migration into the epidural region, the catheter should not be put deeper than 3 cm into the paravertebral space.

8.5.4.3 Ultrasound Technique of Paravertebral Block

Ultrasound approach of PV block (Table 8.5).

8.5.4.4 Troubleshooting

Parasagittal Approach

1. Compared to transverse approach, the parasagittal approach has a lower risk for epidural migration.
2. Real-time injection of drugs prevents neurological injury, vascular injury, and pneumothorax.
3. Do not place the needle too medially or inject a larger volume > 25 ml at one level, as it may cause intrathecal drug spread.

Transverse Approach

1. Avoid puncturing the pleura when needle is placed too lateral from transverse process or entering into epidural or subarachnoid space by placing the needle too medially from transverse process. The ideal needle position is on the lateral one-third side of transverse process. Do not advance the needle blindly.
2. Inadvertent pleural puncture can present as cough, onset of sharp chest pain or shoulder pain or sudden hyperventilation. Sometimes pneumothorax may be delayed and hence an early chest X-ray may not be conclusive.
3. Intravascular injection may be detected with the use of epinephrine containing local anaesthetic solution. Avoid high volumes in upper thoracic paravertebral blocks as the drug may ascend and cause Horner's syndrome due to stellate ganglion block.
4. In lumbar PVB visceral injury or intraperitoneal injection of drug is possible. Motor weakness may occur if the L2 spinal nerve is blocked.

Table 8.5 Ultrasound approach of PV block

Position	Sitting or lateral or prone position	
USG Scanning Landmark	The selected PVB space is prepared under strict asepsis and high frequency linear (10–15 MHz) probe in average built and a low-frequency curvilinear (2–5 MHz) probe in obese patients is used.	
	Parasagittal approach—Probe is placed in craniocaudal orientation over the spinous process of the target paravertebral space. The probe is moved laterally in paramedian sagittal position (2–3 cm lateral to the midline) 1. *In thoracic* region and various structures identified from skin inwards are skin subcutaneous tissue trapezius muscle, Rhomboid muscle, erector spinae muscle, and hyperechoic transverse processes showing acoustic shadow anterior to it. An acoustic window is produced by reflections from the Superior costo transverse ligament and intertransverse ligaments, the paravertebral space and its contents between two adjacent transverse processes. From posterior to anterior external and internal intercostal muscles, the hyperechoic parietal pleura (sliding sign is seen), and lung tissue are seen between ribs (Fig. 8.6a–d) ↓ The needle is placed in a caudal to cephalad trajectory for in-plane technique. The superior costotransverse ligament must be traversed once the needle has made contact with the transverse process. One will experience a "pop" or loss of resistance -For out-of-plane technique, needle tip position can be identified by tissue hydrosection 2. *In lumbar spine*, laminar process is seen as a "saw tooth" or "Horse Heads" and the hyperechoic line is not continuous. Moving more laterally, transverse process in lumbar area is seen as "Trident sign" representing as finger-like shadows behind the transverse process (Fig. 8.6e–g). The needle is inserted, touches the transverse process, and then dips into the paravertebral space, penetrates, and a loss of resistance or "pop" will be felt	*Transverse approach*—The probe is kept in the transverse and partial oblique plane in midline spine of the target paravertebral space 1. *In thoracic* region from posterior to anterior the paraspinal muscles, the hyperechoic transverse process, lateral to transverse process hyperechoic pleura showing "lung sliding sign" is seen The apex of thoracic paravertebral space is visualised as hypoechoic space between parietal pleura and internal intercostal muscle which continues medially with superior costotransverse ligament. This space communicates with posterior intercostal space hence drugs once injected can spread laterally ↓ A slight cephalad or caudad movement of ultrasound probe results in disappearance of ribs and the image shows only transverse process and pleura. After stabilising the hand, the needle is quickly entered from lateral (approximately 4 cm from midline) to medial so that the tip is underneath the transverse process traversing internal intercostal muscles and if it is not identified needle tip is positioned just posterior to parietal pleura (Fig. 8.6h–k) For *out-of-plane* technique probe is not moved cranially or caudally needle is inserted from middle of probe in a slight cephalad direction till needle tip is just lateral to transverse process positioned just posterior to parietal pleura 2. In *lumbar spine*, probe is placed horizontally over vertebral spinous process of target area and moved laterally, lamina is seen as hyperechoic flat line followed by tip of transverse process covered by erector spinae muscle (Fig. 8.11c) The tip of transverse process is marked on skin and probe is rotated to 90^0 (craniocaudal direction) keeping the transverse process in midpoint and identify the "Trident sign" and follow steps as in parasagittal lumbar approach (Fig. 8.6e–g)
	(Tips—Whilst transverse processes seem flat, with squared-off acoustic shadows and less apparent surrounding pleura, ribs appear circular, thin, and surrounded by pleura Avoid too lateral movement as the ribs are seen as rounded shadows and pleura can be seen as sliding signs—Needle should not be advanced beyond 1–1.5 cm below the transverse process. When superior costotransverse ligament is not seen the needle is placed just posterior to parietal pleura Needle may not be visible even in "in plane" technique as the angle is very steep, so tissue hydrosection with normal saline to identify the tip of needle Incorrect placement of the needle tip results in a lack of anterior movement of the parietal pleura after local anaesthetic injection)	

(continued)

Table 8.5 (continued)

POE	Needle is inserted in either in-plane (caudal to cephalad) or out-of-plane approach (visualised only as a bright spot)	Needle is inserted in either in-plane (lateral to medial) or out-of-plane approach (visualised only as a bright spot)
Needle	A 22-G Touhy needle or a 10-cm long, short-bevel echogenic, insulated stimulating needle	
PNS stimulation	Can be used along with USG (0.5 mA, 0.1 ms)	
End point	Feeling of "POP", motor stimulation of intercostal/paraspinal muscles associated with sensory stimulation or paresthesia in the respective area, widening of the contiguous paravertebral spaces/pushing of parietal pleura anteriorly in real-time imaging by LA	
Drug dosage	After negative aspiration, in a single shot block 2.5 ml for one level or 10 ml for 2–3 thoracic levels is administered. Drugs used are 0.25–0.5% bupivacaine or levobupivacaine, 0.2–0.5% ropivacaine, 1–2% lignocaine with epinephrine 1:2,00,000–1:4,00,000 It is estimated that 4–6 dermatomes will be blocked with an injection of 20 ml local anaesthetic	
Mechanism of action	Exact mechanism is unclear. The drug may remain in the paravertebral space or spread into intercostal space laterally, medial epidural space, or in in contiguous space above and below or in combination	
Highlights	A continuous technique may be used by putting an epidural catheter or commercial perineural catheter preferably done in "in plane" technique. For catheter technique, an initial priming of the paravertebral space is required with 5–10 ml of normal saline or 5% dextrose An initial bolus of 5 ml is followed by an infusion of 0.1–0.2 ml/kg/h of local anaesthetic with sensory dosage, which may last for 3–4 days If significant area analgesia is necessary, it is advised to do multiple-level paravertebral blocks a few segments apart rather than quantities greater than 25 ml at a single level Bilateral thoracic PVB can be done if needed like in patients on anticoagulants	

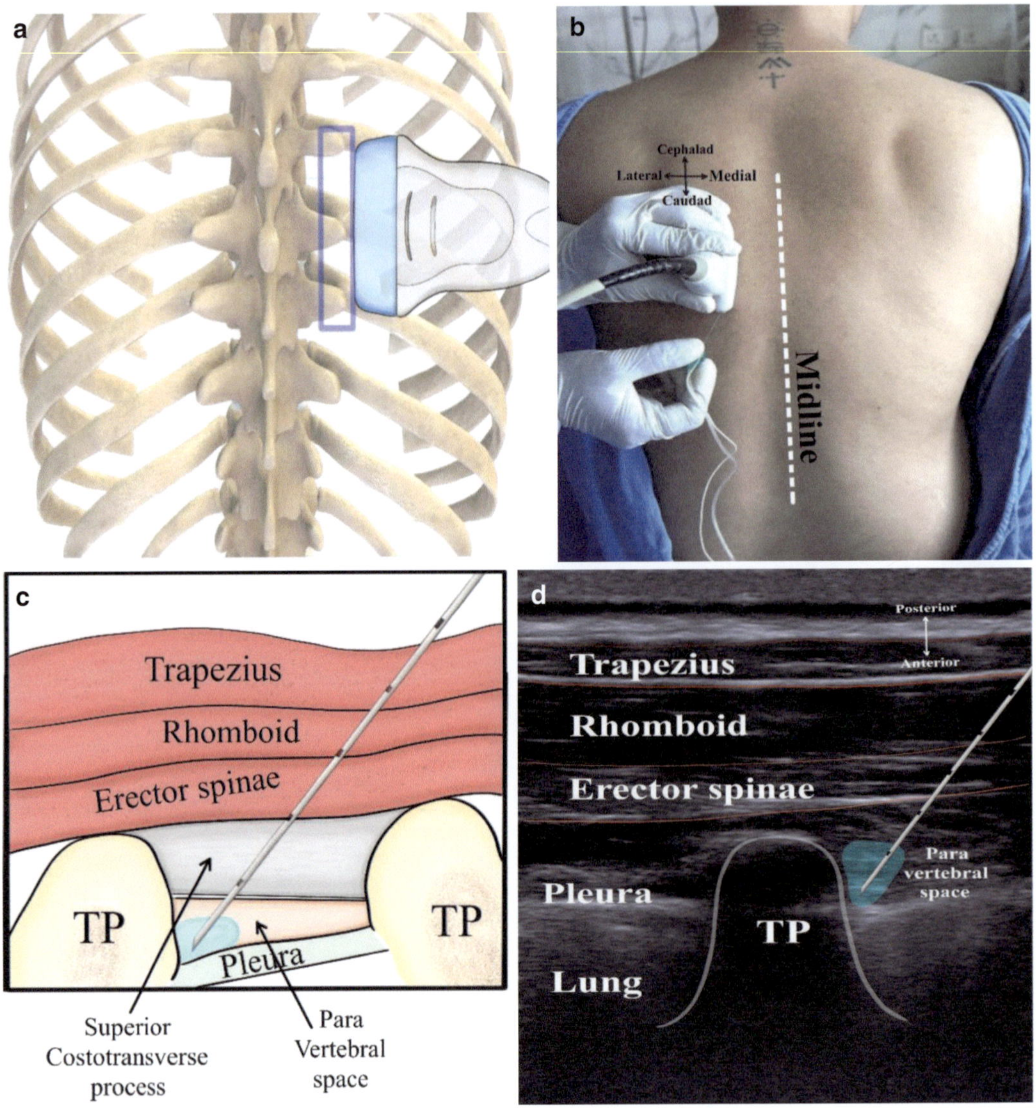

Fig. 8.6 (**a**) Anatomy of thoracic vertebrae with parasagittal probe position. (**b**) Probe position for Paravertebral block via parasagittal approach in thoracic region, (**c**) Schematic representation of parasagittal position of probe showing transverse process(TP) and pleura, paraspinal muscles, and needle is inserted with caudal to cranial trajectory via in-plane approach in paravertebral space (PVS). (**d**) USG image of needle in PVS in parasagittal plane. (**e**) Anatomy of lumbar spine with probe position in lateral position. (**f**) Probe position in parasagittal plane. (**g**) Sonoanatomy showing trident sign with transverse process and erector spinae muscle above it and psoas major muscle between the two transverse processes. Position of needle and drug is seen in in-plane technique. (**h**) Anatomy of thoracic vertebrae and probe position posteriorly in transverse approach, (**i**) Probe position on patient, (**j**) The probe is kept in the transverse plane in midline spine and the ultrasound image shows spinous process (SP), lamina and transverse process (TP), (**k**) On moving the probe laterally transverse process (TP), costotransverse ligament, intercostal muscles is visualised along with the paravertebral space. The needle penetrates the superior costotransverse ligament to enter paravertebral space

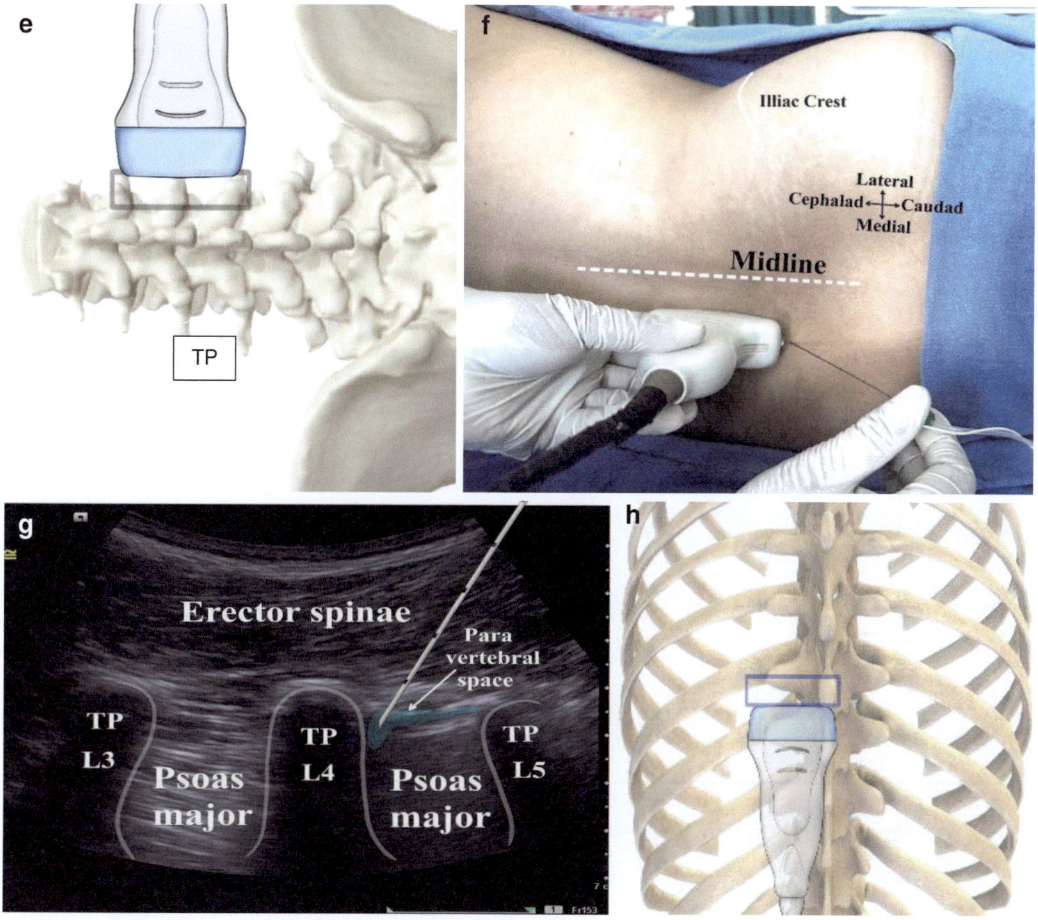

Fig. 8.6 (continued)

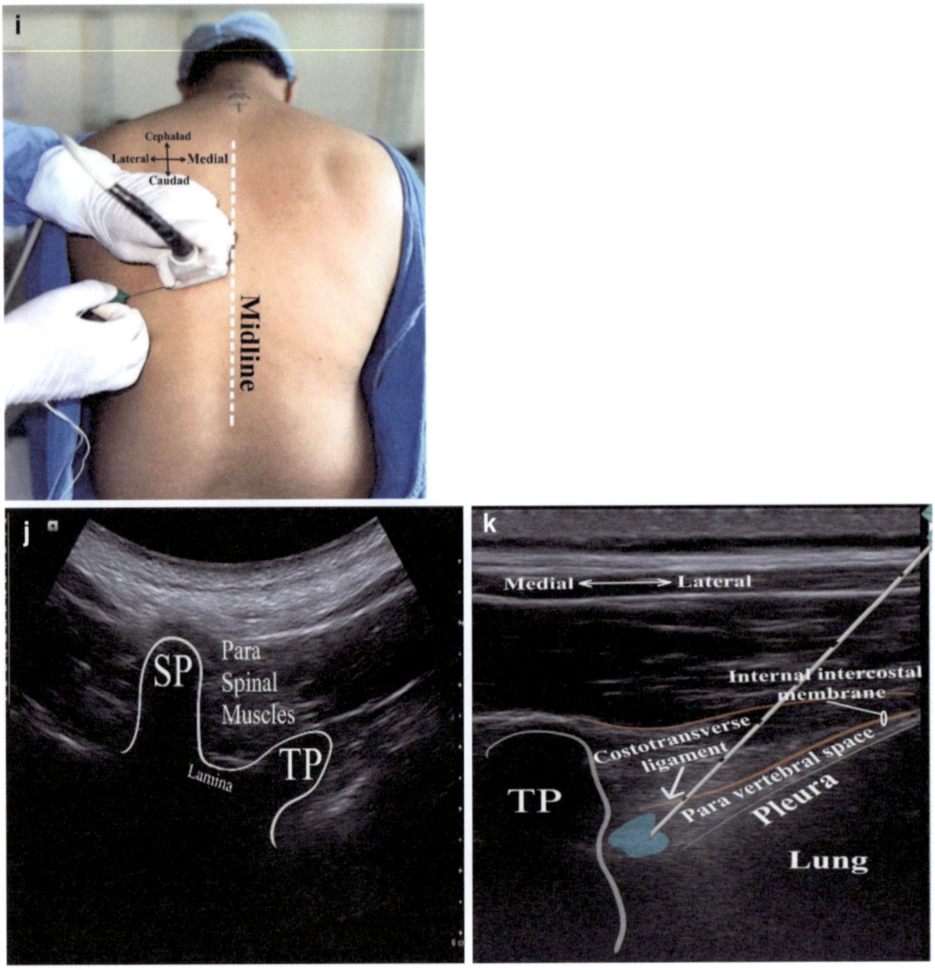

Fig. 8.6 (continued)

8.5.5 Complications

Complications are low from 2.6% to 5%.

- Hypotension—Though relatively low in normovolemic patients as sympathetic block occurs unilaterally.
- Vascular injury can lead to LAST which can be prevented by aspirating and giving drugs in small aliquots and using epinephrine-containing local anaesthetic solution.
- Pleural puncture.
- Pneumothorax.
- Intrathecal or epidural spread.
- Transient ipsilateral Horner syndrome due to cephalad spread.

8.6 Erector Spinae Muscle Plane (ESP) Block

ESP is a confluence of three muscles starting from medial to lateral spinalis, longissimus, and iliocostalis muscles. The muscle is covered with an intermediate layer of TLF on anterior surface and posterior layer of TLF on the posterior surface of erector spinae muscle. ESP can be performed at thoracic, lumbar, and sacral levels. The most commonly used level in thoracic ESP is at or above T5 for thoracic surgeries, T9 level for lower thoracic and upper abdominal surgeries. A level of L3 and sacral S2 level can be used in patients presenting with chronic pain and for patients who are not willing or having contraindications to neuraxial procedures.

8.6.1 Indications

Indications of ESP block (Table 8.6).

8.6.2 Contraindications

Same as Table 8.3.

8.6.3 Block Approaches

8.6.3.1 Landmark and PNS Technique of ESP Block

Landmark and PNS technique of ESP block (Table 8.7).

8.6.3.2 USG-Guided ESP Block

Ultrasound approach of ESP block (Table 8.8).

Table 8.6 Indications of ESP block

Acute pain	Chronic pain
Rib fractures Ventral hernia Thoracotomies Abdominal surgeries: Laparoscopic cholecystectomy, laparotomies, gastric bypass, PCNL, renal transplant, caesarean section Thoracic surgeries: VATS, breast surgeries, cardiac surgeries Sacral ESPB–analgesia for perineal surgeries and radicular pain Spine surgeries	Shoulder pain Refractory headache Lumbar pain as an alternative to anterior epidural block for patients having radiculopathy pain, facet joint pain etc. Complex Regional Pain Syndrome Neuralgias Myofascial pain

Table 8.7 Landmark and PNS technique of ESP block

Position	Sitting, lateral, or prone position
Landmark (Fig. 8.7)	Under all aseptic precautions palpate and identify the spinous process and draw a vertical line joining the vertebral spinous processes (Line 1) Draw a line parallel to line 1 on either side at a distance of 2.5–3 cm (Line 2 and Line 3) Required vertebral level can be identified by counting above from tuffier line (L4 level) or counting below from C7 (the most prominent cervical vertebra) Then at the required level transverse line is drawn transecting all three lines (Line 4) Insert the needle perpendicularly at junction where Line 4 intersects with Line 2 and Line 3 and hit the transverse process of corresponding vertebra (Tips Maximum depth is 3–4 cm in the thoracic transverse process and 5–6 cm in the lumbar transverse process If there is no bony contact, redirect the needle slightly cranial or caudal until you hit a bony structure Multiple manipulations should not be done and avoid greater depth)
POE	POE is 2.5–3 cm lateral to spinous process on the side to be blocked
Needle	A 5–10 cm long, 21–22 gauge short-bevel needle
PNS stimulation	Nerve stimulator set at a current intensity of 1.5 mA (2 Hz, 0.1–0.3 msec)
End point	To hit the corresponding transverse process and subsequently on motor stimulation, paraspinal muscle movement occurs at a current of 0.5 mA. After negative aspiration, 20 ml of local anaesthetic solution is injected in 5 ml aliquots, and observe reduction in muscle twitches
Drug dosage	20 ml of drug injected after negative aspiration.0.25–0.5% bupivacaine or levobupivacaine, 0.2–0.5% ropivacaine, 1–2% lignocaine with epinephrine 1:2,00,000–1:4,00,000
Highlights	Level chosen for thoracic indications is between T2 and T5, for abdominal pelvic indications between T7 and T10, for Spine surgery (mid-point of levels involved), for total hip replacement at L4 or L5 The volume of solution required to cover one vertebral level in thoracic region is 2.5 ml and 5 ml in the lumbar region. On an average, 3.3 ml of solution will cover one vertebral level during ESPB

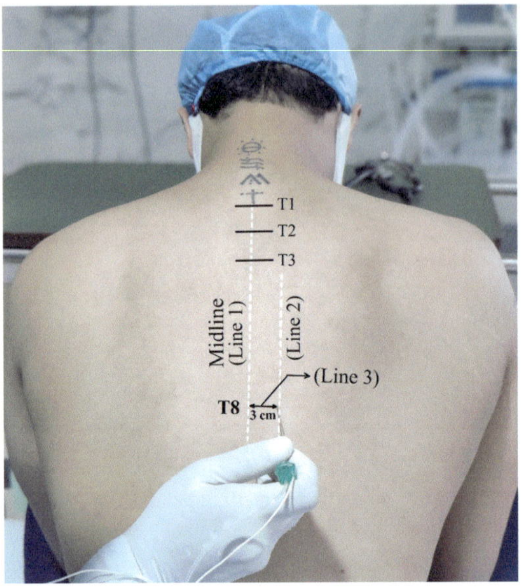

Fig. 8.7 Landmark/PNS-guided ESP block

8.6.4 Other Modifications of Lumbar ESP Block

1. *Aksu technique (Transverse subcostal approach)*: It involves placing the patient in a lateral decubitus position, and using "Shamrock" technique needle is inserted from the lateral to medial side in in-plane approach, and final position of the needle is anterior to the erector spinae muscle (Fig. 8.9a, b).
2. *Tulgar approach*: With the patient in a lateral decubitus position, the medication is deposited between the transverse process and the psoas muscle in addition to classical deposition of drug between TP and erector spinae muscle. This has the additional benefit of being close to the lumbar plexus (Fig. 8.10a, b).

8.6.5 Troubleshooting

- In high-risk patients with coagulopathy who are contraindicated to more invasive operations such as neuraxial procedures, ESP block is safer and is linked with lower risk than PVB.
- If the bony transverse process is not felt within 3–4 cm in thoracic and 5–6 cm in lumbar area then reposition the needle cranial or caudal until the transverse process is hit.

8.6.6 Continuous ESP Block

Indicated for prolonged analgesia in rib fractures, cardiac and thoracic surgeries, and in chronic pain syndromes.

Technique—The catheter is placed using the same technique as mentioned above by putting catheter through the needle using a Touhy needle or catheter over the needle.

Tips

- The angle of needle should be steeper than single shot technique for smooth insertion of catheter.
- The needle bevel should face up after hitting the TP which helps in advancing catheter beyond needle tip.
- Before introducing the catheter 1–3 ml of saline is given for hydrodissection which lifts the erector spinae fascia and helps in easy negotiation of catheter.
- The catheter is advanced 2–5 cm beyond needle tip.
- Always confirm the placement of catheter tip by giving saline under USG guidance.

Infusion Drug Dose

Ropivacaine 0.2% 8–12 mL per hour, with or without a 10-mL patient demand dosage, with a 60-min lockout interval.

8.6.7 Complications

Complications are rare. Likely complications are:

- Pneumothorax after thoracic ESP block.
- Local anaesthetic systemic toxicity (LAST). It occurs due to the high vascularity of the erector spinae muscle, substantial volumes of drug used, large area of drug spread making more tissue contact. Close proximity of the block to the intercostal spaces in the thoracic region lead to increased chances of drug absorption.

Table 8.8 Ultrasound approach of ESP block

Position	Sitting or lateral or prone position	
USG scanning landmark	The selected space is prepared under strict asepsis and high frequency linear (10–15 MHz) probe in average built and low frequency curvilinear (2–5 MHz) probe in obese patients are used	
	Parasagittal approach—Probe is placed in craniocaudal orientation over the spine of the target paravertebral space. The probe is moved laterally in a paramedian sagittal position (2–3 cm lateral to the midline) 1. *In thoracic* region, various structures identified from skin inwards are skin subcutaneous tissue trapezius muscle, Rhomboid muscle, erector spinae muscle, and hyperechoic ribs with external and internal intercostal muscle in between ribs. The hyperechoic pleura is seen below the ribs and internal intercostal muscle Probe is moved from lateral to medial direction until triangular-shaped costotransverse joint is identified. With slight further medial movement of probe, there is clear transition from rounded rib shadow to a flat transverse process with paraspinal muscles over it. (Fig. 8.8a–c) The needle is placed in a caudal to cephalad and vice versa trajectory for in-plane technique till it hits the target transverse process For out of plane technique needle tip position can be identified by tissue hydrosection 2. *In lumbar spine*, laminar process is seen as "saw tooth" or "Horse Heads" and the hyperechoic line is not continuous. Moving more laterally, transverse process in lumbar area is seen as "Trident sign" representing as finger-like shadows behind the transverse process. The needle is inserted in an in-plane or out-of-plane technique till it hits the transverse process (Fig. 8.8d–g)	*Transverse approach* -: The probe is kept in the transverse and partial oblique plane in midline spine of the target space. 1. *In thoracic* region, from posterior to anterior the paraspinal muscles, the hyperechoic transverse process, and lateral to transverse process hyperechoic pleura show "lung sliding sign" is seen. When both transverse process and ribs are seen simultaneously a slight cephalad or caudad movement of ultrasound probe results in disappearance of ribs and image shows only transverse process and pleura The needle is inserted in in-plane technique from lateral to medial direction till it contacts with lateral end of transverse process, withdrawn 1–2 mm, and inject the drug (Fig. 8.8h,i) 2. In *lumbar spine*, probe is placed horizontally over vertebral spinous process of target area and moved laterally, lamina is seen as hyperechoic flat line followed by tip of transverse process covered by erector spinae muscle (Fig. 8.11c) The tip of transverse process is marked on skin and probe is rotated to 90^0 (craniocaudal direction) keeping the transverse process in midpoint. "Trident sign" of transverse process is seen and the needle is inserted in an in-plane or out-of-plane technique till it hits the transverse process (Fig. 8.8g)
	(Tips—Whilst transverse processes seem superficial, flat, with squared-off acoustic shadows and less apparent surrounding pleura, ribs will be dipper, appear circular, thin, and surrounded by pleura. Identification of target thoracic transverse process can be done by counting ribs starting from first rib keeping USG probe in parasagittal plane in cranio caudal direction at a distance of 5–6 cm from midline. Avoid too lateral movement as then ribs are seen as rounded shadows and pleura can be seen as sliding sign. Too medial placement of probe will show hyperechoic flat vertebral lamina. Needle should not be advanced beyond the transverse process. Sometimes needle may not be visible even in "in plane" technique as the angle is very steep, so tissue hydrosection with normal saline to identify the tip of needle).	
POE	Needle is inserted in either in-plane (cephalad to caudal) or out-of-plane approach (visualised only as a bright spot)	Needle is inserted in an in-plane approach from lateral to medial direction
Needle	A 22 G Touhy needle or a 10-cm long short-bevel 22 G echogenic stimulating needle	
PNS stimulation	Can be used along with USG (0.5 mA, 0.1 ms)	

Table 8.8 (continued)

End point	Drug to be deposited between anterior fascial sheath of erector spinae muscle and transverse process in 3–5 ml aliquots whilst visualising LA lifting the erector spinae muscle Motor stimulation of intercostal/paraspinal muscles associated with sensory stimulation or paresthesia in the respective area
Drug dosage	After negative aspiration, in a single shot block 20 ml of drug is injected. Drugs used are 0.25–0.5% bupivacaine or levobupivacaine, 0.2–0.5% ropivacaine, 1–2% lignocaine with epinephrine 1:2,00,000–1:4,00,000.
Mechanism of action:	Firstly, the drug enters the paravertebral space. Secondly, the drug may enter the fascial plane between the muscles and block the posterior rami of spinal nerves.
Highlights	A single bolus of 20–30 ml blocks 4 lumbar or 8 thoracic levels. Continuous infusion is given as 0.2% 8–10 ml/h with initial bolus of 5 ml and lock out interval of 60 min. The volume of solution required to cover one vertebral level in thoracic region is 2.5 ml and 5 ml in lumbar region. On an average, 3.3 ml of solution will cover one vertebral level during ESPB. In lumbar ESPB the transverse process is deeper and lateral as bulk of erector spinae muscle increases as compared to thoracic muscle. Bilateral ESPB can be done if needed like in patients on anticoagulants.

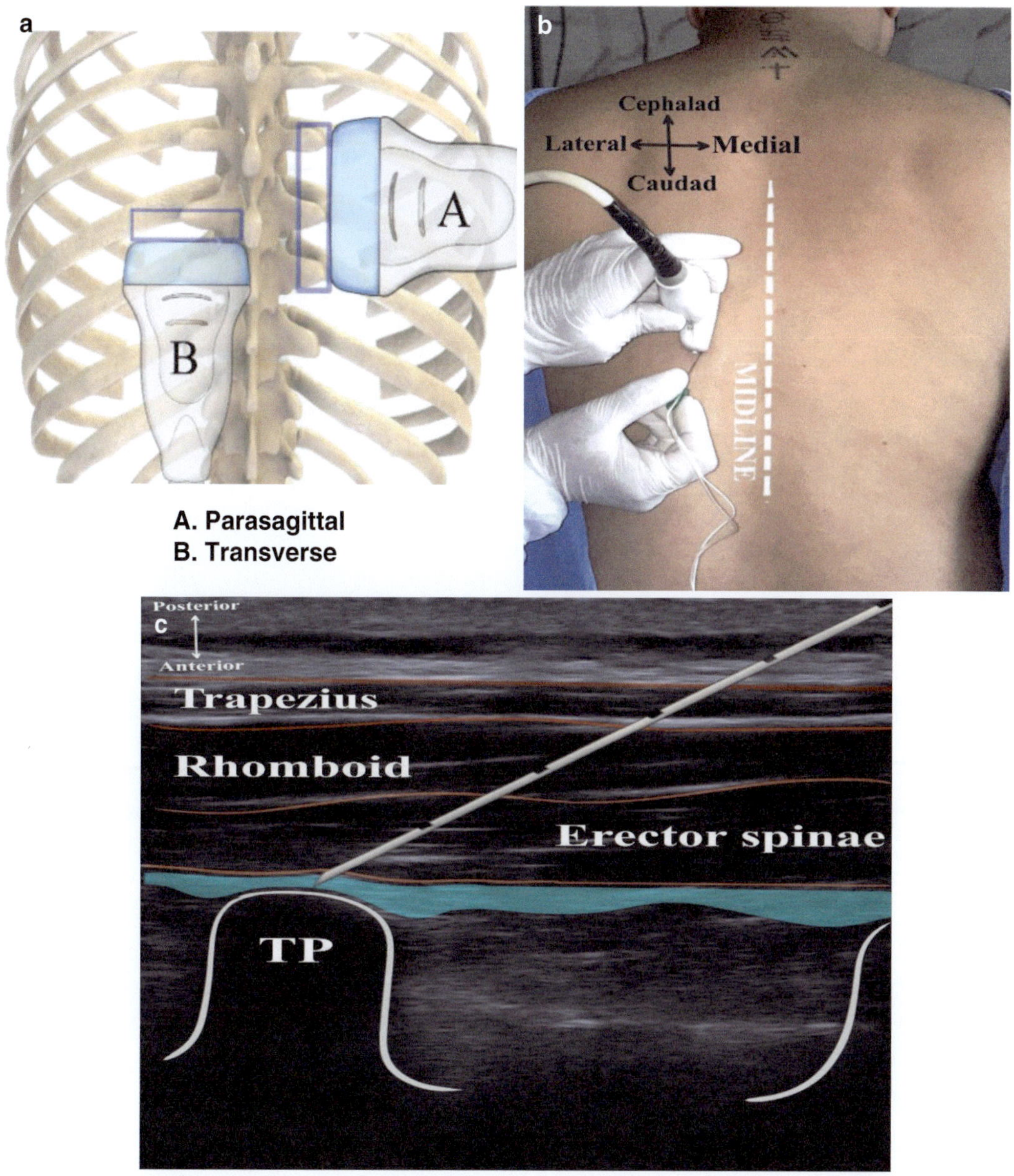

Fig. 8.8 (**a**) Anatomy of thoracic vertebrae and probe position (A. Parasagittal, B. Transverse). (**b**) Parasagittal probe position for parasagittal approach of ESP block. (**c**) USG image showing transverse process (TP), paraspinal muscles, and needle is inserted with caudal to cranial trajectory in in-plane technique just below anterior sheath of erector spinae muscle and above TP. (**d**) Anatomy of lumbar vertebrae and probe position posteriorly in parasagittal plane (A. Parasagittal, B. Transverse). (**e**) Probe position on patient for lumbar parasagittal ESPB. (**f**) Schematic representation of parasagittal position of probe showing erector spinae muscle and needle anterior to ES. (**g**) USG image showing "trident sign" of lumbar transverse process and needle is inserted from caudal to cranial direction in in-plane approach hitting the transverse process and depositing drug for parasagittal approach of ESP block. (**h**) Probe position on patient for thoracic transverse ESP approach. (**i**) USG image showing Transverse process (TP) with paraspinal muscles and pleura. The needle is inserted with caudal to cranial trajectory in in-plane approach hitting over the transverse process

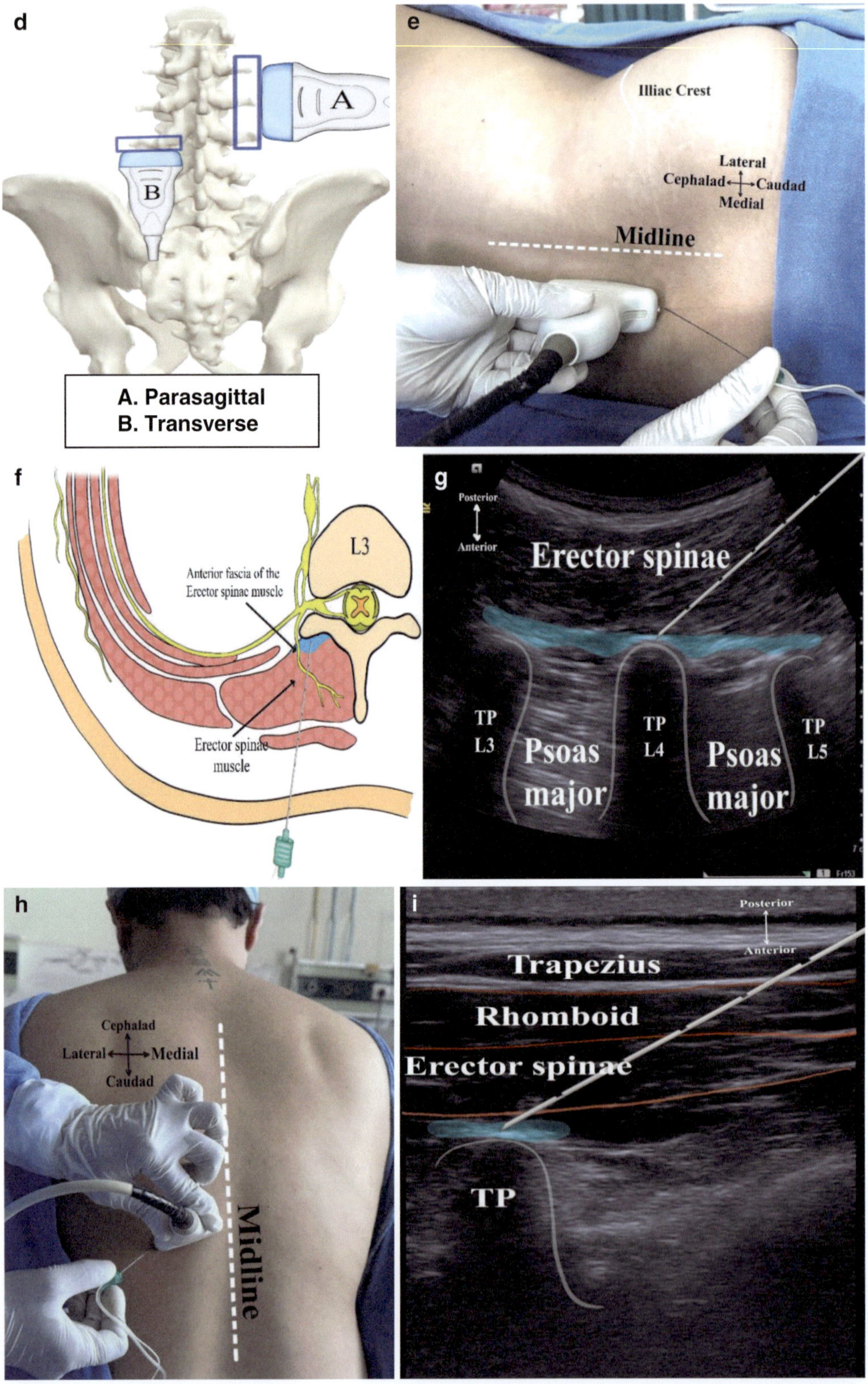

Fig. 8.8 (continued)

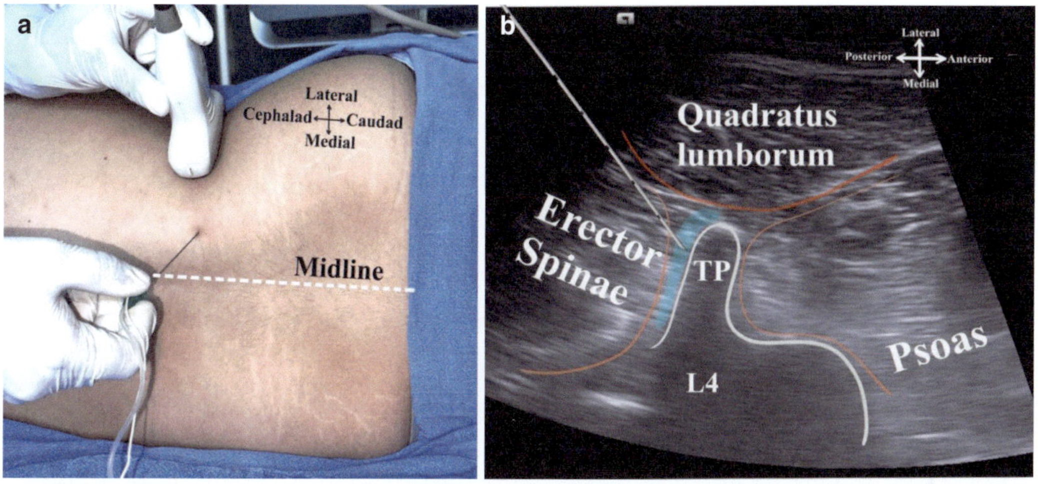

Fig. 8.9 (**a**) Probe and needle position in lateral position of patient for ESPB (*Akshu approach*). (**b**) Sonoanatomy showing erector spinae muscle and needle position with local anaesthetic shown in blue colour (*TP* transverse process)

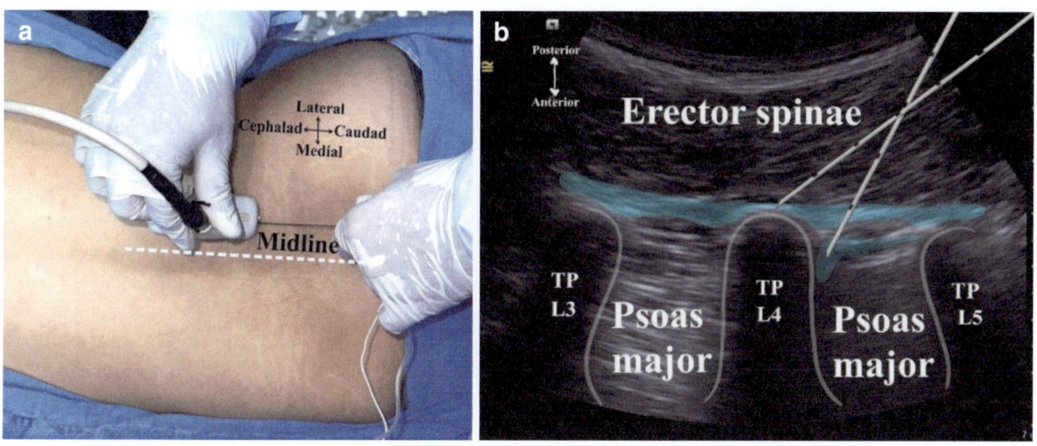

Fig. 8.10 (**a**) Probe and needle position in lateral position of patient for ESPB (*Tulgar approach*). (**b**) Sonoanatomy showing trident sign with transverse process (TP) and ES muscle above it and psoas major muscle between the two TPs. In the Tulgar approach, needle is inserted in plane from caudal to cranial direction and the drug is deposited both anterior to ES and between TP and the psoas major muscle

(The addition of epinephrine to the block solution reduce systemic absorption.)
- Bleeding.
- Infection.
- Sympathectomy is probably because of paravertebral spread.
- Harlequin syndrome (hemifacial erythema) may occur transiently with upper extremity.
- Diaphoresis and concomitant hypotension after a T3 level ESP block.
- Priapism due to bilateral paravertebral spread after a lumbar ESP block.

8.7 Retrolaminar Block (RLB)

Pfeiffer et al. introduced RLB, a more recent paravertebral strategy, in 2006. It is a method of local anaesthesia used to block the interfascial plane whilst using ultrasound imaging. The two pathways by which it functions are the paravertebral pathway, which involves both ventral and dorsal rami, and the lateral pathway, which involves the lateral cutaneous branch and tiny branches of intercostal nerves. Compared to paravertebral block and thoracic epidural anaesthesia, it has a benefit. By avoiding getting the needle tip too close to the spinal nerve roots or pleura, the treatment is made simpler and the danger of injury to those structures is decreased.

8.7.1 Indications

- Rib fractures.
- Thoracic surgery.
- Abdominal surgery.
- Thoracic/Lumbar spine surgery.

8.7.2 Contraindications

Same as Table 8.3.

8.7.3 Block Approaches

8.7.3.1 Landmark Technique RLB

Position: Lateral or prone position of patient.

Procedure: Under strict asepsis block needle is inserted perpendicular at a distance of 1–1.5 cm lateral to target spinous process and LA is injected on the lamina. At the T5 level, 20 ml has approximately 6–9 vertebral levels. Comparison of landmark technique of Retrolaminar block, Erector spinae plane block, and Paravertebral block (Table 8.9).

Drug: 0.25–0.5% bupivacaine or levobupivacaine, 0.2–0.5% ropivacaine, 1–2% lignocaine with epinephrine 1:2,00,000–1:4,00,000.

8.7.3.2 Ultrasound-Guided RLB

Ultrasound approach of RLB block (Table 8.10).

Table 8.9 Comparison of landmark technique of Retrolaminar block, Erector spinae plane block, and Paravertebral block

Parameters	Retrolaminar block	Erector spinae plane block	Paravertebral block
Needle placement	Needle is inserted perpendicular 1–1.5 cm lateral to spinous process and LA is injected on the lamina	Needle is inserted perpendicular 2–3 cm lateral to the spinous process and LA is injected on transverse process	Needle is inserted perpendicular 2–3 cm lateral to the spinous process, then needle is moved 10–15° cranial or caudal to walk off the transverse process and enter the paravertebral space
Costotransverse ligament	Does not pierce the costotransverse ligament	Does not pierce the costotransverse ligament	Pierces the costotransverse ligament
Spread of drug	The surface of the transversospinalis muscle, spread medially to the intertransverse ligament. At T5 level, 20 ml has craniocaudal spread approximately 6–9 vertebral levels	The surface of the external intercostal muscle, spread to iliocostalis muscle. At T5 level, 20 ml has craniocaudal spread of approximately 8–10 vertebral levels and in lumbar it is approximately 4–5 vertebral levels	20 ml has craniocaudal spread approximately 3–-7 vertebral levels
Nerve blocks	Dorsal rami occasionally ventral rami	Dorsal rami	Dorsal and ventral rami
Complications	Rare	Rare	Hypotension, pneumothorax, haematoma

Table 8.10 Ultrasound approach of RLB block

Position	Sitting, lateral, or prone position of patient
USG Scanning Landmark (Fig. 8.11)	Under all aseptic precautions, high-frequency linear (10–15 MHz) probe in average built and low-frequency curvilinear (2–5 MHz) probe in obese patients is placed in sagittal paramedian orientation 5–6 cm lateral to spinous process over the desired area of interest 1. Probe is moved from lateral to medial direction till triangular shaped costotransverse joint and transverse process are identified and with further medial movement of probe vertebral lamina comes into view as flat hyperechoic structures with facet joint as interposed notches. It can be performed by keeping probe in a transverse plane over target spinous process. Craniocaudal tilting of probe helps in identifying transverse process, lamina, and spinous process from lateral to medial direction. RLB can be done in both thoracic and lumbar regions (Fig. 8.11a–c) (Tip—In the thoracic region whilst transverse processes seem flat, with squared-off acoustic shadows and less apparent surrounding pleura, ribs appear circular, thin, and surrounded by pleura Identification of target thoracic transverse process can be done by counting ribs starting from first rib keeping USG probe in parasagittal plane in craniocaudal direction at a distance of 5–6 cm from midline)
POE	Needle is inserted in "in-plane approach" from caudal or cephalad direction till it contacts with lamina in the paramedian sagittal approach and from lateral to medial direction in transverse approach
Needle	A 10-cm long, 22 gauge short-bevel echogenic needle
End point	Drug is deposited between lamina and deep paraspinous muscles in 3–5 ml aliquots whilst visualising LA spread in real time and if there is resistance needle is withdrawn 1–3 mm and again drug is injected
Drug dosage	20 ml of 0.25–0.5% bupivacaine or levobupivacaine, 0.2–0.5% ropivacaine, 1–2% lignocaine with epinephrine 1:2,00,000–1:4,00,000 not to exceed maximum permissible dose for the patient
Mechanism of action	Injectate has variable anterior spread, posteriorly it spreads beneath the paraspinal muscles, median lateral spread is approximately 2.5 cm, and longitudinally median cephalad spread is 3.5 cm with a caudal spread of 10.7 cm from the retrolaminar space
Highlights	The area is determined as per the analgesia requirement. Most commonly described spine level areas are Thoracic T2 level and below and L1–L5 Correct needle tip position was confirmed by the injection of 5 ml of 0.9% normal saline and visualisation of linear fluid spread that distended the fascial plane between the erector spinae muscle and the lamina

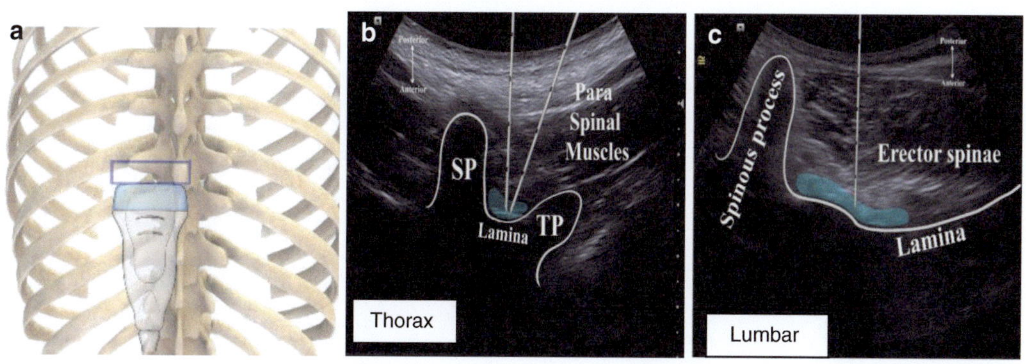

Fig. 8.11 (**a**) Patient position can be sitting or prone with probe in transverse position over target spine as shown in thorax region (similar approach for lumbar region). (**b**, **c**) Sonoanatomy of thorax and lumbar region in transverse orientation of probe and needle trajectory is seen perpendicular (out plane). The hyperechoic line seen is lamina LA is injected over lamina. In-plane approach can also be used (*SP* Spinous process, *TP* Transverse process)

8.7.4 Advantages

- RLB can be performed easily and safely under ultrasound guidance.
- No major vessels at the site of injection.
- Theoretically, RLB could reduce the risk of epidural haematoma, spinal cord and nerve injury, pneumothorax, and incidental epidural injection of local anaesthetics.

8.8 Intercostal Nerve Block

Intercostal nerve (ICN) is a mixed nerve and provides band-like analgesia. Intercostal nerve block anatomically provides similar pain relief as PVB but requires blocking of intercostal nerves at each level. The number of intercostal nerve blocks is determined by at least one rib above and one rib below the optimal location.

8.8.1 Anatomy

Inferior edge of the ribs can be used as a landmark to block intercostal nerves which lie at the angle of lower ribs 6–8 cm and 4–7 cm in upper ribs from the spinous process. The advantage is that at this site the rib is the most superficial and subcostal groove is the widest. In the subcostal groove of a rib the neurovascular bundle is arranged from most superior to inferior as intercostal vein, artery and nerve. This is sandwiched between internal intercostal and innermost intercostal muscle (Fig. 8.12).

8.8.2 Indications

- Rib fractures.
- Chest wall surgery.
- Upper abdominal surgery (somatic pain).
- Herpetic neuralgia.
- Chronic cancer pain.

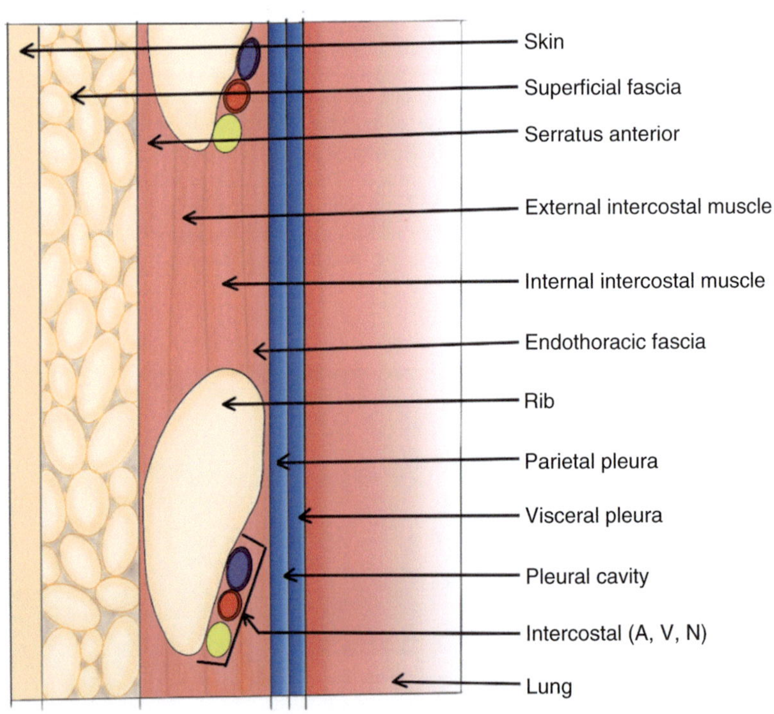

Fig. 8.12 Parasagittal anatomy of intercostal space

8.8.3 Contraindications

Same as Table 8.3.

8.8.4 Block Approaches

8.8.4.1 Landmark Technique of Intercostal Nerve Block

Landmark/PNS-guided Intercostal nerve block (Table 8.11).

Troubleshooting

- Do not advance the needle too deep (the average distance between rib and pleura is 8 mm) after hitting the inferior border of rib to prevent pneumothorax.
- To avoid misplacement of needle tip, it is advisable to attach an extension to the needle and aspiration is done by an assistant.
- T1–7 blocking of intercostal nerve block is technically challenging, due to presence of scapula and rhomboid muscle. So, an average distance for point of needle entry from spinous process taken is 4–6 cm.

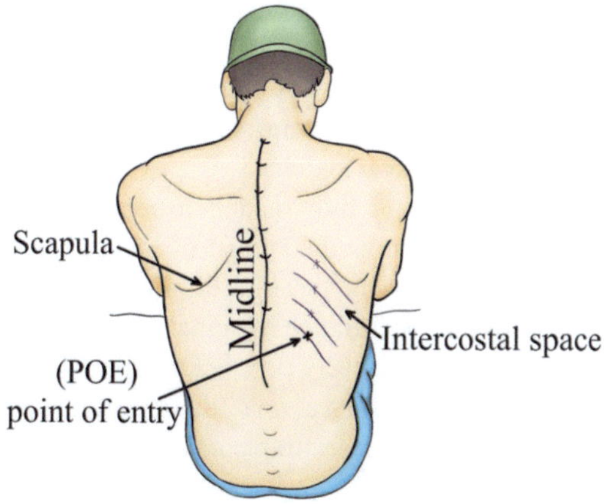

Fig. 8.13 Figure showing anatomical landmarks and POE of needle for Intercostal nerve block

Table 8.11 Landmark/PNS-guided Intercostal nerve block

Position	Sitting with leaning forward, lateral with block side up, or prone with arm hanging by the side
Landmark (Fig. 8.13)	Under all aseptic precautions palpate and identify the spinous process (T4 level) and inferior edge of scapula (T7 level) to mark the thoracic level At the required thoracic level, the rib is identified in parasagittal plane at a distance of 6–8 cm from spinous process or posterior midclavicular line or at the angle of rib The neurovascular bundle is found in groove on inferior border of ribs with a nerve in most inferior portion of groove after intercostal artery (Fig. 8.13) (Tips Lateral cutaneous branch of spinal nerve originates proximal to midaxillary line so ICN can be blocked anywhere proximal to it The subcostal groove is the widest at the angle of the rib, and also the rib is superficial and easy to palpate there)
POE and Technique	A 5-cm long, 21–22 gauge short-bevel needle is inserted at 20°, bevel facing cephalad and after hitting the lower border of rib it is advanced gently to "walk off" the rib a few "mm" to reach the subcostal groove. A "pop" is felt before entering the needle in subcostal groove due to piercing the fascia of the internal intercostal muscle
PNS stimulation	Nerve stimulator set at a current intensity of 1.5 mA (2 Hz, 0.1–0.3 msec)
End point	To feel the "pop" and subsequently on motor stimulation, thoracic muscle movement occurs at a current of 0.5 mA. After negative aspiration of blood, 3–5 ml of local anaesthetic is injected at each level (Tip—"Pop" may not be felt all the time Average distance from the posterior aspect of the rib to the pleura averages 8 mm, so avoid advancing the needle beyond a few mm to prevent the risk of pneumothorax)
Drug dosage	0.25–0.5% bupivacaine or levobupivacaine, 0.2–0.5% ropivacaine, 1–2% lignocaine with epinephrine 1:2,00,000–1:4,00,000
Highlights	Rib counting can be done by from below lower most rib as 12th rib. From lower angle of scapula, the corresponding vertebrae is T7, and this can be used to trace seventh rib

8.8.4.2 USG Technique of Intercostal Nerve Block

USG-guided intercostal nerve block (Table 8.12).

Troubleshooting

- Avoid crossing the maximum permissible dose of local anaesthetics. In combinations do not reach upper limit of both local anaesthetics, instead use adjuvants to avoid local systemic anaesthetic toxicity.
- Avoid injecting into medial aspect of ribs closer to spine as the spread of local anaesthetics may occur through dural sleeve and lead to rare occurrence of spinal block.
- Need to aspirate every time before injecting in small aliquots of local anaesthetic solution to avoid intravascular, intrapleural, or intrathecal injection.
- Patient should be monitored for up to 30 min to ensure absence of any complications and also establishment of analgesia following intercostal nerve block.

8.8.5 Complications

- Haematoma.
- Pneumothorax (1% cases), usually asymptomatic, needs reassurance and observation Rarely needs intercostal drainage.
- Risk of penetrating the peritoneum and abdominal viscera whilst performing lower ICN block.
- Local anaesthetic toxicity-Absorption from the intercostal space is rapid; arterial plasma concentration peaks in 5–10 min.
- Nerve damage and muscle trauma.
- Spinal cord injury may occur due to epidural or spinal spread or uptake of neurolytic agents like alcohol.
- Infection.

Table 8.12 USG-guided intercostal nerve block

Position	Sitting with leaning forward, lateral with block side up, or prone with arm hanging by the side
Landmark (Fig. 8.14a–c)	Under all aseptic precautions palpate and identify the required thoracic level as mentioned in landmark-guided technique The high-frequency linear probe is placed in the longitudinal axis in the midline and moved laterally approximately 4 cm till flat surface of transverse process changes to rounded shadow of ribs. The probe is placed in such a way that two ribs are seen in cross-sectional view Identify the external intercostal (EI) and internal intercostal (II) muscles in between the two ribs. At the inferior border intercostal vessels can be visualised. Anterior to ribs hyperechoic shadows of pleura with sliding sign is seen
POE (Fig. 8.14b, c)	The needle is inserted in plane (caudal to cranial direction) to transducer and the final needle tip is positioned between internal and innermost intercostal muscle or deep into internal intercostal muscle. Individual-level intercostal nerves need to be blocked
Needle	A 5–10 cm long, 21–22 gauge short-bevel needle
PNS stimulation	Nerve stimulator set at a current intensity of 1.5 mA (2 Hz, 0.1–0.3 msec)
End point	After negative aspiration 3–5 ml of LA is deposited at each level to be blocked between internal and innermost intercostal muscle
Drug dosage	0.25–0.5% bupivacaine or levobupivacaine, 0.2–0.5% ropivacaine, 1–2% lignocaine with epinephrine 1:2,00,000–1:4,00,000
Highlights	Rib counting can be done by from below lower most rib as 12th rib. From lower angle of scapula, corresponding vertebrae as T7, and this can be used to trace seventh rib

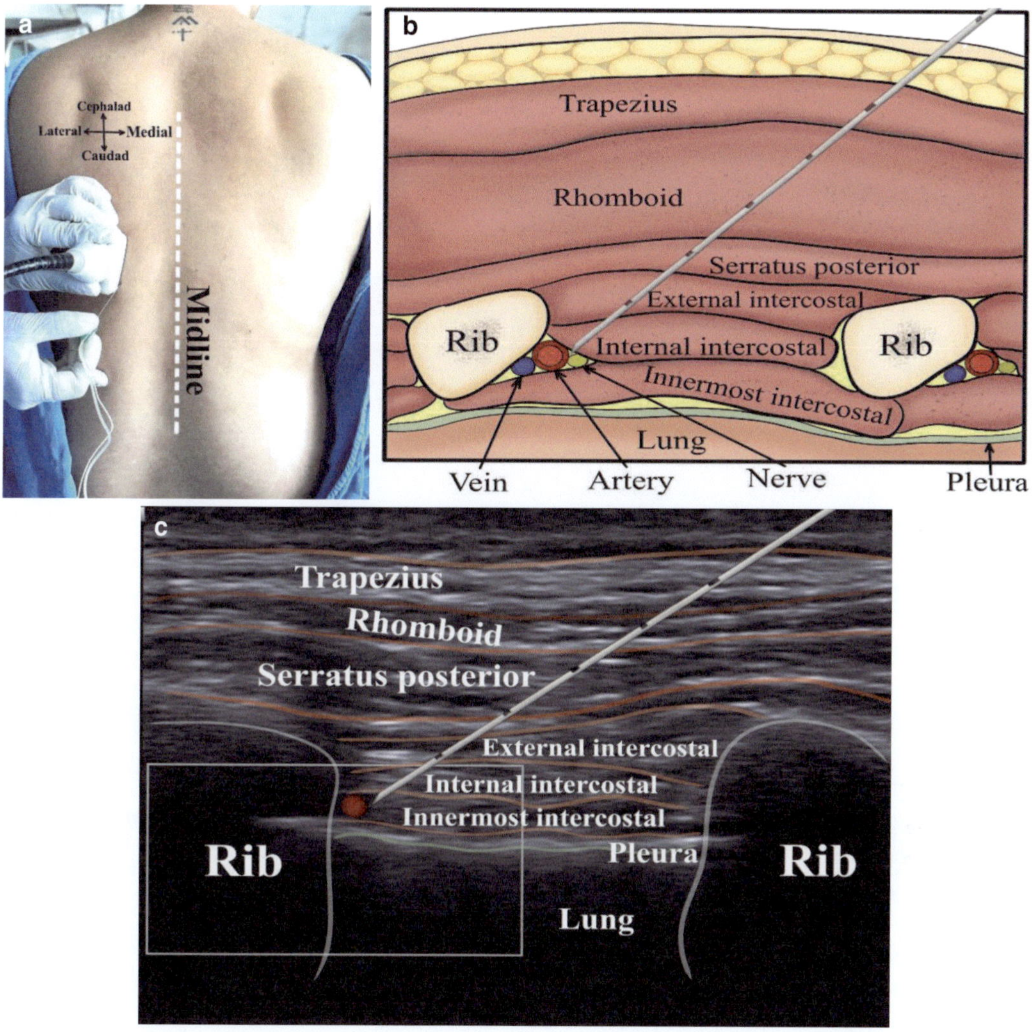

Fig. 8.14 (**a**) Patient and probe position for Intercostal nerve block. (**b**) Illustration of anatomy of intercostal muscles and nerve and needle position. (**c**) USG image of intercostal nerve block with final needle position

8.9 Quadratus Lumborum (QL) Block

The posterior transversus abdominis plane (TAP) block, sometimes referred to as the QL block, is a relatively novel method of regional analgesia. Blanco initially spoke of it in the year 2007.

8.9.1 Clinical Anatomic Correlation

The thoracolumbar fascia has three layers (Fig. 8.15).

- Anterior thoracolumbar fascia—encircles the anterior aspect of the QL and psoas muscles and continues laterally as the transversalis fascia.
- Intermediate/Middle thoracolumbar fascia—lies between the posterior surface of the QL muscle and the anterior surface of the erector spinae muscle.
- Posterior thoracolumbar fascial surrounds the erector spinae muscle. Transversus abdominis is traced more posteriorly till the transversus aponeurosis arises after recognising the three layers of abdominal wall muscles.

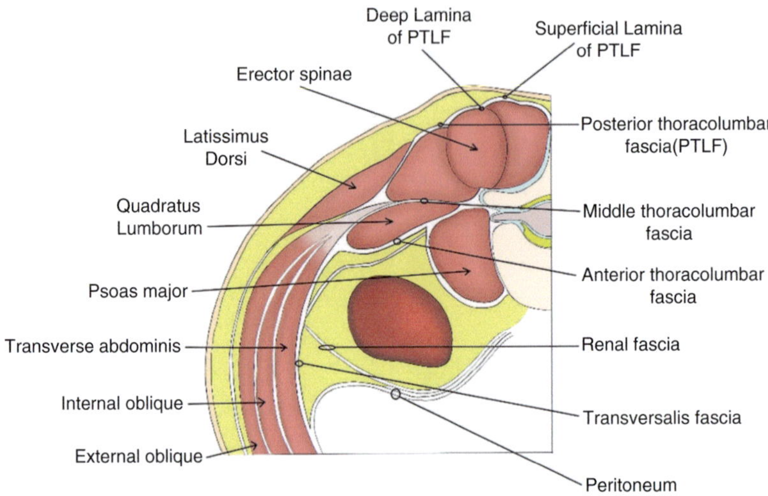

Fig. 8.15 Clinical anatomic correlation of QL muscle

The Lateral Interfascial Triangle (LIFT) is formed by:

Base by the lateral margin of the erector spinae muscle, sides by the deepest lamina of the posterior layer called the paraspinal retinacular sheath (PRS) with overlying posterior and middle layers of the TLF, and apex by the lateral raphe (Fig. 8.15).

The Shamrock sign and dorsi-planter flexion on stimulation of the same side of the block are used to identify the QL muscle.

According to the most recent research, there are four alternative methods for performing a QL block, namely a QL1 or lateral QLB, QL 2 block or posterior QLB, QL 3 block or an anterior (trans-muscular) QLB, and QL 4 or intramuscular QLB.

Table 8.15 shows different dermatomes covered by Quadratus Lumborum (QL) block.

8.9.2 Indications

The QLB produces a broad sensory coverage of approximately T6-L1 and may extend up to T4 in cephalad direction and can spread caudally till L3. QLBs can therefore be utilised to relieve abdominal and pelvic pain following surgery.

Indications for QLB (Table 8.13).

Table 8.13 Indications for QLB

Acute pain	Chronic pain
Rib fractures Ventral hernia Thoracotomies Abdominal surgeries: Laparoscopic cholecystectomy, laparotomies, gastric bypass, PCNL, renal transplant, caesarean section Thoracic surgeries: VATS, breast surgeries, cardiac surgeries Sacral ESPB—analgesia for perineal surgeries and radicular pain Spine surgeries	Shoulder pain Refractory headache Lumbar pain as an alternative to anterior epidural block for patients having radiculopathy pain, facet joint pain etc. Complex Regional Pain Syndrome Neuralgias Myofascial pain

Table 8.14 Contraindications of QLB

Absolute	Relative
Patient refusal Local site infection Allergy to local anaesthetics	Coagulopathy or bleeding disorder Caution in kyphoscoliosis or spine deformity

8.9.3 Contraindications

Contraindications of QLB (Table 8.14).

8.9.4 Block Approach

8.9.4.1 Ultrasound-Guided Approach to QL Block

Position: Sitting, lateral, supine with a lateral tilt or prone position.

Needle: 20–22 G, 10 cm long short beveled echogenic needle.

Probe: For posterior QL a high-frequency linear ultrasound probe is required but for obese and anterior QL block a low-frequency ultrasound probe would be better.

Technique

The probe is positioned transversely above the iliac crest (Fig. 8.16a, b). When the rectus abdominis and three layers of the abdominal wall muscles are identified and traced posteriorly, the deep fascia of the transversus abdominis and the thoracolumbar fascia are linked. The QL and latissimus dorsi muscles can be traced medially or posteriorly to the transversus aponeurosis. The probe is then advanced medially to the transverse process, the erector spinae muscle is visible posteriorly, and the psoas major is seen anteriorly to the transverse process as "Shamrock Sign" which consists of the transverse process of L4 as the "stem" and psoas major, QL, and erector spinae as "3 cloves of the shamrock (Fig. 8.16c, d). The needle entry for various approaches for QLB and drug deposition is summarised in Table 8.15.

8.9.5 Continuous Catheter Placement Technique

Catheter can be placed in a similar technique as a single shot injection using a Tuohy needle. The correct placement of catheter is confirmed by injecting 2–3 ml of normal saline and 3–6 cm of catheter is kept beyond needle tip.

Table 8.15 Needle entry for various approaches for QLB and dermatomes covered

Type of QL block	Needle entry and drug deposition	Dermatomes covered
Lateral QL block/posterior transversus abdominis plane block (QLB 1) (Fig. 8.16c, d)	-Needle inserted in-plane with anterior/lateral to posterior/medial direction - Drug is deposited lateral to the QL muscle, between the aponeuroses of internal oblique and transversus abdominis muscles	T6–7 to L1
Posterior QL block (QLB 2) (Fig. 8.16c, d)	-Needle inserted in-plane with lateral/anterior to medial/posterior direction - Drug is deposited posterior to the QL muscle inside the middle layer of the TLF close to the LIFT, in the plane between the QL and either the latissimus dorsi or erector spinae muscles	T6–7 to L1
Anterior/Transmuscular/Subcostal (QLB 3) (Fig. 8.16c, d)	-Needle is inserted in-plane in a posterior/medial to anterior/lateral direction through the QL muscle -Drug is deposited medial to the QL muscle, between the QL and psoas major muscles	T10 to L3
Intramuscular (QLB 4) (Fig. 8.16c, d)	-Needle is inserted in-plane in anterior/lateral to posterior/medial direction -Drug is deposited into the QL muscle itself	T7 to T12

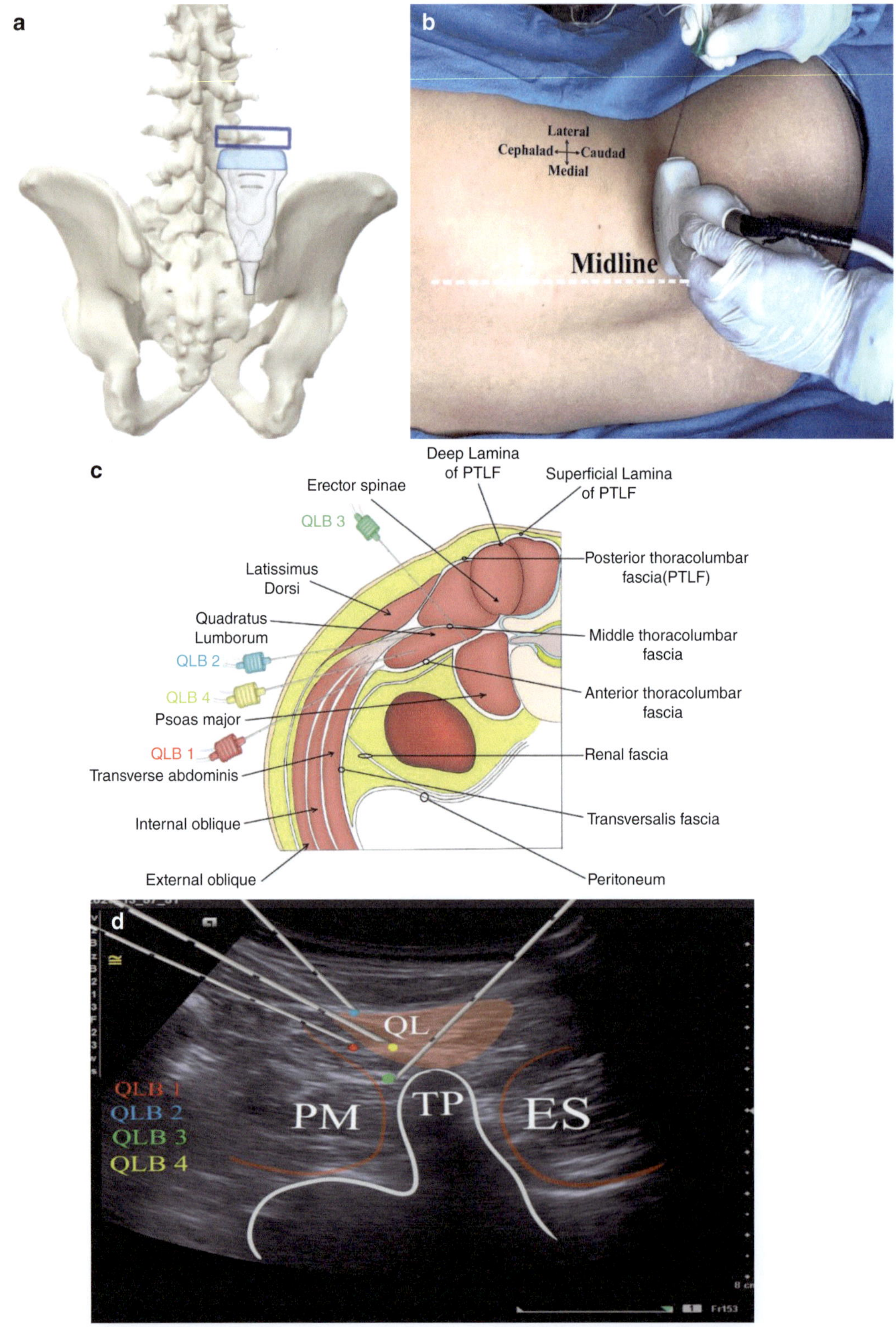

Fig. 8.16 (**a**, **b**) Illustration of anatomy and Probe position for QLB. (**c**, **d**) The three muscle layers of the abdominal wall and QL muscle, ES muscle, PM lumbar vertebrae with TP seen as "Shamrock Sign" in anterolateral view. The different approaches for the block are shown as per needle tip placement with respect to quadratus lumborum muscle. *QL* Quadratus lumborum, *TP* Transverse Process, *ES* Erector spinae, *PM* Psoas Major

Drug

- After negative aspiration and hydro dissection with 5.0 ml of normal saline, the placement of the needle is verified. After confirmation 20 ml of 0.25–0.5% bupivacaine or levobupivacaine, 0.2–0.5% ropivacaine, 1–2% lignocaine with epinephrine 1:2,00,000–1:4,00,000 is injected.
- For continuous infusion bolus injection as for single block followed by continuous infusion of 0.1–0.2% levobupivacaine or ropivacaine, or 0.125%bupivacaine at the rate of 5–10 ml/h.

8.9.6 Salient Features

- It has been noted that posterior and lateral QL blocks result in more thorough anaesthesia and analgesia of the anterior abdominal wall as compared to posterior TAP block.
- A broader analgesic distribution is ensured by anterior QL, which produces analgesia from T12-L4 dermatomes. A cadaveric study showed that the injectate consistently spread to the genitofemoral, iliohypogastric, and subcostal nerves as well as to varying degrees to the lateral cutaneous and ilioinguinal nerves. The diffusion of the injectate to the lumbar plexus and potential analgesia to the lower limbs are additional benefits of anterior QL block. As evidenced by the fact that patients may walk after intraperitoneal and retroperitoneal procedures, QL block relieves both somatic and visceral discomfort.
- According to reports, paravertebral drug distribution occurs after a QL block between the fifth and tenth thoracic vertebrae.
- QL block has been shown to reduce postoperative analgesics and pain scores up to 24–48 hours post-operatively. The close proximity of QL block to vertebral column leads to spread of drug to paravertebral space, resulting in both visceral and somatic pain relief.

8.9.7 Troubleshooting

The precautions during QL block are required to prevent damage to peritoneum, abdominal organ injuries like kidney and local anaesthetic systemic toxicity.

8.9.8 Complications

Complications are mostly related to the lack of ultrasonographic anatomical understanding and experience in needle manipulation.

- Hypotension may be due to the spread of drugs into paravertebral space causing sympathetic block.
- Bleeding and Needle trauma of surrounding retroperitoneal structures (e.g. pleura, kidney, liver, and spleen) are possible, especially in QL1 and QL3. In QL1 and QL3 approaches bleeding can occur as fascial planes contain branches of lumbar arteries (Fig. 8.17).
- Lower limb/quadriceps weakness especially in QL3 block (reported in QL1 and QL3 block).

  Spread to Lumbar plexus, especially in QL3 block.
- Because there was a significant amount of local anaesthetic administered for the block and the block space is quite vascular, local anaesthetic systemic toxicity (LAST) can occur. Although peak plasma concentration of LA is lower as compared to TAP block.
- Infection.

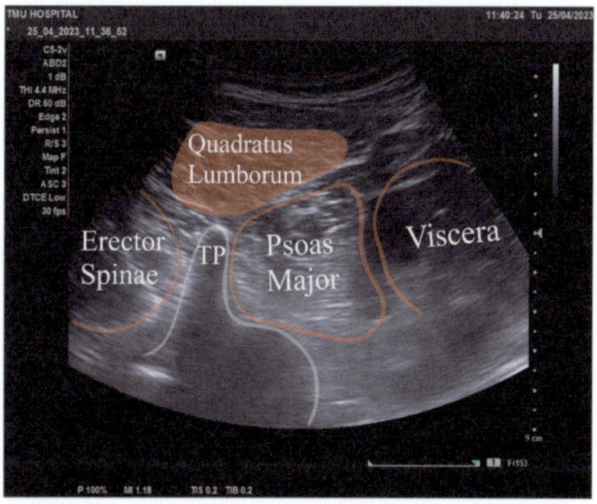

Fig. 8.17 Complications due to visceral injury can occur whilst performing blocks at L3 or higher levels in posterior truncal blocks when patient is in lateral decubitus position

8.10 Thoracolumbar Interfacial Plane Block (TLIP)

8.10.1 Anatomy

The spinal nerve is divided into the ventral motor root and the dorsal sensory root. At the intersection of the superior articular process and transverse process, dorsal rami appear. The posterior ramus surrounds the facet joints and provides cutaneous supply for the whole back region, from the vertex to the coccyx, as well as branches that feed ligaments, joints, and all of the segmental spinal muscles. The sensory portion of the dorsal rami of the thoracolumbar nerves is blocked by thoracolumbar interfacial plane block (TLIP). In 2015, Hand et al. published the first description of an ultrasound-guided TLIP block.

8.10.2 Indication

- Post-operative pain following spine surgery.
- Since TLIP primarily targets the dorsal rami, the usefulness of this block resides in the advantage of doing awake spine procedures. Monitoring of neurophysiology is unaffected by TLIP.

8.10.3 Contraindications

Same as Table 8.3.

8.10.4 Block Approach

Ultrasound-guided approach of TLIP block (Table 8.16).

8.10.5 Troubleshooting

Aspirate each time before injecting drug. Use increments of 3 ml each time before injecting

Table 8.16 Ultrasound approach of Thoracolumbar interfacial plane (TLIP) block

Position	Prone or lateral position
USG Scanning Landmark (Fig. 8.18a–c)	Under all aseptic precautions, low-frequency curvilinear (2–5 MHz) probe is used to identify L3 spinous process Probe is placed in transverse plane and moved in a lateral direction to identify multifidus, Longissimus, and iliocostalis muscles, respectively The fascial plane between the multifidus and longissimus muscles is from the point of the spinous process to the tip of the superior articular process (Tips Compared to the longissimus muscle, the echotexture of the multifidus muscle is distinct. The lateral border of the multifidus muscle is rounded at the L2 level. Multifidus muscle size is significantly less at lower lumbar level.)
POE (Fig. 8.18b, c)	Needle is inserted at 30° angle from the skin in "in plane approach" from lateral to medial direction through bulk of longissimus muscle towards multifidus muscle and needle tip is directed to interfascial plane between two muscles
Needle	A 10-cm long, 22 gauge short-bevel needle
End point	Drug is deposited between longissimus and multifidus muscle interface near superior articular process. Hydro dissection is done after negative aspiration in 3–5 ml aliquots whilst visualising local anaesthetic spread in real time
Drug dosage	20 ml 0.25–0.5% bupivacaine or levobupivacaine, 0.2–0.5% ropivacaine, 1–2% lignocaine with epinephrine 1:2,00,000–1:4,00,000 on either side of spine
Highlights	Modified TLIP involves placement of needle tip between iliocostalis and longissimus muscle and injecting 5–6 ml of local anaesthetic. On depositing 5–6 ml of drug superficial to the thoracolumbar fascia and erector spinae muscle can provide pain relief in skin and subcutaneous area of the paraspinal muscle

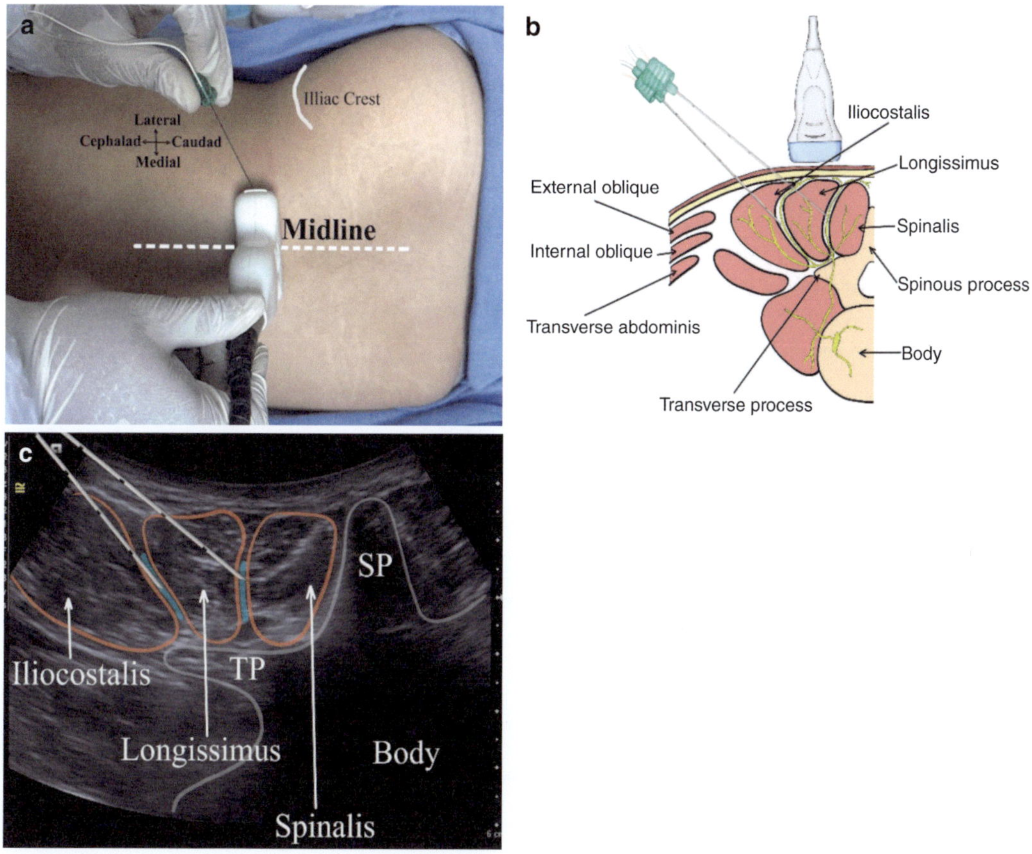

Fig. 8.18 (**a**) Probe and patient position for TLIP block. (**b**) Muscles from medial to lateral Spinalis/multifidus, Longissimus, and iliocostalis with needle insertion from lateral to medial direction. (**c**) Sonoanatomy showing midline transverse probe placement with spinous process, lamina and transverse process, medial to lateral multifidus, Longissimus, and iliocostalis muscles. The needle is inserted lateral to medial in plane and drug is injected between spinalis/ multifidus and longissimus block, close to the superior articular process, and modified TLIP block includes withdrawing the needle and depositing of drug between longissimus and iliocostalis muscles

drug. Look for spread of drug under real time. Do not keep needle too medial to avoid entering the intervertebral foramen. Avoid any vascular injury.

8.10.6 Complications

- Haematoma.
- Accidental neuraxial anaesthesia.
- Infection.

8.11 Conclusion

Posterior truncal blocks require expertise and precision as the structures lie close to the neuraxial spine. The learning curve with ultrasound-guided plane blocks can be improved with good knowledge of anatomy and at least initial blocks placed under the guidance of a supervisor or faculty who has expertise in regional nerve blocks. The advantages of posterior truncal blocks under ultrasound guidance include not disturbing the surgical planes when surgery is performed on the anterior abdomen or anterior part of chest wall, providing both sensory and visceral analgesia in majority of the blocks and the spread of drug in real time.

Further Reading

Ardon AE, Lee J, Franco CD, Riutort KT, Greengrass RA. Paravertebral block: anatomy and relevant safety issues. Korean J Anesthesiol. 2020;73(5):394–400.

Balocco AL, López AM, Kesteloot C, Horn JL, Brichant JF, Vandepitte C, et al. Quadratus lumborum block: an imaging study of three approaches. Reg Anesth Pain Med. 2021;46(1):35–40.

Boezaart AP, Lucas SD, Elliott CE. Paravertebral block: cervical, thoracic, lumbar, and sacral. Curr Opin Anaesthesiol. 2009;22(5):637–43.

Bogduk N. The innervation of the lumbar spine. Spine (Phila Pa 1976). 1983;8(3):286–93.

Bogduk N. Functional anatomy of the spine. Handb Clin Neurol. 2016;136:675–88.

Chen N, Qiao Q, Chen R, Xu Q, Zhang Y, Tian Y. The effect of ultrasound-guided intercostal nerve block, single-injection erector spinae plane block and multiple-injection paravertebral block on postoperative analgesia in thoracoscopic surgery: a randomized, double-blinded, clinical trial. J Clin Anesth. 2020;59:106–11.

Chin KJ, El-Boghdadly K. Mechanisms of action of the erector spinae plane (ESP) block: a narrative review. Can J Anaesth. 2021;68(3):387–408.

Chin KJ, Versyck B, Elsharkawy H, Rojas Gomez MF, Sala-Blanch X, Reina MA. Anatomical basis of fascial plane blocks. Reg Anesth Pain Med. 2021;46(7):581–99.

Christopher S, Gopal TVS, Vardhan V. Thoracolumbar interfascial plane block, way forward for awake endoscopic laminectomies. Indian J Anaesth. 2020;64(5):436–7.

Dam M, Moriggl B, Hansen CK, Hoermann R, Bendtsen TF, Børglum J. The pathway of injectate spread with the transmuscular quadratus lumborum block: a cadaver study. Anesth Analg. 2017;125(1):303–12.

Elias E, Nasser Z, Elias C, Rahman A, Nunna R, Oskouian RJ, et al. Erector spinae blocks for spine surgery: fact or fad? Systematic review of randomized controlled trials. World Neurosurg. 2022;158:106–12.

Elkhashab Y, Wang D. A review of techniques of intercostal nerve blocks. Curr Pain Headache Rep. 2021;25(10):67.

Farag E, Seif J. Thoracolumbar interfascial block (TLIP): a new technique of interfascial plane blocks. J Clin Anesth. 2020;61:109640.

Frost BA, Camarero-Espinosa S, Foster EJ. Materials for the spine: anatomy, problems, and solutions. Materials (Basel). 2019;12(2):253.

Gadsden JC. The role of peripheral nerve stimulation in the era of ultrasound-guided regional anaesthesia. Anaesthesia. 2021;76(Suppl 1):65–73.

Guerra-Londono CE, Privorotskiy A, Cozowicz C, Hicklen RS, Memtsoudis SG, Mariano ER, et al. Assessment of intercostal nerve block analgesia for thoracic surgery: a systematic review and meta-analysis. JAMA Netw Open. 2021;4(11):e2133394.

Ishizuka K, Sakai H, Tsuzuki N, Nagashima M. Topographic anatomy of the posterior ramus of thoracic spinal nerve and surrounding structures. Spine (Phila Pa 1976). 2012;37(14):E817–22.

Kamel AAF, Elhossieny KM, Hegab AS, Salem DAE. Ultrasound-guided retrolaminar block versus thoracic epidural analgesia for pain control following laparoscopic cholecystectomy. Pain Physician. 2022;25(6):E795–803.

Kim SH. Anatomical classification and clinical application of thoracic paraspinal blocks. Korean J Anesthesiol. 2022;75(4):295–306.

Kot P, Rodriguez P, Granell M, Cano B, Rovira L, Morales J, et al. The erector spinae plane block: a narrative review. Korean J Anesthesiol. 2019;72(3):209–20.

Koutp A, Sadoghi P, Petritsch J, Skias C, Grechenig P, Andrianakis A, Feigl GC. Anatomic-topographic investigation of the branches of the dorsal ramus of thoracic spinal nerves. Pain Med. 2022;23(11):1869–74.

Niazi AU, Peng PW, Ho M, Tiwari A, Chan VW. The future of regional anesthesia education: lessons learned from the surgical specialty. Can J Anaesth. 2016;63(8):966–72.

Onishi E, Toda N, Kameyama Y, Yamauchi M. Comparison of clinical efficacy and anatomical investigation between retrolaminar block and erector spinae plane block. Biomed Res Int. 2019;2019:2578396.

Rendina EA, Ciccone AM. The intercostal space. Thorac Surg Clin. 2007;17(4):491–501.

Saadawi M, Layera S, Aliste J, Bravo D, Leurcharusmee P, Tran Q. Erector spinae plane block: a narrative review with systematic analysis of the evidence pertaining to clinical indications and alternative truncal blocks. J Clin Anesth. 2021;68:110063.

Turbitt LR, Mariano ER, El-Boghdadly K. Future directions in regional anaesthesia: not just for the cognoscenti. Anaesthesia. 2020;75(3):293–7.

Turhan Ö, Sivrikoz N, Sungur Z, Duman S, Özkan B, Şentürk M. Thoracic paravertebral block achieves better pain control than erector spinae plane block and intercostal nerve block in thoracoscopic surgery: a randomized study. J Cardiothorac Vasc Anesth. 2021;35(10):2920–7.

Ueshima H, Otake H, Lin JA. Ultrasound-guided quadratus lumborum block: an updated review of anatomy and techniques. Biomed Res Int. 2017;2017:2752876.

Urits I, Ostling PS, Novitch MB, Burns JC, Charipova K, Gress KL, Kaye RJ, Eng MR, Cornett EM, Kaye

AD. Truncal regional nerve blocks in clinical anesthesia practice. Best Pract Res Clin Anaesthesiol. 2019;33(4):559–71.

Yang HM, Park SJ, Yoon KB, Park K, Kim SH. Cadaveric evaluation of different approaches for quadratus lumborum blocks. Pain Res Manag. 2018;2018:2368930.

Ye Y, Bi Y, Ma J, Liu B. Thoracolumbar interfascial plane block for postoperative analgesia in spine surgery: a systematic review and meta-analysis. PLoS One. 2021;16(5):e0251980.

Approach and Troubleshooting to Lower Limb Blocks

9

Mukesh Kumar Prasad and Payal Jain

Abstract

Regional Anesthesia for lower limb surgeries has been in practice for centuries.

Slowly and steadily with evolving equipment, techniques, and anesthetic agents a new chapter of peripheral nerve block in the ever-growing textbook of regional anesthesia opened, overcoming the shortcomings of central neuraxial block thus, expanding the horizon of application of anesthesia in critically ill patients. This chapter includes the approaches and troubleshooting toward blocking all the major peripheral nerves of the Lower Limbs via Blind, Nerve Stimulator Guided, Ultrasound-Guided techniques. Nerves can be blocked as a single shot or as a continuous injection. The major obstacles one can encounter during the block performance which can lead to partial success or complete failure are dealt with ease and explanation for enhancement of one's skill. This chapter includes Lumbar plexus block, Sacral plexus block, Sciatic nerve block, Femoral nerve block, Obturator nerve block, Lateral femoral cutaneous nerve block, Fascia iliaca compartment block, Saphenous nerve block, Popliteal fossa block, Ankle block, PENG block and iPACK block.

Keywords

Lumbar · Sacral · Sciatic · Femoral · Saphenous · Nerve blocks · Ankle block · IPack

9.1 Lumbar Plexus Block (PSOAS Compartment Block)

9.1.1 Introduction

Lumbar plexus alone and in combination with sacral plexus/sciatic nerve is used for anesthesia and analgesia of most lower limb surgeries aptly called one-legged anesthesia. These blocks prevent the systemic effects/complications of general anesthesia and central neuraxial blocks and are extremely helpful in patients with comorbidities. Lower extremity blocks are used as a part of multimodal analgesia and also prevent the development of chronic pain and post-amputation pain. These blocks are found to be cost-effective at times as compared to general anesthesia and can be used effectively, especially in low-resource settings.

M. K. Prasad (✉) · P. Jain
Department of Anaesthesiology, Teerthanker Mahaveer Medical College and Research Centre, Moradabad, India
e-mail: mukeshkumar2002@gmail.com

M. K. Prasad, S. J. S. Bajwa (eds.), *Steps to Successful Regional Anesthesia*,
https://doi.org/10.1007/978-981-97-4098-7_9

9.1.2 Anatomy

Lumbar plexus originates from ventral rami of L1-L4 (contribution from T12 to L5) and it passes through the psoas major muscle and comes out as various branches (Terminal nerves—iliohypogastric (L1, ±T12), ilioinguinal (L1), and genitofemoral nerves (L1 and L2)).

The lumbar plexus then divides into an anterior division giving rise to the obturator nerve (L2-L4), and a posterior division from which the femoral (L2-L4) and lateral femoral cutaneous nerves (L2, L3) arises (Fig. 9.1).

9.1.3 Indications

Lumbar plexus block in combination with Sacral plexus or Sciatic nerve block can be used for providing anesthesia and analgesia for all lower limb surgeries including proximal hip fracture, intertrochanteric, subtrochanteric, trochanteric, hip arthroscopy, total hip arthroplasty, and total knee arthroplasty.

9.1.4 Contraindications

Contraindications of lumbar plexus block (Table 9.1).

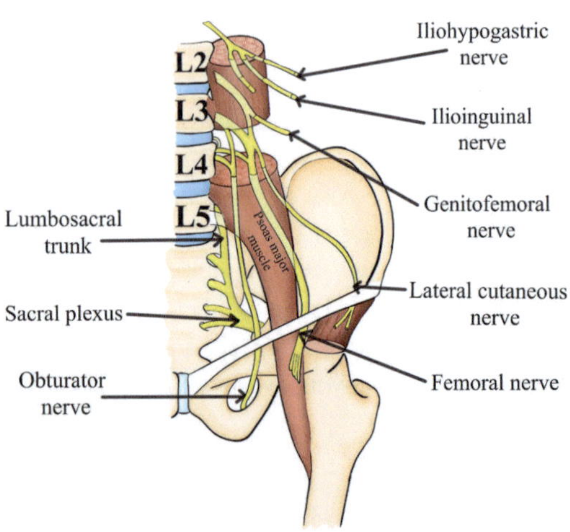

Fig. 9.1 Anatomy of Lumbar plexus

9.1.5 Preparations

Preparation of lumbar plexus block (Table 9.2).

9.1.6 Drugs

Drugs used for lumbar plexus block (Table 9.3).

Table 9.1 Contraindications of lumbar plexus block

Absolute	Relative
Patient refusal Local site infection Allergy to Local anesthetics INR > 1.5 or < 12 h post LMWH cessation as a posterior approach to lumbar plexus is comparable to central neuraxial blockade	Anticoagulation or bleeding disorders Femoral nerve neuropathy Pre-existing neurological deficit Systemic sepsis, especially for catheter placement Major spine injury or deformity Fixed cardiac output or cardiac compromised patients since chances of epidural or total spinal is present

Table 9.2 Preparation of block

Pre-requisites	Equipment/materials required
Informed consent NPO status Optimal sedation if necessary Emergency, resuscitation drugs, and equipment Secure IV access Appropriate sedation, monitoring (HR, NIBP, Spo2, ECG, RR, etc.), and oxygen supply Site and side of block should be marked and confirmed	Sterile towels and 4 inches × 4 inch gauze packs 10–20 ml syringes with Local anesthetic Sterile gloves, marking pen, and surface electrode One 1.5 in., 25-gauge needle for skin infiltration A 10-cm long, 21–22 gauge short-bevel, insulated stimulating needle Peripheral nerve stimulator Injection pressure monitor USG machine with curvilinear transducer (2–5 MHz), sterile sleeve, and gel

9.1.7 Block Approaches

9.1.7.1 Landmark, PNS Approaches

Landmark, PNS Approaches for lumbar plexus block (Table 9.4).

Tips

- Lumbar spinous process should be palpated and taken as midline and not the gluteal crease as it usually sags and may not correspond to midline.
- In obese patients and patients with high iliac crest, it is difficult to identify iliac crest moreover most of the time it does not correspond to L4 spinous process.
- Palpate ASIS and follow laterally and posteriorly for highest point of pelvic bone.
- Avoid eliciting contraction beyond 0.5 mA where there is a chance of placement of needle in dural sleeve which can lead to epidural or total spinal anesthesia.
- PNS and fluoroscopy-guided approach to overcome in absence of USG.

Table 9.3 Drugs used for lumbar plexus block

Drug	Onset (min)	Anesthesia (h)	Analgesia (h)
2% Lignocaine	10–20	2–5	3–8
0.5%Ropivacaine	15–30	4–8	5–12
0.75%Ropivacaine	10–15	5–10	6–24
0.5%Bupivacaine	15–30	5–15	8–30

9.1.7.2 PNS + Fluoroscopy-Guided Lumbar Plexus Block

PNS + fluoroscopy-guided Lumbar Plexus block (Table 9.5).

Table 9.4 Landmark, PNS Approaches for lumbar plexus block

	Winnie's	Capdevilla	Chayen's	Dekrey's
Position	Lateral decubitus with side to be blocked upside			
Landmark and technique (Fig. 9.2)	Line 1 is horizontal line (Tuffiers line, intercristal line) joining both iliac crests Line 2 (midline) is line joining lumbar spinous processes Line 3 is parallel to Line 2 starting from PSIS moving cranially intersecting Line 1 Line 4 is drawn from the center of the L4 spinous process laterally intersecting line 3			
POE (Fig. 9.2)	Junction of Line 1 and Line 3	Junction of medial two-third and lateral one-third on Line 4	Line was drawn 3 cm below from point of intersection of Line 1 and Line 2 and then 5 cm lateral	3 cm–4 cm lateral to L3 spinous process
Needle	A 10-cm PNS needle was inserted perpendicular at POE hitting transverse process of (L4-L5 in Winnie's, L4 in Capdevilla's, L5 in Chayen's, L3 in Dekrey's), then withdrawn slightly and redirected either cephalad or caudad 5°–10° (except in Dekrey's approach Caudally) not beyond 2 cm (Trick—If above maneuver does not work withdraw and redirect needle medially 10° –15°)			
PNS stimulation	Peripheral nerve stimulation starts with initial current setting of 1.5 mA (2 Hz, 0.1–0.3 ms) and continues till quadriceps contraction is elicited by impulses of 0.5 mA			
End point	Quadriceps femoris muscle contraction (Patellar twitch/dancing patella)			
Drug dosage	25 ml–35 ml (individual Local anesthetic or in combination) Surgical anesthesia (0.5–0.75% ropivacaine, 0.25–0.5% bupivacaine, 0.25–0.5% levobupivacaine,1–2% Lidocaine with or without epinephrine) Analgesia (0.2–0.375% ropivacaine, 0.1 25–0.25% bupivacaine, 0.125–0.25% levobupivacaine,0.5%–1% lidocaine with or without epinephrine)			
Highlights		Most acceptable	More chances of medial/epidural spread	More chances of visceral injury (especially kidney) Less acceptable

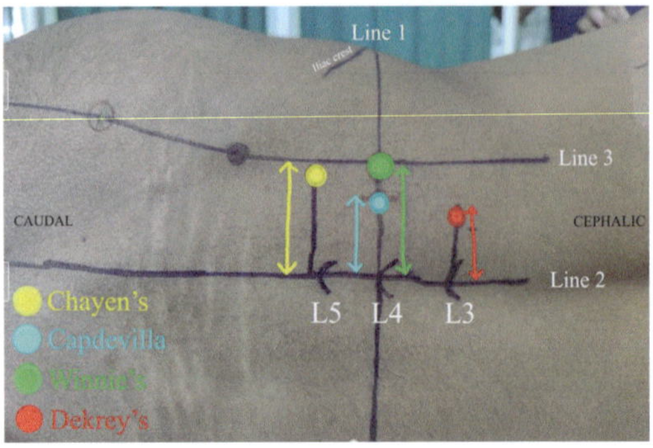

Fig. 9.2 Landmark for various approaches to lumbar plexus block. Line 1 is a horizontal line (Tuffiers line, intercristal line) joining both iliac crests. Line 2 (midline) is line joining lumbar spinous processes Spinous processes. Line 3 is parallel to Line 2 starting from PSIS moving cranially intersecting Line 1

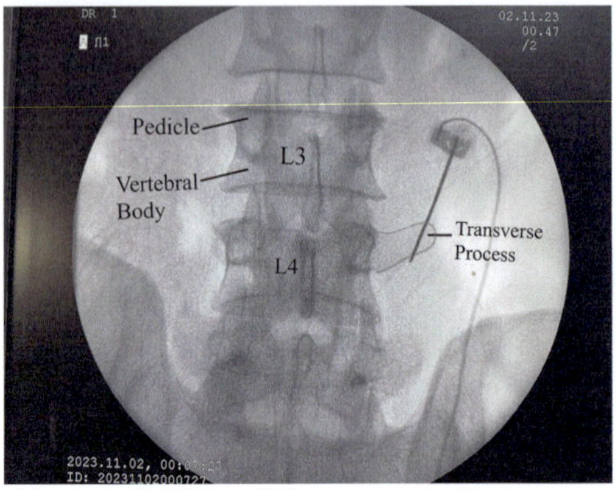

Fig. 9.3 Fluoroscopy-guided Lumbar Plexus block

Table 9.5 PNS + fluoroscopy guided Lumbar Plexus block

Position	Lateral Decubitus with side to be blocked upside
Landmark and technique	Identify L4 vertebra with a fluoroscope in anteroposterior view by gradually moving from sacrum upward. Identify the L4 transverse process. A 10-cm PNS needle inserted from lateral end of transverse process after skin infiltration with Local anesthetics. Needle advanced toward transverse process under fluoroscopy guidance till needle hit it. The needle is withdrawn 0.5 cm and redirected caudad to transverse process not beyond 2 cm (Fig. 9.3).
End point	Response is seen as a contraction of quadriceps muscle (Patellar twitch/ dancing patella)
Advantages	Can be used in patients with poorly defined landmarks and absence of USG

9.1.7.3 USG Approaches

1. *Karmakar Parasagittal Approach.*
   Karmakar parasagittal approach (Table 9.6).
2. *Modified Intertransverse Approach (Taha/Karmakar).*
   Modified Taha/Karmakar intertransverse approach (Table 9.7).
3. *Shamrock/Subcoastal Approach.*
   Shamrock/subcoastal approach (Table 9.8).

Table 9.6 Karmakar parasagittal approach

Position	Lateral Decubitus
Probe	Curvilinear (2–5 MHz) kept in parasagittal plane about 3–4 cm from midline
USG scanning landmark (Fig. 9.4a)	Under all aseptic precautions, probe is placed in paramedian position lateral to midline in lumbar region. Facet joint seen as bright echogenic bumps. Identify sacrum and L5 transverse process by hyperechoic reflection and dark shadow below them, then move upward toward L4 and mark it (Fig. 9.4a) Move slight laterally, identify transverse process (Bright echoes with dropout shadow beneath them). Three transverse processes (L2, L3, and L4) can be seen as Trident. Psoas muscle is seen in between prongs of trident (Fig. 9.4b) (Trick: Slight medial tilt (10–15°) of probe usually helps in focusing the facet and transverse process easily)
POE	A 10-cm echogenic insulated needle can be inserted in either in plane (cephalad to caudad direction) or out-of-plane (lateral or medial side of probe) approach
PNS stimulation	Can be used along with USG (decrease current till 0.5 mA, 0.1 ms)
End point	Needle tip is kept in posterior one-third of Psoas muscle and contractions of Quadriceps / patellar twitch are seen if nerve stimulation is used
Drug dose	20–25 ml of Local anesthetic with or without adjuvants after negative aspiration

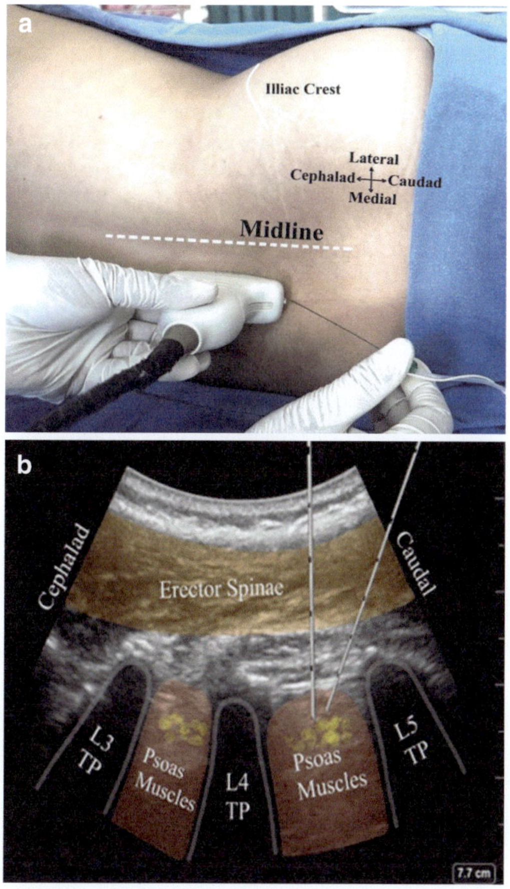

Fig. 9.4 (**a**) Probe and needle position in patient. (**b**) USG image showing "Trident sign" and final needle position

Tips

- Patient need to be positioned properly for good landmark identification and marking and better USG image visibility.
- In lateral position skin sags down, especially in elderly and obese patients, so, identification of midline should be done judiciously. In continuous Lumbar plexus block catheter should be kept 5–6 cm deep in order to prevent displacement during movement.
- Since Lumbar Plexus is deep block and uncomfortable for patients, appropriate sedation/ Local anesthetic infiltration is necessary.
- Avoid connecting the Local anesthetic syringe while advancing and manipulating the needle, dural puncture or intravascular placement of

Table 9.7 Modified intertransverse approach (Taha/ Karmakar)

Position	Lateral with operative side up with hips and knees slightly flexed
USG probe	Low-frequency curvilinear (2–5 MHz), in L3-L4 intertransverse space moved medially
Landmark and technique	Place the probe in a paramedian plane in lumbar region, lateral to midline Identify the facet joints or articular processes (raised bumps as bright echogenic reflections). Identify L4 vertebra counting up from sacrum At L4, probe is rotated 90° making it perpendicular to midline (transverse position) (Fig. 9.5a) *Identify the transverse process by sliding the probe laterally* (*Trick*—Place the vertebral body at the side of the screen and transverse process with the psoas muscle in the center) *Move probe cephalad and caudad in this transverse view* Place probe between the transverse processes of L3–4 or L4–5 and focus on psoas muscle which is deep to the level of the transverse process. Quadratus lumborum laterally and the erector spinae muscles posteriorly (*Trick*—Identify the wave pattern formed by transverse process, articular process and vertebral body (Fig. 9.5b) *Try to identify the lumbar plexus within the psoas muscle* (Trick—Seen as a white, hyperechoic region usually upper one-third within the muscle) Corresponding nerve root can be identified more medially at the edge of the vertebral body
POE	A 10–15 cm echogenic insulated needle can be used in-plane approach lateral to medial direction crossing Quadratus Lumborum into Psoas muscle (Fig. 9.5b)
PNS stimulation	Can be used along with USG (decrease current till 0.5 mA, 0.1 ms)
End point	Spread of LA within Psoas muscle Patellar twitch/ Patellar snap/ Patella dance sign if nerve stimulation is used
Dose	20–25 ml of Local anesthetic with or without adjuvants after negative aspiration

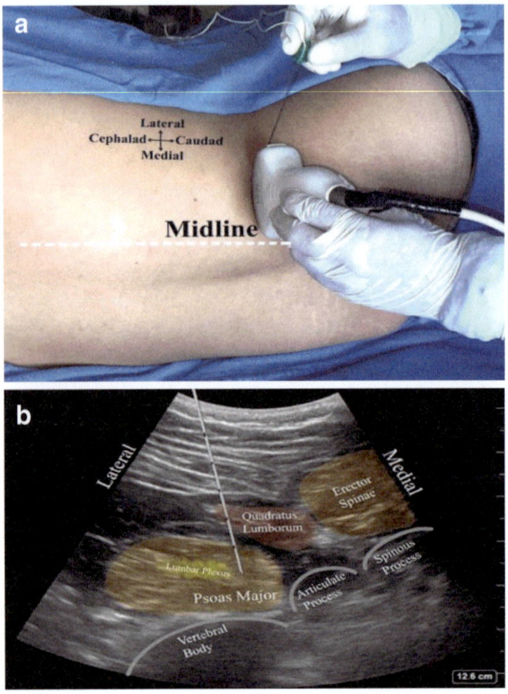

Fig. 9.5 (**a**) Probe and needle position in patient. (**b**) USG image showing Modified Intertransverse Approach and final needle position

needle can be identified as CSF or blood flow from needle, respectively.

- If no twitch is obtained at the identified target point try giving various attempts at same point before changing the target point.
- Fast injection is avoided which may lead to epidural spread or nerve injury.
- Muscle stimulation even after Local anesthetic may suggest needle tip in dural sleeves or intravascular injection. Withdraw and redirect the needle.
- Combination techniques or dual guidance, i.e., ultrasound guidance and nerve stimulation or fluoroscopy and nerve stimulation provide better assessment and placement of needle.

9.1.8 Troubleshooting Lumbar Plexus Block

(INTERPRETATION FOR PNS).

Troubleshooting of PNS Lumbar Plexus Block—Interpretation for PNS (Table 9.9).

Table 9.8 Shamrock/ subcoastal approach

Position	Lateral with operative side up with hips and knees slightly flexed
USG probe	Low-frequency curvilinear (2–5 MHz)
Landmark and technique	Place the probe in subcostal region just above the iliac crest in transverse plane (*Trick*—In obese patients, it is difficult to place the probe between iliac crest and costal margin, keeping a rolled sheet/pillow between bed and opposite flanks opens the space for transducer) Identify abdominal wall muscles then move the transducer posteriorly and caudally to identify L4 transverse process reflections). Identify L4 vertebra counting up from sacrum At L4 transverse process which forms the stem of Shamrock (A three-leaf clover) identify quadratus lumborum (lateral leaf), Erector Spinae muscle (posterior leaf) and Psoas muscle(anterior leaf) in relation to L4 transverse process (*Trick*—In case of poor visibility of Shamrock sign, especially in elderly and repeated interference from transverse process tilt the transducer caudally till transverse process disappears and bulging of vertebral body and Psoas muscle is seen. The needle tip is directed posteromedially inside the interpsoas compartment. Use PNS needle and look for quadriceps contractions)
POE	A 10–15 cm echogenic insulated needle is inserted perpendicular to skin (in-plane) approximately 3–4 cm from the midline in a paramedian plane (Fig. 9.6a, b)
PNS stimulation	Can be used along with USG (decrease current till 0.5 mA, 0.1 ms)
End point	Spread of LA within Psoas muscle Patellar twitch/ Patellar snap/ Patella dance sign
Dose	20–25 ml of Local anesthetic with or without adjuvants after negative aspiration

9.1.9 Complications

Various complications of Lumbar plexus block (Table 9.10).

9.1.10 Recap

Lumbar Plexus Block Recap (Table 9.11).

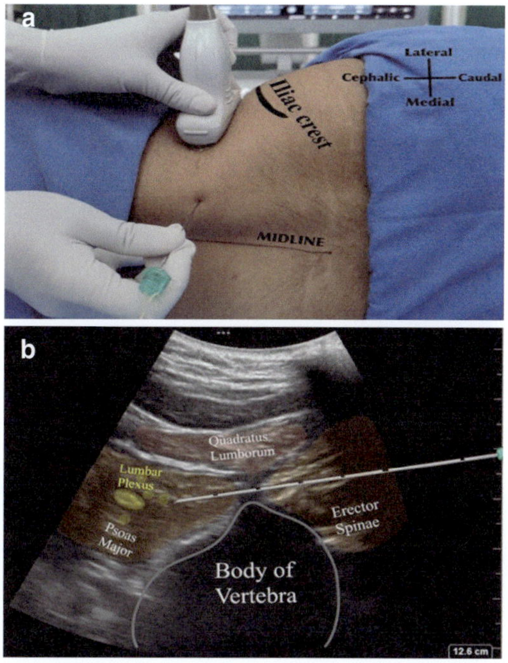

Fig. 9.6 (**a**) Probe and needle position in patient. (**b**) USG image showing " Shamrock sign" and final needle position

Table 9.9 Troubleshooting lumbar plexus block (interpretation For PNS)

Response	Stimulation	Interpretation	Rescue measures
No response	Needle tip not close to Lumbar Plexus	Too lateral or cephalad	Recheck landmarks and redirect needle cephalad / caudal to transverse process and medial
Quadriceps contractions	Stimulation of L3-L4 root	Best response	Decrease current to 0.5 mAmp and administer drug
Abdominal wall contraction	Direct abdominal muscle contractions/ stimulation of iliohypogastricn. (L1 ± T12) (Anterior division)	Too far lateral	Redirect medially
Paraspinal muscles contraction	Direct stimulation of paraspinal muscles	Needle too superficial	Move needle further deep
Hamstrings/Gastrocnemius contraction	Stimulation of L4 or L5 component of Sacral plexus	Too medial and caudal	Withdraw and redirect laterally
Hip joint/Thigh flexion	Direct stimulation of Psoas muscle	Needle too deep	Withdraw needle
Scrotum/Labial paresthesia	Genitofemoral (L1-L2 stimulation)	Too anteromedial	Withdraw and redirect laterally
Thigh adduction	Obturator n. (L2-L4 (Anterior division of ventral rami) stimulation	Too medial	Withdraw and redirect laterally
Contralateral limb twitching	Stimulation of opposite limb	Needle likely intrathecal	Withdraw and redirect laterally
No stimulation after crossing 2 cm of transverse process	Needle far away from lumbar plexus	Too lateral	Recheck landmarks and redirect needle medial and cepalad/ caudal to transverse process
Weakness/numbness of both limbs after injection	Epidural/intrathecal injection	Too medial	Withdraw and redirect laterally
Aspiration of fluid/CSF	Intrathecal needle placement	Too medial	Withdraw and redirect laterally/ abandon procedure

Table 9.10 Various complications of Lumbar plexus block

Due to needle puncture	Due to erroneous Local anesthetic injection	Due to Local anesthetic Local anesthetic systemic toxicity (LAST)
Direct nerve trauma (Trick—Use short beveled needle to avoid direct trauma)	Epidural spread—Unilateral/ Bilateral leading to hemodynamic instability. (hypotension, bradycardia)	Intravascular injection (highly vascular Psoas muscle, Inferior vena cava, aorta) (Tricks—Avoid deep needle insertion beyond 2 cm after reaching transverse process Keep needle end open while advancing needle and look for blood Avoid high pressure and fast injection Give drug in small aliquots of 3–5 ml after aspiration)
Abdominal viscera injury (Renal damage especially from the L3 approach, e.g., Dekrey approach and wrong identification of vertebra due to high iliac crest		
Retroperitoneal hematomas, subcapsular hematoma of the kidney due to noncompressible bleeding (Trick—Avoid multiple needle insertions) Lumbar plexus block can be given in patients on antiplatelet therapy provided there is no spontaneous bleeding but catheter placement needs to be avoided in these patients	Spinal spread—Large volume may lead to total spinal, leading to cardiovascular collapse, apnoea, seizures, and loss of consciousness (Trick—keep needle end open while advancing needle and look for CSF/ blood -Give drug in small aliquots of 3–5 ml after aspiration)	
Neurological damage due to intraneural injection (Trick—Avoid giving injection if patient complains of pain while injecting-Withdraw needle and readjust needle for motor response -Avoid high pressure and fast injection -Avoid giving LA if motor response is obtained below 0.5 mA. Withdraw needle as chances of dural sleeve injection leading to epidural/spinal spread)	Lumbar sympathetic block—May cause hemodynamic instability	
Psoas Abscess due to poor asepsis, continuous catheter placement—Maintain strict asepsis during procedure and maintenance of catheter		

Table 9.11 Lumbar plexus block recap

	Approaches	End point	Drug dose	Highlights
Landmark and PNS	Winnie's classical	Quadriceps contraction	25 ml–35 ml in small aliquots over 2–3 min (individual Local anesthetic or in combination) Surgical Anesthesia- (0.5–0.75% ropivacaine, 0.25–0.5% bupivacaine,0.25–0.5% levobupivacaine,1–2% Lidocaine with or without epinephrine) Analgesia (0.2–0.375% ropivacaine, 0.1 25–0.25% bupivacaine, 0.125–0.25% levobupivacaine, 0.5–1% lidocaine with or without epinephrine)	Needle tip should not be advanced beyond 2 cm of transverse process
	Capdevila			Most acceptable
	Chayen's			More Chances of medial/epidural spread
	Dekrey			More chances of visceral injury (especially kidney) -Response absent at times less acceptable
Fluro +PNS	Fluoroscopy is used to identify L4 vertebra and transverse process with fluoroscope in anteroposterior view	Quadriceps contraction		Can be used in patients with poorly defined landmarks and absence of USG
USG Guided	Parasagittal (Karmakar,2008)	Drug in substance of psoas major muscle and Quadriceps contraction	20 ml–25 ml in small aliquots over 2–3 min (individual Local anesthetic or in combination) Surgical Anesthesia- (0.5–0.75% ropivacaine, 0.25–0.5% bupivacaine,0.25–0.5% levobupivacaine,1–2% Lidocaine with or without epinephrine) Analgesia- (0.2–0.375% ropivacaine, 0.125–0.25% bupivacaine, 0.125–0.25% levobupivacaine, 0.5–1% lidocaine with or without epinephrine)	–
	Modified Intertransverse approach (Taha/ Karmakar,2015)			–
	Subcoastal approach (Gaur A)/ Shamrock (Borglum)			Shorter performance time and fewer needle redirections. Combined US–PNS provides a quicker onset for lumbar plexus blocks

9.2 Sacral Plexus Block

9.2.1 Introduction

The sacral plexus innervates much of the skin and subcutaneous tissue (dermatomes), muscle (myotomes), and bones (osteotomes) of the gluteal, pelvic, posterior thigh, and much of the leg regions. Sacral plexus block in combination with lumbar plexus block can be used for anesthesia and analgesia in most lower limb surgeries.

9.2.2 Anatomy

Sacral plexus is formed by Ventral rami of S1–S4 nerve roots with contribution from the L4 and L5 roots to form Lumbosacral trunk. Ventral rami is divided into anterior and posterior divisions. Sacral plexus is located deep within the pelvis between pyriformis muscle posteriorly and pelvic fascia anteriorly, sacrum medially, and Ischium laterally. Sacral plexus gives rise to 12 nerves of which Sciatic is the largest branch. Other major branches are superior gluteal nerve, inferior gluteal nerve, posterior femoral cutaneous nerve, and pudendal nerve.

Sacral plexus is related to the sigmoid colon, ureter, internal iliac artery, and vein anteriorly. The superior gluteal artery and vein are positioned between the lumbosacral trunk and the first sacral nerve, and the inferior gluteal artery and vein are located between the second and third sacral nerves. The sciatic nerve is formed when the sacral plexus's nerves come together in the pelvis as they descend toward the greater sciatic foramen.

9.2.3 Indication

- Surgeries around and below knee.
- Along with lumbar plexus analgesia and anesthesia for hip surgeries.
- Post-operative pain management thigh/leg amputation, total knee arthroplasty, and popliteal fossa surgery.

9.2.4 Contraindications

Same as for lumbar plexus block (Table 9.1).

9.2.5 Preparations

Refer to Table 9.2.

9.2.6 Drugs

Drugs used for sacral plexus block (Table 9.12).

9.2.7 Block Approaches

9.2.7.1 Landmark and PNS Approaches

Landmark, PNS Approaches Sacral Plexus Block (Table 9.13).

9.2.7.2 USG Approaches

1. *TAHA'S Parasacral Approach.*

   USG-guided Taha's Parasacral Approach (Table 9.14).

Tips

1. The lower lateral boundary of the greater sciatic foramen is formed by PBI (characteristic curved hyperechoic appearance). It can be identified simply at the level of the uppermost point of the Fig. 9.4.
2. In greater sciatic foramen, the sciatic nerve is the most lateral structure emerging and hence it appears just medial to the PBI.
3. Moving caudally orientation of sciatic nerve changes from medial to posterior border of ischium.

Table 9.12 Drugs used for sacral plexus block

Drug	Onset (min)	Anesthesia (h)	Analgesia (h)
2% Lignocaine	10–20	2–5	3–8
0.5%Ropivacaine	15–30	4–8	5–12
0.75%Ropivacaine	10–15	5–10	6–24
0.5%Bupivacaine	15–30	5–15	8–30

Table 9.13 Landmark, PNS approaches sacral plexus block

	Mansour's parasacral approach	Modified Mansour's approach
Position	Lateral decubitus with side to be blocked upside	
Landmark and technique	Line joining PSIS and ischial tuberosity on the side to be blocked (Line 1) Line 1 divided into 3 parts	
Point of Entry (POE)	6 cm from PSIS on the line 1 (Fig. 9.7)	Insertion junction of cephalad one-third and caudad two-third on Line 1 (Fig. 9.7)
Needle	A 22G, 10 cm PNS needle inserted perpendicular at POE (Trick—If the above maneuver does not work withdraw and redirect needle medially/laterally 10° –15°)	
PNS stimulation	Peripheral nerve stimulation starts with an initial current setting of 1.5 mA (2 Hz, 0.1–0.3 ms) and continued till plantar / dorsiflexion of foot is elicited by impulses of 0.5 mA.	
End point *	Response is seen as plantar / dorsiflexion of foot (Most acceptable)	
Drug dosage	20 ml–25 ml (individual Local anesthetic or in combination) Surgical anesthesia (0.5–0.75% ropivacaine, 0.25–0.5% bupivacaine,0.25–0.5% levobupivacaine, 1–2% Lidocaine with or without epinephrine) Analgesia (0.2–0.375% ropivacaine, 0.1 25–0.25% bupivacaine,0.125–0.25% levobupivacaine, 0.5%–1% lidocaine with or without epinephrine)	

* *Various responses to Sacral plexus stimulation*	
Response	*Nerves/muscles stimulated*
Hamstrings contraction	Biceps femoris (Long head by tibial division of sciatic nerve and short head by common fibular division of sciatic nerve), semitendinosus muscles (tibial division of sciatic nerve)
Plantar flexion of foot	Tibial portion of plexus (flexor hallucis longus and brevis (great toe), the flexor digitorum longus (the lateral four toes at the DIP joints), and the flexor digitorum brevis (the lateral four toes at the PIP joints)
Dorsiflexion/ eversion foot/ toes	Peroneal division of plexus (Tibialis anterior, the extensor hallucis longus (EHL), and the extensor digitorum longus (EDL))
Inversion of foot	Both tibial and common peroneal nerves (tibialis anterior, which we have seen already, and tibialis posterior)

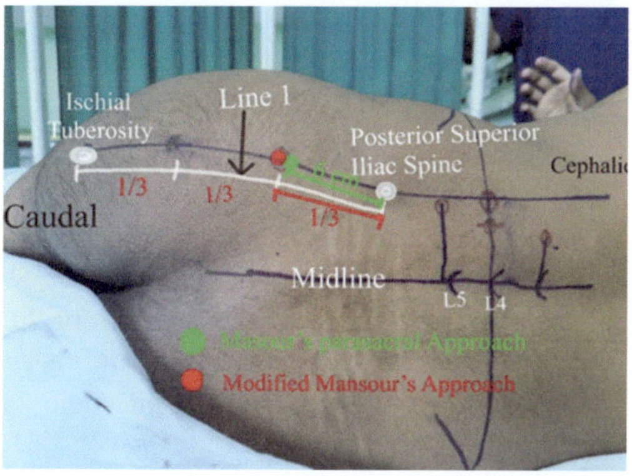

Fig. 9.7 Landmark for various approaches to Sacral plexus block. Line 1—Line joining PSIS and Ischial tuberosity on the side to be blocked. Line 1 divided into three parts

4. In thin patients, Peristaltic movement of bowels can be appreciated in thin patients deep to nerve.

2. *Bendsten's Parasacral Parallel Shift.*

USG-guided Bendsten's Parasacral Parallel Shift (Table 9.15).

Advantages

1. The first advantage is that the injection point is deep into the piriformis muscle, thus ensuring Local anesthetic is deposited sufficiently proximal to block all the lumbar-sacral nerves, especially the superior gluteal nerve.

Table 9.14 USG-guided Taha's parasacral approach

Position	Lateral with operative side up with hips and knees slightly flexed or prone position
Probe	Low-frequency curvilinear (2–5 MHz)
Landmark and technique	From uppermost point of the gluteal cleft 8 cm lateral, place the probe in axial plane (Fig. 9.8a) If the above landmarks are not seen, especially in obese patients or muscular patients Move probe cranially to identify ala of ilium (hyperechoic oblique line descending laterally) Move probe caudally looking for gap formed by greater sciatic notch in an oblique line Tilt probe caudally, the gap widens, posterior body of ilium (PBI) seen and sacral plexus appears as hyperechoic structure medial to PBI (Fig. 9.8b) Sacral plexus is deep and seen anterior to gluteus maximus and pyriformis muscle (*Tricks*—Sciatic nerve is seen triangular (cross-sectional view/short axis view) as probe position is perpendicular to nerve) Slight cauda l tilt improve USG imaging as sciatic nerve runs from deep to superficial surface
POE	The 22G 10–15 cm echogenic insulated needle is advanced inferior to the probe via an out-of-plane approach toward the nerve
PNS stimulation	Can be used along with USG (decrease current till 0.5 mA from 1.5 mA, 0.1 ms)
Drug dose	15–20 ml of Local anesthetic with or without adjuvants after negative aspiration
End point	Drug spread anterior to pyriformis muscle above sciatic nerve Hamstring, leg, or foot contractions

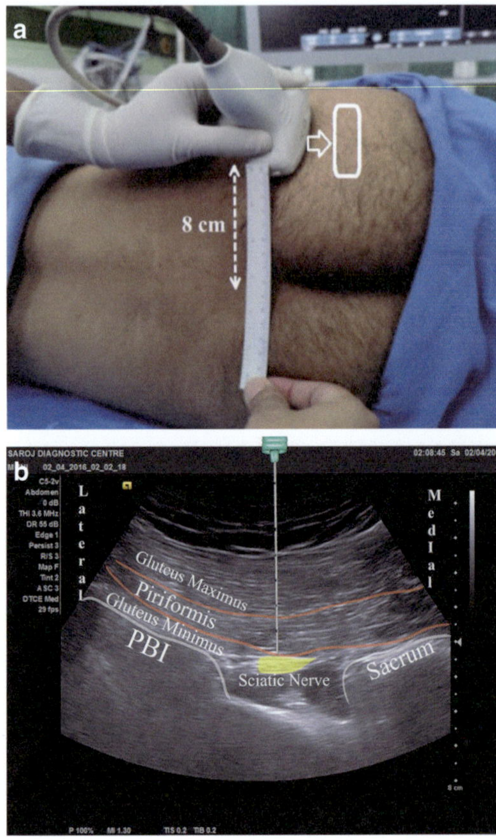

Fig. 9.8 (**a**) Probe and needle position in patient. (**b**) USG image showing and final needle position

2. Sciatic nerve is viewed in axis, which is parallel to the nerve in its length. A slight rotation of the transducer to align more perfectly parallel to the nerve axis perfectly creates the most perfect nerve image.
3. *PIP (Parasacral Ischial Plane) Block.*

   USG-guided parasacral ischial plane (PIP) approach (Table 9.16).

Advantages of PIP Block

1. Ultrasound landmarks are guided by bones which have a congruous relationship with sacral plexus.
2. No need for neurostimulation so can be performed effectively even in above or below-knee amputated patients.
3. Neurovascular structures are away from the point of needle entry and end points and hence intravascular and intraneural injection is avoided.
4. Since End point for the block is a bony landmark, so it is relatively easy to perform even in obese or edematous patients.

Table 9.15 USG-guided Bendsten's parasacral parallel shift

Position	Lateral with operative side up with hips and knees slightly flexed
Probe	Low-frequency curvilinear (2–5 MHz)
Landmark (Fig. 9.9a)	Line drawn from greater trochanter (GT) to posterior superior iliac spine (PSIS) Divided into medial and lateral parts from midpoint
Technique	Place the probe in medial half of GT-PSIS line in parasagittal oblique plane (Fig. 9.9a) Slide probe in caudal and medial direction (Fig. 9.9b) Identify ala of ilium covered by gluteus maximus and gluteus minimus muscle (Fig. 9.9c) Slide probe further in same direction Greater sciatic notch identified as a break in ala and appearance of sacral plexus seen below Gluteus maximus and pyriformis muscle (Fig. 9.9d) (*Tip*—Sciatic nerve is seen flat (longitudinal) as probe position is parallel to nerve (Long axis view) The most ideal nerve image is created by slightly rotating the transducer to align it more completely parallel to the nerve axis Internal pudendal blood vessels are interlaced with nerves and lie deeper into them. So, it is recommended to use the color Doppler to identify their presence)
POE	A 22G, 10 cm long PNS needle is advanced from inferior and lateral sides of the probe via an in-plane approach toward the nerve (Fig. 9.9d) (Trick—Out-of-plane technique can be used if the nerve is not deeper than 5 cm)
PNS stimulation	Decrease current to 0.3–0.5 mA from 1.5 mA
Drug dose	15–20 ml of Local anesthetic with or without adjuvants after negative aspiration
End point	Drug spread anterior to pyriformis muscle above sciatic nerve Hamstring, leg, or foot contractions with PNS stimulation

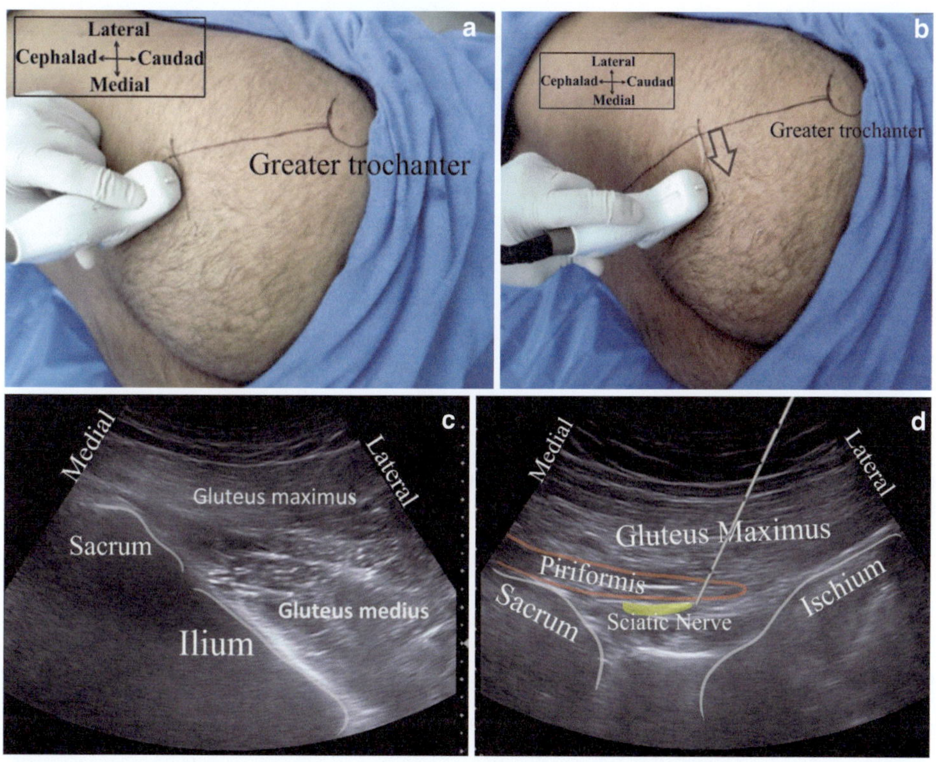

Fig. 9.9 (**a**) Probe position is in medial half of GT-PSIS line. (**b**) Slide probe in caudal and medial direction. (**c**) USG image showing ala of ilium covered by gluteus maximus and gluteus minimus muscle. (**d**) USG image showing sacral plexus seen below Gluteus maximus and pyriformis muscle and final needle position

Table 9.16 USG-guided parasacral ischial plane (PIP) approach

Position	Lateral with operative side up with hips and knees slightly flexed
Probe	Low-frequency curvilinear (2–5 MHz)
Landmark	The piriformis forms the ceiling of the greater sciatic foramen and proceeds laterally to attach to greater trochanter. A fascial plane exists between the muscles and the ischial bone, which connects directly with the sacral plexus. Hence, injecting Local anesthetic immediately superficial to the ischium at the level of the greater sciatic foramen leads to tracking of LA medially toward the sacral plexus Line drawn from greater trochanter to posterior superior iliac spine Probe position along the line and medial edge of probe kept on PSIS
Technique	Probe position along the line drawn connecting PSIS and greater trochanter in such a way that medial edge of probe is kept on PSIS The probe is kept on medial half of GT-PSIS line (Fig. 9.9a) Slide probe in inferomedial direction (Fig. 9.9b) Identify the posteromedial border of Ischium under the pyriformis (Fig. 9.10)
POE	A 22G, 10 cm long PNS needle is advanced from lateral to medial direction in in-plane approach targeting posteromedial part of ischium (Fig. 9.10)
Drug dose	15–20 ml of Local anesthetic with or without adjuvants after negative aspiration
End point	Bony contact with ischium

9.2.8 Troubleshoot in Sacral Plexus Block

Troubleshoot in Sacral Plexus Block (Table 9.17).

9.2.9 Complications of Sacral Plexus Block

Complications of Sacral Plexus Block (Table 9.18).

9.2.10 Recap of Sacral Plexus Block

Sacral Plexus Block Block recap (Table 9.19).

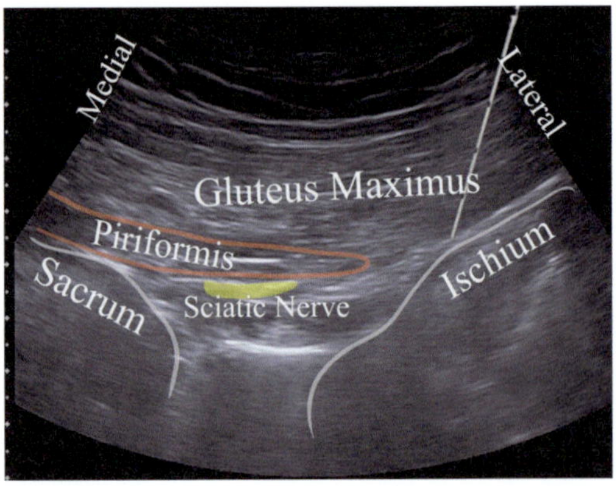

Fig. 9.10 USG image showing needle on posteromedial part of ischium

Table 9.17 Troubleshoot in sacral plexus block

Response	Stimulation	Interpretation	Rescue measures
With only PNS			
No response only bony contact	Needle tip is not close to sacral plexus	Too lateral (Ischium, Ilium),	Recheck landmarks and redirect needle medial, lateral, and caudal
		Too Medial (sacrum)	Recheck landmarks and redirect needle laterally
		Cephalad (if not lateral or medial and landmarks are correct)	Redirect needle caudally
Tensor fascia lata /gluteus medius/minimus contraction	Superior gluteal nerve (*L4*-S1)	Cehalad and lateral	Redirect needle caudal and medial
Gluteus maximus contraction	Inferior Gluteal nerve (L5-S2)	Caudal and medial	Redirect lateral
Genital tingling	Pudendal nerve (S2, S3, S4)	Medial and deep	Redirect lateral and superficial
No response (needle went beyond 10 cm)	Needle tip is not close to sacral plexus	Too inferior crossed the sciatic notch	Withdraw and redirect lateral and cephalad

Table 9.18 Complications of sacral plexus block

<table>
<tr><th>Due to needle puncture</th><th>Due to erroneous Local anesthetic injection</th><th>Due to Local anesthetic
Local anesthetic systemic toxicity (LAST)</th></tr>
<tr><td>Direct nerve trauma
(Trick—Use short beveled needle)</td><td>Sympathetic block due to Proximal volume spread may cause hypotension
(Trick—Avoid large-volume drug
-Avoid high-pressure and fast injection
-Give drug in small aliquots of 3–5 ml after aspiration not more than 20 ml)</td><td rowspan="4">Intravascular injection (,)
(Tricks—Internal pudendal blood vessels—use color Doppler
Inferior gluteal vessels—Avoid going too medial
Keep the needle end open while advancing needle and look for blood
Avoid high-pressure and fast injection
Give drug in small aliquots of 3–5 ml after aspiration)</td></tr>
<tr><td>Abdominal viscera injury (rectum, colon, bladder)
(Trick—Avoid needle advancement 2 cm beyond border of sacrum)</td><td>Urinary retention—During bilateral block or high volume (more than 20 ml) drug due to pudendal nerve and parasympathetic block
(Trick—same as above)</td></tr>
<tr><td>Neurological damage due to intraneural injection.
(Trick—same as Lumbar plexus block)</td><td>Subarachnoid injection (rare) leading to total spinal
(Trick—same as above)</td></tr>
<tr><td></td><td>Numb penis/numb hemi-perineum—Due to pudendal nerve block</td></tr>
</table>

Table 9.19 Sacral plexus block block recap

<table>
<tr><th></th><th>Approaches</th><th>End point</th><th>Drug dose</th><th></th></tr>
<tr><td rowspan="2">Landmark and PNS</td><td>Mansour's parasacral Approach</td><td>Hamstrings contraction/ Dorsiflexion/ plantar flexion</td><td rowspan="5">20–25 ml
0.5% bupivacaine 10 ml +2% lidocaine 10 ml with or without adjuvant
0.75% Ropivacaine 15–20 ml with or without adjuvant
0.75% Ropivacaine 10 ml + 2% Lidocaine 10 ml with or without adjuvant 20 ml</td><td rowspan="2">Avoid needle advancement 2 cm beyond border of sacrum to minimize pelvic organ injury</td></tr>
<tr><td>Modified Mansour's Approach</td><td>Hamstrings contraction/ Dorsiflexion/ plantar flexion</td></tr>
<tr><td rowspan="3">Dual guidance (USG + PNS)</td><td>Taha's Approach</td><td>Hamstrings contraction/ Dorsiflexion/ plantar flexion</td><td>Rapid and highly successful identification and blockade of the sciatic nerve</td></tr>
<tr><td>Bendsten's (Para Sacral Parallel Shift)</td><td>Hamstrings contraction/ Dorsiflexion/ plantar flexion</td><td>The advantage is that the injection point is deep into the piriformis muscle, ensuring that Local anesthetic is deposited sufficiently close to the lumbar-sacral nerves, particularly the superior gluteal nerve</td></tr>
<tr><td>PIP block</td><td>Bony contact with posteromedial border of Ischium</td><td>For analgesia</td></tr>
</table>

9.3 Sciatic Nerve Block

9.3.1 Introduction

It is the largest (5 mm high and 10–15 mm wide), longest nerve of the lower limb. Victor Pauchet, first described it in L'Anesthesie Regionale in 1920, known as the classic approach of Labat. Alon Winnie modified the Labat Approach in 1975, anterior approach described by George Beck in 1963, and lithotomy approach described by Prithvi Raj in 1975 to allow sciatic nerve block to be performed in supine position. Recently, subgluteal and parasacral approach was introduced by Pia di Benedetto and Philippe Cuvillon. The relationship of sciatic nerve to the pelvis is constant throughout the life.

9.3.2 Anatomy

Anatomy of sciatic nerve (Table 9.20).

9.3.3 Indications

- Lower limb surgeries (combined with either femoral nerve block, obturator nerve block, saphenous nerve block, or psoas compartment block depending on the site of surgery).
- Analgesia before transport.
- For definitive orthopedic surgical repair of lower leg or ankle fractures.
- Patients in whom it may be desirable to avoid the sympathectomy accompanying neuraxial block.

9.3.4 Contraindications

Contraindications to sciatic nerve block (Table 9.21).

9.3.5 Drugs

Drugs used for sciatic nerve block (Table 9.22).

Table 9.20 Anatomy of sciatic nerve

Sciatic nerve—The course of the sciatic nerve can be estimated by drawing a line on the back of the thigh beginning from the apex of the popliteal fossa to the midpoint of the line joining the ischial tuberosity to the apex of the greater trochanter (Fig. 9.11)		
Roots	L4-L5, S1-S3 (Fibers from both anterior primary rami of lumbosacral plexus)	
Course (Fig. 9.11)	It is presented Inferior to Piriformis muscle Passing through greater sciatic foramen It lies between greater trochanter of femur and ischial tuberosity Present between gluteus maximus (Post.) and Quadratus femoris (Ant.) Moves along posteromedial aspect of femur 4–10 cm above popliteal crease divides into Tibial nerve and Common Peroneal nerve	
Innervations/Actions	Muscle supply	Posterior compartment of thigh—Biceps femoris, Semimembranosus, Semitendinosus, Ischial portion of adductor magnus
	Motor	Knee flexion, hip adduction
	Cutaneous	Skin of foot and lower leg (except medial leg) (Fig. 9.12)
	Joint	Hip joint (posterior part of capsule)

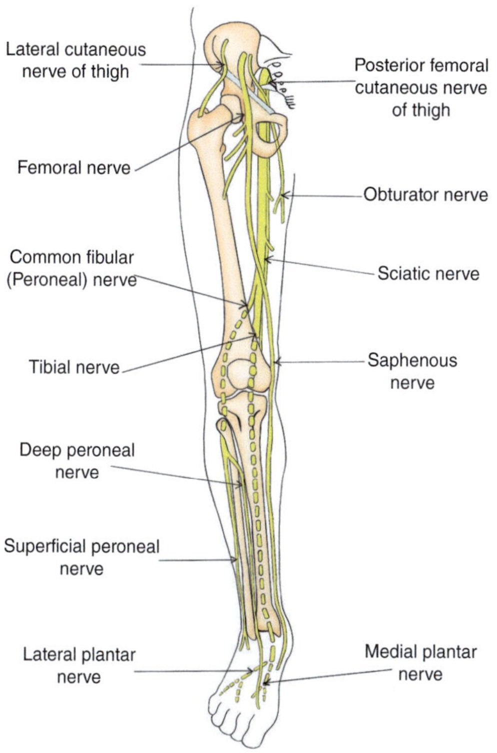

Fig. 9.11 Course of Sciatic nerve

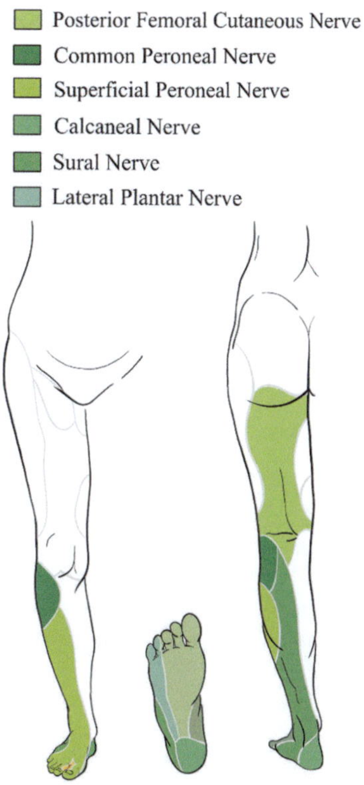

Fig. 9.12 Dermatomal distribution of Sciatic nerve

Table 9.21 Contraindications to sciatic nerve block

Absolute	Relative
Patient refusal	Anticoagulation or bleeding disorders
Local site infection	Sciatic nerve neuropathy
Allergy to Local anesthetics	Large inguinal lymph nodes/tumor
	Avoid/discuss with surgeon if compartment syndrome suspected

Table 9.22 Drugs used for sciatic nerve block

Drug	Onset (min)	Anesthesia (h)	Analgesia (h)
2% Lignocaine	10–15	5–6	5–8
0.5% Ropivacaine	15–20	6–12	6–24
0.75% Ropivacaine	10–15	8–12	8–24
0.5% Bupivacaine	15–30	8–16	10–48

9.3.6 Preparations

Refer to Table 9.2.

9.3.7 Block Approaches

Various approaches for sciatic nerve block (Table 9.23).

9.3.7.1 Landmark and PNS-Guided Technique

1. *Posterior Approach—Transgluteal Approach/ Posterior Approach/Classic Approach of Labat.*

Transgluteal approach, Posterior approach, Classic approach of Labat for sciatic nerve block (Table 9.24).

Table 9.23 Various approaches to sciatic nerve block

Blocks (Subtypes)	Position	Where in course
Classic approach of Labat	Lateral decubitus	SN exits the greater sciatic foramen, deep to piriformis
Mansour's parasacral approach	Lateral	
Sub-gluteal approach	Lateral decubitus	Midway between greater trochanter and ischial tuberosity
Raj approach	Lithotomy	
Beck's anterior approach	Supine	Medial to the lesser trochanter
Sukhani's infragluteal approach	Prone	Lateral to the tendon of biceps femoris (Upper thigh)
Guardini's subtrochanteric approach	Supine	Under the belly of biceps femoris (Mid-thigh)
Popliteal fossa approach	Prone/supine / lateral/lithotomy	4–10 cm above popliteal crease, bounded by biceps femoris laterally, and semitendinosus and semimembranosus medially

Table 9.24 Transgluteal approach, Posterior approach, Classic approach of Labat (for surgery on knee, calf, achilles tendon, ankle, and foot)

Position	Lateral position (Sim's) with operative site up with foot over-dependent leg and thigh maximally flexed with adequate knee flexion and a forward tilt with palpating hand firmly pressed on gluteus muscle to decrease skin-to-nerve distance
Landmark (Fig. 9.13)	Line 1—Line joining greater trochanter to posterior superior iliac spine Line 2—Line joining greater trochanter to sacral hiatus Line 3—Line drawn perpendicular from midpoint of Line 1 intersecting Line 2
POE	Under all aseptic precautions, a line is drawn from midpoint of Line 1 till it intersects Line 2 or POE is 5 cm caudal on this line
Needle	22 Gauge (10–12 cm long insulated) in a perpendicular direction is inserted in the direction toward an imaginary point where femoral vessels pass through inguinal ligament
PNS stimulation	Initial set to deliver 1–1.5 mA (2 Hz,100 μsec)
End point	Twitches of the hamstrings, calf muscles, foot, or toes at 0.3–0.5 mA (approx. Occurs at depth 5–8 cm)
Drug dosage	15–25 ml of Local anesthetic injected after negative aspiration of blood

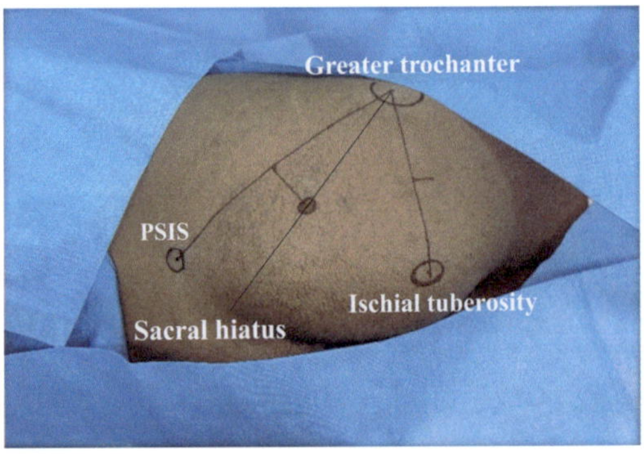

Fig. 9.13 Surface landmark for sciatic nerve block in the posterior approach

Tips

1. Keep the palpating hand firmly, small movements can bring substantial change in needle position because of high mobility of soft tissue in gluteal region.
2. Inadequate skin anaesthesia despite proper block, can need local infiltration at the site of incision.
3. Resistance to injection, withdraw the needle by 1 mm, still persistent check the needle for patency.

Table 9.25 Troubleshooting for Sciatic Nerve Block in posterior approach

Response	Stimulation	Interpretation	Rescue measures
No response	None	Reassess the point of entry	Redirect the needle 5–10 degrees cranially/caudally to initial plane
Twitch of gluteal muscle	Direct stimulation of muscle	Needle is too shallow	Advance the needle further
Needle contacts bone without twitch	Needle hitting sacral or iliac bone	Needle is medial and cephalic directed	Redirect laterally and caudally
Needle contacts bone with twitch	Needle hitting the Hip joint/ischial bone	If Hip joint (needle is too lateral) If Ischial bone (needle is too medial)	Withdraw and redirect laterally or medially
Needle to a depth of 8–10 cm but neither bone contact nor twitch	Needle too deep	Needle has crossed the Sciatic notch	Redirect the needle laterally and cephalic
Paresthesia of genital organs	Pudendal nerve stimulated	Needle is too inferior and medial	Withdraw and redirect the needle in the opposite direction

Troubleshooting
Troubleshooting for Sciatic Nerve Block in posterior approach (Table 9.25).

Continuous Sciatic Nerve Block
Tuohy needle is inserted using the same landmarks in a slight caudal direction, i.e., needle tip is pointing toward the patient's foot. After the response 15–25 ml of Local anesthetic is injected followed by catheter insertion around 5 cm beyond the needle tip. Catheter is secured and clearly marked and checked for inadvertent intravascular placement. Continuous infusion is started at 5–10 ml/hr. using 0.1% Ropivacaine, 0.25% Bupivacaine.

2. *Posterior Approach—Parasacral Approach.*

Parasacral approach for sciatic nerve block (Table 9.26).

Troubleshooting
Troubleshooting sciatic nerve block in parasacral approach (Table 9.27).

Continuous Parasacral Sciatic Nerve Block
The technique is similar to the single shot injection with slight caudal angulation of the needle

Table 9.26 Parasacral approach (anesthesia and analgesia when combined with femoral or psoas compartment block)

Distribution	Posterior thigh, hamstrings, biceps femoris, part of hip and knee joint, and entire leg below knee except medial part of leg
Position	Lateral decubitus, dependent limb is kept straight, limb to be blocked is flexed at both hip and knee
Landmark and technique (Fig. 9.14)	Posterior-Superior iliac spine (PSIS) and ischial tuberosity (IT) ↓ Line is drawn between the points
POE	Under all aseptic conditions 2 ml of 0.1% lignocaine is infiltrated followed by needle insertion 6 cm caudad to the PSIS on this line
Needle	10 cm insulated needle advanced in sagittal plane
PNS stimulation	Initial set to deliver 1–1.5 mA (2 Hz, 100 μsec)
End point	Visible or palpable twitches of hamstrings, calf muscles, foot, or toes at 0.3–0.5 mA (usually at a depth of 6–8 cm)
Drug dosage	20–25 ml of Local anesthetic with intermittent aspirations
Highlights	Best for continuous infusion of Local anesthetic, anesthesia of entire sacral plexus plus obturator nerve block

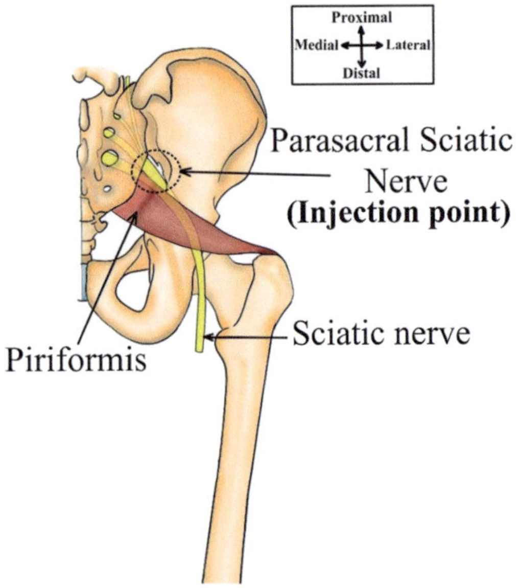

Fig. 9.14 Landmark for sciatic nerve block in parasacral approach

Table 9.27 Troubleshooting sciatic nerve block in parasacral approach

Response	Stimulation	Interpretation	Rescue measures
Needle contact with bone	Superior or near greater sciatic notch	Needle not to be advanced 2 cm beyond this point, as chances of pelvic viscera injury increases	Needle directed caudally and laterally

with tip facing distally, to facilitate threading of the catheter. After obtaining the motor response 20 ml of drug is injected followed by catheter insertion 3–5 cm beyond the needle tip.

Tips

1. Winnies double injection technique (to block peroneal and tibial nerve separately) was more time consuming with similar anesthesia characteristics than parasacral approach.
2. For confirmation of catheter placement, contrast media can be injected through the catheter, presence of a spindle 2–3 cm in length with an oblique orientation crossing the sciatic notch on the anteroposterior radiograph and/or shadowing of the sacral roots are considered to indicate injection into correct plane and adequate placement of the catheter. After securing an infusion of ropivacaine 0.2% at 5 ml/hr. should be started.
3. *Posterior Approach—Subgluteal Approach.*

Subgluteal approach for sciatic nerve block (Table 9.28).

Table 9.28 Subgluteal approach for sciatic nerve block

Position	Lateral decubitus, dependent limb is kept straight, limb to be blocked is flexed at both hip and knee
Landmark and technique	A line is drawn between the greater trochanter of the femur and Ischial tuberosity
POE	Under all aseptic precautions, a perpendicular line is drawn 4 cm caudal from midpoint of this line (Fig. 9.15)
Needle	20 Gauge, 10 cm needle
PNS stimulation	Initial set to deliver 1–1.5 mA (2 Hz, 100 μsec)
End point	Visible or palpable twitches of hamstrings, calf muscles, foot, or toes at 0.3–0.5 mA (usually at a depth of 6–8 cm)
Drug dosage	20 ml of Local anesthetic with intermittent aspiration
Highlights	Reduces patient discomfort, ultrasound-guided technique can be used

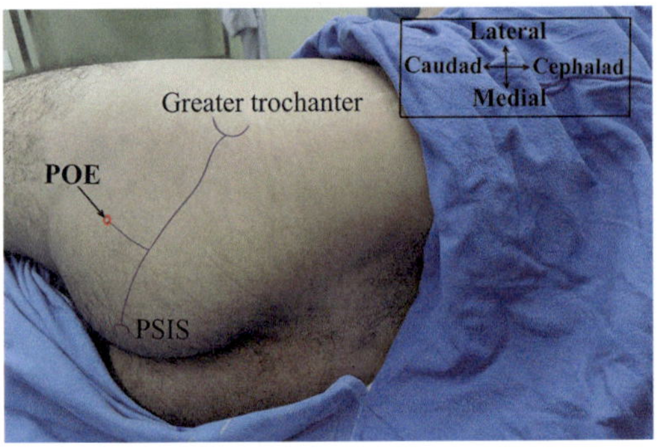

Fig. 9.15 Subgluteal approach to sciatic nerve block

Tips

1. The soft tissues should not be over stretched when marking the needle insertion site as sub-

sequent recoil of the tissues will occur, causing distance to the nerve to be underestimated.

2. Explain the need for frequent repositioning to avoid stretching and ischemia of the anesthetized nerve. Heel pads to avoid bed sores.
4. *Anterior approach.*

Anterior approach for sciatic nerve block (Table 9.29).

Troubleshooting

Troubleshooting anterior approach for sciatic nerve block (Table 9.30).

9.3.7.2 Complications

Complications of posterior approach for sciatic nerve block (Table 9.31).

9.3.7.3 Ultrasound-Guided Sciatic Nerve Block

It reduces the risk of vascular puncture.

Table 9.29 Anterior approach for sciatic nerve block

Distribution	Surgery on the leg below the knee, particularly ankle and foot except medial strip of skin
Position	Supine with leg extended
Landmark and technique (Fig. 9.16a, b)	Femoral crease, Femoral artery pulse ↓ Line passing through the pulse of the femoral artery and perpendicular to the femoral crease
POE	4–5 cm distally on the line
Needle	Perpendicular to the skin plane
PNS stimulation	Set to deliver current at 1.5 mA
End point	Visible or palpable twitches of calf muscles, foot, or toes at 0.3–0.5 mA (at a depth of 8–12 cm)
Drug dosage	20 ml of Local anesthetic deposited
Highlights	Use is much less clinically because distribution is limited and higher level of skill is required Not suitable for catheter insertion because of deep location and perpendicular angle of needle insertion required, best reserved for patients who have spinal injuries or positioning difficulties

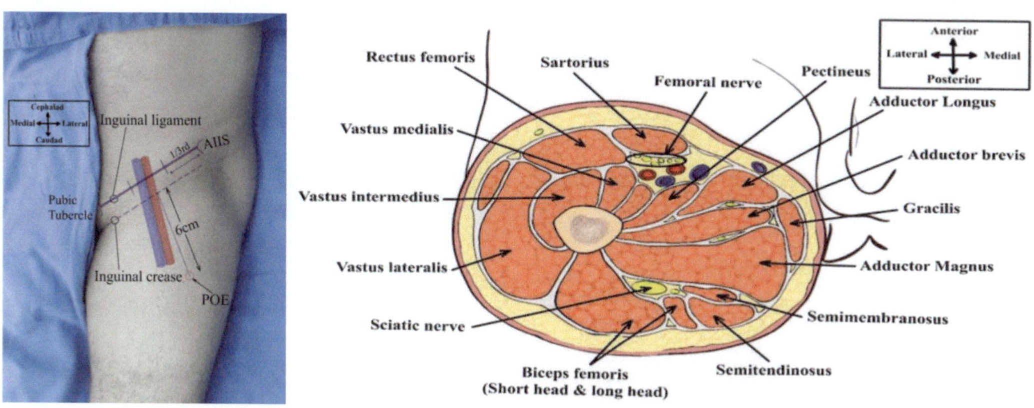

Fig. 9.16 (**a**) Landmark for anterior sciatic nerve block. (**b**) Cross section of landmark-guided sciatic nerve block. *AL* Adductor longus, *AB* Adductor brevis, *AM* Adductor magnus, *SM* Semitendinosus, *SM* Semimembranosus, *BF* Biceps femoris

Table 9.30 Troubleshooting anterior approach for sciatic nerve block

Response	Stimulation	Interpretation	Rescue measures
Twitch of Quadricep muscles		Needle superficial	Advance the needle further
Local twitch at femoral crease	Direct stimulation of iliopsoas, pectineus	Needle too superficial	Reassess the landmark
No bony contact / twitch till 12 cm			Redirect laterally
Bony contact (lesser trochanter)			Foot to be laterally rotated, if it fails redirect needle medially
Twitch of hamstrings		Unreliable end point as branches of hamstrings depart the main nerve at the level of needle insertion	Withdraw and redirect needle 5–10 degrees either medially or laterally

1. *Anterior Approach.*

   USG-guided Anterior approach sciatic nerve block (Table 9.32).

Approaches	Transducer position
Anterior approach	Transverse on proximal medial thigh
Transgluteal approach	Transverse on posterior buttock between ischial tuberosity and greater trochanter
Subgluteal approach	Transverse on gluteal crease Sciatic Nerve Block

Tips

1. If nerve not visualized move the transducer proximally/distally to clearly visualize it.
2. Dorsiflexion/Planter flexion of ankle to move the nerve within the intermuscular plane, facilitating identification.

Table 9.31 Complications of landmark-guided sciatic nerve block

Due to needle puncture	Due to Local anesthetic	Due to catheter
Hematoma (Tip—Avoid multiple needle insertions)	Local anesthetic systemic toxicity (LAST)—Correct dose and volume to be calculated, with frequent aspirations	Infection (Tip—Remove the catheter within 72 hrs)
Nerve injury—2–4/10,000 (Tip—Do not inject drug if response present at <0.3 mA)	Falls (Tip—Patient to wear knee immobilizer)	
Infection (Tip—Strict adherence to aseptic measure)	Pudendal nerve block (Due to diffusion of drug)	
Vascular Puncture (Avoid deep insertions beyond 2 cm of bony contact to avoid pelvic vessels)	Nerve ischemia (due to Torniquet, Local anesthetic, and epinephrine in combination)	
Perforation of pelvic organs (Advance the needle in medial)		

An in-plane approach may be difficult due to steep angle of the needle and use of curved.

2. *Transgluteal/Subgluteal approach* The preference for one approach over the other is based on the patient's anatomical characteristics and the operator's personal preference. The subgluteal approach may be a better choice for most patients and indications, including obese patients.

   Subgluteal approach is performed just a few centimeters more distally than transgluteal approach, and is technically simpler to perform.

Sonoanatomy	Transgluteal	Subgluteal
	Sciatic nerve is blocked between greater trochanter and ischial tuberosity	The nerve is just below the level of the gluteal crease where the nerve lies more superficial
Probe used	Curvilinear probe	Linear probe

Sonoanatomy	Transgluteal	Subgluteal
Location of nerve	Located immediately deep to the gluteus maximus muscle and superficial to the quadratus femoris muscle	Positioned between the long head of the biceps femoris muscle and the posterior surface of the adductor magnus

USG-guided Subgluteal approach/ Transgluteal approach (Table 9.33).

Continuous Ultrasound-Guided Subgluteal Block

Advancement of the needle in plane in a lateral-to-medial direction until the tip is adjacent to the nerve and deep to the gluteus maximus fascia and quadratus femoris muscle, ensure appropriate catheter location.

Alternatively, the catheter can be inserted using a longitudinal view. With this approach, after successful imaging of the sciatic nerve in the cross-sectional view, the transducer is rotated 90° so that the sciatic nerve is visualized in the longitudinal view. However, this approach requires significantly greater US imaging skills.

Proper placement of the needle also can be confirmed by obtaining a motor response of the calf or foot, at which point 4–5 mL of local anesthetic is injected. This small dose of local anesthetic serves to ensure adequate local anesthetic distribution as well as to make the catheter advancement easier.

The catheter is secured by either taping it to the skin or tunneling. A common infusion strategy consists of ropivacaine 0.2% at a rate of 5 mL/min with a patient-controlled bolus of 5 mL/h.

Tips

1. Tilting the transducer proximally or distally can help improve the contrast and bring the nerve "out of the background" of the musculature.
2. Often, the nerve is better imaged after the injection of local anesthetic.
3. Alternatively, sliding the transducer slightly proximal or distal can improve the quality of the image and allow for better visualization.
4. Needle tip is difficult to visualize due to the steep angle and depth of the needle placement.
5. The inferior gluteal artery is a useful land mark to locate the sciatic nerve which is seen medial to the nerve.

Table 9.32 Anterior approach

Position	Supine with slight external rotation and abduction, with hip and knee slightly flexed
Landmark (Fig. 9.17a)	Low-frequency probe is placed in transverse position on proximal medial thigh Sciatic nerve is imaged at the level of lesser trochanter, anteromedial aspect of the thigh (at a depth of 6–8 cm) Skin and subcutaneous tissue Femoral artery (beneath the sartorius muscle) Musculature of three fascial compartments of the thigh (anterior, medial, posterior) Adductor Longus, Adductor Brevis, Adductor Magnus (Superior to inferior) Sciatic nerve is a hyperechoic oval structure sandwiched between adductor magnus and bicep femoris
POE	Transducer is transverse and 10 cm needle is inserted in plane from medial/lateral aspect of thigh or out of plane (Fig. 9.17b)
Needle	Once tip is in proper position (PNS guidance can be used) 1–2 ml of injectate to confirm deposition of drug in sciatic sheath and delineation of the nerve (Fig. 9.17c)
Dose	10–15 ml of Local anesthetic
End point	Hydrodissection or spread of drug within the sheath.
Highlight	No lateral position needed, not well suited for catheter insertion as needle transverses through many muscles, plus position is cumbersome, and perpendicular insertion is challenging

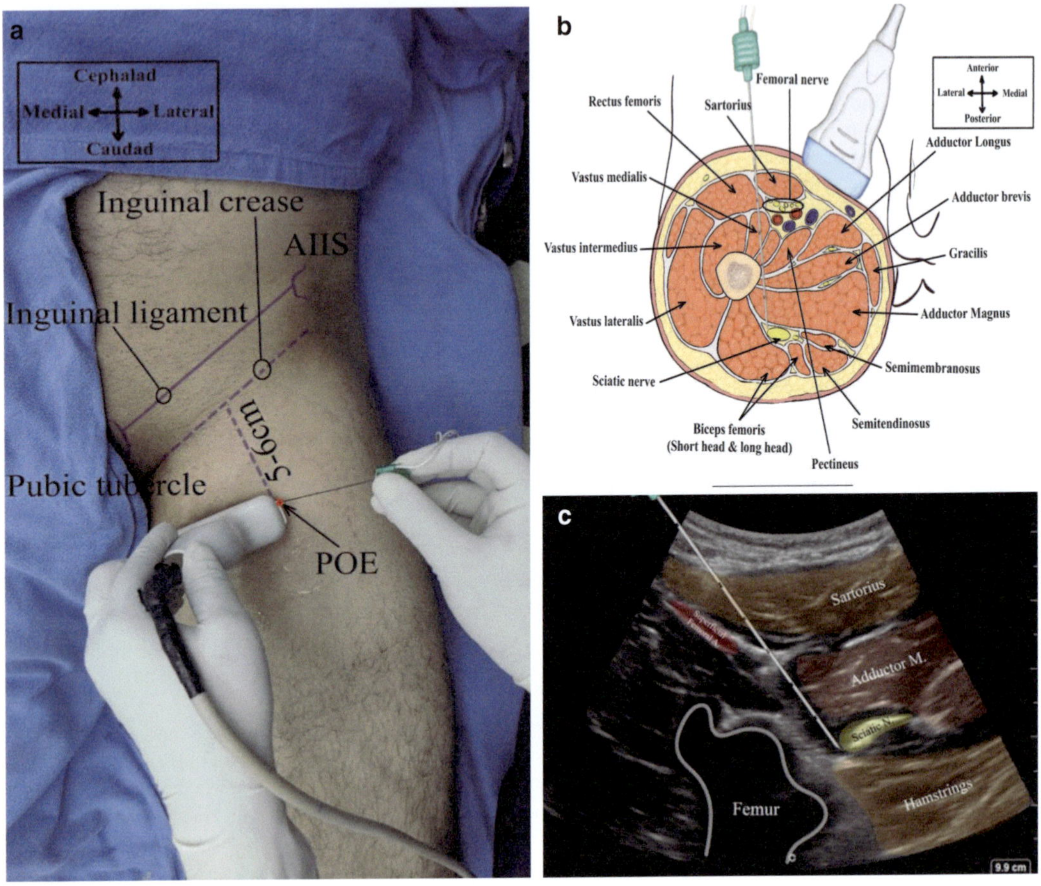

Fig. 9.17 (**a**) Probe position for anterior sciatic nerve block. (**b**) Cross section of proximal thigh with sciatic nerve block. (**c**) USG image of anterior sciatic nerve block

Table 9.33 Subgluteal approach/Transgluteal approach

Position	Lateral, with the side to be anesthetized up and with the hip and knees flexed
Landmark (Fig. 9.18a)	Line drawn between greater trochanter and the ischial tuberosity The initial transducer position is in the depression between the two bony structures
POE	Ultrasound probe was positioned parallel to the line with its orientation marker directed laterally (i.e., directed toward the greater trochanter, so as to provide a transverse scan of the subgluteal space and the sciatic nerve) (Fig. 9.18a) Subgluteal space (It extended from the greater trochanter laterally to the ischial tuberosity medially) is seen as a hypoechoic area between gluteus maximus and the quadratus femoris muscles The sciatic nerve was seen as an oval hyperechoic nodule
Needle	In-plane needle is inserted typically from the lateral aspect of the transducer, and advanced toward the sciatic nerve (Table 9.18b)
Dose	15–20 ml of Local anesthetic is injected
End point	The goal is to place the needle tip adjacent to the sciatic nerve, deep into the gluteus maximus muscle

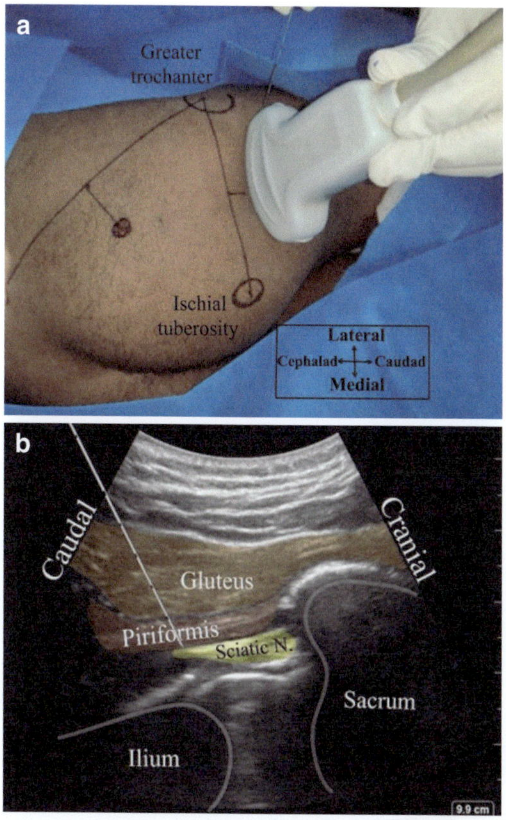

Fig. 9.18 (**a**) Probe position for Subgluteal approach. (**b**) USG images of transgluteal sciatic nerve block with in-plane needle insertion

9.4 Femoral Nerve Block

9.4.1 Introduction

A femoral nerve block is relatively simple to learn and administer, and has a low risk of complications. The femoral nerve block can be used for surgical anesthesia and post-operative pain management for cases involving anterior thigh and knee. Femoral nerve block can be used as a sole technique or in combination with lateral femoral cutaneous nerve, obturator nerve, and sciatic nerve block for various surgeries involving hip, thigh, knee, leg, and foot.

9.4.2 Anatomy

Femoral nerve anatomy (Table 9.34).

9.4.3 Indications

- Surgery on anterior aspect of thigh and for superficial surgery on the medial aspect of the leg below the knee.
- Prolonged analgesia for fracture on the femoral neck or shaft, total knee arthroplasty—Continuous technique, highly useful in emergency rooms and to facilitate physical and radiological examinations.
- Supplemental with sciatic or popliteal block to provide complete anesthesia of the lower leg and ankle.

9.4.4 Contraindication

Contraindications of Femoral nerve block (Table 9.35).

9.4.5 Preparations

Refer to Table 9.2.

9.4.6 Drugs

Drugs used Femoral Nerve Block (Table 9.36).

9.4.7 Block Approaches

9.4.7.1 Landmark and PNS-Guided Technique

Landmark and PNS-Guided Femoral Nerve Block (Table 9.37).

Table 9.34 Femoral nerve anatomy

Roots	Originates from dorsal divisions of the anterior rami of the L2, L3, and L4 spinal nerves		
Course	The femoral nerve travels through the pelvis in the groove between the psoas and the iliacus muscles (Fig. 9.19) Emerges at the junction of middle and lower thirds of lateral border of Psoas muscle Enters thigh posterior to inguinal ligament Lateral and posterior to Femoral artery Deep to both fascia lata and fascia iliaca Into thigh it divides into anterior and posterior branches (4 cm below the inguinal ligament)		
Innervations/ Actions	*Muscle supply*	*Anterior branch* Hip flexors—Pectineus, Iliacus, and Sartorius Knee extensors-Quadriceps femoris, Rectus femoris	*Posterior branch* Branches to Quadriceps femoris Saphenous nerve (sensory branch)
	Motor	Hip flexion, Knee extension	
	Cutaneous	Anterior cutaneous branches—skin of anteromedial thigh Saphenous nerve—skin of the medial leg and foot (Fig. 9.20)	
	Joint	Anterior wall of Hip joint, Anterior Femur, Anteromedial knee joint	

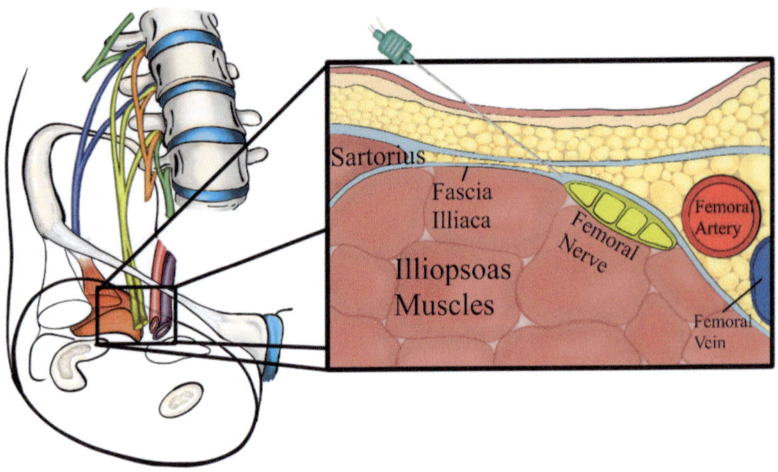

Fig. 9.19 Schematic representation and cross section of the femoral nerve in the groin area

Tips

1. Sensory block was checked on the anterior and medial aspect of thigh and on medial aspect of lower leg. Motor block by checking the ability to elevate the foot from table.
2. USG Adductor canal block is preferred over femoral nerve block because of the impaired knee extension and weight bearing associated with FNB.
3. Knee immobilizers should be used while ambulation to prevent falls after FNB.
4. Paraesthesia should not be sought as the preferred method for giving FNB.

Troubleshooting of Landmark-Guided Femoral Nerve Block

Troubleshooting of landmark-guided femoral nerve block (Table 9.38).

Continuous Femoral Nerve Block

Catheter is inserted 5 cm beyond tip of the needle. After negative aspiration 10 ml of LA is injected followed by 5 ml/h (0.2% Ropivacaine).

Tips

If resistance is felt during catheter insertion withdraw to the skin and reinsert.

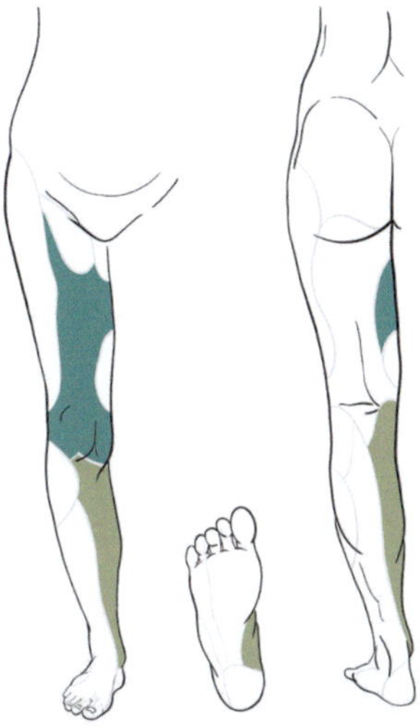

Fig. 9.20 Sensory distribution of the femoral nerve

Table 9.35 Contraindications of femoral nerve block

Absolute	Relative
Patient refusal Local site infection Allergy to local anesthetics	Anticoagulation or bleeding disorders Femoral nerve neuropathy Peritoneal infection Large inguinal lymph nodes/tumor Avoid/discuss with surgeon if compartment syndrome suspected Femoral vascular graft Previous ilioinguinal surgery /burn

Table 9.36 Drugs used femoral nerve block

Drug	Onset (min)	Anesthesia (h)	Analgesia (h)
2% Lignocaine	10–20	2–5	3–8
0.5% Ropivacaine	15–30	4–8	5–12
0.75% Ropivacaine	10–15	5–10	6–24
0.5% Bupivacaine	15–30	5–15	8–30

Complications

Complications of landmark-guided femoral nerve block (Table 9.39).

Table 9.37 Landmark and PNS-guided femoral nerve block

Position	Supine with slight abduction 10–20°, slight external rotation (Tip—In obese patients with difficult anatomy flat pad can be placed under the patient's buttocks in order to expose the inguinal region)
Landmark (Fig. 9.21a)	Under all aseptic precautions Line is drawn connecting the anterior superior iliac spine (ASIS) and the pubic tubercle (PT) and femoral artery is palpated on it
POE	POE is 1.5 cm lateral to the femoral artery and 1 cm below the inguinal ligament at 30–45-degree angle to the skin in a cephalad direction (Fig. 9.21b) ↓ Needle pierces through Fascia Lata above and Fascia Iliaca below with a feeling of "double pop" Needle to be positioned below the Fascia Iliaca
Needle	A 5-cm long, 21–22 gauge short-bevel, insulated stimulating needle
PNS stimulation	Nerve stimulator is set at a current intensity of 1 mA (2 Hz, 0.1–0.3 msec)
End point	Quadriceps muscle contraction (Patellar twitch) at current of 0.3 mA–0.5 mA
Drug dosage	15–20 ml of drug injected after negative aspiration
Highlights	Multiple injection techniques where individual muscle twitches were observed and drugs given at multiple sites have been abandoned

9.4.7.2 Ultrasound-Guided Femoral Nerve Block

Ultrasound-guided Femoral nerve block (Table 9.40).

Tips

1. Femoral nerve can be identified by slight tilting cranially or caudally over the iliacus muscle.
2. Optimum transducer pressure has to be applied to avoid obscuring femoral vein as well as inter fascial plane, to enhance optimum spread of drug.

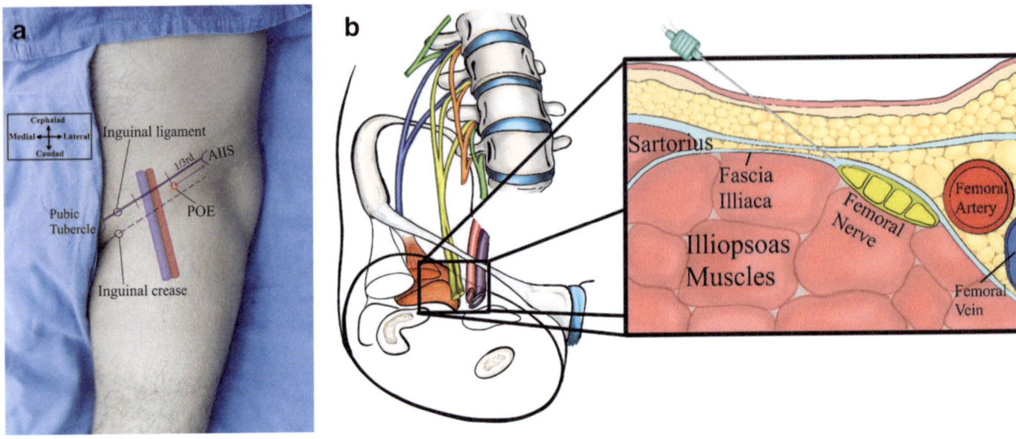

Fig. 9.21 (**a**) Landmark for femoral nerve block. (**b**) Cross section of landmark guided femoral nerve block

Table 9.38 Troubleshooting of landmark-guided femoral nerve block

Response	Stimulation	Interpretation	Rescue measures
No response	None	Needle too lateral or too medial	Reassess landmarks and reinsert needle
Bone is contacted (Superior ramus of pubic bone or Femur)	None,	Needle is too deep	Withdraw and reinsert
Vascular puncture	None	Needle is inserted too medially	Withdraw and move the needle laterally by 1 cm
Sartorius muscle twitch—Band-like thigh contraction without patella movement	Nerve to Sartorius muscle	Needle tip anterior and medial	Move the needle laterally and go 1–3 mm deeper
Flexion of thigh/external rotation of thigh	Stimulation of Iliopsoas/Pectineus muscle	Needle is too deep	Withdraw and reinsert the needle

Table 9.39 Complications of landmark-guided femoral nerve block

Due to needle puncture	Due to Local anesthetic	Due to catheter
Hematoma (Tip—Withdraw the needle and redirect laterally, press the puncture site for 2–3 mins)	Local anesthetic systemic toxicity (LAST)	Infection (Tip—Remove the catheter within 72 h)
Nerve injury—2-4/10,000 (Tip—Do not inject drug if response present at <0.3 mA)	Falls (Tip—Patient to wear knee immobilizer)	
Infection (Tip—Strict adherence to aseptic measure)		

3. Try to identify the fascia Lata, as drug beneath wrong sheath could lead to block failure.
4. Never inject against high resistance as it may mean intrafascicular placement.
5. Following surgery like hip surgeries landmarks may be displaced due to fluid extravasation, with arteries and nerves deeper than usual position.

Continuous US-Guided Femoral Nerve Block

It includes placement of the catheter just deep to fascia iliaca near the femoral nerve. Needle is inserted in plane, after confirming the needle placement, catheter is advanced 2–4 cm beyond the tip to inject the full dose (0.2% Ropivacaine at a rate of 5 ml/h).

Table 9.40 Femoral nerve block (USG approach)

Position	Supine with affected limb abducted and externally rotated
Landmark (Fig. 9.22a)	Under all aseptic precautions, high-frequency linear (10–15 MHz) transducer placed transversely on femoral crease ↓ Identify femoral artery and vein in short axis view(cross-section) and fascia lata and iliaca above it ↓ Moved probe medial to lateral to identify the nerve as triangular/oval hyperechoic structure sandwiched between two layers of fascia iliaca above the iliacus muscle lateral to femoral artery
POE	Once identified, a skin wheal of LA is made 1–1.5 cm away from the lateral edge of the transducer (Fig. 9.22a) ↓ Needle inserted in-plane from lateral to medial side just lateral to femoral artery (Fig. 9.22b) (Tip-Out-of-plane approach can be used and needle is inserted perpendicular to the skin, caudal to probe in cephalad direction following the needle tip toward the femoral nerve.)
Needle	A 5-cm long, 21–22 gauge short-bevel, insulated stimulating/ needle
PNS stimulation	Can be used along with USG (0.5 mA, 0.1 msec).
End point	Drug to be deposited below the fascia iliaca posterolateral or anteriorly displacing the femoral nerve as hypoechoic spread deep to the fascia iliaca and around the nerve
Drug dosage	1–2 ml of drug injected to identify the correct position of the needle; 10–15 ml of drug deposited

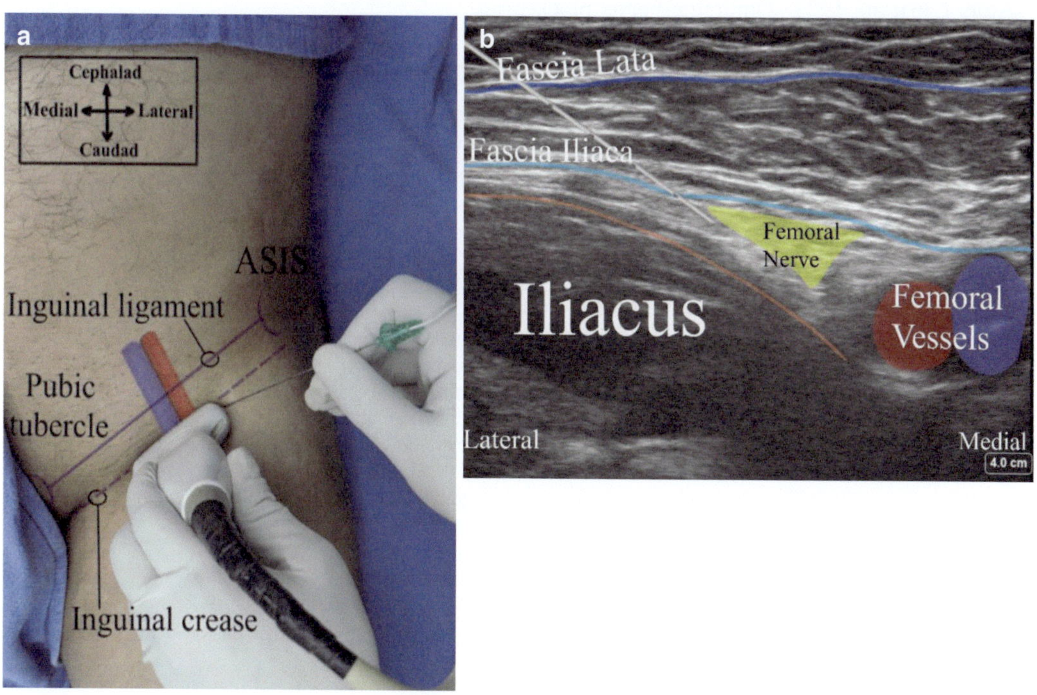

Fig. 9.22 (**a**) Probe and needle position for femoral nerve block. (**b**) In plane needle position for femoral nerve block

Tips

1. Out-of-plane approach increases the chances of vascular injury if needle tip is not visible all the time.
2. Non-stimulating catheters are used for US-Guided technique as proper catheter placement is confirmed by deposition of drug in proper fascial plane and not the motor response.
3. Femoral catheter dislodgement is very common due to shallow placement of nerve along with highly mobile adipose tissue, so the needle should be inserted a bit too laterally so that a good length of catheter is placed inside iliacus muscle to avoid displacement.

9.5 Obturator Nerve Block

9.5.1 Introduction

Obturator nerve block was first described by Gaston Labat in 1922. Obturator nerve block along with femoral nerve and sciatic nerve can be used to anesthetized the entire lower limb. Labat's classic technique has been modified by Parks and Wassef. In 1973, Alon Winnie introduced the 3 in 1 block technique via paravascular inguinal injection but further studies showed it to be unreliable for obturator nerve block.

9.5.2 Anatomy

Obturator nerve Anatomy (Table 9.41).

9.5.3 Indications

1. To treat hip joint pain.
2. Relief of adductor muscle spasm.
3. Combine sciatic nerve block with femoral nerve block for procedures distal to proximal third of the thigh.
4. Improve tourniquet tolerance.
5. Improve quality of post-operative analgesia.
6. Suppress obturator reflex during Transurethral resection of bladder tumor (TURBT).
7. Diagnosis and treatment of chronic pain states secondary to knee arthrosis or pelvic tumors.

9.5.4 Contraindications

Contraindications of Femoral nerve block (Table 9.42).

Table 9.41 Obturator nerve anatomy

Roots	Anterior primary rami of L2, L3, and L4		
Course	Originates from Anterior division of Ventral Primary Rami of L2-L4 roots Descends to pelvis on the medial side of psoas muscle Common obturator nerve, runs between the pectineus and obturator externus muscles immediately after the nerve emerges from the obturator canal Exits the pelvis through obturator foramen after dividing into Anterior and Posterior branch At the level of femoral crease Anterior branch lies between Adductor longus and Brevis Posterior branch between Adductor brevis and Magnus		
Innervations / Actions	Muscle supply	Anterior division- Adductor longus, Adductor brevis and Gracilis, innervates femoral artery	Posterior division- Obturator externus and Adductor magnus (except the hamstring part), innervates popliteal artery
	Motor	Adduction of thigh, Lateral rotation of thigh (Obturator externus)	
	Cutaneous	Cutaneous branch supplies skin of posteromedial aspect of the inferior third of the thigh (Fig. 9.23)	
	Joint	Anterior branch—Anteromedial aspect of the hip joint Posterior branch—Posterior aspect of knee joint	

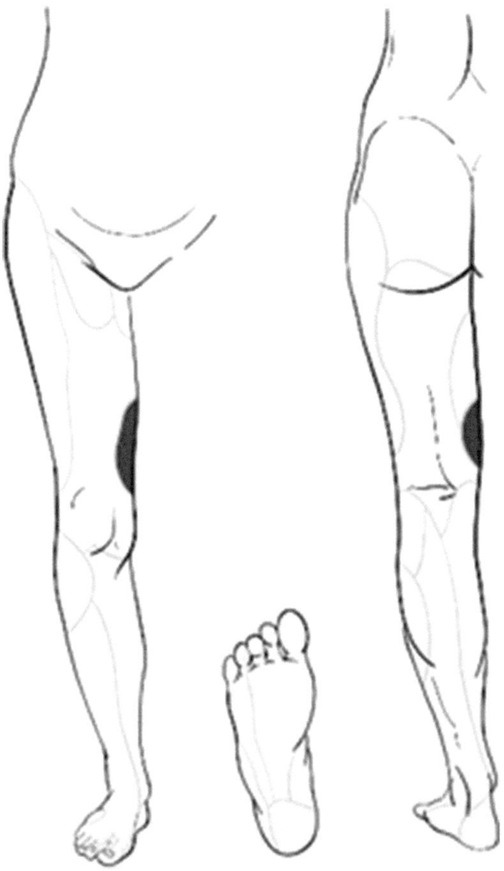

Fig. 9.23 Cutaneous innervation of Obturator nerve

Table 9.42 Contraindications of Femoral nerve block

Absolute	Relative
Patient refusal Local site infection Allergy to local anesthetics	Anticoagulation or bleeding disorders Obturator nerve neuropathy Large inguinal lymph nodes/Tumor Avoid/discuss with surgeon if compartment syndrome suspected

9.5.5 Preparations

Refer to Table 9.2.

9.5.6 Drugs

Drugs used for Femoral nerve block (Table 9.43).

Table 9.43 Drugs used for Femoral nerve block

Drug	Surgery type	Onset of motor block (min)	Duration (H)
1–2% Mepivacaine	TURBT (for adductor muscle spasm)	15	3–4
1–2% Lidocaine	TURBT (for adductor muscle spasm)		
0.25–0.5% Ropivacaine	Lower limb surgeries	25	8–10
0.25–0.5% Bupivacaine	Lower limb surgeries		
0.25–0.5% Levobupivacaine	Lower limb surgeries		

9.5.7 Block Approaches

9.5.7.1 Landmarks and PNS-Guided Approach

The common landmarks to all the approaches:

- Anterior superior iliac spine (ASIS) and Pubic tubercle (PT).
- Femoral artery, Femoral crease.
- Tendon of adductor longus muscle.

Older Techniques

Various techniques of obturator nerve block (Table 9.44).

Labat's Classic Technique

Labat's Obturator Nerve Block (Table 9.45).

Paravascular Selective Inguinal Block

Paravascular Selective Inguinal Block (Table 9.46).

9.5.7.2 Ultrasound-Guided Obturator Nerve Block

Ultrasound approach to Obturator nerve block (Table 9.47).

Table 9.44 Various techniques of obturator nerve block

Name of the technique	Brief explanation	Success rate
3 in 1 Block Technique	Distal compression is given to a large volume of drug that is injected beneath the fascia iliaca with the presumption of its spread to the lumbar plexus or obturator nerve	Not successful
Iliofascial Block technique	More lateral approach to 3 in 1 Block technique	More successful block of lateral femoral cutaneous nerve than obturator nerve
Psoas compartment block	Posterior approach to lumbar plexus	Complete lumbar plexus block with single injection Femoral nerve block close to 100% Obturator nerve block 88–93%
Parasacral Sciatic Block (plexus block)	Parietal peritoneum and Pelvic fascia anatomically surrounding sacral plexus are separated from obturator nerve	Complete block of sacral plexus, not reliable for obturator nerve

Tips

1. Out-of-plane approach by Taha—A needle is inserted from the point indicated by the yellow circle in an anterior-to-posterior direction ultrasound guidance. In the approach used by Lin et al. a needle is inserted from the point indicated by the red circle, in a lateral-to-medial direction, using in-plane ultrasound.
2. Alternatively, the common nerve can be blocked at the level between Pectineus (Lower Border) and Adductor Brevis using an Out-of-plane technique from the given above insertion point with 5–10 ml of Drug. Nerves appear as hyperechoic, flat, thin, fusiform

Table 9.45 Labat's obturator nerve block

Position	Supine with 30-degree abduction of limb to be blocked
Landmark (Fig. 9.24)	Line 1–1.5 cm line from pubic tubercle laterally in horizontal plane Line 2–1.5 cm long line is drawn caudally from lateral end of Line 1
POE	Needle is inserted perpendicular to skin from distal end of Line 2 till bony contact is encountered (depth of 1.5–4 cm) of superior pubic rami ↓ Needle is withdrawn 1 cm and redirected cephalad and laterally at 45° to the obturator foramen 2–3 cm deeper than initial bony contact
Needle	22 Gauge 10 cm long
PNS stimulation	At a current intensity of 1.5 mA (2 Hz, 0.1–0.3 msec)
End point	Sustained Adductor muscle contractions at 0.3 mA–0.5 mA
Drug dosage	Fractionated dose of 10–15 ml
Highlights	If the block is performed more distally, only one of the divisions may be blocked, leaving the medial thigh skin (anterior division) or posterior knee capsule (posterior division) unblocked

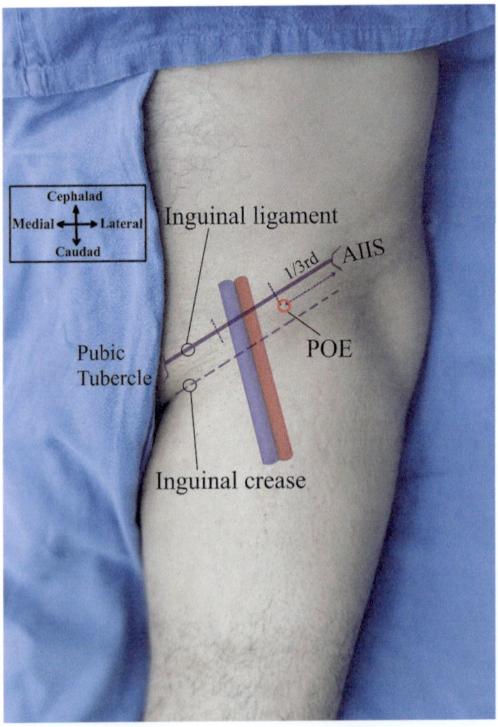

Fig. 9.24 Landmark for obturator nerve block

Table 9.46 Paravascular selective inguinal block

Position	Supine with 30-degree thigh abduction and external rotation
Landmark	Identify femoral artery at inguinal crease and tendon of adductor longus at pubic tubercle (Tip—For adductor longus tendon identification, extreme leg abduction is required)
POE	21G insulated needle is inserted at the midpoint of the line drawn over the inguinal crease from the femoral artery to the tendon of the adductor longus in a 30° cephalad direction ↓ At a depth of 2–3 cm via adductor longus muscle and twitches are seen on posteromedial aspect of thigh where 5–7 ml of drug is deposited ↓ Needle is advanced further and slightly laterally 0.5–1.5 cm over adductor brevis and twitches are seen posteromedially where 5–7 ml of drug is deposited
Needle	21/22 Gauge, 5–10 cm long
PNS stimulation	At a current intensity of 1.5 mA (2 Hz, 0.1–0.3 msec) decreased to 0.4–0.5 mA
End point	(a) Twitch at 0.5 mA due to adductor longus and gracilis stimulation (anterior branch) (b) Twitch at 0.5 mA due to adductor magnus stimulation (posterior branch)
Drug dosage	5–7 ml of drug at both the levels
Highlights	Selective block of anterior and posterior branches of obturator nerve, easier to perform, needle is away from intrapelvic structures, articular branches to hip joint are not blocked

Table 9.47 Ultrasound approach to Obturator nerve block

Position	Supine with 30-degree abduction of limb to be blocked.
Landmark	The US transducer is kept transversally at the level of femoral crease (Fig. 9.25a, c) Identify the femoral vessels Transducer is moved medially to locate pectineus and the adductor muscles
POE	Needle is inserted 1–2 cm medial to femoral vein either at the femoral crease or 1–3 cm inferior to inguinal crease on medial aspect
Needle	In plane technique (a) Needle is advanced between Adductor Longus and Adductor Brevis and 5–10 ml of Drug given in this fascial plane (b) Needle is advanced further to position needle tip between Adductor Brevis and Magnus and 5–10 ml of Drug given in this fascial plane
PNS stimulation	Can be used at a current intensity of 1.5 mA (2 Hz, 0.1–0.3 msec) decreased to 0.5 mA
End point	In-plane approach—Needle tip between Adductor longus and Brevis and between Adductor Brevis and magnus Out-of-plane approach—Needle tip between pectineus and Obturator externus (Fig. 9.25b, d)

shaped structures invested in fascia of the adductor muscles.

3. Peripheral nerve stimulator can be used as an adjunct to elicit contraction of the adductor muscles.

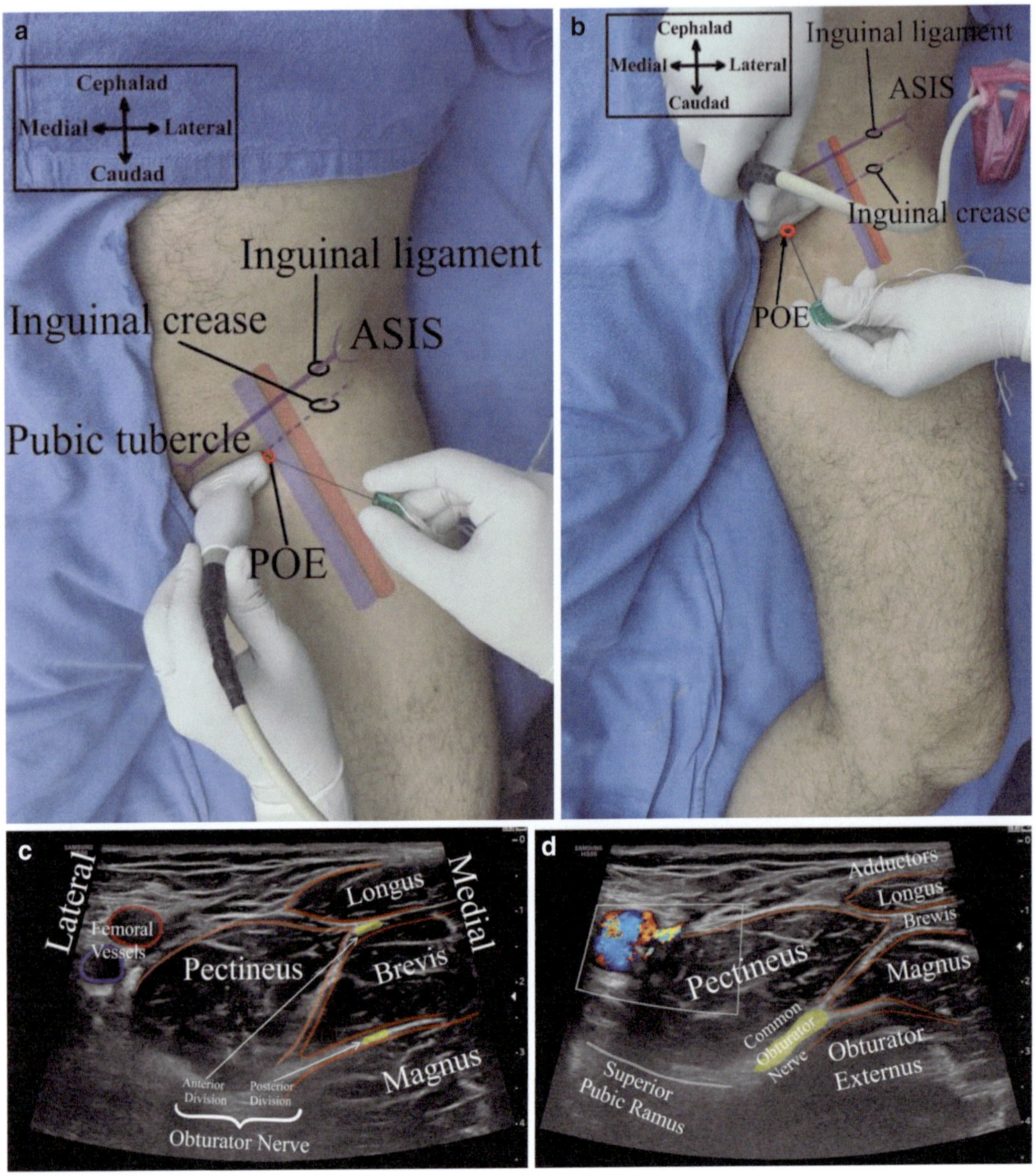

Fig. 9.25 (**a**) Probe position for obturator nerve block (in plane). (**b**) USG image of obturator nerve block (in plane). (**c**) Probe position for obturator nerve block (out of plane). (**d**) USG image of obturator nerve block (out of plane)

9.6 Lateral Femoral Cutaneous Nerve Block/Lateral Cutaneous Nerve of the Thigh

9.6.1 Introduction

Lateral Femoral cutaneous nerve (LFCN) block is a sensory block, which supplies the lateral thigh. LFCN is usually used in combination with other nerves like femoral, obturator, and sciatic. LFCN is superficial nerve having variable presentation and can be blocked using landmark, nerve stimulation, and ultrasound assistance.

9.6.2 Anatomy

Lateral femoral cutaneous Nerve originates from posterior division of L2 and L3. It travels from lateral border of psoas major muscle, crosses the iliacus muscles toward anterior superior iliac spine (ASIS), and passes behind or through the lateral portion of the inguinal ligament. Then it traverses in front of or through the sartorius muscle descending deep into the fascia lata and gives cutaneous supply to lateral thigh. Owing to its variable anatomy landmark guided block has variable success rate, however, peripheral nerve stimulator and ultrasound assistance have increased the success rate. The dermatomes supplied by LFCN are shown in Fig. 9.26.

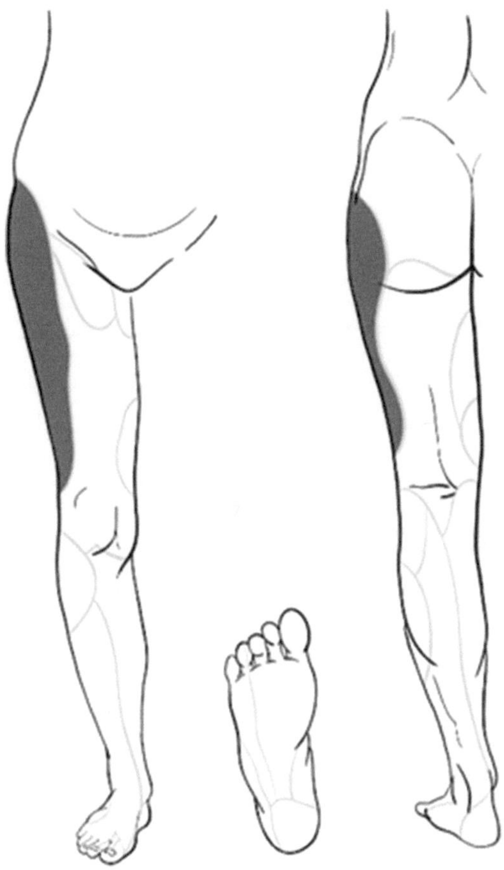

Fig. 9.26 Dermatomal distribution of Lateral femoral cutaneous nerve

9.6.3 Indications

- Lateral femoral cutaneous nerve block is usually used in combination.with other nerve blocks like femoral, obturator, or sciatic nerves and can be used various leg procedures.
- Reduce tourniquet pain.
- Superficial procedures on the lateral thigh like skin graft harvesting.
- As diagnostic and therapeutic block for neuralgia involving the lateral femoral cutaneous nerve known as meralgia paresthetica.

9.6.4 Contraindications

Contraindications for Lateral femoral cutaneous nerve (Table 9.48).

9.6.5 Preparations

Refer to Table 9.2.

9.6.6 Block Approaches

9.6.6.1 Landmark Approach

Landmark Approach—Lateral femoral cutaneous nerve (Table 9.49).

9.6.6.2 USG Approach

USG Approach of Lateral femoral cutaneous nerve (Table 9.50).

Table 9.48 Contraindications for Lateral femoral cutaneous nerve

Absolute	Relative
Patient refusal Local site infection Allergy to local anesthetics	Coagulation disorders Previous femoral bypass surgery

Table 9.49 Landmark approach—lateral femoral cutaneous nerve

Position	Supine position
Landmark and technique	Line 1 is a 2-cm horizontal / vertical line from ASIS Line 2 is a 2-cm line drawn perpendicular downward/horizontal from distal end of line 1
POE	Distal end of line 2 (Fig. 9.27)
Needle	A 5-cm needle is inserted perpendicular at POE until a loss of resistance is encountered. This first POP is felt when needle pierces fascia lata (Trick—Since loss of resistance is inconsistent and may not be perceived all the time, a fanwise infiltration of local anesthetic from medial to lateral direction increase the success rate)
PNS stimulation and end point	Though lateral femoral cutaneous nerve is sensory, nerve stimulator induced current (2 mA, 1 msec) can elicit paresthesia in the area of nerve supply
Drug dosage	10 ml of local anesthetic (individual or in combination) Surgical anesthesia (0.5–0.75% ropivacaine, 0.25–0.5% bupivacaine, 0.25–0.5% levobupivacaine, 1–2% Lidocaine with or without epinephrine) Analgesia- (0.2–0.375% ropivacaine, 0.125–0.25% bupivacaine, 0.125–0.25% levobupivacaine, 0.5%–1% lidocaine with or without epinephrine) In children, 0.15 mL/kg per side is adequate for adequate analgesia

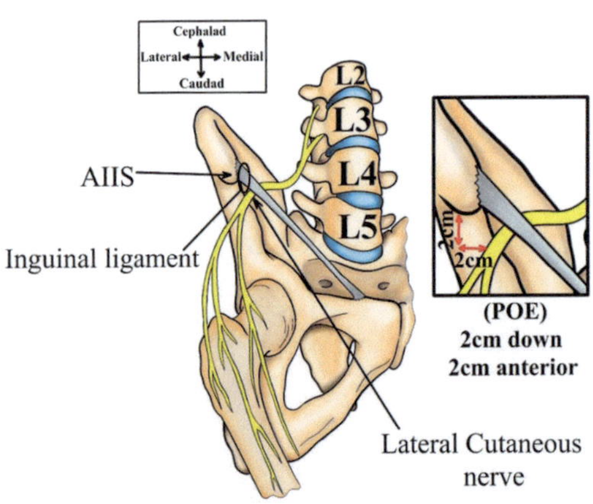

Fig. 9.27 Schematic representation of lateral femoral cutaneous nerve block

Table 9.50 USG Approach of Lateral femoral cutaneous nerve

Position	Supine position
Probe	High-frequency linear (10–15 MHz) probe
USG scanning landmark (Fig. 9.28a)	Under all aseptic precautions, place immediately medial and inferior to ASIS and parallel to inguinal ligament after aseptic skin preparation (Fig. 9.28a) Identify Sartorius muscle medially and Tensor Fascia lata laterally in short axis view LFCN identified as hypoechoic structure between the muscles
POE	Needle inserted using in-plane technique from lateral side of probe through subcutaneous tissue and tensor fascia lata muscle (Fig. 9.28b) (Tip—Needle can be inserted from medial side keeping in mind not to damage femoral vessels) Out-of-plane approach can also be used, however, final needle tip position is achieved by intermittent injecting LA in small aliquots (1 ml) Needle tip is positioned between tensor fascia lata and sartorius muscle and position is confirmed by injecting 1–2 ml of LA (Tip—If intramuscular LA spread is seen, a few mm needle tip movement in either direction and injection of 1–2 ml of LA is used to confirm the final needle position)
End point	Spread of LA in between tensor facia lata and sartorius and nerve is seen as a small oval hypoechoic structure floating in LA
Drug dose	A total of 5–10 ml drug is deposited

Potential Problems

The superficial nature of this block allows one to avoid most problems associated with regional blocks.

Tips

– Sometimes tendinous part of sartorius muscle is confused with LFCN. A proximal dynamic scan toward ASIS can differentiate LFCN in the fat-filled space below the ASIS.

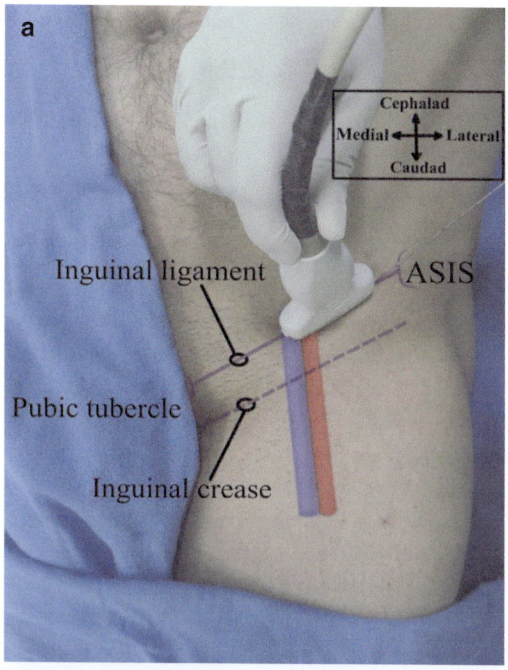

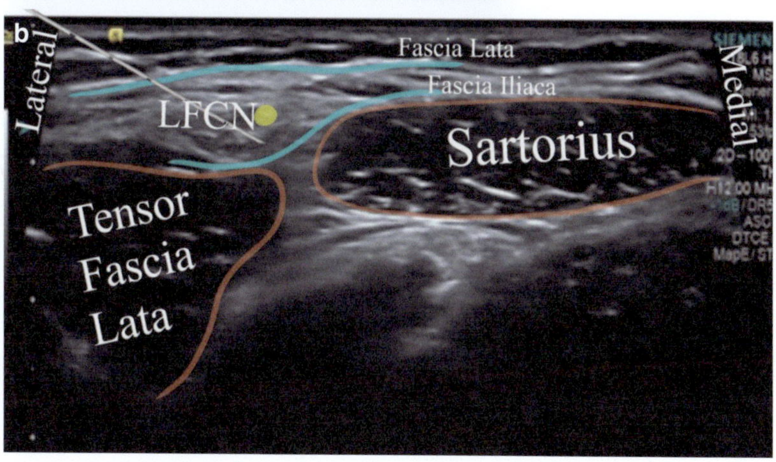

Fig. 9.28 (**a**) Probe and needle position of lateral femoral cutaneous nerve block. (**b**) USG image of lateral femoral cutaneous nerve block

– -Since this block is used in combination with other nerves and volume of drug required is more as compared to solitary required for nerve block so it is advisable to use a lower concentration (0.2% ropivacaine/0.125% bupivacaine) of drug for LFCN Block.

9.6.7 Complications

The potential complications of LFCN blockade are direct nerve puncture, intraneural injection, unintentional motor blocks of femoral and obturator nerve involvement, and intravascular injections.

However, with ultrasound guidance these complications can be minimized.

9.7 Fascia Iliaca Compartment Block

9.7.1 Introduction

Initially described by Dalens et al., Fascia Iliaca compartment allows for sufficient volume deposition and spread to at least femoral and lateral femoral cutaneous nerve and may be to Obturator nerve. This block is technically easy and cost–effective, especially the landmark approach. It is opioid sparing but does not provide complete analgesia.

9.7.2 Anatomy

The iliac fascia or Abernethy's Fascia is fascia present in region of ilium of the pelvis.

Fascia Iliaca Attaches

Anteriorly—External iliac vessels, posterior part of inguinal ligament, fascia Lata.
Posteriorly—Nerves of Lumbar Plexus.
Medially—It forms the posterior wall of the femoral sheath (lacuna vasorum), containing femoral vessels, and femoral branch of genitofemoral nerve.
Laterally—Forms Roof of Lacuna musculorum containing psoas major and iliacus muscles and femoral nerve.

Fascia Iliaca Compartment (Fig. 9.29) Is a Potential Space Between

Anteriorly—Posterior surface of fascia Iliaca that covers illiacus and psoas major muscle.
Posteriorly—Anterior surface of Iliopsoas muscle.
Medially—The vertebral column.
Craniomedially—Continuous with the space between quadratus lumborum muscle and its fascia.
Craniolaterally—Inner lip of the iliac crest.

9.7.3 Indications

1. Perioperative analgesia for Hip, Femur, and Knee surgeries (along with Sciatic nerve Block).
2. Analgesia for plaster applications in children.
3. Analgesia for lower leg tourniquet pain during awake surgery.

   *Check the safe dose, if required decrease the concentration rather than volume.

9.7.4 Contraindications

Contraindications for Fascia Iliaca Compartment block (Table 9.51).

9.7.5 Preparation

Refer to Table 9.2.

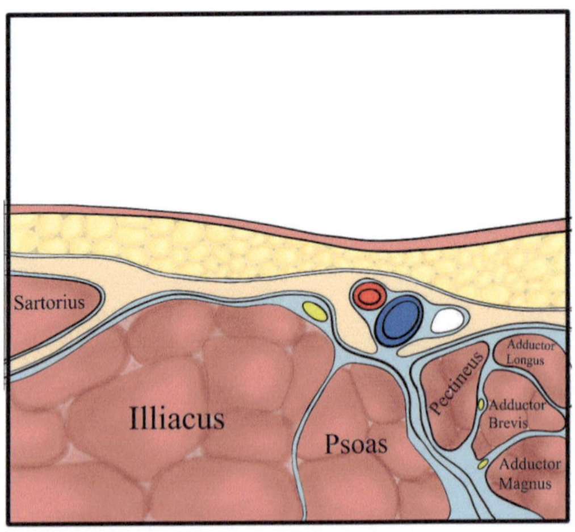

Fig. 9.29 Cross-sectional anatomy of the fascia iliaca compartment

Table 9.51 Contraindications or Fascia Iliaca Compartment block

Absolute	Relative
Patient refusal Local site infection Allergy to local anesthetics	Coagulation disorders Previous femoral bypass surgery

9.7.6 Block Approaches

9.7.6.1 Landmark-Guided Technique

Landmark-guided Fascia Iliaca Compartment block (Table 9.52).

Tips

1. Femoral arterial pulse can be palpated where medial and middle third of the inguinal ligament meet.
2. The needle insertion point is mid-way between Femoral nerve and Lateral Femoral Cutaneous Nerve allowing local anesthetic to spread and block these two nerves.
3. As Obturator nerve is separated from other two nerves by muscle bulk so its block via this approach is unreliable.
4. The second Pop is subtle in feel.

Table 9.52 Landmark-guided Fascia Iliaca compartment block

Position	Supine position
Landmark (Fig. 9.30a)	Identify anterior superior iliac spine (ASIS) and the pubic tubercle (PT) of the side to be blocked - Draw a line between ASIS and PT Divide the above line into three parts
POE (Fig. 9.30a)	1 cm caudal from the junction of the lateral and middle third after Local infiltration (Femoral pulse should be palpable 1.5–2 cm medial to the POE)
Needle (Fig. 9.30b)	Pierce the skin at 90 degrees with blunt-tipped/short beveled needle ↓ Once the skin is pierced redirect and advance the needle tip 60 degrees cranially observing for 2 pops (First pop—Perforates Fascia Lata, Second pop—Perforates Fascia Iliaca) ↓ Reduce the angle between needle and skin surface to 30 degrees and advance the needle 1–2 mm
Drug dosage	If no resistance is felt give 5 ml drug in aliquots (total 20 ml) after negative aspiration
Highlights	Genitofemoral nerve runs on anterior aspect of the psoas muscle, posterior to fascia iliaca thus FICB can block this nerve too

5. If no distinct pops are felt during needle placement, then withdraw the needle, check landmarks, and change angle to be more perpendicular.
6. If resistance comes readjust the needle as it might be hitting Iliacus muscle.
7. If bone is being hit, needle is too deep, withdraw and redirect cranially.
8. Blood on aspiration, remove the needle and apply pressure for at least 5 mins, reinsert more laterally.
9. When the syringe is de-attached from the needle back flow of LA must be seen, if not then either the needle is blocked or not in space.
10. Do not inject drug if pain or paresthesia is encountered.
11. For continuous technique, Cannula (Contiplex Cannula) is preferred over a catheter as the insertion of catheter in fascial plane cannot be controlled with blind technique.

9.7.6.2 Ultrasound-Guided Approach

Below/Infra Iliaca Block

USG-Guided below/Infra Iliaca block (Table 9.53).

Tips

1. If the branches of femoral artery are seen, move the probe cranially.
2. If resistance is felt during drug injectate, withdraw the needle (needle in muscle tissue).
3. Slight pain on injection is normal, severe pain means intraneural injection, withdraw and redirect.
4. No pain relief after 30 min advocates use of 15–20 ml half the concentration of drug.
5. Successful block of LFCN and ON depends on the proximal spread of drug as these nerves lie superior to fascia iliaca.

Supra Inguinal Fascia Illiaca Block

USG-guided supra inguinal approach to FICB (Table 9.54).

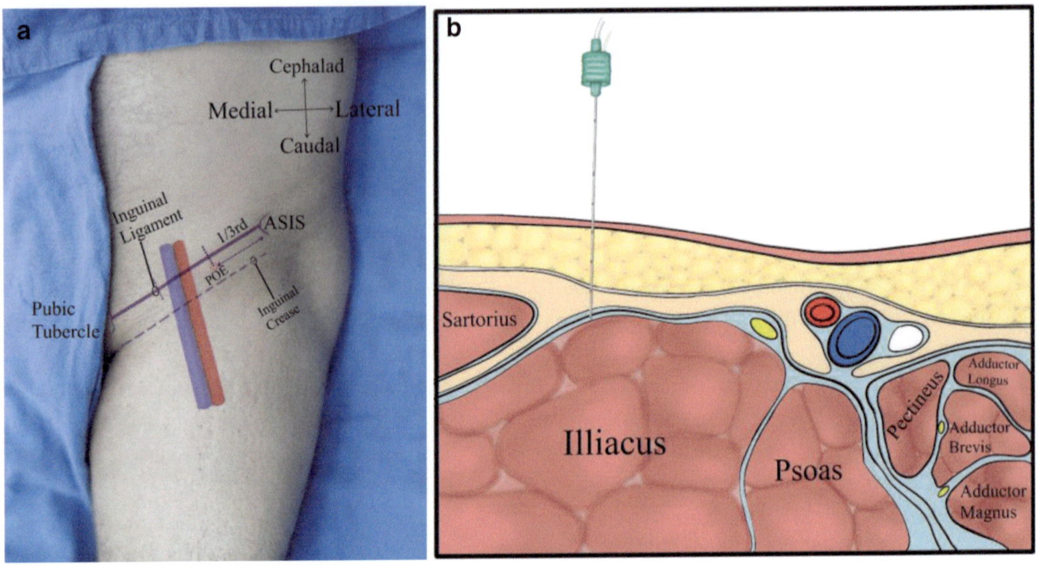

Fig. 9.30 (**a**) Landmark for FICB (ASIS—Anterior superior iliac spine). (**b**) Cross section of FICB showing the point of entry and drug spread

Table 9.53 USG-Guided below/Infra Iliaca block

Position	Supine
Landmark	Use high-frequency probe (13–18 MHz, Linear Array) Probe kept transversely over the anterior thigh below the inguinal ligament (Fig. 9.31a) Identify the femoral artery and iliopsoas muscle laterally (hypoechoic) with overlying hyperechoic fascia Iliaca (Fig. 9.31b) Hyperechoic femoral nerve is seen lying between iliopsoas and fascia iliaca at depth of 2–4 cm Moving Laterally triangular-shaped sartorius muscle is identified and further lateral ASIS is present
POE	In-plane/out-of-plane technique is used (Fig. 9.31c)
Needle	Advance the needle (50–100 mm) until tip is placed below the fascia iliaca around lateral third of line joining ASIS and Pubic tubercle
End point	Separation of fascia iliaca from iliopsoas muscle with LA spreading toward femoral nerve medially and Iliac crest laterally
Drug dosage	30–40 ml of 0.2% ropivacaine/0.25% bupivacaine/levobupivacaine
Highlights	More volume less concentration is given thus not good for dense blocks Out-of-plane technique is difficult

Table 9.54 USG-guided supra inguinal approach to FICB

Position	Supine
Landmark	High-frequency probe (6–14 MHz, Linear Array) is placed in the sagittal plane to obtain image of ilium and iliacus muscle (Fig. 9.32a) Identify the femoral Artery Probe is moved laterally and superiorly along the inguinal ligament toward the ASIS to lie laterally to Femoral Nerve (Fig. 9.32b) Deep circumflex artery is identified around 1–2 cm cephalad to inguinal ligament
POE	In-plane technique used. 2–4 cm caudad to inguinal ligament aiming toward deep circumflex artery, i.e., cephalad to inguinal ligament (Fig. 9.32a)
Needle	Advance the needle (50–10 cm) until the tip is placed below the fascia iliaca
End point	LA spread between fascia iliaca and iliacus muscle into the iliac fossa, with upward movement of deep circumflex artery or spread of LA is observed cranial to the point where the iliac muscle passes under the abdominal muscle (Fig. 9.32b)
Drug dosage	30–40 ml of 0.2% ropivacaine/0.25% bupivacaine/levobupivacaine
Highlights	This is a large volume block and spread of drug should be ensured in proper plane under USG guidance for success of the block

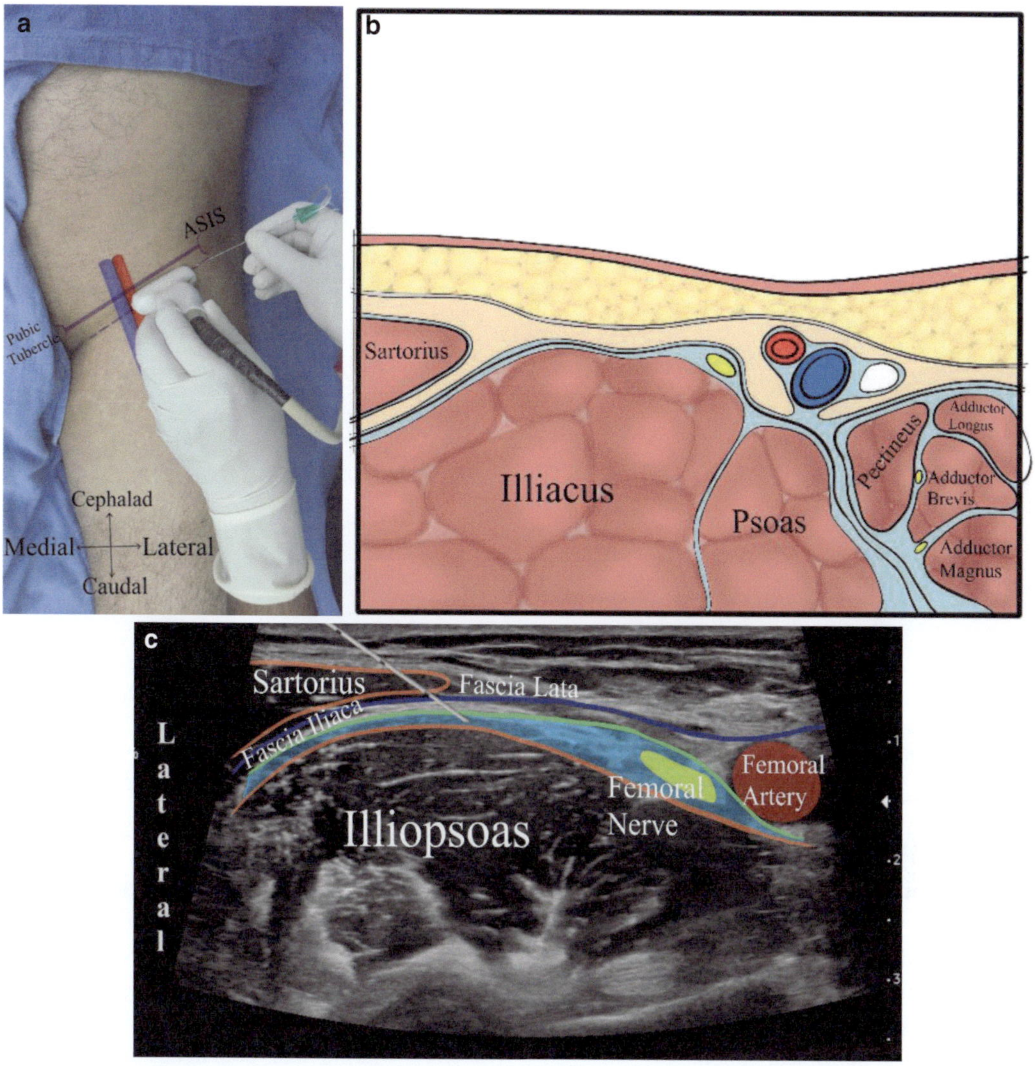

Fig. 9.31 (**a**) Probe kept transversely below the inguinal ligament. (**b**) Cross section of infra iliaca fascia block. (**c**) USG image showing in plane of plane needle insertion

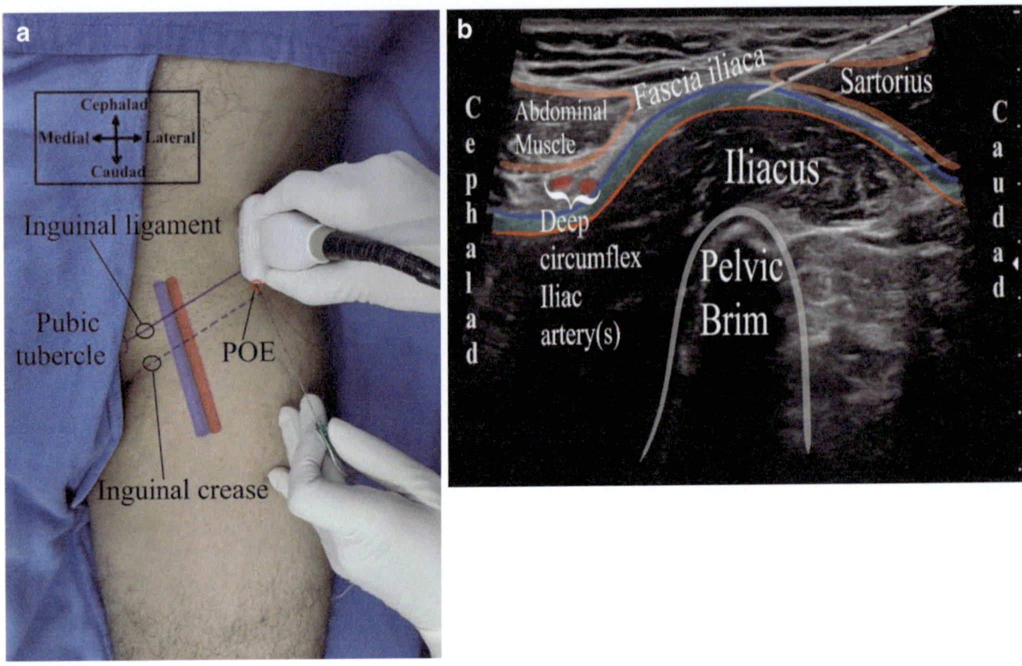

Fig. 9.32 (**a**) Probe kept in sagittal plane above the inguinal ligament moving toward ASIS. (**b**) USG image showing in plane needle insertion between fascia iliaca and iliacus muscle. *ASIS* Anterior superior iliac spine, *IM* Iliopsoas muscle

9.7.7 Complications

1. Block failure.
2. Hematoma.
3. Quadricep weakness.
4. Bladder and peritoneal puncture.
5. Neuropraxia.

9.8 Saphenous Nerve Block

9.8.1 Introduction

Historically, saphenous nerve block was given as subcutaneous injection using above knee femoral Para-condylar approach or below knee using a great saphenous vein as landmark. In 1993, Van derwal demonstrated a more proximal technique. Studies have shown that proximal Trans-sartorial approach to be 80% successful as compared to more distal approaches (65% for Para condylar and 40% for saphenous vein landmark).

Horn and colleagues demonstrated its consistent course with the saphenous branch of saphenous branch of the descending genicular artery (SDGA). Marian and colleagues showed that USG AC block lateral to the superficial femoral artery (SFA) proximally is more successful than distally.

A recent cadaveric study conducted by injection of 10 ml dye into proximal adductor canal (AC) block showed that it may result in significant analgesia to the knee joint through blockade of the saphenous nerve, posteromedial branch of the nerve to vastus medialis, superior medial genicular nerve, and genicular branch of obturator nerve, whereas distal AC was associated with greater motor sparing.

It is advantageous over femoral nerve block because of its motor sparing effect.

9.8.2 Adductor Canal Anatomy

Adductor canal is located in the distal portion of the middle third of the thigh. It is a gateway for neurovascular structures from the femoral triangle to popliteal fossa.

Proximal Border—Apex of the femoral triangle (medial border of the adductor longus muscle).
Antero Lateral Wall—Fascia of Vastus Medialis.
Posteromedial Wall—Fascia of Adductor Longus and Magnus.
Medially (Roof)—Vaso adductor membrane immediately deep into the sartorius muscle.
Distal border—Adductor hiatus (Opening within the Adductor Magnus Muscle).

Structures Passing Through Adductor Canal

1. Superficial femoral artery.
2. Femoral vein.
3. Saphenous nerve (small, round, hyperechoic structure anterior to artery) (Table 9.55 *Saphenous Nerve anatomy*).
4. Saphenous branch of descending genicular artery.
5. Genicular branch of obturator nerve.

Landmarks for adductor canal (AC)—Few centimeters distal to the midpoint between Anterior Superior Iliac Spine and the Patellar base corresponds to the proximal end of the AC/ distal femoral triangle blocks.
Advantage of Adductor canal Block—A properly performed block anesthetizes the anterior group of sensory nerves and along with other block techniques could target the posterior group of nerves without affecting the motor nerves, thus accelerating pain-free post-operative ambulation and enhances recovery.

9.8.3 Indications

1. Analgesia for knee surgery.
2. Along with other nerve blocks for Medial Ankle/Foot Surgeries.
3. Saphenous nerve stripping or harvesting.

Distribution of Anesthesia

Sensory block of leg—Medial aspect of leg from Tibial Tubercle to medial malleolus (MM).
Sensory block of foot—MM to 2 cm proximal to the base of great toe.

9.8.4 Contraindications

Contraindications for Saphenous Nerve block (Table 9.56).

Table 9.55 Saphenous nerve anatomy

Roots	L3-L4 Largest cutaneous branch of Femoral nerve (Posterior branch)		
Course	Branches from Femoral nerve in proximal third of thigh Nerve is lateral to the femoral sheath in the Adductor canal (Hunter's canal/Sub-sartorial canal) It crosses SFA anteriorly and then medially before emerging from the Adductor Canal with the Saphenous branch of descending genicular artery Nerve pierces Fascia Lata between Gracilis and Sartorius muscles dividing into Infrapatellar branch and Distal saphenous branches It is lateral to great saphenous vein		
Innervations / Actions	Cutaneous	Infrapatellar branch—Anterior inferior knee capsule and skin below patella.	Distal saphenous branch—Skin of the lower leg medially and a branch to medial ankle

Table 9.56 Contraindications for Saphenous nerve block

Absolute	Relative
Patient refusal Local site infection Allergy to local anesthetics	Anticoagulation or bleeding disorders Obturator nerve neuropathy Large inguinal lymph nodes/Tumor Avoid/discuss with the surgeon if compartment syndrome suspected

9.8.5 Preparations

Refer to Table 9.2.

9.8.6 Block Approaches

The ideal injection site seems to be the midportion of the adductor canal (the midpoint between the proximal and distal ends) as it is high enough to block the saphenous nerve and trans-muscular branches of the nerve to Vastus medialis (NVM), but distal enough to avoid spread to the femoral triangle.

Saphenous nerve can be blocked by various approaches. With the advent of USG, the Landmark approaches have been used to a lesser extent due to difficulty in interpretation.

9.8.6.1 Landmark, PNS-Guided Saphenous Nerve Block

1. *PNS-Guided Saphenous Nerve Block (Peri Femoral Approach).*

   PNS-guided Peri femoral approach for Saphenous Nerve Block (Table 9.57).
2. *Saphenous Nerve Block (Trans Sartorial Approach).*

   PNS-guided Trans sartorial approach for Saphenous Nerve Block (Table 9.58).

Tips
Identification of sartorius muscle is enhanced by elevating the extended leg by 5–10 cm.

3. *The various other approaches to Saphenous Nerve Block are as Follows:*

   Other approaches to Saphenous Nerve Block (Table 9.59).

Table 9.57 Saphenous Nerve Block (Peri femoral approach)

Position	Supine with thigh abducted and externally rotated
Landmark	Inguinal crease and femoral artery Nerve to vastus medialis runs alongside the saphenous nerve
POE	4 cm below the inguinal crease and 0.5 cm lateral to femoral artery
Needle	A 5–10 cm long, 21–22 gauge short-bevel, insulated stimulating needle
PNS stimulation	At a current intensity of 1.5 mA (2 Hz, 0.1–0.3 msec) decreased to 0.4–0.5 mA
End point	Contraction of medial aspect of thigh and movement of patella at current of 0.3 mA–0.5 mA
Drug dosage	5–10 ml (Approximate depth of nerve is 2–4 cm)
Highlights	Indirect indicator as saphenous nerve is a pure sensory nerve

Table 9.58 PNS-guided Saphenous Nerve Block (Trans sartorial approach)

Position	Supine position
Landmark	Sartorius muscle, Patella
POE	3–4 cm superior and 6–8 cm posterior to superomedial border of patella
Needle	A 5-cm long, 21–22 gauge short-bevel, insulated stimulating needle was inserted at 45° caudally and posteriorly (Fig. 9.33)
PNS stimulation	At a current intensity of 1.5 mA (2 Hz, 0.1–0.3 msec) decreased to 0.4–0.5 mA
End point	Contraction of medial aspect of thigh and movement of patella at current of 0.3 mA–0.5 mA
Drug dosage	5–10 ml (At a depth of 3–5 cm)

9.8.6.2 Ultrasound-Guided Saphenous Nerve Block

Saphenous nerve can be blocked at various points.

1. Junction of middle and distal third of thigh (Table 9.60).
2. Below the knee at level of tibial tuberosity (Table 9.61).
3. At Ankle (Table 9.74).

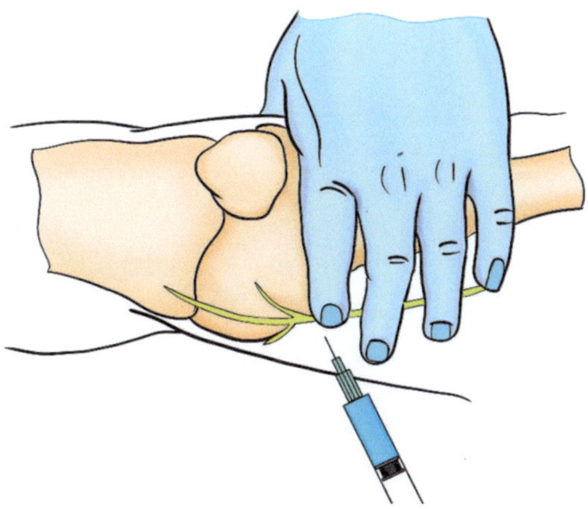

Fig. 9.33 Trans sartorial approach for Saphenous nerve block

Table 9.59 Other approaches to Saphenous nerve block

Approach	Goal
Medial femoral condyle (MFC)	Condyle is palpated, LA is injected in a fan-wise direction between skin and periosteum slightly posterior to MFC
Paravenous / Below the knee field block	A linear subcutaneous infiltration of LA; 3–4 cm distal to tibial condyle anterior-to-posterior direction (Adjacent to saphenous nerve)
At the medial malleolus	LA is injected subcutaneously above and anterior to medial malleolus around saphenous vein

Table 9.60 USG-guided Saphenous Nerve Block Junction of middle and distal third of thigh

Position	Supine with thigh abducted and externally rotated
Landmark (Fig. 9.34a)	High-frequency transducer is placed transversely on the anteromedial aspect of thigh Above Knee—Between Sartorius and Vastus medialis muscle Saphenous nerve is hyperechoic circle anterolateral to the femoral artery
Technique and POE	Under all aseptic conditions identify the femoral artery at the inguinal crease then probe is moved distally to trace artery as it becomes popliteal artery at adductor hiatus (approximately mid-thigh) or Probe is kept at popliteal crease and traced back 5–7 cm proximally till hyperechoic appearance of vastoadductor membrane fades femoral artery is identified

(continued)

Table 9.60 (continued)

Needle	A 5–10 cm long, 21–22 gauge short-bevel, insulated stimulating needle in in-plane approach from lateral to medial direction (Fig. 9.34b, c)
PNS stimulation	At a current intensity of 1.5 mA (2 Hz, 0.1–0.3 msec) decreased to 0.4–0.5 mA
End point	LA spread anterolateral to femoral artery
Drug dosage	5–10 ml (At a depth of 2–3 cm)
Highlights	Adductor canal block can lead to partial motor block, nerve can be confused with posteromedial branch of nerve to vastus medialis Out-of-plane approach can be used

Tips

1. The injection should surround the nerve and vessel in its aponeurotic plane circumferentially rather in the linear horizontal direction.
2. Move the probe axially to find SFA and caudally to find the vastus medialis and adductor muscles.

Saphenous Nerve Block at Ankle joint can be performed both by landmark and USG guidance described in Sect. 9.10 (Table 9.74).

Tips

1. Transducer is to be applied gently to avoid compression of the saphenous vein.
2. If a large volume of LA is given in sub sartorial space, then partial motor block of vastus medialis can also occur due to nerve block of NVM supplying this muscle. Thus, be cautious regarding unsupported ambulation after block.
3. To avoid any motor block the nerve is distally below sartorius as feasible.
4. Always use 1–2 ml of drug to confirm the needle position.
5. Color Doppler can be used to identify vessels—femoral artery, descending geniculate artery (saphenous branch), and saphenous vein.
6. An out-of-plane technique can also be used through the sartorius muscle but aliquots of LA have to be used to confirm the needle direction.

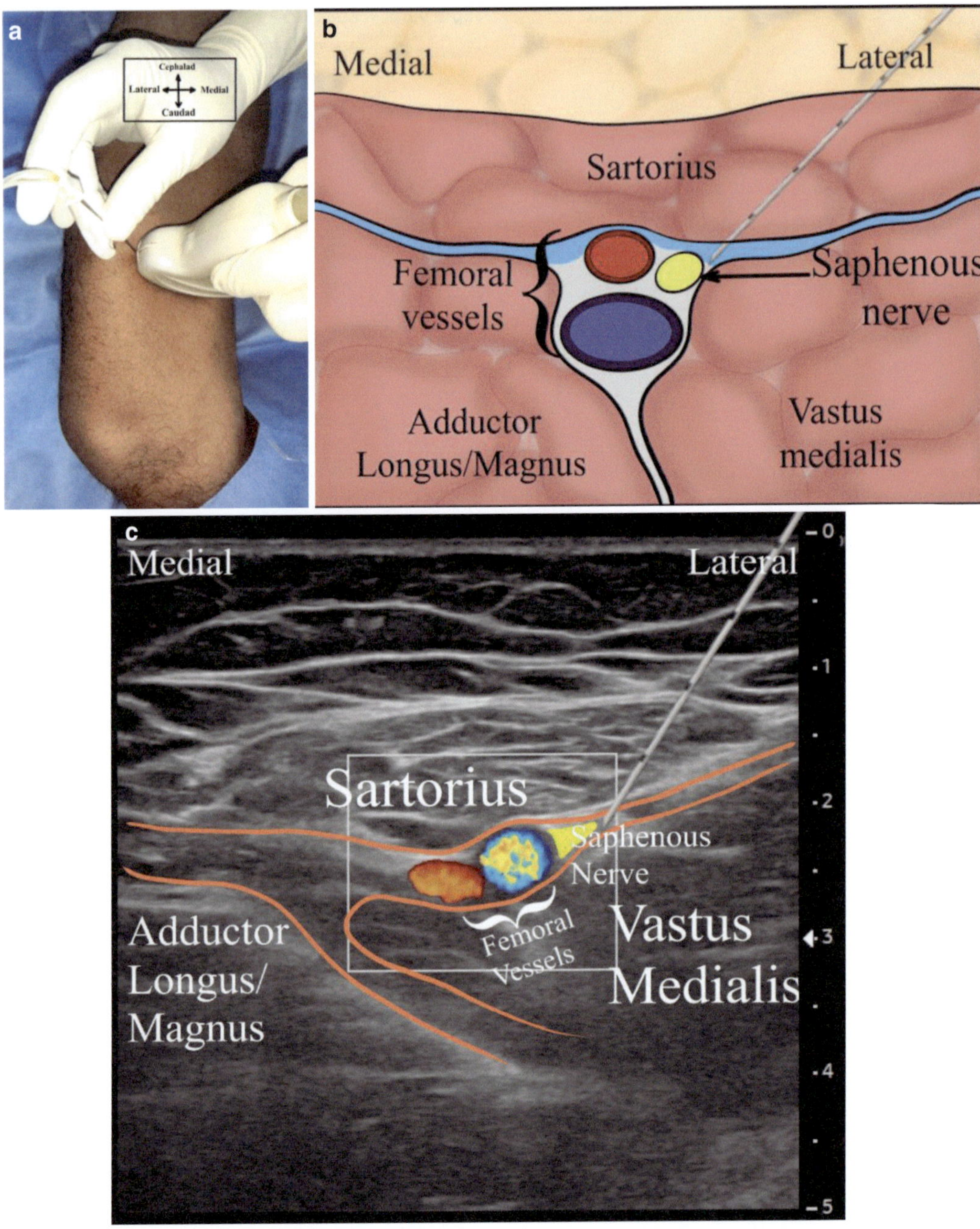

Fig. 9.34 (**a**) Probe position and in-plane approach needle insertion for nerve block. (**b**) Schematic diagram of saphenous nerve block above knee. (**c**) USG image of in-plane needle position for saphenous nerve block

7. Nerve may not always be delineated So, 5–10 ml of LA in plane between Sartorius and Vastus medialis should suffice.
8. Increment dosing and frequent aspiration are important when giving the block because of the close proximity with vessels.

9.8.7 Complications

1. Infection at the site.
2. Nerve injury.
3. Pain on injection.
4. Allergic reaction.
5. Local anesthetic systemic toxicity.
6. Bleeding.

Table 9.61 USG-guided Saphenous nerve block below knee

Position	Supine with leg straight
Landmark	Below knee—Along Tibial side of leg, adjacent to saphenous vein Linear transducer is placed at level of tibial tuberosity (Fig. 9.35a)
POE	LA is infiltrated between saphenous vein and fascia Lata (short axis view)
Needle	In plane from Lateral to Medial Direction (Fig. 9.35b)
End point	LA spread adjacent to saphenous vein (Below knee)
Drug dosage	5–10 ml (At a depth of 2–3 cm)
Highlights	Below knee it can be blocked by subcutaneous infiltration of plane just medial to tibial tuberosity

9.9 Popliteal Fossa Block

9.9.1 Introduction

It is the blockade of Sciatic nerve in the Popliteal Fossa before the division into Tibial nerve and Common Peroneal Nerve. The Posterior approach was described by Duane Keith Rorie and Lateral approach by Jerry Vloka. Posterior approach is preferred because of ease of nerve scanning rest both approaches provide similar results and ease of catheter insertion. Popliteal Fossa Block is superior as it helps to maintain knee flexion.

9.9.2 Anatomy

Popliteal Fossa—Boundaries (Fig. 9.36)

Supero laterally—Posterior knee of Biceps Femoris.
Supero medially—Semitendinosus.
Inferiorly—Lateral and Medial heads of gastrocnemius.

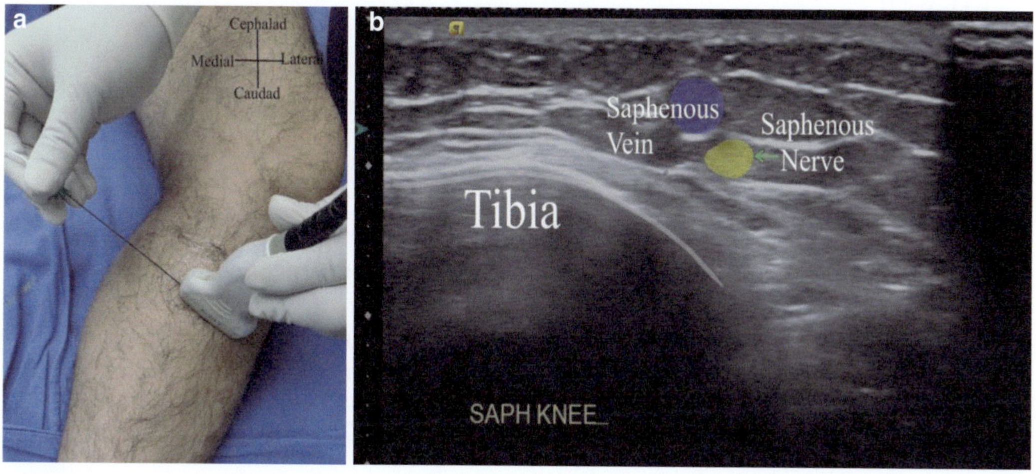

Fig. 9.35 (**a**) Probe position for saphenous nerve block below knee. (**b**) USG image showing Saphenous nerve below knee

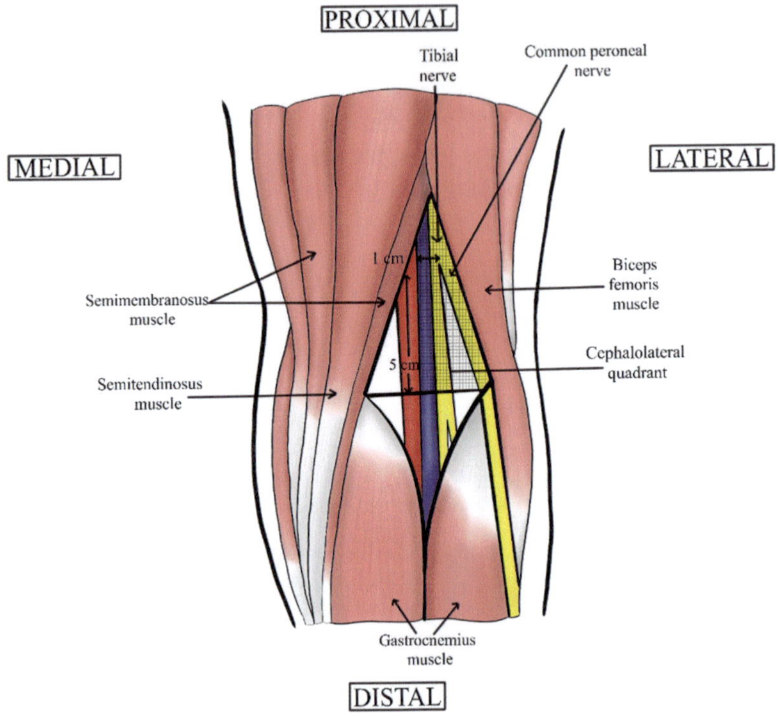

Fig. 9.36 Boundaries of popliteal fossa

Sciatic nerve and Popliteal vessels are not enveloped by same paraneural sheath thus, they do not form a neurovascular bundle.

Contents

- Tibial nerve, common fibular nerve (also known as the common peroneal nerve).

Course of Tibial Nerve and Peroneal Nerve (Table 9.63)

- Popliteal vein.
- Popliteal artery (a continuation of the femoral artery).
- Small saphenous vein (termination).
- Popliteal lymph nodes and vessels.

9.9.3 Indications

1. Surgeries of lower leg; distal two-third (tibia, fibula, ankle, and foot). Blocking of femoral nerve and saphenous nerve may be required for complete anesthesia.
2. Analgesia lasts for 12–24 h with long-acting anesthetics.
3. Analgesia for Calf torniquet.
4. Anesthesia for short saphenous vein stripping.

9.9.4 Contraindications

Contraindication for popliteal fossa block (Table 9.64).

9.9.5 Preparations

Refer to Table 9.2.

9.9.6 Block Approaches

9.9.6.1 Landmark, PNS-Guided Approaches

Landmark, PNS-guided approaches to popliteal fossa block (Table 9.65).

Table 9.63 Course of Tibial nerve and peroneal nerve

Tibial Nerve—Largest Terminal Branch of Sciatic nerve Branches off at the superior angle of Popliteal Fossa, crossing the popliteal vessels lateral to medial At the inferior angle of popliteal fossa, it passes deep to soleus to enter back of leg. Downward and medially to posteromedial side of ankle. Midway between medial malleolus and medial tubercle of calcaneum. Terminates deep to flexor retinaculum by dividing into medial and lateral plantar nerves		
Root Value	Tibial Nerve—Anterior division of anterior rami of Sciatic Nerve (L4-S3) Branches—Lateral and Medial Plantar nerve, anastomotic branch of Sural nerve	
Course	Encased in a common fascial sheath these divide around 8–10 cm above popliteal fossa	
Innervations/ Actions	*Muscle supply*	In popliteal fossa—Posterior compartment of leg (Gastrocnemius, Soleus, Plantaris, and Popliteus) Back of leg—Tibialis posterior, flexor digitorum longus, flexor hallucis longus and deep part of soleus. In the foot—Medial plantar nerve- Abductor hallucis, flexor digitorum brevis, flexor hallucis brevis, and first lumbrical Lateral Planter Nerve— Flexor digitorum accessories and Abductor digiti minimi. Flexor digiti minimi, third and fourth interossei, second, third, and fourth lumbricals, first and second plantar interossei, and adductor hallucis
	Motor	Plantarflexion of ankle, Flexion of knee, Lateral rotation of thigh, flexion of great toe, flexion of digits, inversion of foot
	Cutaneous	In the popliteal fossa—Medial sural cutaneous nerve (Posterolateral aspect of leg) Back of leg—Medial calcaneal nerve (skin of back and lower surface of the heel) Skin on the heel of foot (Lateral and Medial Plantar nerve) Foot—Medial planter nerve supplies medial sole and medial three and one-half toes Lateral Plantar Nerve—Skin of the sole, skin of lateral side of toe, interdigital cleft
	Joint	In the Popliteal fossa—Superior medial genicular nerve Middle genicular nerve Inferior genicular nerve Back of Leg—Supplies ankle joint Foot—Bones of tarsus and metatarsus

Common Peroneal Nerve—At Apex of Popliteal Fossa sciatic nerve bifurcates into tibial and common fibular nerve. Follows the medial border of biceps femoris. Lateral and inferior direction over the gastrocnemius Nerve wraps around neck of fibula to enter the lateral compartment of leg Between attachments of fibularis longus muscle Divides into superficial fibular and deep fibular nerve		
Root Value	Common Peroneal Nerve—Posterior Divisions of anterior rami of Sciatic nerve(L4-S3)	
Course	Encased in a common fascial sheath these divide around 8–10 cm above popliteal fossa	
Innervations/ Actions	*Muscle supply*	Main branch—Short head of the biceps femoris Superficial Fibular Nerve—lateral compartment of leg-Fibularis Longus and Brevis Deep Fibular Nerve—Muscle of anterior compartment of the leg, Tibialis anterior, extensor digitorum Longus and Extensor Hallucis Longus
	Motor	Flexion of knee, Foot eversion, Dorsiflexion of foot, and extension of digits
	Cutaneous	Common Fibular nerve— Sural Communicating nerve—Skin over lower posterolateral leg Lateral Sural cutaneous nerve—Skin over upper lateral leg Superficial fibular nerve—Skin of anterolateral leg, Dorsum of foot Deep fibular Nerve—Skin between first and second toes

Table 9.64 Contraindication for popliteal fossa block

Absolute	Relative
Patient refusal Local site infection Allergy to local anesthetics	Anticoagulation or bleeding disorders Femoral nerve neuropathy Neurological deficit

Table 9.65 Landmark, PNS guided approaches to popliteal fossa block

	Posterior approach, Inter tendinous approach	Lateral approach
Position	Prone Position with operative leg supported below the knee Knee to be slightly bent and foot resting free on the bed Palpating hands-on Biceps femoris	Supine position Knee to be slightly flexed and foot resting free on the bed Leg to be internally rotated at the hip joint Foot at 90-degree angle to horizontal plane
Landmark	Popliteal Triangle and Popliteal crease (Fig. 9.37)	Popliteal Crease, vastus laterialis muscle, and Biceps femoris/ Iliotibial tract (If BF atrophied) (Fig. 9.38)
POE	7 cm Proximal to Popliteal Crease and 1 cm Lateral to Apex of popliteal triangle. (Between bicep femoris and semitendinosus tendon)	8–10 cm Proximal to Popliteal Crease (between Vastus laterialis and BF)
Needle	21 Gauge, 10 cm insulated needle 18 Gauge, 10 cm insulated Tuohy needle if catheter placement required Perpendicular insertion to skin f/b 45–60 degree tilt to skin in cephalad direction	Inserted in horizontal plane between two muscles and advanced to contact the femur bone Withdraw and redirect 30 degrees posterior to horizontal plane of contact (1–2 cm)

(continued)

Table 9.65 (continued)

	Posterior approach, Inter tendinous approach	Lateral approach
PNS stimulation	Peripheral nerve stimulation starts with initial current setting of 1.5 mA (2 Hz, 0.1–0.3 ms) and continued till response is elicited by impulses of 0.5 mA	
*End point**	Best response is Inversion of Foot and Dorsiflexion of foot. (At 0.2–0.5 mA) At low current sometimes the response of only great toe is left	
	Depth: 3–5 cm	Depth: 5–7 cm
Drug dosage	35–40 ml of LA	20–25 ml of LA
Highlights	The chances of vascular puncture are less because of the superficial and lateral relation of nerves to vessels	No prone position, stimulation of common peroneal nerve obtained first as this nerve is more superficial and lateral

**Various responses to stimulation*

Response	*Nerves stimulated*
Inversion of foot	Tibial and deep peroneal nerve
Eversion of foot	Superficial peroneal nerve
Plantar flexion	Posterior tibial nerve
Dorsiflexion	Deep peroneal nerve

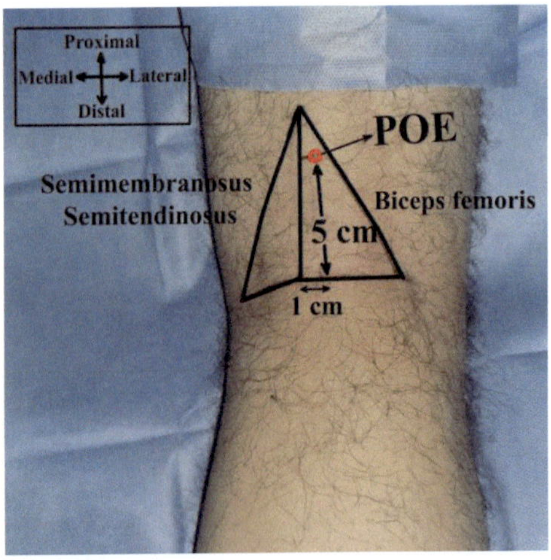

Fig. 9.37 Surface landmark for popliteal sciatic nerve block in posterior approach

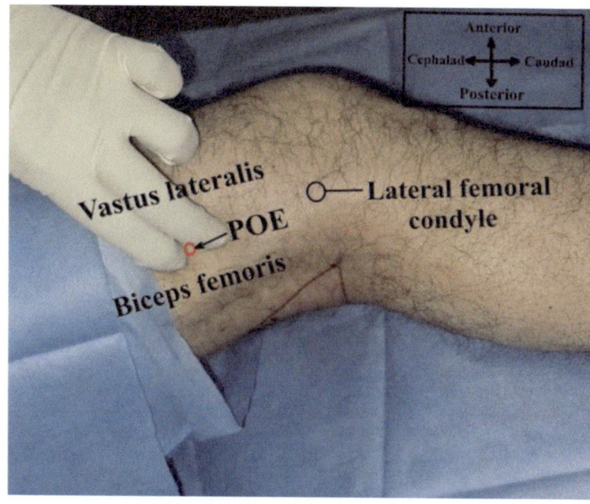

Fig. 9.38 Surface landmark for popliteal sciatic nerve block in lateral approach

Tips

1. Popliteal Fossa can be accentuated by making the patient bend the knee against resistance, relying on tendon is more precise approach.
2. Give the block as cephalad as possible before the division of sciatic nerve.
3. The foot should be allowed to protrude out of the bed.
4. In patients with peripheral neuropathy or systemic illness like diabetes and sepsis end point at 1 mA is also acceptable.
5. To confirm the correct proximal needle placement a small redirection of needle of 1–2 mm will lead to a change in motor response from planter flexion to dorsiflexion.
6. Breach of sciatic nerve comes with a fascial click.
7. The injection pressure must not be too high when injecting the drug as chances of intrafascicular injury are too high because of large fascicles.
8. Too deep insertion can lead to contact with Femur bone—withdraw the needle.
9. Ensure ergonomic position for the person performing the block.
10. Keep the fingers of palpating hands as firm as possible to avoid injection of drug outside the sciatic sheath.

Troubleshoot

Troubleshooting for Landmark, PNS-Guided Approaches to popliteal fossa block (Table 9.66).

Continuous Popliteal Block

Slight cephalad angulation of needle is necessary to facilitate needle insertion. After obtaining an appropriate response inject 10–15 ml of drug and advance the catheter 5 cm beyond the needle tip and start the infusion at 5 ml/h of ropivacaine 0.2% or similar along with rescue analgesia for breakthrough pain. Same technique for Lateral and posterior approach, just for lateral approach use a 10-cm length needle.

9.9.6.2 Ultrasound-Guided Approach for Popliteal Sciatic Nerve Block

Ultrasound-Guided Approach for Popliteal Sciatic Nerve Block (Table 9.67).

Tips

1. Tilting the probe caudally is necessary to bring out the nerve from the adipose tissue.
2. To confirm the nerve patient is asked to dorsiflex and plantar flex the ankle which makes the two branches move in relation to each other.
3. Block the common sciatic nerve, i.e., within Vloka's sheath, not individual nerves. If individual nerves are seen slide the probe cranially till they join.

Table 9.66 Troubleshooting for Landmark, PNS-Guided Approaches to popliteal fossa block

Response	Interpretation	Rescue measures
No response	Anterior and cranially placed	(1) Visualize the anatomical landmarks mentally (2) Redirect the needle 5–10° posteriorly beyond plane of the skin femur distance (3) After around 30–40° if still no response reinsert the needle 1–2 cm inferior to initial insertion site
Twitch at Biceps Femoris	Needle too lateral	Redirect the needle medially
Local twitch of semitendinosus and semimembranosus	Needle too medial	Redirect laterally by 15°
Local twitch of calf muscles	Needle outside sciatic sheath	Continue insertion
Inadvertent vascular puncture	Too medial and deep attempts	Withdraw and redirect laterally
Bone contact (Femur)	Too deep	Withdraw superficially
Local twitch of Biceps Femoris	Too shallow	Insert further
Local twitch of Vastus laterialis	Needle is anteriorly directed	Withdraw and redirect posteriorly

Table 9.67 Ultrasound-guided approach for popliteal sciatic nerve block

	Posterior	Lateral
Position	Prone/Lateral Position with operative leg supported below the knee Knee to be slightly bent and foot resting free on the bed	Supine/Lateral Position Foot to be rested on an elevated footrest Flexing the knee while stabilizing the foot and ankle on bed
Landmark (Fig. 9.39a, b)	Probe Transversely at popliteal crease (Parallel to it), aided with color Doppler. Move the probe cranially 5–10 cm from crease	
POE	Locate Popliteal artery and Popliteal vein (at a depth of 3–4 cm), vein is superficial (posterior) to the artery Nerve seen superficial and lateral to the vein/artery, as hyperechoic, oval, or round structure with honeycomb pattern, tilt the probe proximal or distal (Fig. 9.39c)	
Needle (Fig. 9.39a, b)	In plane from lateral to medial or out of plane (Fig. 9.39c)	In plane 2–3 cm above the lateral edge of transducer in horizontal direction (to reduce the angle between the needle and footprint of transducer)
End point	After penetration of sciatic sheath inject 20–30 ml of LA	
Drug dosage	20–30 ml of LA (Do not inject against high pressure)	
Highlights	Goal is to deposit the local anesthetic within the Vloka's sheath	

4. The presence of adipose tissue makes the nerve visibility a challenge, so keep adjusting the depth, gain, focus, and direction of US beam.
5. Out-of-plane technique in posterior approach is less painful as the needle passes through skin and adipose tissue and less on muscles.

Continuous USG Popliteal Sciatic Nerve Block

Needle is placed in the epineural sheath of the nerve and the catheter is inserted 4–5 cm beyond needle tip with correct placement ensured by the spread of the drug within the sheath. Continuous infusion of ropivacaine 0.2% at 5 ml/h has to be started with as required boluses of 5 ml.

Lateral Approach Is More Preferred Over Posterior Approach for Catheter Placement

1. Subcutaneous placement of catheter in posterior approach is more prone to displacement in comparison to Biceps femoris stability in lateral approach.
2. Mobility of lateral aspect of thigh is less in comparison to back of knee.
3. Access to catheter is more convenient in lateral approach.

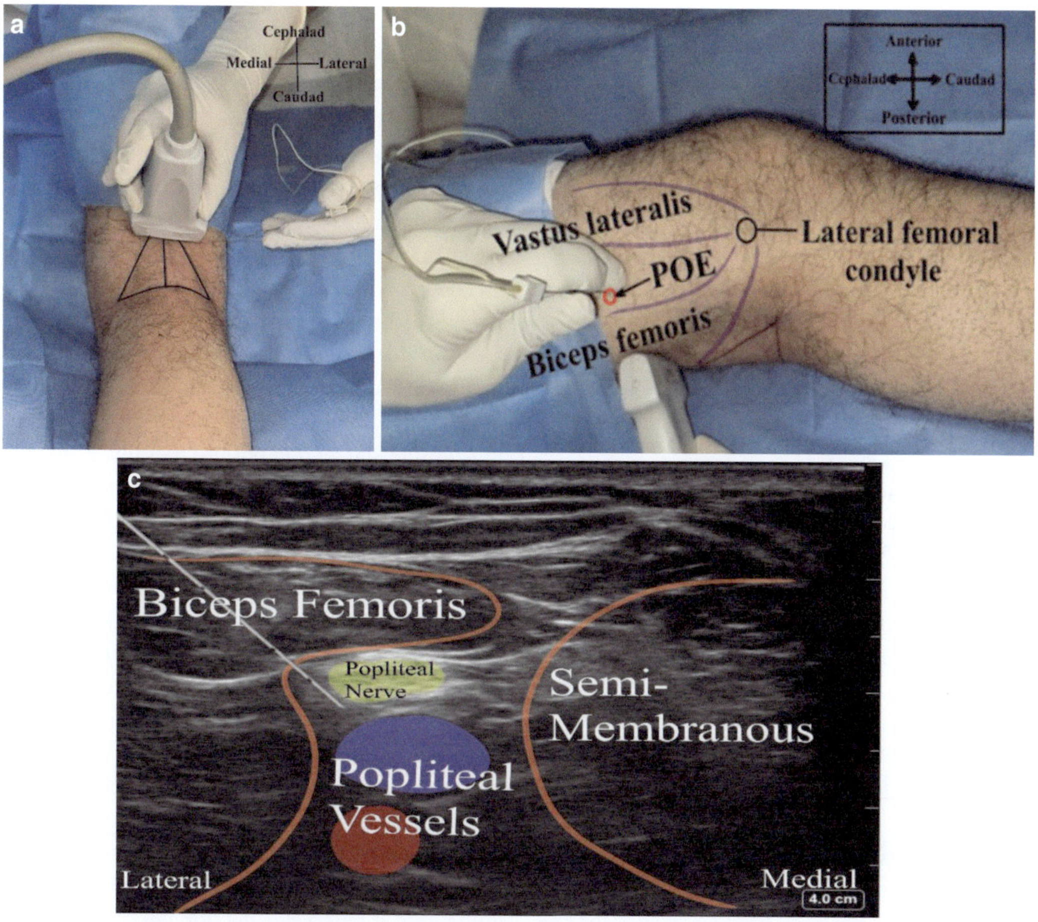

Fig. 9.39 (**a**) Probe and needle position during popliteal sciatic nerve block in posterior approach. (**b**) Probe and needle position during popliteal sciatic nerve block in lateral approach. (**c**) USG image of popliteal sciatic nerve block in posterior or lateral approach

9.9.7 Complications

Complications popliteal fossa block (Table 9.68).

Table 9.68 Complications popliteal fossa block

Due to needle puncture	Due to local anesthetic	Due to catheter
Hematoma (Tip—Avoid deep and multiple punctures)	Local anesthetic systemic toxicity (LAST)	Infection (Tip—Remove the catheter within 72 h)
Vascular puncture (Tip—Avoid medial insertion and going beyond 2 cm after bicep femoris twitch)		
Nerve injury—2-4/10,000 (Tip—Do not inject drug if response present at <0.3 mA)	Pressure necrosis of heel (Tip—Heel padding and frequent repositioning)	
Infection (Tip—Strict adherence to aseptic measure)		

9.10 Ankle Block

9.10.1 Introduction

The ankle block has been used since ages for providing anesthesia and analgesia below ankle joint. The ankle block constitutes a blockade of terminal branches of sciatic and femoral nerves which includes three superficial and two deeper nerves. Though sciatic and femoral nerve block at the level of thigh or knee joint (adductor canal/ subsartorial saphenous blocks and popliteal sciatic block) can be used for ankle anesthesia and analgesia when lesser calf muscle involvement is desired ankle block can be used as preferred choice. The ankle block can be solely performed as superficial ring block by skin infiltration to nerve stimulator and ultrasound-assisted individual nerve blocks with success.

9.10.2 Anatomy

Five nerves need to be blocked to make ankle block a complete success. Out of five nerves, four are branches from Sciatic nerve and one is terminal of femoral nerve. From medial to lateral Posterior tibial nerve (L4-S3) superficial (L4-S1) and deep (L4–5) Peroneal (fibular) nerve, and sural nerve (S1–2) are branches of sciatic nerve. Saphenous nerve (L3–4) is terminal branch of femoral nerve. The knowledge that out of five nerves three are superficial to facia (Superficial peroneal, sural, and saphenous) and two nerves are deep (posterior tibial and deep peroneal) to facia is essential for successful ankle block.

Posterior tibial nerve is found posterior to medial malleolus and is usually placed anterior-to-posterior tibial vessels and flexor hallucis longus muscle and tendon posterolaterally. It divides into lateral and medial plantar nerves and provides sensation to the calcaneum and plantar surface (sole) of the foot.

Deep peroneal nerve, a branch of common peroneal nerve is found between tibialis anterior and extensors (hallucis longus and digitorum longus) tendons of big toe lateral to anterior tibial artery above the ankle joint. It corresponds to the posterior interosseous nerve of the forearm It innervates the first web space of the foot.

Superficial peroneal nerve, the second branch of common peroneal nerve runs deep to peroneal muscles in lateral aspect of leg. At the level of ankle joint it innervates the dorsum of foot.

Sural nerve formed by cutaneous branches of tibial and common peroneal nerves at middle or proximal leg. At the ankle joint, it becomes superficial travels posterior to lateral malleolus and innervates the lateral ankle and foot.

Saphenous nerve is terminal extension of femoral nerve which travels on medial aspect of leg near ankle joint and innervates the medial aspect of the ankle and foot.

Figure 9.40 Dermatomal distribution of *Posterior tibial nerve, Deep peroneal nerve, Superficial peroneal nerve, Sural nerve, and Saphenous nerve.*

9.10.3 Indications

1. Surgical procedures for foot.
2. Supplement lumbosacral plexus anesthesia.
3. Post-operative analgesia for below-ankle surgery.

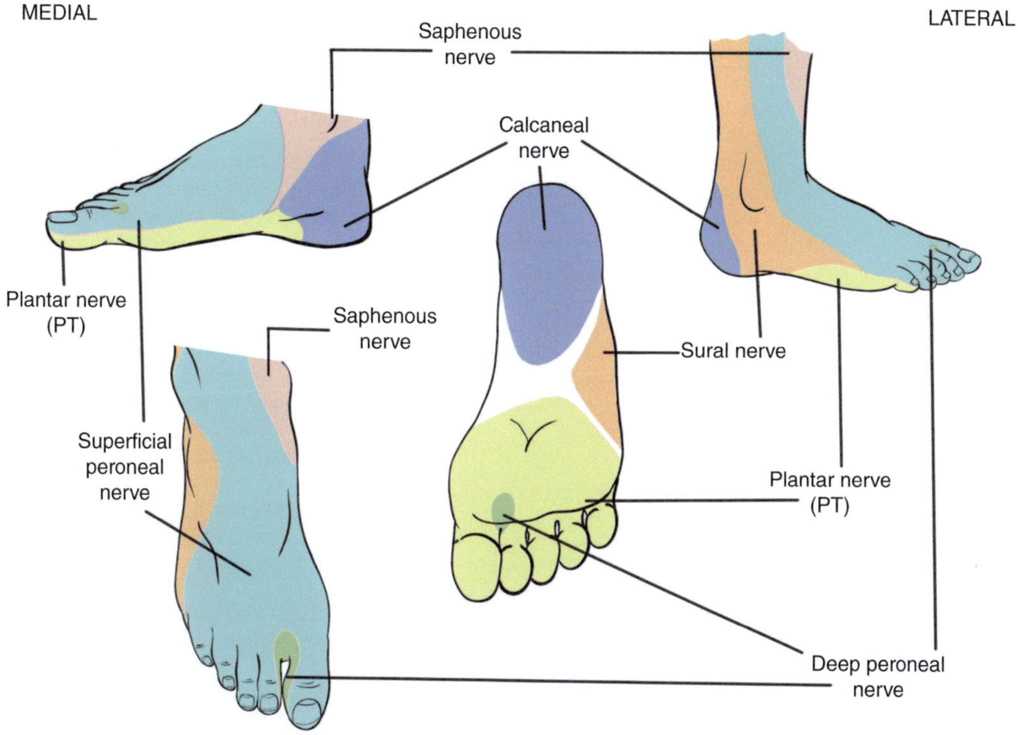

Fig. 9.40 Dermatomal distribution of posterior tibial, deep peroneal, superficial peroneal, sural, and saphenous nerve

Table 9.69 Contraindication for ankle block

Absolute	Relative
Patient refusal Local site infection Allergy to local anesthetics	Anticoagulation or bleeding disorders Neuromuscular disease/damage in contralateral limb in ambulatory patient

9.10.4 Contraindications

Contraindication for ankle block (Table 9.69).

9.10.5 Preparations

Refer to Table 9.2.

9.10.6 Block Approaches

9.10.6.1 Landmark, PNS, and USG Approach

1. *Posterior Tibial Nerve.*
   Different approaches to posterior tibial nerve block (Table 9.70).
2. *Deep Peroneal Nerve.*
   Different approaches to deep peroneal nerve block (Table 9.71).
3. *Superficial Peroneal Nerve Block.*
   Different approaches to superficial peroneal nerve block (Table 9.72).
4. *Sural Nerve.*
   Different approaches to sural nerve block (Table 9.73).

Table 9.70 Different approaches to posterior tibial nerve block

	Landmark	PNS	Ultrasound guided
Position	Patient is supine with the foot elevated and supported on pillows, preferably at the edge of the OT table, and the ankle rotated with semi flexed knee as needed for needle placement, or the operator can change position as needed		
Landmark technique and POE and end point (Fig. 9.41)	The posterior tibial artery is palpated behind the medial malleolus and needle is inserted posterior to it till it touches the bone. The needle is withdrawn 2–3 mm and drug is deposited (Fig. 9.42a) Another 1–2 mL of LA is fanned from medial to lateral direction to enhance the success rate of the block	4 fingers /6–8 cm above medial malleolus and posterior to posterior tibial artery Plantar flexion of the toes elicited	High-frequency linear (10–15 MHz) transducer is placed between medial malleolus and achillis tendon creating a transverse image (short axis view) (Fig. 9.42b) Identify pulsatile posterior tibial artery and the nerve typically appears posterior to the artery with mixed echogenicity From anterior to posterior tibialis posterior, flexor digitorum longus, posterior tibial artery, posterior tibial nerve, and flexor hallucis longus are identified On proximal movement of probe flexor hallucis longus which lies medial and posterior to the nerve can be confirmed by observing the movement by moving the great toe Both in-plane (from posterior side) and out-of-plane approaches can be used (Fig. 9.42c)
Needle	22G, 4-cm needle	22G, 50 mm long needle	22G, 50 mm long echogenic needle
Drug dosage	3–5 mL of LA 0.75% or 0.5% ropivacaine, or 0.5% bupivacaine		

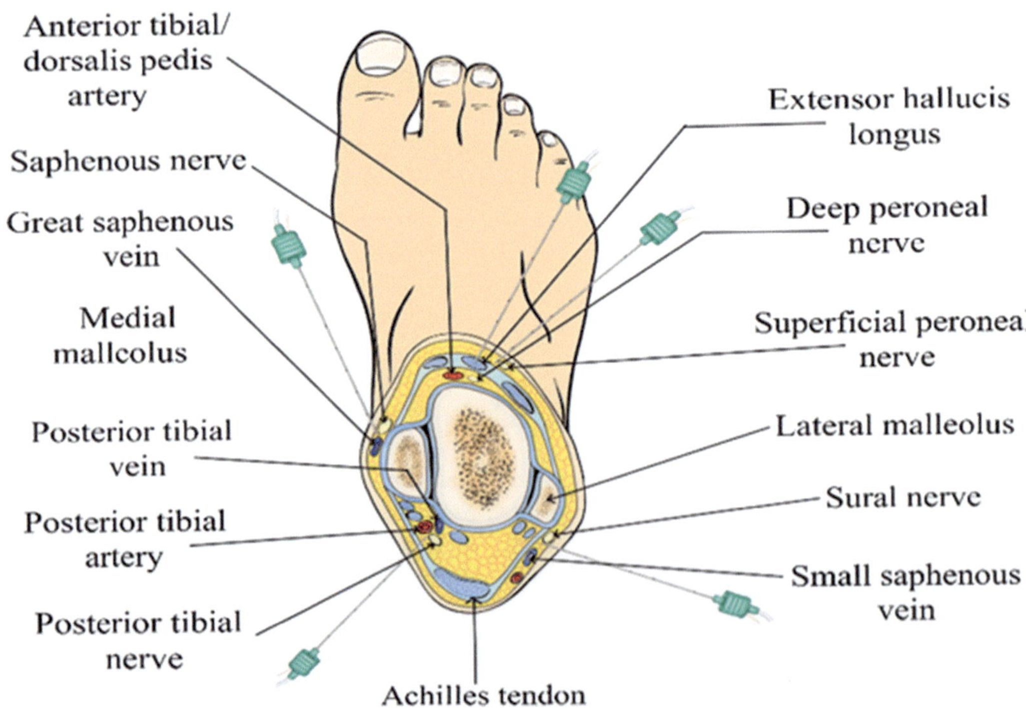

Fig. 9.41 Landmark/PNS-guided ankle block

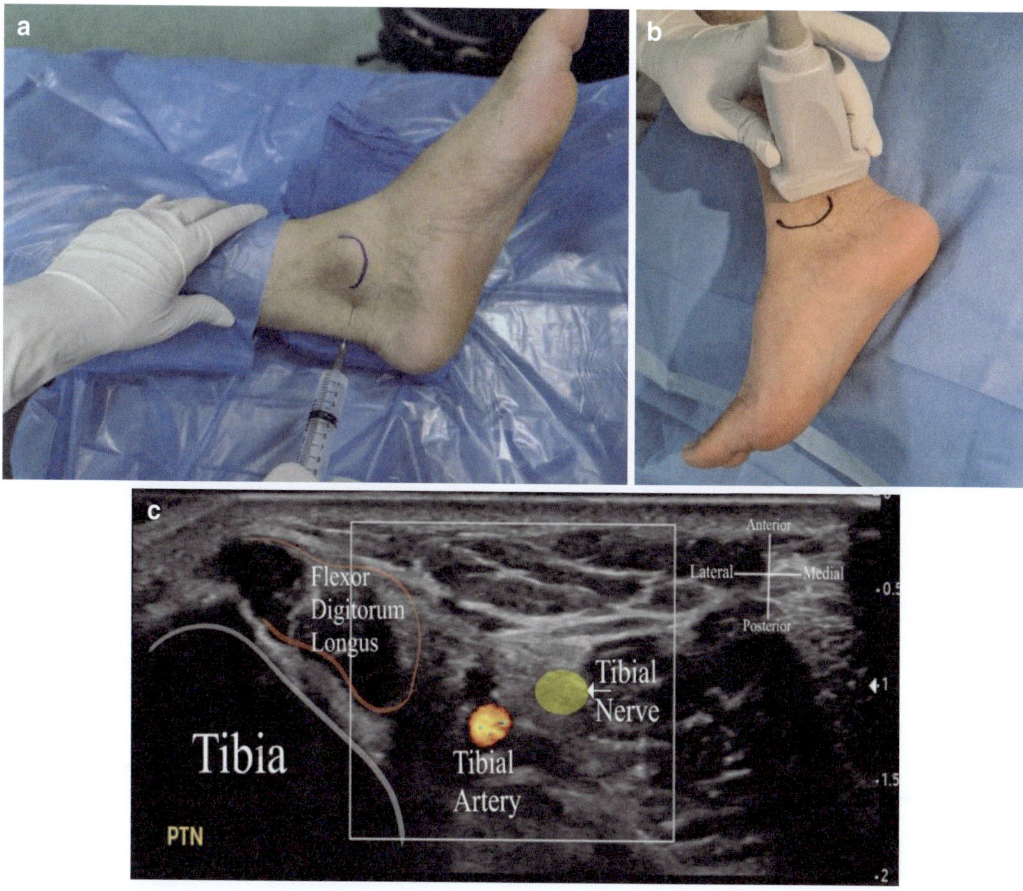

Fig. 9.42 (**a**) Landmark-guided infiltration for posterior tibial nerve block. (**b**) Ultrasound probe position for posterior tibial nerve block. (**c**) Ultrasound image showing posterior tibial nerve posterior to posterior tibial artery

Table 9.71 Different approaches to deep peroneal nerve block

	Landmark	PNS	Ultrasound guided
Position	Patient is supine with the foot elevated and supported on pillows, preferably at the edge of the OT table, and the ankle rotated with semi-flexed knee as needed for needle placement, or the operator can change position as needed		
Landmark technique POE and end point (Fig. 9.41)	On dorsum of foot along the intermalleolar line the dorsalis pedis artery is palpated between the extensor hallucis longus (medial) and extensor digitorum longus tendons (lateral), which can be made prominent by flexing the great toe. The needle is withdrawn 2–3 mm and drug is deposited (Fig. 9.43a)	On dorsum of foot and anterior leg 4 fingers /6–8 cm above ankle crease between tibialis anterior (medial) and the extensor hallucis longus and extensor digitorum longus (lateral) tendons lateral to anterior tibial artery - Dorsiflexion of the toes is elicited	- High-frequency linear (10–15 MHz) transducer is placed across the dorsal aspect of the patient's ankle joint in intermalleolar line (short axis view) (Fig. 9.43b) Identify the dorsalis pedis artery. The DPN is typically located lateral to the vessels with hypo- or mixed echogenicity. Both in-Plane (from lateral side) and out-of-plane approaches can be used (Fig. 9.43c)
Needle	22G, 4-cm needle	22G, 50 mm long needle	22G, 50 mm long echogenic needle
Drug dosage	3–5 mL of LA 0.75% or 0.5% ropivacaine, or 0.5% bupivacaine		

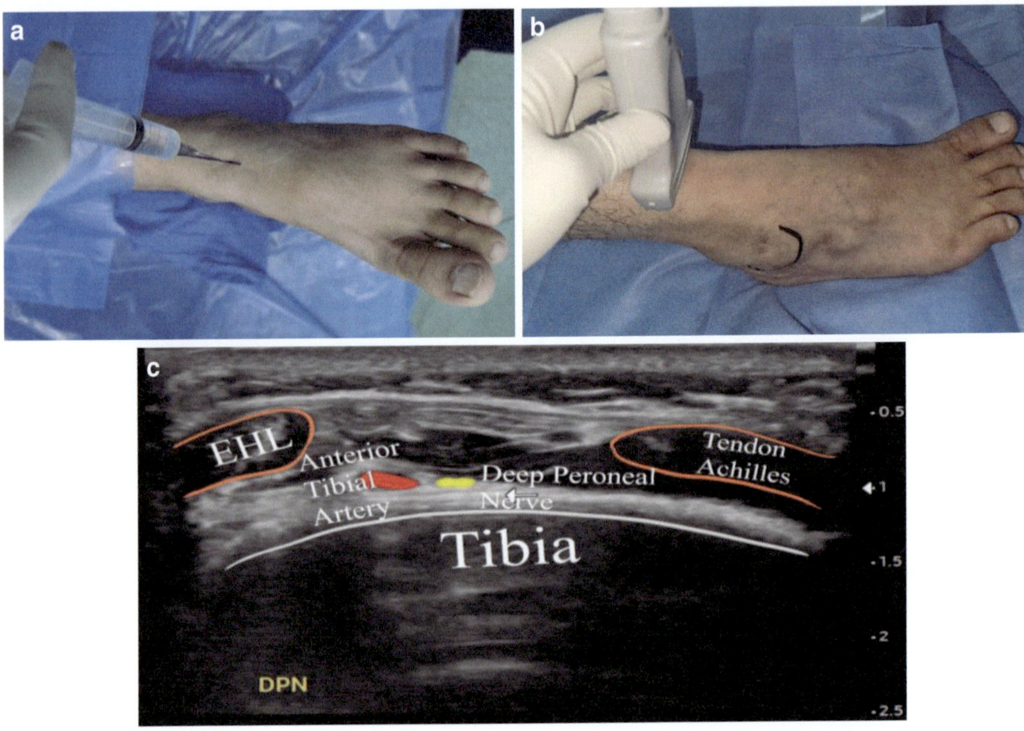

Fig. 9.43 (**a**) Landmark-guided infiltration for deep peroneal nerve block. (**b**) Ultrasound probe position for deep peroneal nerve block. (**c**) Ultrasound image showing deep peroneal nerve lateral to anterior tibial artery

Table 9.72 Different approaches to superficial peroneal nerve block

	Landmark	PNS	Ultrasound guided
Position	Patient is supine with the foot elevated and supported on pillows, preferably at the edge of the OT table, and the ankle rotated with semi-flexed knee as needed for needle placement, or the operator can change position as needed		
Landmark technique POE and end point	Subcutaneous infiltration between the lateral malleolus and the anterior border of the tibia from same entry point used for deep peroneal nerve (Fig. 9.44a) (Tip—In swollen ankle a targeted block in distal leg above fibula is more successful)	Junction of lower two-third and one-third of the line joining lateral tibial condyle and lateral malleolus is identified It lies between Extensor digitorum longus anteriorly and peroneus brevis muscle posteriorly. Drug is deposited when eversion of foot is elicited below 0.5 mA	High-frequency linear (10–15 MHz) transducer is placed transversely just above the lateral malleolus and moved proximally along the fibula making the muscles of lateral and anterior compartments more pronounced (Fig. 9.44b) Around 5–10 cm above the lateral malleolus superficial peroneal nerve can be seen as a honeycomb structure lying in the grove within the intermuscular septum separating extensor digitorum longus and peroneus longus/brevis Both in-plane and out-of-plane approaches can be used (Fig. 9.44c)
Needle	22G, 4-cm needle	22G, 50 mm long needle	22G, 50 mm long echogenic needle
Drug dosage	5–7 mL of LA 0.75% or 0.5% ropivacaine, or 0.5% bupivacaine		

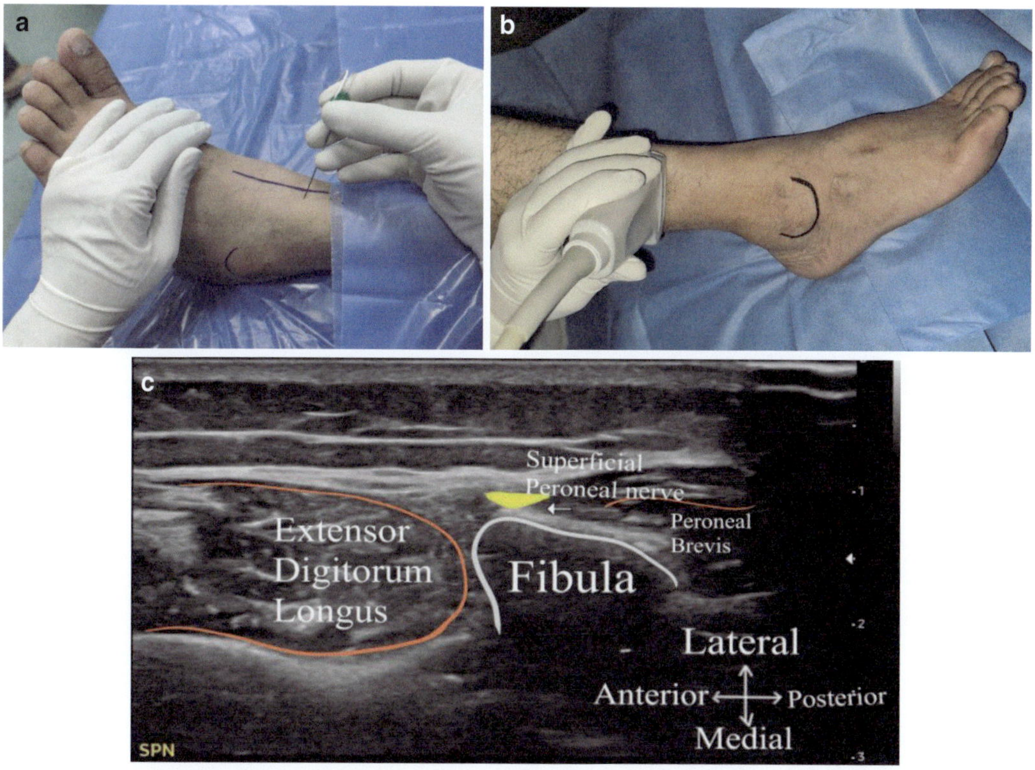

Fig. 9.44 (**a**) Landmark-guided infiltration for Superficial peroneal nerve block. (**b**) Ultrasound probe position for Superficial peroneal nerve block. (**c**) Ultrasound image showing Superficial peroneal nerve

Table 9.73 Different approaches to sural nerve block

	Landmark	Ultrasound guided
Position	Patient is supine with the foot elevated and supported on pillows, preferably at the edge of the OT table, and the ankle rotated with semi-flexed knee as needed for needle placement, or the operator can change position as needed	
Landmark technique POE and end point (Fig. 9.41)	The nerve is blocked by injecting LA along the lateral border of the Achilles tendon around the lateral aspect of the ankle at the cephalad border of the lateral malleolus. The needle is advanced anteriorly toward the fibula if paraesthesia is felt inject 3–5 ml LA (Fig. 9.45a) If paraesthesia not elicited inject 5–7 ml LA as the needle is withdrawn after hitting fibula as subcutaneous wheal	High frequency linear (10–15 MHz) transducer is placed in a transverse orientation just above the lateral malleolus of the ankle (Fig. 9.45b) Identify lesser saphenous vein The nerve appears as a small hyperechoic structure next to the lesser saphenous vein LA is injected around the vein Both In-Plane (from anterior side) and out-of-plane approaches can be used (Fig. 9.45c)
Needle	22G, 4-cm needle	22G, 50 mm long echogenic needle
Drug dosage	3–7 mL of LA 0.75% or 0.5% ropivacaine, or 0.5% bupivacaine	
Highlights		Tip-To confirm the nerve, when probe is moved proximally both nerve and vein comes above achillis tendon)

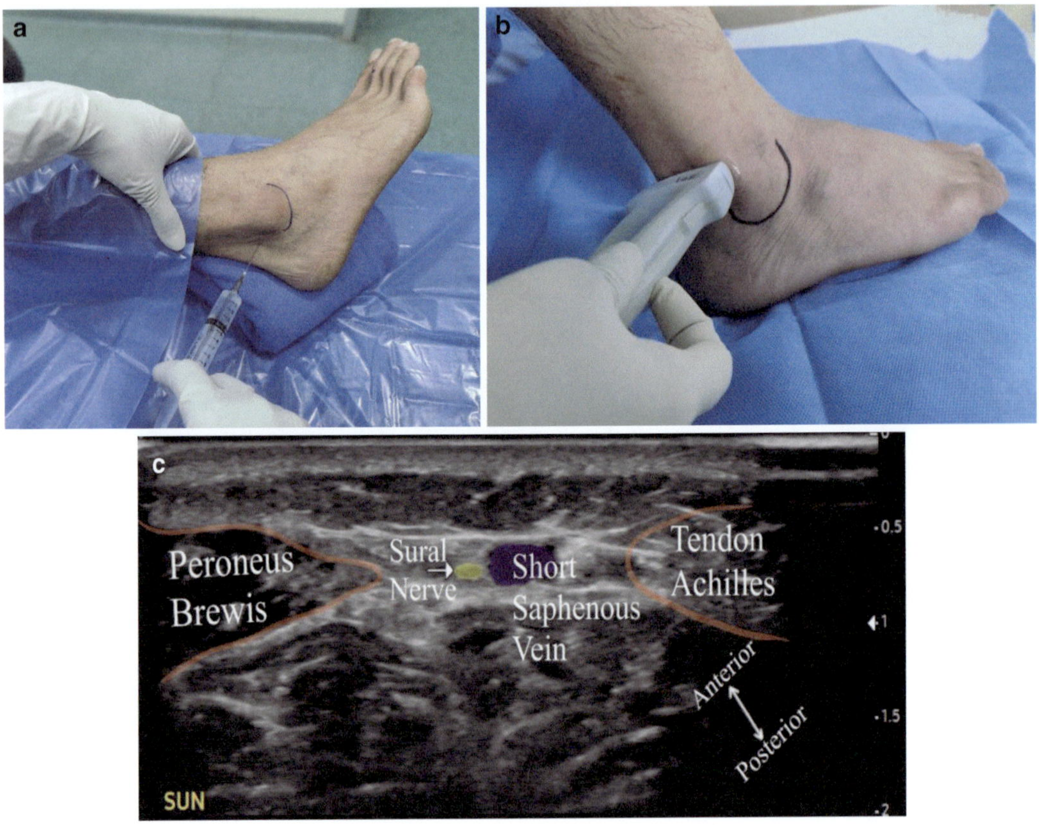

Fig. 9.45 (**a**) Landmark-guided infiltration for sural nerve block. (**b**) Ultrasound probe position for sural nerve block. (**c**) Ultrasound image showing sural nerve next to the lesser saphenous vein

5. *Sural Nerve Block.*

   Different approaches to sural nerve block (Table 9.74).

Tips

Dynamic scan or trace back technique is useful tool to differentiate between nerve and tendon as during proximal scan tendon can be seen changing as muscle. Moreover, muscle movement can be appreciated while patient moves his ankle or toe.

9.10.7 Complications

1. Hematoma—If there is a vascular puncture then withdraw the needle and press the puncture site for 2–3 min.
2. LAST—It is rare as local anesthetic plasma levels are relatively low following an ankle block and toxicity can result from direct intravascular injection. Aspiration prior to injection avoids this complication.
3. Nerve injury—No drug should be injected if motor response present <0.3 mA, or high resistance felt on injection.

Table 9.74 Different approaches to saphenous nerve block

	Landmark	Ultrasound guided
Position	Patient is supine with the foot elevated and supported on pillows, preferably at the edge of the OT table, and the ankle rotated with semi-flexed knee as needed for needle placement, or the operator can change position as needed	
Landmark technique POE and end point	Subcutaneous infiltration medial and superior to the medial malleolus and directed posteriorly toward the Achilles tendon (Fig. 9.46a)	High-frequency linear (10–15 MHz) transducer is placed just above the medial malleolus (Fig. 9.46b) Identify the long saphenous vein Saphenous nerve is usually identified medial to vein (Fig. 9.46c)
Needle	22G, 4-cm needle	22G, 50 mm long needle
Drug dosage	3–7 mL of LA 0.75% or 0.5% ropivacaine, or 0.5% bupivacaine/levobupivacaine	
Highlights		Tips—Apply very light pressure with the transducer as the long saphenous vein is easily compressible Saphenous nerve may not be consistently present at this level

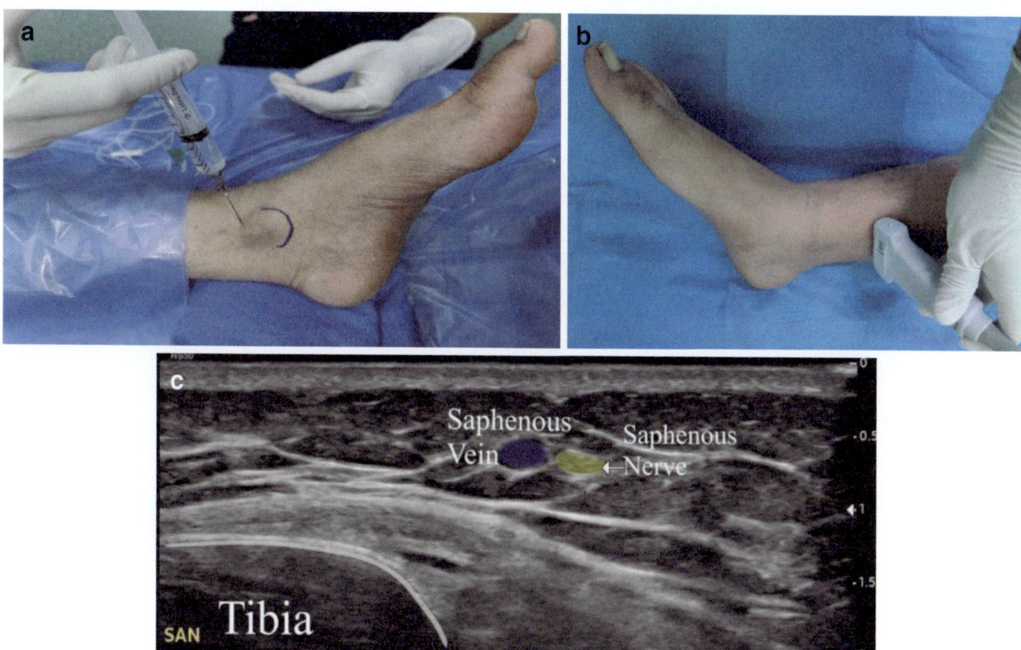

Fig. 9.46 (**a**) Landmark-guided infiltration for saphenous nerve block. (**b**) Ultrasound probe position for saphenous nerve block. (**c**) Ultrasound image showing saphenous nerve next to great saphenous vein

4. Neuropathy—Due to accidental intraneuronal injection or pinning the nerve against the bones with the needle at the time of injection.
5. Achilles tendon avulsion—very rare.

9.11 PENG Block

9.11.1 Introduction

Intertrochanteric femur fracture which consists of almost 45–50% of hip fractures is one of the most common causes of severe perioperative pain. In this patient population, effective perioperative analgesia that reduces the requirement for opioids and their associated side effects. Fascia iliaca block (FIB), 3 in 1 block, lumbar plexus block, epidural, and femoral blocks are used commonly for analgesia of hip fracture. These modalities are associated with sparing of pain and weakness of quadriceps. Girón-Arango et al. originally reported the PEricapsular nerve group (PENG) block as an ultrasound-guided regional anesthetic approach focused on blocking hip articular branches. PENG block is used to block articular branches of femoral, obturator, and accessory obturator nerves providing sensory supply to anterior hip capsule avoiding weakness of limbs.

9.11.2 Anatomy

The joint capsule of hip joint which is mainly supplied by the femoral, sciatic, and obturator nerves is responsible for majority of the pain experienced during any breach in the hip joint. A complex network of articular branches supplies the joint capsule (Fig. 9.47).

Two articular branches are derived from the femoral nerve supplying the pectineus and iliopsoas muscles besides articular branches from the obturator nerve which innervates the inferior and anteromedial aspect of the hip joint. The nerve to the quadratus femoris and sciatic nerves is also likely to have contributions in the posteromedial portion of the joint capsule. Since these articular branches arise proximally, distal blocking of femoral nerve leads to incomplete analgesia. Moreover, blocking femoral, sciatic, and obturator nerves in proximal positions results in significant weakness of the leg.

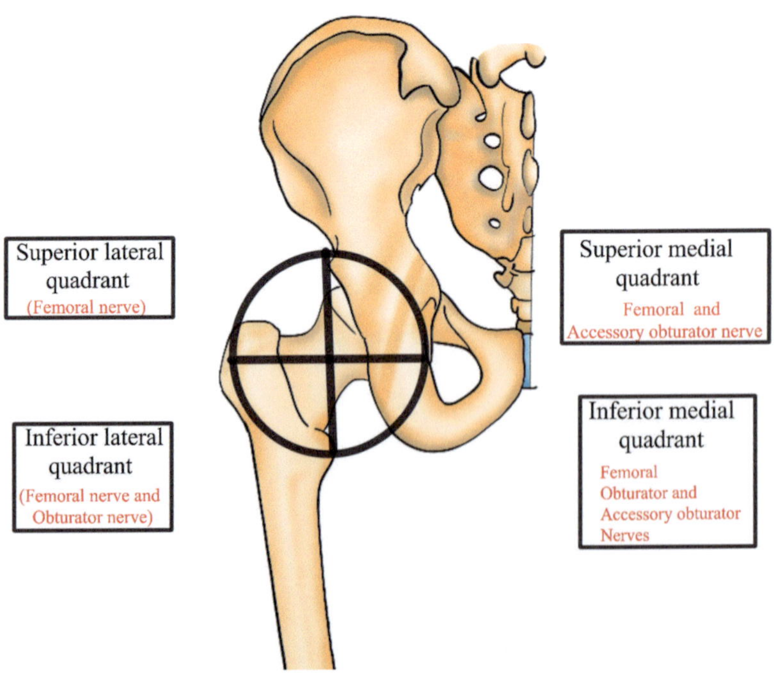

Fig. 9.47 Clinical anatomy of PENG block

Table 9.75 USG approach to PENG block

Position	Supine with affected limb abducted and externally rotated
Landmark	Anterior superior iliac aspine (ASIS), Anterior inferior iliac spine (AIIS), illiopubic eminence (IPE), psoas tendon
Technique	Under all aseptic precautions, curvilinear (2–5 MHz) transducer was placed parallel and over to inguinal crease at the level of ASIS. The probe is gradually rotated approximately 45 downward and inferior to identify the anterior inferior iliac spine, the iliopubic eminence, and the psoas tendon (Fig. 9.48a, b)
Needle	A 10-cm long, 21–22 gauge short-bevel needle
POE	A skin wheal of LA is made 1–1.5 cm away from the lateral edge of the transducer. Needle inserted in-plane from lateral to medial direction and the needle tip is placed between iliopsoas tendon anteriorly and the pubic ramus posteriorly between the anterior inferior iliac spine and iliopubic eminence using hydrodissection (Fig. 9.48b, c). (Tip-Out-of-plane approach can be used and needle is inserted perpendicular to the skin, caudal to probe in cephalad direction following the needle tip between AIIS and IPE Advantage—lateral femoral cutaneous nerve injury is avoided)
End point	LA spread is seen between psoas tendon and pubic ramus
Drug dosage	15–20 ml of drug deposited in 5 ml aliquots (0.2%/0.375% Ropivacaine, 0.25% bupivacaine/ levobupivacaine)

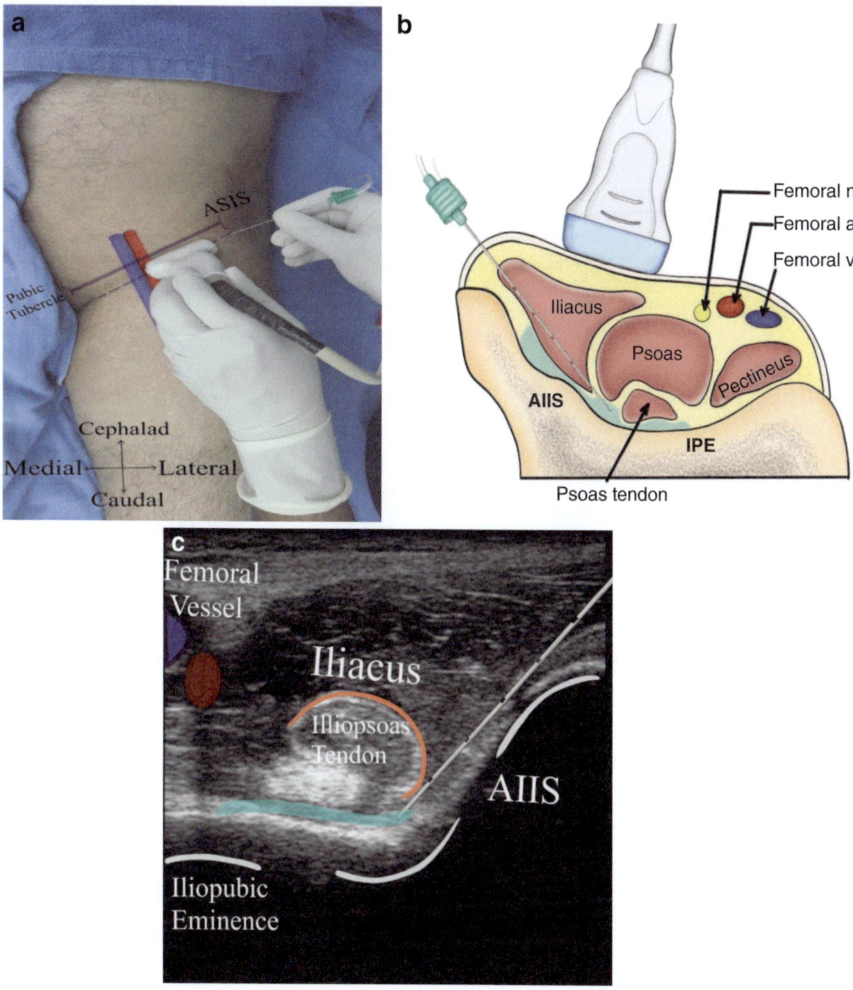

Fig. 9.48 (**a**, **b**) Probe and needle position for in-plane approach of needle insertion. (**b**) schematic diagram of PENG Block. (**c**) USG image of in-plane needle position for PENG block

The anterior capsule is the most densely innervated part of the joint, implying that these nerves should be the primary targets for hip analgesia. Previous anatomic investigations have revealed that the anterior hip capsule is innervated by the ON, axilliary obturator nerve (AON), and FN. PENG block primarily targets these nerves and aids in providing analgesia for hip fractures.

9.11.3 Indications

Post-operative pain management after hip joint surgeries.

Post-traumatic pain management with fractures involving proximal femur/femoral head.

9.11.4 Contraindications

Refer to Table 9.51.

9.11.5 Preparations

Refer to Table 9.2.

9.11.6 Block Approaches

USG approach to PENG block (Table 9.75).

Tips

- Not particularly helpful in intraarticular conditions of hip joint causing pain.
- Injection into iliopsoas muscles can be identified by increased injection pressure and pain on injection.
- To prevent motor blockade due to involvement of femoral nerve, which is in close proximity to iliopsoas muscle always better to avoid intramuscular injection and reposition the needle deep through iliofemoral ligament.
- In association with lateral femoral cutaneous nerve block, PENG Block can be used for analgesia of surgery involving lateral part of thigh along with fractured neck femur.

9.11.7 Complications

- General complications include infection, bleeding, neuropathy, and local anesthetic systemic toxicity.
- Quadriceps muscle weakness may occur secondary to the femoral nerve blockade.

9.12 iPACK

9.12.1 Introduction

Total knee arthroplasty (TKA) is one of the most commonly performed knee surgeries worldwide. TKA is associated with extreme pain post-operatively compromising early mobilization and speedy rehabilitation. Many regional nerve blocks like femoral, sciatic, and saphenous have been tried with variable success and side effects like motor weakness, delayed ambulation, and incomplete analgesia. These blocks also had the limitation of sparing popliteal plexus supplying the posterior aspect of knee. A novel regional anesthetic technique, originally described by Dr. Sanjay Sinha for posterior knee analgesia is ultrasound-guided local anesthetic infiltration between popliteal artery and posterior capsule of the knee (iPACK). In theory, the iPACK block has less of a motor and sensory blockade below the knee than the more distal sciatic nerve block because it targets the sensory articular branches originating from the sciatic, tibial, and common peroneal nerves, and the posterior division of the obturator nerve innervating the posterior aspect of the knee joint.

9.12.2 Anatomy

Behind the knee joint is a fine mesh of nerves called popliteal plexus which originates from articular branches of superior and inferior branches of tibial nerve, posterior branch of obturator nerve,

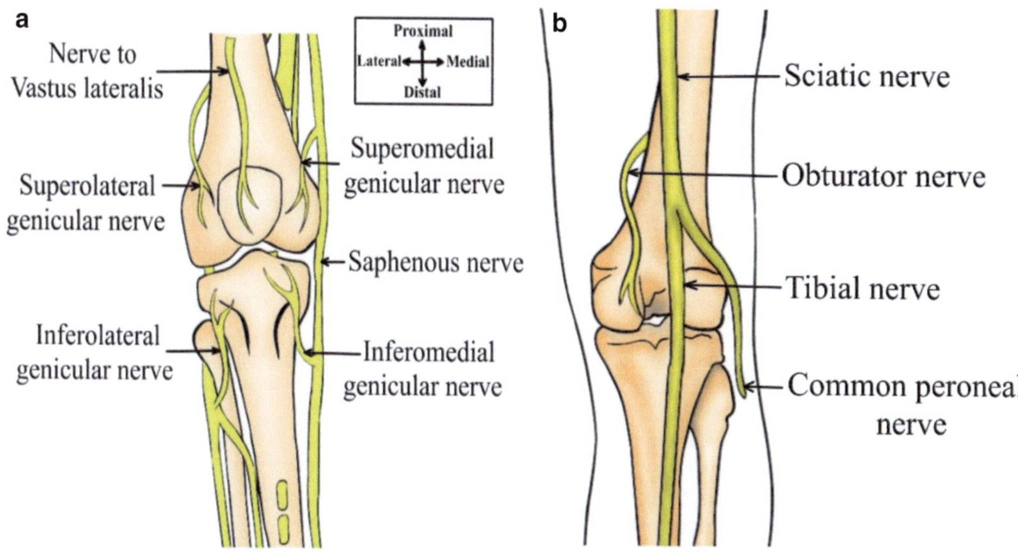

Fig. 9.49 (**a**, **b**) Articular branches supplying anterior part and posterior capsule of knee

and branches from common peroneal nerve. These articular branches innervate the posterior capsule of the knee, traveling through a tissue space between the popliteal artery and the femur. (Fig. 9.49a, b). Under ultrasound guidance, local anesthetic solution can be injected into this tissue plane to block these articular branches. This block provides posterior knee analgesia without compromising sensorimotor function of the leg/foot.

9.12.3 Indications

- Reduce the post-operative pain after total knee arthroplasty.
- Procedures involving the posterior aspect of the knee.
- Post-operative analgesia after Anterior Cruciate Ligament repair.

9.12.4 Contraindications

The absolute contraindications are patient refusal, local site infection, allergy to local and relative contraindication is coagulation disorder.

9.12.5 Preparations

Refer to Table 9.2.

9.12.6 Block Approaches

USG-guided Ipack Approach (Table 9.76).

9.12.7 Complications Limitations and Specific Risks

1. Intravascular injection.
2. Saphenous nerve injury during medial-to-lateral approach.
3. Sciatic nerve injury as it is close to posterior knee capsule.

Limitations

1. iPACK is used as a supplemental block with adductor canal /saphenous nerve block in knee arthroplasty as it provides analgesia only for posterior aspect of knee.

Table 9.76 USG-guided Ipack Approach

Position	Prone, Supine, or supine position with the lower extremity flexed at the knee and abducted at the hip and a pillow is placed under the thigh as support (frog leg position)
Probe	High-frequency linear (10–15 MHz) or Low-frequency curvilinear (2–5 MHz) probe depending on patient physique. Low-frequency probe is preferred as it covers a wide scanning view
USG scanning landmark	Under all aseptic precautions, place the probe on medial side of lower third of thigh (Fig. 9.50a) Identify femur and femoral vessels in short axis view as continuous hyperechoic lines and pulsating artery, respectively (Fig. 9.50b, c) Move probe downward till femoral artery appears in popliteal fossa through adductor hiatus as popliteal artery The transducer is now moved and positioned inferiorly and posteriorly to view the space between popliteal artery and the femur shaft just above the femoral condyles
POE	A 10–15 cm echogenic insulated needle is via in-plane approach from the anterior end of the transducer parallel to femur from medial to lateral direction between the popliteal artery and the femur (Fig. 9.50b, c) (TIP—Lateral to medial approach is also possible especially in prone or in supine position when knee is semi-flexed and leg is adducted and probe is placed in posteriorly in popliteal fossa)
End point	Tip of needle is moved 2 cm beyond the lateral border of the popliteal artery and LA is injected in 3 ml aliquots while withdrawing the needle back. (TIP—Avoid advancing needle tip beyond 2 cm which may lead to blockade of common peroneal nerve leading to foot-drop)
Drug dose	A total of 15–20 ml 0.25% Bupivacaine/ levobupivacaine, 0.2%/0.375%/0.5% Ropivacaine is deposited between femur and popliteal artery

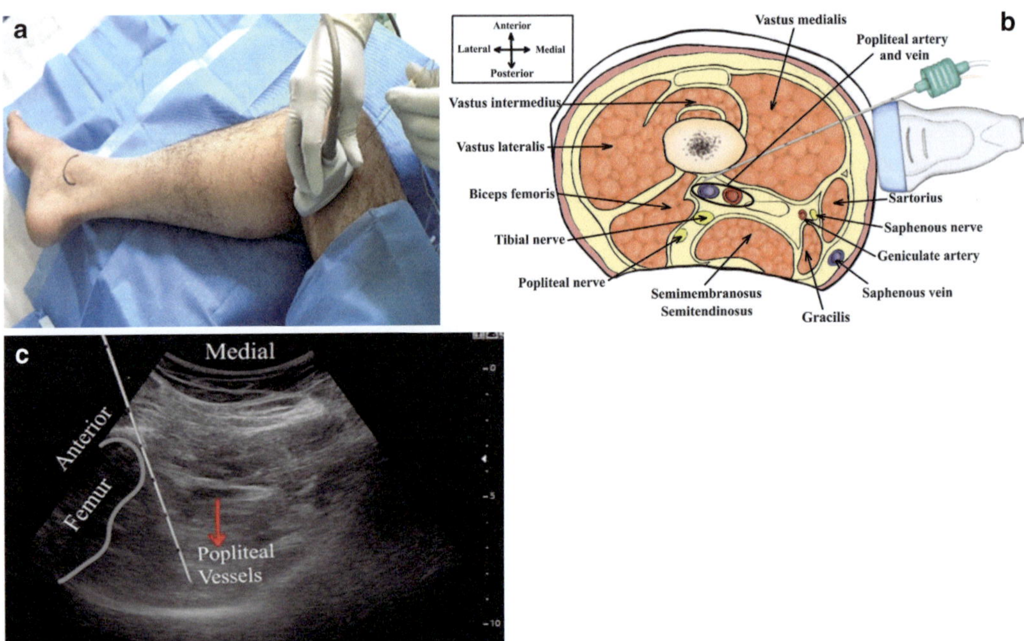

Fig. 9.50 (**a**) Probe position for ipack block. (**b**) Cross-section image of in-plane needle position for iPack block. (**c**) USG image of in-plane needle position for iPack block

2. This block is ultrasound dependent as it is performed in close proximity to major nerves and vessels.
3. Probe placement is difficult in obese patients, especially in supine and knee flexed position.

Further Reading

Aaron Hanyu-Deutmeyer DO, Pritzlaff SG. Peripheral nerve stimulation for the twenty-first century: sural, superficial peroneal, and tibial nerves. Pain Med. 2020;21(Suppl):S64–7.

Albaqami MS, Alqarni AA. Efficacy of regional anesthesia using ankle block in ankle and foot surgeries: a systematic review. Eur Rev Med Pharmacol Sci. 2022 Jan;26(2):471–84.

Bendtsen TF, Lönngvist PA, Jspsen KV, Petersen M, Knudsen L, Børglum J. Preliminary results of a new ultrasound-guided approach to block the sacral plexus: the parasacral parallel shift. Br J Anaesth. 2011;107:278–80.

Bendtsen TF, Pedersen EM, Moriggl B. Anatomical considerations for obturator nerve block with fascia iliaca compartment block. Reg Anesth Pain Med. 2021;46(9):806–12.

Capdevila X, Coimbra C, Choquet O. Approaches to the lumbar plexus: success, risks, and outcome. Reg Anesth Pain Med. 2005;30:150–62.

Desmet M, Vermeylen K, van Herreweghe I, et al. A longitudinal supra-inguinal fascia iliaca compartment block reduces morphine consumption after total hip arthroplasty. Reg Anesth Pain Med. 2017;42(3):327–33.

Di Benedetto P, Pinto G, Arcioni R, De Blasi RA, et al. Anatomy and imaging of lumbar plexus. Minerva Anestesiol. 2005;71:549–54.

Et T, Korkusuz M, Basaran B, Yarımoğlu R, Toprak H, Bilge A, Kumru N, Dedeli İ. Comparison of iPACK and periarticular block with adductor block alone after total knee arthroplasty: a randomized clinical trial. J Anesth. 2022 Apr;36(2):276–86.

Fusco P, Di Carlo S, Paladini G, Scimia P, Petrucci E, Marinangeli F. The perpendicular sacral plexus block: an alternative approach to the sacral plexus. Minerva Anestesiol. 2019 May;85(5):562–3.

Girón-Arango L, Peng PWH, Chin KJ, Brull R, Perlas A. Pericapsular nerve group (PENG) block for hip fracture. Reg Anesth Pain Med. 2018;43(8):859–63.

Guo J, Hou M, Shi G, Bai N, Huo M. iPACK block (local anesthetic infiltration of the interspace between the popliteal artery and the posterior knee capsule) added to the adductor canal blocks versus the adductor canal blocks in the pain management after total knee arthroplasty: a systematic review and meta-analysis. J Orthop Surg Res. 2022, Aug 12;17(1):387.

Hadzic A, Vloka JD. Anterior approach to sciatic nerve block. In: Hadzic A, Vloka J, editors. Peripheral nerve blocks. New York: McGraw-Hill; 2004.

Hansen J, Netter F. Netter's atlas of human anatomy. 6th ed. Philadelphia: Sanders Elsevier; 2014. p. 486–9.

Karmakar MK, Li JW, Kwok WH, et al. Sonoanatomy relevant for lumbar plexus block in volunteers correlated with cross-sectional anatomic and magnetic resonance images. Reg Anesth Pain Med. 2013a:391–7.

Karmakar MK, Shariat AN, Pangthipampai P, Chen J. High-definition ultrasound imaging defines the paraneural sheath and the fascial compartments surrounding the sciatic nerve at the popliteal fossa. Reg Anesth Pain Med. 2013b;38:447–51.

Kwofie MK, Shastri UD, Gadsden JC, Sinha SK, Abrams JH, Xu D, Salviz EA. The effects of ultrasound-guided adductor canal block versus femoral nerve block on quadriceps strength and fall risk: a blinded, randomized trial of volunteers. Reg Anesth Pain Med. 2013;38(4):321–5.

Lin J-A, Nakamoto T, Yeh S-D. Ultrasound standard for obturator nerve block: the modified Taha's approach. Br J Anaesth. 2015;114(2):337–9.

Lin D-Y, Morrison C, Brown B, et al. Pericapsular nerve group (PENG) block provides improved short-term analgesia compared with the femoral nerve block in hip fracture surgery: a single-center double-blinded randomized comparative trial. Reg Anesth Pain Med. 2021;46(5):398–403.

Liu Y, Ke X, Wu X, Mei W. Ultrasound-guided lumbar plexus block in supine position. Anesthesiology. 2018 Apr;128(4):812.

Lopez-Lopez D, Reza PC, Vazquez MG, Garcia PD. PENG block: advantages of out-of-plane approach. Indian J Anaesth. 2021;65:563–4.

Luftig J, Dreyfuss A, Mantuani D, Howell K, White A, Nagdev A. A new frontier in pelvic fracture pain control in the ED: successful use of the pericapsular nerve group (PENG) block. Am J Emerg Med. 2020;38(12):2761.e5–9.

Marsland D, Dray A, Little NJ, Solan MC. The saphenous nerve in foot and ankle surgery: its variable anatomy and relevance. Foot Ankle Surg. 2013;19(2):76–9.

Nagel EM, Gantioque R, Taira T. Utilizing ultrasound-guided femoral nerve blocks and fascia iliaca compartment blocks for proximal femur fractures in the emergency department. Adv Emerg Nurs J. 2019;41(2):135–44.

Nwawka OK, Meyer R, Miller TT. Ultrasound-guided subgluteal sciatic nerve perineural injection: report on safety and efficacy at a single institution. J Ultrasound Med. 2017;36(11):2319–24.

Ochroch J, et al. Analgesic efficacy of adding the IPACK block to a multimodal analgesia protocol for primary total knee arthroplasty. Reg Anesth Pain Med. 2020;45(10):799–804.

Reilly O, Desmet M, Kearns R. Fascia iliaca compartment block. BJA. 2019;19(6):191–7.

Sakamoto J, Manabe Y, Oyamada J, Kataoka H, Nakano J, Saiki K, et al. Anatomical study of the articular branches innervated the hip and knee joint with reference to mechanism of referral pain in hip joint disease patients. Clin Anat. 2018;31(5):705–9.

Saranteas T, Anagnostopoulos D, Kostroglou A, Souvatzoglou R. The "Shamrock method" for ultrasound-guided lumbar plexus nerve block in the supine position. J Clin Anesth. 2021 Aug;71:110249.

Sauter AR, Ullensvang K, Niemi G, et al. The Shamrock lumbar plexus block: a dose finding study. Eur J Anaesthesiol. 2015;32:764–70.

Shevlin S, Johnston D, Turbitt L. The sciatic nerve block. Br J Anes. 2020;20(9):312–20.

Standring S. Gray's anatomy the anatomical basis of clinical practice. 40th ed. Elsevier Health Sciences UK; 2008. p. 2533–4.

Steenberg J. Møller Systematic review of the effects of fascia iliaca compartment block on hip fracture patients before operation. Br J Anaesth. 2018;120(6):1368–80.

Thybo KH, Mathiesen O, Dahl JB, Schmidt H, Hagi-Pedersen D. Lateral femoral cutaneous nerve block after total hip arthroplasty: a randomised trial. Acta Anaesthesiol Scand. 2016;60(9):1297–305.

Wang AZ, Fan K, Zhou QH, Wang C, Niu Q, Chan Y. A lateral approach to ultrasound-guided sacral plexus block in the supine position. Anaesthesia. 2018;73:1043–4.

Wiederhold BD, Garmon EH, Peterson E, Stevens JB, O'Rourke MC. StatPearls [Internet]. Treasure Island: StatPearls Publishing; 26 Sep 2022. Nerve Block Anesthesia.

Yektaş A, Balkan B. Comparison of sciatic nerve block quality achieved using the anterior and posterior approaches: a randomised trial. BMC Anesthesiol. 2019;19:225.

Yoshida T, Nakamoto T, Hashimoto C, Aihara S, Nishimoto K, Kamibayashi T. An ultrasound-guided lateral approach for proximal sciatic nerve block: a randomized comparison with the anterior approach and a cadaveric evaluation. Reg Anesth Pain Med. 2018;43:712–9.

Approach and Troubleshooting to Central Neuraxial Blocks

10

Madhuri S. Kurdi, Sukhminder Jit Singh Bajwa, and Saurabh Barde

Abstract

Central neuraxial block is a very commonly used useful technique for a variety of surgeries. Traditionally, it has been a blind technique and hence has been associated with several incidences of failure or inadequate block. Nowadays, with the advent of modern technology including ultrasound, fluoroscopy and other techniques, the troubleshooting during the administration of central neuraxial block can be prevented or overcome. This chapter describes the various technical approaches to central neuraxial block and some useful methods to overcome troubleshooting when it occurs.

Keywords

Caudal · Central neuraxial block · Epidural anaesthesia · Failed · Spinal anaesthesia · Ultrasonography

M. S. Kurdi (✉)
Department of Anaesthesiology, Karnataka Medical College and Research Institute (KMC RI), Hubballi, Karnataka, India

S. J. S. Bajwa
Department of Anaesthesiology & Critical Care, Gian Sagar Medical College & Hospital, Patiala, Punjab, India

S. Barde
Faculty at Datta Meghe Medical College and SMHRC, Nagpur, Maharashtra, India

10.1 Introduction

Central neuraxial block is a generally preferred technique in anaesthesia practice and chronic pain management mainly because it is simple to perform and it provides rapid onset and dense block. It includes spinal, epidural, combined spinal-epidural and caudal-epidural block.

Neuraxial anaesthesia includes placement of local anaesthetic in or around the central nervous system. The local anaesthetic in spinal anaesthesia is placed directly in the intrathecal space, whereas in epidural anaesthesia, it is placed in the epidural space.

10.2 Brief Relevant Anatomy of the Central Neuraxis

The vertebral column consists of 33 vertebrae: 7 cervical, 12 thoracic, 5 lumbar, 5 fused sacral and 4 coccygeal. It has 4 curves. The cervical and lumbar curves are convex anteriorly whereas the thoracic and sacral curves are convex posteriorly. The curves have a significant effect on the spread of local anaesthetic in the subarachnoid and epidural space. The vertebral column is bounded together by several ligaments which gives it stability and elasticity. These include the supraspinous ligament, interspinous ligament, ligamentum flavum and the longitudinal ligament. The vertebral column articulates superiorly with the skull,

M. K. Prasad, S. J. S. Bajwa (eds.), *Steps to Successful Regional Anesthesia*,
https://doi.org/10.1007/978-981-97-4098-7_10

and inferiorly, with the two hip bones. A typical lumbar vertebra is made up of the body, the vertebral arch, the transverse process, the spinous process, superior and inferior articular processes. The dural sac is mostly constituted by the outer layer of dura and the inner layer called arachnoid membrane, which regulates diffusion of drugs into the intrathecal space. The pia mater surrounding the spinal cord is a permeable structure allowing the passage of drugs through intercellular spaces. The epidural space is a semi-circular space which lies between the spinal dura and the spinal periosteum. It extends from the base of the skull to the sacrococcygeal membrane and has direct communications with the paravertebral space. It is bounded superiorly by the foramen magnum and inferiorly by the sacral hiatus and sacrococcygeal membrane. Ligamentum flavum completes the posterior wall in direct continuity with the periosteum of the spinal canal. The epidural space is potentially an empty space with negative pressure and contains spinal nerve roots, epidural vessels, fat and lymphatics.

10.3 Approaches to Central Neuraxial Block

There are several approaches to central neuraxial block. A knowledge of these approaches and the problems that can be encountered in them is essential in clinical practice, both to increase practitioner confidence and comfort, and patient comfort. There are different major approaches that can be adopted for central neuraxial blockade. These include:

(a) Landmark-based approach
(b) Fluoroscopy-guided approach
(c) Ultrasound-guided approach

10.3.1 Landmark-Based Approach

Midline Approach
This is well known and commonly practised. It is usually used for lumbar/lower thoracic epidural/spinal block. The spinal/epidural needle is introduced into the skin in the midline, angled slightly cephalad. The structures traversed include skin, subcutaneous tissue, supraspinous ligament, interspinous ligament, ligamentum flavum and dura mater for spinal block (Fig. 10.1). For epidural block, the feeling of resistance of the ligamentum flavum indicates entry into the epidural space and dura mater is not traversed. In case the needle encounters bone at a shallow depth, it could be hitting the cephalad spinous process, and if it encounters bone at a deeper depth, it could be walking down the inferior spinous process. In such a situation, the needle should be redirected slightly cephalad and reinserted.

Vertebral Level Landmark

C7	Bony knob at base of neck
T7-8	Lower limits of scapulae
L2	Terminal point of 12th ribs
L4	Line across iliac crests
S2	Posterior iliac spines

The indicators for identification of the epidural space by landmark technique include the tactile method, visual method, mechanical method and ultrasonography. In the tactile method, the thumb of the anaesthesiologist rests

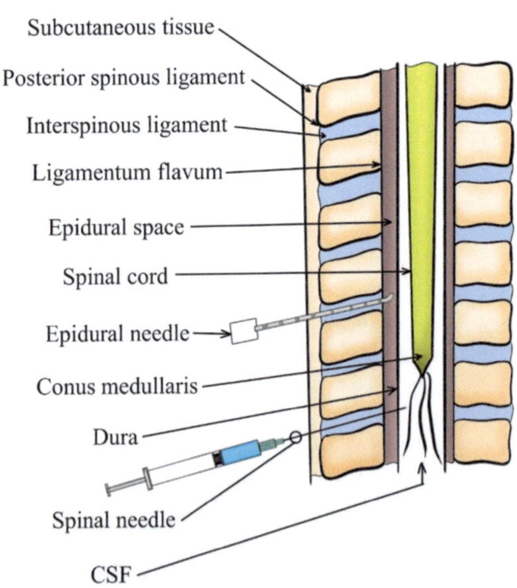

Fig. 10.1 Various structures traversed during midline and paramedian approach

on the end of the piston of a small syringe containing air or saline. The sudden loss of resistance that is felt as the needle crosses the ligamentum flavum indicates entry of needle tip into the epidural space. Saline is preferred to air as liquid will transmit the pressure changes more accurately. The thicker the needle shaft, the better will be the tactile change in sensation.

The visual method depends on recognition of negative pressure in the epidural space. In Gutierrez's hanging drop method, a drop of saline is placed on the hub of the advancing needle and it gets sucked into the needle when the needle tip enters the epidural space. The hanging drop technique can be used in the sitting position. Odom's capillary tube is another device that uses this negative pressure principle. Mechanical devices can also be used in place of the anaesthesiologist's thumb.

Lateral Paramedian Approach

It is adopted if midline ligaments are calcified. The needle is inserted 1 cm lateral and 1 cm caudal to spinous process 10–15 degrees off the sagittal plane in a cephalo-medial plane (Fig. 10.2). The spinous process, supraspinous and infraspinous ligaments are circumvented leading to a more direct path. This approach is preferred in the mid and high thoracic regions. The spinous processes are more acutely angled in the thoracic region. Hence, the needle has to be inserted at a more acute angle and pass through more distance to reach the epidural space in the midline and thoracic regions compared to the lumbar region.

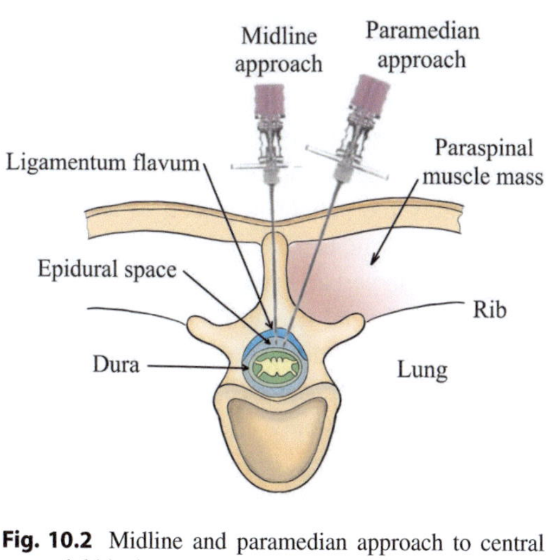

Fig. 10.2 Midline and paramedian approach to central neuraxial blocks

Caudal-Epidural Approach

It involves placing the needle through the sacral hiatus. It is used in paediatric and patients with chronic pain. Patient is placed in prone or lateral decubitus. By palpating sacral cornua as two bony prominences, the sacral hiatus can be identified as a dimple in between. A needle is inserted at 45 degree to the sacrum and redirected if the posterior of sacral bone is contracted. A subjective feeling of 'give' or loss of resistance suggests piercing the sacrococcygeal ligament, but is associated with a miss rate up to 26% even in experienced hands. The 'whoosh test', performed by auscultation at the thoracolumbar region with a stethoscope while injecting 2 mL of air, has a sensitivity of 80% and a specificity of 60% in adults. Palpating for subcutaneous bulging on rapid injection of 5 mL air or saline is also another confirmatory test.

Median Approach to Trans-Sacral Epidural Block

It is an alternate to caudal block in adults. It is used for surgery, patients with cancer pain affecting rectal, anal or urethral region. The catheter is placed 5 cm cephalad at S2-S3 with a 19G Tuohy needle by median approach.

Taylor's Approach

It is a modification of paramedian approach. It is used in patients with deformities like scoliosis, kyphoscoliosis or arthritis. A spinal needle is inserted in a cephalo-medial direction through skin wheal raised 1 cm medial and 1 cm caudal to the lowermost prominence of the posterior superior iliac spine (Fig. 10.3). The procedure can be done with the patient in the sitting/lateral/prone position.

Combined Spinal-Epidural Block

This technique consists of inserting a fine needle into the epidural space, and after injecting local anaesthetic, pushing needle into the subarachnoid space to administer further local anaesthetic.

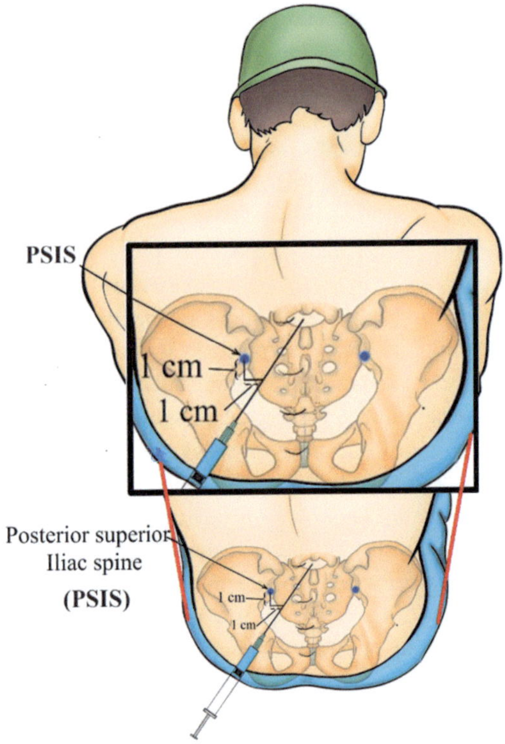

Fig. 10.3 Taylor's approach for central neuraxial blocks

Techniques

- Single Needle—Single Interspace Method
- Double Needle—Double Interspace Method
- Double Needle—Single Interspace Method
- Needle Beside Needle—Single Interspace Method

The needle-through-needle technique is the most preferred technique. It is used in caesarean section and orthopaedic surgeries.

Sequential Combined Spinal-Epidural Anaesthesia

A small spinal dose which is inadequate for the surgery is initially used and the block is then extended cephalad with epidural drug. It is most commonly used in obstetric anaesthesia practice and in patients undergoing orthopaedic surgery. Haemodynamic stability will be more balanced in this technique.

An 18 G Tuohy needle with epidural catheter is passed in the upper space for example, L2-L3, and subarachnoid block is administered at L3-L4 space with a 27 G Quincke needle with 1.2 mL of 0.5% hyperbaric bupivacaine. This is further advanced with titrated doses of 0.25% isobaric bupivacaine.

Another method would be the passing of a 25G Whitacre needle through a Tuohy needle and 2 mL (10 mg) of 0.5% hyperbaric bupivacaine is injected into the subarachnoid space over 30 s. 19 G epidural catheter is inserted 4–5 cm into the epidural space. If the desired spinal level is not achieved after 10 min of block, incremental epidural top-up dose with isobaric bupivacaine 0.5% 2 mL for every unblocked segment is calculated and given through the catheter till T10 level is reached.

Segmental Spinal Block

Here, a limited number of number of nerve roots are bathed by an anaesthetic solution within the subarachnoid space, providing anaesthesia in the surgical field dermatomes.

The block is performed via a single puncture with a cutting tip/pencil point tip spinal needle (27 G Quincke or Whitacre) with 45–60 degree angulation or through combined epidural spinal anaesthesia with intrathecal injection followed by passage of epidural catheter. It is administered as single shot or continuous spinal.

Thoracic spine magnetic resonance imaging has shown that there is a space between the dura and spinal cord and there is a greater depth of post subarachnoid space at mid thoracic levels than at lumbar and upper thoracic levels and it is safe to administer the block in this region with no resultant neurological damage.

Both isobaric and hyperbaric local anaesthetic solutions can be used. Hyperbaric solutions produce longer lasting block. The puncture can be performed in the sitting or lateral position, and immediately the patient is placed in a cephalacline position with isobaric solution and cephalodecline with hyperbaric solution. The injection of drug through spinal needle should be very slow and cautious until dural puncture is confirmed with free flow of cerebrospinal fluid (CSF) through the needle; only after this can the local anaesthetic be injected. Bupivacaine, levobupivacaine and ropivacaine are the local anaesthetics that can be used. Opioids, dexamethasone, midazolam, dexmedetomidine, clonidine and ketamine can be used as adjuvants.

Both the median and paramedian approach can be used. The needle insertion point and local anaesthetic volume can be as follows (Table 10.1):

This approach has been used in for radical cystectomy, lower segment caesarean section, laparoscopic cholecystectomy, breast cancer surgery, gastrostomies, hepatectomy, open abdominal surgeries for malignancies, resection of colonic tumours especially in patients with comorbidities like chronic obstructive pulmonary disease/bronchial asthma/lung carcinoma, geriatric patients with comorbidities and impaired pulmonary function where general anaesthesia would be risky (Table 10.2).

Continuous Spinal Anaesthesia (CSA)

It is not a much commonly used technique. It can be performed with a paediatric Tuohy epidural needle of 19 G, and a paediatric epidural catheter of 22 G can be inserted and fixed at 6 cm. A standard Tuohy needle of 16 G with 18G epidural catheter is also feasible for the purpose. Spinal microcatheters can also be used for the purpose. The most commonly used CSA set is a catheter-through-needle set that comes with 22G Sprotte needle and 25G nylon catheter. Some use Tuohy epidural set for CSA which has 18G Tuohy needle and 20G nylon catheter. The backflow of cerebrospinal fluid is looked for and the drug, initially a small dose e.g. 1.5 mL of 0.5% hyperbaric bupivacaine is administered over a minute. Spinal effect is looked for by testing in the concerned region. Based on the assessment of block height, top-up volumes of 0.5 mL of 0.5% bupivacaine can be administered to titrate block height and maintain haemodynamic stability.

The shortcomings of this technique include difficulty in threading microcatheters, catheter kinking, failed continuous spinal anaesthesia (low failure rate because placement of the Tuohy needle in the subarachnoid space can be easily confirmed by the escape of CSF), spinal infections, post-dural puncture headache especially with epidural catheters, catheter breakage during removal especially with microcatheters, cauda equina syndrome and neurological complications. Catheter breakage can be prevented by removing the CSA catheter with the patient's spine in a flexed position, slow removal of the catheter and pulling out the catheter as close to its insertion point as possible.

Epidural Volume Extension Technique

It is a modified method of combined spinal epidural. Low dose spinal anaesthesia is given and is immediately followed by epidural volume extension in which saline is injected into the epidural space. In this technique, there is thecal compression of subarachnoid space due to volume effect, which promotes cephalad displacement of local anaesthetic in the CSF.

Table 10.1 Local anaesthetic volume with respect to needle insertion level

	Needle insertion space	Local anaesthetic solution	Dose	Adjuvant
1.	T9–T10	Bupivacaine isobaric/hyperbaric	5–10 mg	Fentanyl 20 μg
2.	T5–T6	Bupivacaine isobaric	5–8 mg	Morphine 50 μg/fentanyl20 μg
3.	T10–T11	Bupivacaine hyperbaric	7.5 mg (1.3–2 mL)	Fentanyl 20 μg

Table 10.2 Local anaesthetic volume according to surgeries

	Type of surgery	Spinal needle insertion level	Local anaesthetic volume range (mL)
1.	Colonic resection	T4–T5	1.7
2.	Laparoscopic cholecystectomy	T8–T11	1.5–3.5
3.	Breast surgery	T5–T6	1.1–4
4.	Gastrectomy Gastrostomy	T6–T8 T8–T9	0.9–1.2 1

The epidural space is identified with a 17 G Tuohy epidural needle, and then the dura is punctured with a 25G Whitacre needle through the Tuohy needle. 10 mg of bupivacaine heavy is then injected into the subarachnoid space after the free flow of CSF is noted. Then, a 19G epidural catheter is inserted up to 4–5 cm into the epidural space, after which 10 mL of saline is injected into the epidural space. The epidural volume expansion should preferably be done 5 min after intrathecal injection to produce an increase in the sensory level of block. Increased time interval between intrathecal injection and epidural volume expansion can lead to failure of increase in sensory height. The technique can be used in high risk cardiac/pulmonary cases to reduce haemodynamic disturbances of routine spinal anaesthesia.

Fractionated Injection Technique

A half dose of the mixture, e.g., 25 µg fentanyl plus 15 mg bupivacaine 0.5% mixture, is injected intrathecally, and then, the other half is injected after 45 seconds while the needle is still in place. The patient who till now is in the sitting position is then immediately laid down in the supine position. In some studies, 2/3rd of the total calculated dose has been given initially followed by 1/3rd dose after 90 s with both doses administered at a rate of 0.2 mL/s. Studies have shown that fractional spinal anaesthesia leads to a longer duration and more favourable levels of sensory blockade compared to the bolus method. In addition, haemodynamic changes and complications occur less frequently following this technique.

10.3.2 Fluoroscopy-Guided Central Neuraxial Blockade

10.3.2.1 Indications

Fluoroscopy-guided central neuraxial blockade though not routinely performed can be used in obese patients with difficult spine anatomy like kyphoscoliosis, ankylosing spondylitis or failed attempts to landmark-guided approach in absence of ultrasound or expertise of using ultrasound (Table 10.3).

Table 10.3 Fluoroscopy-guided central neuraxial block

Position	Prone, sitting or left-lateral decubitus position with the arms at the side of the body or the arms elevated to avoid obstruction during fluoroscopy imaging
Landmark	C-arm projection—Obtain true anteroposterior view of the target lumbosacral spine so that spinous process is equidistant from both the pedicles and squaring of the vertebral endplates by variable degrees of lateral and oblique C-arm rotation. (Tip—Adjust the vertebral disk endplates so that they appear as a single line, with disk spaces clearly visible, by using craniocaudal C-arm adjustments till vertebral body has a 'box' appearance, with the spinous process along the midline (Fig. 10.4). In lateral–lateral position of C-arm adjust the disk endplates so as to superimpose the pedicles by using craniocaudal C-arm movement (Fig. 10.5). Adjust the posterior wall so as to superimpose the articular processes by using right left C-arm movement. If properly done, the vertebral body has a box appearance and the foramina are clearly visible)
Point of Entry and technique	Under all aseptic precautions and after local anaesthetic infiltration, needle is inserted on lower border of vertebral body just medial to pedicle immediately inferior to the target interlaminar space (like for L3-L4 interlaminar space L4 lower border is targeted) in a anteroposterior view (Fig. 10.6). The needle is advanced slightly medially until it made contact with the lamina, and then was redirected in a more medial and cephalad direction till the interlaminar space is identified using loss of resistance technique for epidural needle placement. (Tip—In thoracic level the entry angle is approximately 30–40 degree to skin in medial and cephalad direction till it makes contact with upper border of lamina. Then the C-arm is rotated in lateral direction and the needle is advanced in lateral view just crossing the facet line simultaneously identifying the epidural space using loss of resistance technique) (Fig. 10.7)
End point	In anteroposterior (AP) view, needle tip just crossed the upper border of the lamina in lumbar region; however, in thoracic region needle tip may cross midline. (Tip—Can be confirmed by injecting dye and seeing the spread going up and down in posterior epidural space)

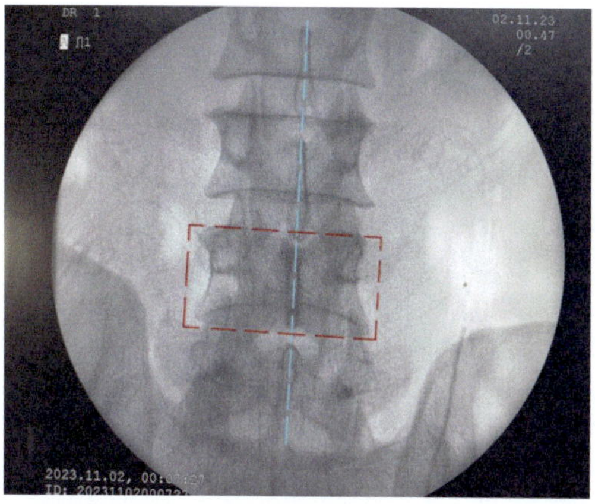

Fig. 10.4 AP view shows the vertebral body appearing as a box with spinous processes in the midline

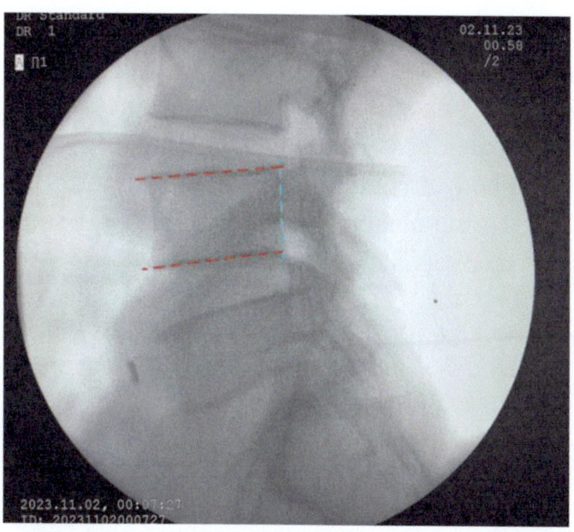

Fig. 10.5 The lateral view shows profiled disk endplates and the posterior vertebral wall

Advantages—It is simple to see the precise intervertebral space and needle manipulation can be done in real-time and can be performed with both hands as compared to ultrasound.

Disadvantages—Cannot be used in pregnant patients, are ineligible for this technique, exposure to radiation to both practitioner and patient

Complications—Bleeding, haematoma, nerve injury

10.3.3 Ultrasound-Guided Central Neuraxial Blockade

Traditionally, as the spinal/epidural needle would advance, the anaesthesiologist would appreciate

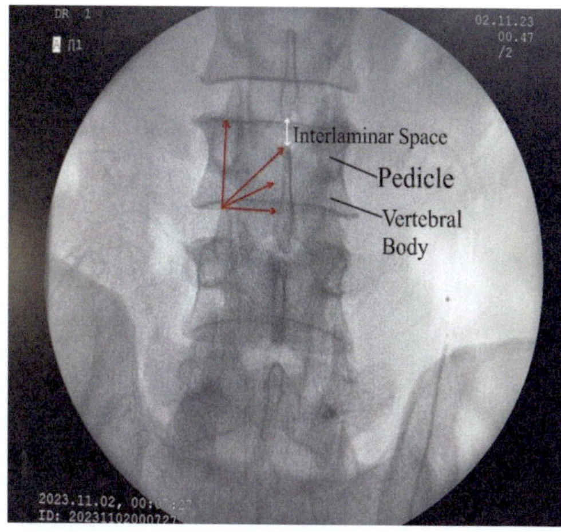

Fig. 10.6 Red solid dot showing the skin insertion site in AP view at the junction of a line parallel to the vertebral column that pass through the middle of the pedicle and the lower border of vertebral body immediately inferior to the target interlaminar space at thoracic and lumbar level

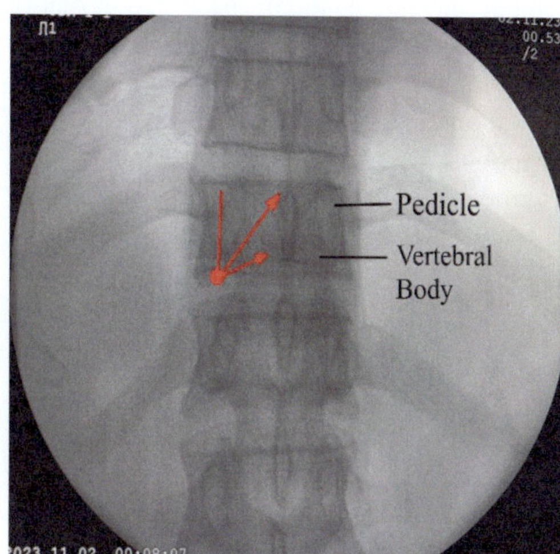

Fig. 10.7 The entry angle is approximately 30–40 degree to skin in medial and cephalad direction till it makes contact with upper border of lamina in the thoracic level

changes in tissue resistance and get a mental picture of where the needle tip lies. Nowadays, this has been revolutionised by ultrasound.

Spinal ultrasound is challenging because the structures that are needed to be imaged are protected by a very complex, articulated encasement of bones through which there exists a very limited acoustic window for the ultrasound beam. Also, the structures that are to be visualised are located deep.

The equipment needed for this technique includes an ultrasound machine with a curved ultrasound probe of low frequency (2–5 MHz).

10.3.3.1 Clinically Relevant Sono-Anatomy of Central Neuraxis

The patient can be in the sitting, left-lateral or prone position. It is usually done pre-procedure. The scanning planes can be as follows:

Longitudinal Axis (Sagittal Scanning)

The lumbar spine is flexed and the transducer is placed at distance of 1–2 cm lateral to the spinous process (midline) in a longitudinal orientation. It is tilted to direct the beam medially. The probe is then oriented towards the midline to the desired vertebral level. The image of a 'saw' will appear. Two echogenic linear structures will be seen in the gaps. The superficial line represents the ligamentum flavum, epidural space and posterior dura and is termed as the posterior complex. The deeper line includes the anterior dura, posterior longitudinal ligament and the posterior aspect of the vertebral body on the intervertebral disc and is termed the anterior complex. The intervening dark space between the anterior and posterior complexes corresponds to the intrathecal space. The longitudinal scanning helps to identify the intervertebral level and intervertebral space.

Transverse Axis

The transducer is positioned in the transverse plane on the spinous process of the vertebral body. The 'tower' sign will now be seen where the spinous process will appear like a tower (Fig. 10.8a, b). The probe is then rotated caudally in the space so that the tower sign disappears and the 'flying bat' sign emerges (Fig. 10.9a, b).

The identification of the spinous process in the transverse plane determines the midline, which is marked as a dot on the skin at the midpoint of the ultrasound probe when the image is centred on the screen. The image of an interspace visualising the ligamentum flavum, ventral and posterior dura mater, posterior longitudinal ligament, vertebral body, transverse process and articular process can be obtained by moving the probe in a caudal or cephalad direction.

Once the best image of the interspace is obtained, a mark is made on the skin at the width

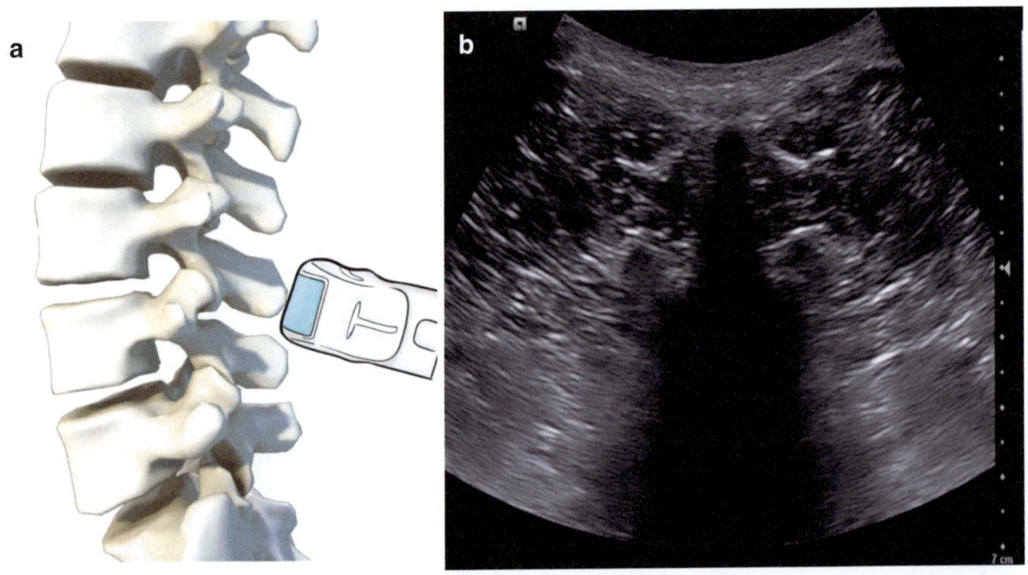

Fig. 10.8 (**a**) Probe position for transverse spinous process approach through L3-4 interspace showing tower like appearance of spinous process. (**b**) USG image of transverse spinous process approach through L3-4 interspace showing tower like appearance of spinous process

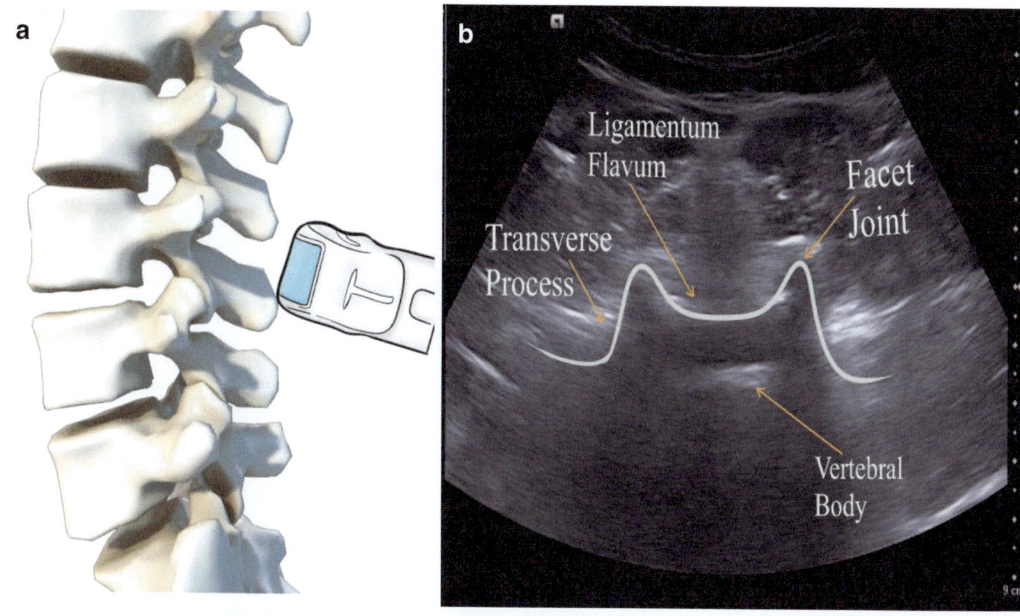

Fig. 10.9 (**a**) Probe position for transverse interspinous view at L3-4. (**b**) USG image of transverse interspinous view at L3-4 showing 'Flying Bat' appearance

of the probe, which represents the interspace. The ideal needle insertion point for central neuraxial blockade can be marked on the skin by joining the vertical line intersecting the midline point and a horizontal line intersecting the interspace point. The needle insertion depth can be estimated by measuring the depth from the skin to the posterior complex using the electronic calipers of the ultrasound machine.

10.3.3.2 Five Basic Ultrasound Views

Parasagittal Transverse Process View

The ultrasound probe is placed in a parasagittal orientation 3–4 cm lateral to the midline and just above the upper border of sacrum. Here the transverse processes of successive lumbar vertebrae are visualised. These appear as short hyperechoic curvilinear structures with pronounced 'finger-like' acoustic shadowing beneath, an appearance that has been described as the 'trident sign' (Fig. 10.10a, b).

Parasagittal Articular Process View

The probe is slided medially from parasagittal transverse view until a continuous hyperechoic line of 'humps' is seen. Each hump represents the facet joint between the superior and inferior articular process of successful vertebrae (Fig. 10.11a, b).

Parasagittal Oblique(Interlaminar) View

From the parasagittal articular process view, the probe is tilted to angle the beam in a lateral to medial direction towards the median sagittal plane, 'saw tooth' appearance is obtained (Fig. 10.12a, b).

Transverse Spinous Process View

From parasagittal oblique view, probe is rotated 90 degree into a transverse orientation and centred on neuraxial midline (Fig. 10.13a, b).

Transverse Interlaminar View

From the transverse spinous process view, the probe is slided in a cephalad/caudal direction to align the beam with the interspinous and interlaminar space. This provides a transverse interlaminar view of the contents of the vertebral canal (Fig. 10.14).

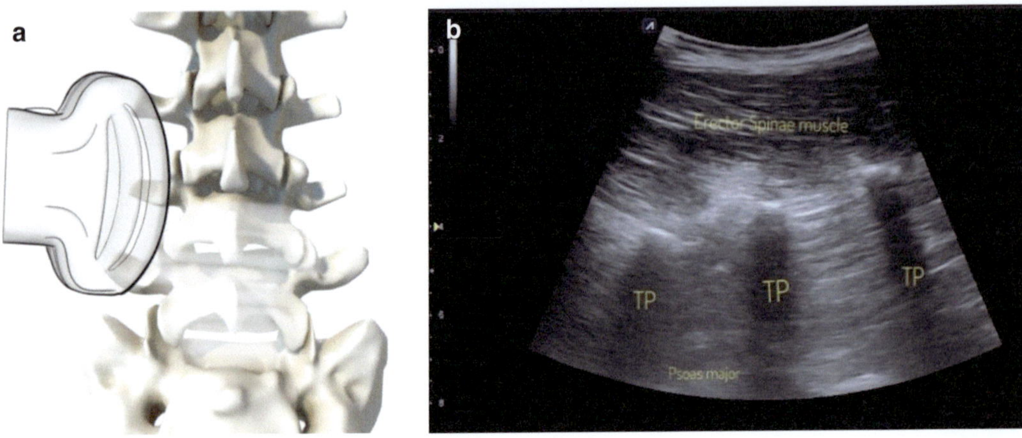

Fig. 10.10 (**a**) Parasagittal transverse process view: Placement of probe in vertical orientation 3–4 cm lateral to midline. (**b**) USG image showing finger-like long acoustic shadows (Trident sign) seen formed by adjacent transverse processes

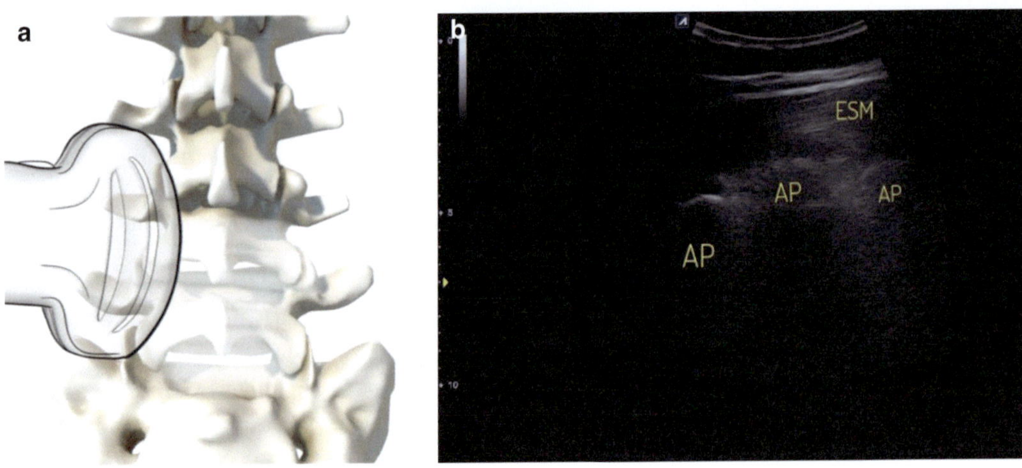

Fig. 10.11 (**a**) Parasagittal articular surface view: Probe from parasagittal transverse process view position is moved medially. (**b**) USG showing shallower acoustic shadows formed by articular processes of adjacent vertebrae similar to continuous camel hump

10.3.3.3 Which View and Plane to Choose for Scanning?

- It is better to scan in both transverse and longitudinal planes as they complement each other during ultrasound scanning of spine.
- The two most useful sonographic views are the parasagittal oblique view and the transverse midline inter-spinal-laminar view.
- The intervertebral space can be identified and visualised by parasagittal oblique view. The depth of needle insertion can be estimated in transverse interlaminar view.

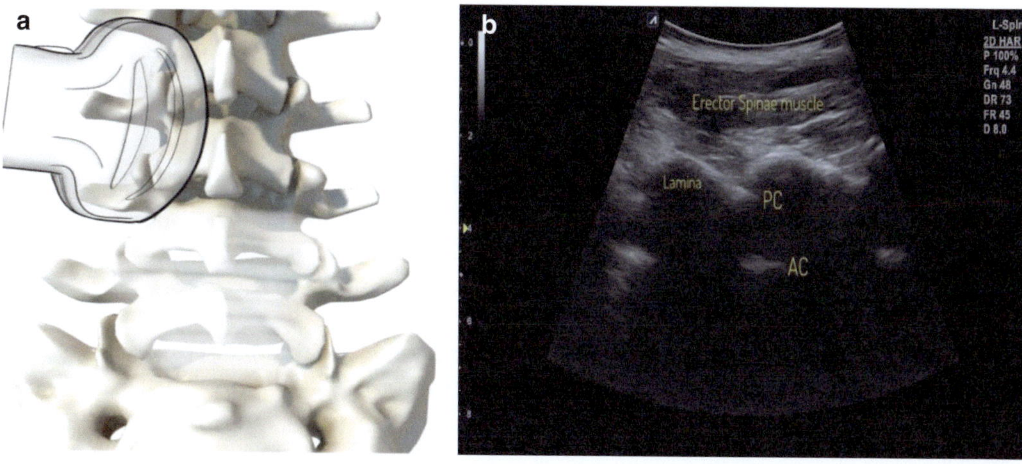

Fig. 10.12 (**a**) Parasagittal oblique(interlaminar) view: Probe from parasagittal articular surface view position is tilted to look from lateral to medial direction into vertebral canal. (**b**) Continuous hump like shadows are replaced by intermittent saw tooth like shadows of adjacent laminae

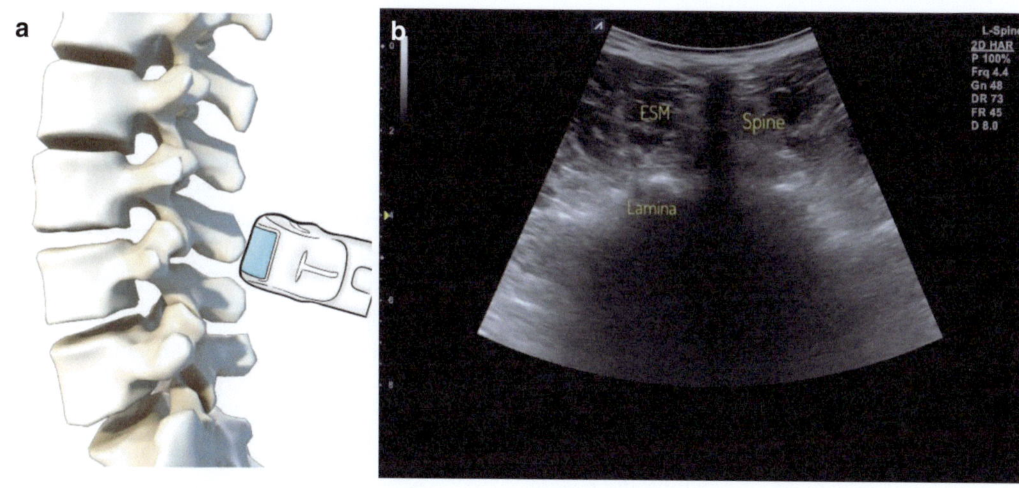

Fig. 10.13 (**a**) Transverse spinous process view: Placement of probe in horizontal orientation on spinous process of the vertebra. (**b**) USG showing pointed, hyperechoic shadow with dark anechoic shadow underneath formed by spine and laminae bilaterally

10.3.3.4 When Is Ultrasound-Guided Central Neuraxial Blockade Useful?

- In patients with an atypical spine like scoliosis, those with obesity, pregnancy, wherein the landmarks are not palpable. The intervertebral level, ideal needle insertion point and needle insertion depth can be estimated in such cases with ultrasonography.

10.3.3.5 Advances in Ultrasound-Guided Central Neuraxial Block

A machine learning real-time system that uses a deep convolutional neural network and successfully identifies lumbar vertebral levels to classify transverse images of the lower spine is available. Landmarks obtained from novel automated spinal landmark identification technique may be commonly used in the future.

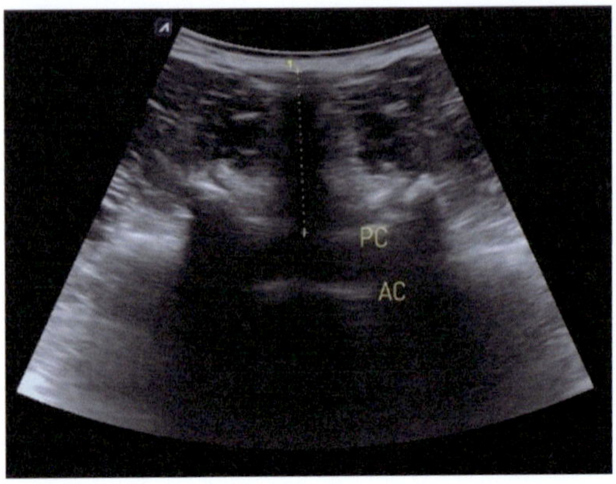

Fig. 10.14 Transverse interlaminar view: Placement of probe in horizontal orientation in between two adjacent spinous processes. Hyperechoic posterior complex (PC) formed by posterior dura and ligamentum flavum with epidural space in between and anterior complex (AC) formed by vertebral body, posterior longitudinal ligament and anterior dura seen. The distance of posterior complex from the skin can be measured using caliper tool

Real-time ultrasonography-guided paramedian spinal anaesthesia—The interspinous space is identified by using the real-time images in posterior sagittal oblique view, and the needle can be visualised breaching into the spinal space. The sacrum is the first structure to be identified, after which the probe is advanced cephalad with an angle of 20° tilted towards the midline. Then, the lumbar lamina is identified along with a target space. The probe is then further rotated 25° towards the midline to achieve a classical oblique parasagittal approach. This approach provides the ergonomic advantage of handling the needle and the probe together.

In spite of all the different approaches and aids to central neuraxial blockade, troubleshooting can occur during central neuraxial blockade.

10.4 Troubleshooting During Central Neuraxial Blockade Procedure

This can include (1) Failed spinal block (2) Failed epidural block (3) Unilateral/patchy/inadequate spinal or epidural block (4) Allodynia, paresthesias (5) Bloody tap (6) Dry tap (7) Accidental placement of the catheter in the subarachnoid or intravascular space (8) Accidental dural puncture.

10.4.1 Failed Spinal Anaesthesia/ Partial Block (Insufficient Height, Quality or Duration)/ Patchy Block

It can occur due to the following reasons/ following situations:

- Faulty clinical technique, inexperience (especially the unsupervised trainee), failure to appreciate the need for a meticulous approach.
- Insufficient preparation and check of equipment and drugs.
- Failed lumbar puncture or 'Dry tap'—This is failure of appearance of CSF at the spinal needle hub when there is possible confirmed placement of needle tip in the subarachnoid space denoted by 'give away' feel of dura even after waiting for adequate time. The causes of dry tap include:
  - (a) Dehydration resulting in low CSF pressure.
  - (b) Blocked needle, needle in wrong space (lumbar interspace not matching the surgical intervention), incorrect needle insertion.
  - (c) Poor positioning of the patient. Correct patient positioning may not be possible due to (i) abnormalities of the spine such as kyphosis, scoliosis (ii) calcification of ligaments (iii) osteoporosis (iv) obesity (v) patient anxiety (vi) inexperienced operation theatre assistant.
  - (d) Previous spinal surgery, severe spinal canal stenosis.
  - (e) Narrowing of thecal sac because of lipomatosis or arachnoiditis and iliopsoas abscess extending to epidural space.
- Loss of injectate due to leakage of dry solution through defect at the junction of needle hub and shaft.

easily create a false loss of resistance by pushing too hard during the process of needle advancement. For the supervisor, it is also hard to know whether the trainee feels true loss of resistance when visually supervising the whole process.

- Equipment and device problems—The orifice of the catheter when lateral or anterior in the epidural space can put the local anaesthetic more on one side, thus producing a unilateral block. Manufacturing errors such as faulty markings on epidural catheters can lead to wrong depth of placement. Knotting of catheter (internal/external) can cause obstruction. Debris in catheter can cause epidural failure.
- Incorrect choice of dose, concentration and volume of local anaesthetic.
- Midline approach may be more associated with difficulties in localisation of epidural space and in catheter insertion both in lumbar and thoracic region. A thoracic epidural block is a relatively more difficult procedure than procedures used in other regions, because the spinous process of the thoracic vertebra is longer than that of the lumbar vertebra, and the area through which the needle can approach the epidural space is relatively smaller due to an acute angle and larger distance between the skin and the epidural space. Therefore, the success rate of thoracic epidural intervention is only about 68% under a blind technique due to inadequate position of the needle tip, misplacement, occlusion and migration of the catheter.

10.4.1.5 Prevention and Management of Epidural Failure

1. **Epidural catheter related tips**
    - Use of a soft tipped, flexible epidural catheter can result in fewer paraesthesia. It curls up or changes the course as it brushes against nerve roots/other obstacles.
    - Catheter materials that soften at body temperature decrease the rate of paraesthesia.
    - Softer, single hole catheters and flexible wire-reinforced polyurethane catheters are associated with a lower incidence of intravascular catheterisation.
    - Inserting the catheter at least 4 cm into epidural space can achieve a higher success rate. Werster recommends that 3 cm is the ideal length of the Portex catheter (with side holes) to be inserted into the epidural space.
    - Tunnelling the epidural catheter for 5 cm/suturing of epidural catheter is associated with less migration of catheter.
    - There is considerable movement of the skin and soft tissues over the lumbar spine with change of position in an obese patient. So, the epidural catheter can be inserted and then, the patient's position can be changed before applying the fixative dressing (either sitting to left lateral or left lateral to sitting).
    - Multi-orifice epidural catheters are said to be better than single orifice catheters.
2. **Use of technical devices**

    There are many devices designed to help identify the epidural space and to differentiate false loss of resistance from true loss of resistance during epidural puncture. They allow the anaesthesiologist to grip the epidural needle with both hands, to omit pushing the barrel of the syringe with the other hand and to make the procedure more controlled and hence safer. These commercially available methods include Epimatic®, Episure Autodetect® and Epidrum® techniques of loss of resistance.

    Devices such as CompuFlo® epidural instrument and cheaper techniques such as loss of resistance using 3-way stopcock and two syringes can also be used. Air-refill test with a B Braun air syringe Perifix® can be used as a supplementary test alongside conventional loss of resistance. The test can be used in air-refill positive cases. When the test is positive (it will usually be positive in labouring women), we can be strongly confident about the correct needle location.

    Older methods include spring loaded technique, Macintosh balloon, Brooks device, vertical tube of Dawkins, Oxford epidural space indicator, Odom's capillary tube method, manometer technique and many more. Newer methods include Doppler guidance, pressure transducer-guided method and auditory amplification of sound made by the epidural needle as it traverses the interspinous ligament and ligamentum flavum. Ultrasound is the most advanced technical aid that can be used.

3. **Use of epidural test dose**

   Administration of a small volume of local anaesthetic with epinephrine to rule out unintended intravascular, subdural or intrathecal placement of epidural needle or catheter tip is called as test dose. An ideal test dose should help a clinician to detect placement of every epidural needle or catheter tip in the intravascular/intrathecal space without any false positive alarms leading to unnecessary manipulation or reposition. Also, an ideal test dose should not cause any serious side effects or complications.

   The epidural test dose includes drug choices and doses as follows-1) For combined intrathecal and intravenous catheter tip detection: a) Lignocaine 1.5% or bupivacaine 0.25% with epinephrine 5 μg /ml(1:200000)3 ml. Positive intravascular test dose is indicated by an increase in heart rate of 20 beats/min within 1 min. Positive intrathecal test is indicated by motor blockade in 3–5 min. 2) For intravenous catheter tip detection: a) Lignocaine 100 mg/bupivacaine 25 mg b) Fentanyl 100 μg. Positive test is indicated by tinnitus, circumoral numbness and dizziness with lignocaine/bupivacaine and dizziness and/drowsiness within 5 min after fentanyl injection. 3) For intrathecal catheter tip detection: Lignocaine 40–50 mg/bupivacaine 7.5 mg. Positive test is indicated by motor blockade at 3–5 min.

   The test dose for labour epidural is controversial and the best policy is to consider each dose as a test dose and keep giving not more than 5 ml of the solution prepared (0.1% or lower concentration of bupivacaine). Alternatively, one can give 3 ml of 1.5% lignocaine with epinephrine. It is better not to use lignocaine if one is planning for a 'walking epidural'.

   Epinephrine can cause utero-placental insufficiency; so it is not much preferred in pregnant women. Injection fentanyl 100 μg wehen given as an epidural test dose will cause sedation within 5 min in the parturient if the catheter tip is intravascularly placed. Doppler precordial auscultation will detect intravascular tip after injection of 10 ml agitated saline as epidural test dose.

   Profound sensory and motor block after test dose injection of local anaesthetic indicates unintended intrathecal or subdural location of the epidural catheter tip. Smaller divided volumes of test dose should be given when epidural catheter is placed in higher thoracic region to avoid high spinal or total spinal anaesthesia and subsequent haemodynamic and respiratory instability.

4. **Use of adjuvants**—Addition of opioids/epinephrine to epidural solution can decrease local anaesthetic dose and improve the quality of analgesia.

10.4.1.6 Tips for Epidural Needle Puncture, Catheter Insertion and Removal

- If there is an entrapped wire-reinforced catheter, it can be removed by placing the patient in the lateral decubitus position/original insertion position and removal in 30–60 min or applying gentle, continuous traction.
- Blunt-tipped multiport catheter is less traumatic with less chances of intravascular cannulation.
- Limiting the amount of catheter threaded into the epidural space may reduce the risk of knotting the catheter.
- Using the correct angle of epidural needle puncture. Studies have shown that when the epidural needle is inserted at an angle of 50–60 degrees, catheter advancement is more successful than when an angle of 90 degrees is used, both in thoracic and lumbar epidurals.
- Ultrasound can assist with planning spinal/epidural needle insertion, trajectory and depth, especially in a difficult spine.

10.4.1.7 Complications of Epidural Catheter

These can occur due to direct needle trauma to the nerve, impingement of nerve by an epidural catheter or direct local anaesthetic toxicity. They can occur after soon after needle puncture before passing the catheter, after giving test dose or when threading the catheter or after passing the catheter. Paraesthesia is more commonly seen in pregnant women. Radiating pain can occur during spinal or epidural needle insertion and catheter placement. These can be a warning sign of nerve injury. Female gender, the midline approach and the use of Portex catheter are more associated with paraesthesia during central neuraxial block procedure. Paraesthesia can be reduced by using the paramedian approach presumably because of the straighter and more midline course taken by the catheter in this approach. Undue pressure should never be used while injecting a drug through an epidural catheter.

Bloody Tap

Sometimes, blood is visible at the spinal needle hub instead of CSF when the needle tip hits any of the vein in the epidural plexus. Possibility of bloody tap is more in pregnant women because of fullness of valveless epidural veins caused by retrograde pressure generated in the abdomino-pelvic venous system by the weight of gravid uterus. Risk factors for bloody tap include traumatic/bloody previous lumbar puncture performed within the past 2 weeks, low platelet count (possibly≥70,000/mL which is associated with the risk of spinal-epidural haematoma) and interval of less than 15 days or less between lumbar punctures. In case of bloody tap, the needle can be redirected, repositioned or withdrawn if advanced too far for clear CSF flow.

Accidental Placement of the Catheter in the Subarachnoid/Intravascular Space

Subarachnoid Space

The epidural catheter can enter the subarachnoid space usually during insertion despite a negative syringe aspiration test, especially if undue force is used to pass the catheter. Migration of a working catheter in the later period has also been reported.

Undetected occurrence of migration of epidural catheter in the subarachnoid space can be disastrous as the injection of large amount of local anaesthetic can lead to extensive block involving cranial nerves as well resulting in cardiorespiratory arrest. Migration is considered clinically significant if movement is more than 1 cm into the space. The presence of catheter tip in the subarachnoid space should be suspected if there is free flow of clear fluid after aspiration with syringe or after lowering the proximal end below the insertion site. The suspicion should also arise if there is unexpected and unintended extensive block within 10–15 min even after a small dose of local anaesthetic injection.

In case of accidental placement of epidural catheter in subarachnoid space and drug injection, haemodynamic instability and respiration should be supported till the recovery from block is complete. The catheter in the subarachnoid space can be used for spinal anaesthesia technique.

Tunnelling of epidural catheter under the skin may prevent migration of the catheter from its original place.

Intravascular Space

The epidural catheter can enter the epidural veins during insertion or may migrate later on. Blood seen in the catheter that is lying outside the skin with or without aspiration indicates epidural venous puncture. However, sometimes the catheter tip may be intravascular, but aspiration using a syringe can be negative due to collapse of the vein by negative pressure. Holding the catheter tip below the level of insertion and checking for free flow of blood into the catheter may be more reliable to rule out intravascular placement. Test dose administration can confirm the intravascular location of the catheter tip. Large dose of local anaesthetic can result in local anaesthetic systemic toxicity.

The incidence of unintended intravascular epidural catheter is reported to be more common in pregnant women in whom placement is done for either labour analgesia or for caesarean delivery. Paediatric patient population may also have incidence close to 5%. Single orifice catheters are likely to have higher chances of going into intravascular space compared to multi-orifice catheters. If intravascular placement is detected during insertion, the catheter may be withdrawn few centimetres and confirmed with either aspiration or a test dose. Continuous aspiration of blood even after adequate withdrawal of catheter necessitates complete withdrawal and relocation in other intervertebral space. Injection of 5–6 mL volume of normal saline before threading of the catheter may displace the veins from its path and prevent venous injury.

10.4.2 Accidental Dural Puncture

Every anaesthesiologist will experience accidental dural puncture by the epidural needle in his/her lifetime. The chances are more during training period, with multiple attempts, anxiety, difficult spine or sudden movement by the patient. The incidence is about 1% and is more common in labouring women. Post-dural puncture headache develops in 60–80% after unintentional dural puncture. Appearance of free flowing CSF in the hub of epidural needle confirms the dural puncture. If unintentional dural puncture occurs, the depth should be noted from the markings on the epidural needle that might be helpful in performing therapeutic epidural blood patch which is the gold standard for post-dural puncture headache.

Further action depends on the indication of the epidural procedure. The needle may be withdrawn and the procedure is abandoned if that was for steroid injection. Another space may be chosen if catheter placement is necessary in the epidural space, especially in the thoracic region when it is being used for analgesia in patients with multiple ribs fracture. The epidural catheter may be threaded into the subarachnoid space for anaesthesia technique. Keeping the epidural catheter in situ for at least 24 h after accidental dural puncture can help in reducing the chances of CSF leak and post-dural puncture headache.

10.4.3 Inability to Thread the Epidural Catheter and Dealing With It

Usually, the epidural catheter should pass at least 3–5 cm beyond the epidural needle tip. Sometimes, even after correctly locating the epidural space, there is difficulty in advancement of the catheter to the desired depth. This may happen due to abutting of catheter tip against blood vessel or a nerve root or bone. To overcome this issue, patient can be asked to take deep breath which increases negative pressure in the epidural space and may help in further advancement of the catheter. Administration of 5–6 mL of normal saline may expand the epidural space and help threading of the catheter.

10.5 Summary

Success in central neuraxial blockade depends on:

1. A good assessment of the spine before the procedure. This includes looking for the alignment of the vertebrae, location of iliac crests, lumbar spinous processes and interspaces.
2. Correct angle of the needle during puncture and identification of correct intervertebral space.
3. A good knowledge of neuraxial anatomy and sono-anatomy.
4. Absence of conditions such as spine abnormalities including lordosis and kyphosis, subcutaneous oedema of the back as in pregnancy-induced hypertension, increased subcutaneous tissue as in obesity.
5. Good knowledge of anatomical changes of pregnancy in the spine such as increased length of interlaminar space, shallow posterior dura mater with ascending spinal interspace.
6. Use of different approaches when the traditional approach fails.

Further Readings

Carvalho LP, Agarwal A, Kashiwagi FT, Corrêa I, Pereira JE, El Dib R. Commonly-used versus less commonly-used methods in the loss of resistance technique for identification of the epidural space: a systematic review and meta-analysis of randomized controlled trials. J Clin Anesth. 2017;38:41–51.

Chin KJ, Karmakar MK. Ultrasonography of the adult thoracic and lumbar spine for central neuraxial blockade. Anesthesiology. 2011;114:1459–85.

Derakhshan P, Faiz SHR, Rahimzadeh P, Salehi R, Khaef G. A comparison of the effect of fractionated and bolus dose injection on spinal anesthesia for lower limb surgery: a randomized clinical trial. Anesth Pain Med. 2020;10(5):e102228.

Gray H, Williams PL, Bannister LH. Gray's anatomy: the anatomical basis of medicine and surgery. 38th ed. New York: Churchill Livingstone; 1995. p. 2092.

Gurudatt CL. Unintentional dural puncture and postdural puncture headache-can this headache of the patient as well as the anaesthesiologist be prevented? Indian J Anaesth. 2014;58:385–7.

Gvalani SK, Keskar M. Title predictors of difficult sub-arachnoid block. Int J Res Med Sci. 2016;4:3783–8.

Hakim KYK. Comparative study between sequential combined spinal epidural anesthesia versus epidural volume extension in lower limb surgery. Ain-Shams J Anesthesiol. 2020;12:4.

Halder B, Narayan AK, Shandilya AS. Taylors approach as a savior in difficult spine anatomy. Indian J Clin Anaesth. 2020;7:700–2.

Hermanides J, Hollmann MW, Stevens MF, Lirk P. Failed epidural: causes and management. Br J Anaesth. 2012;109:144–54.

Hetherington J, Brohan J, Rohling R, Gunka V, Abolmaesumi P, Albert A, et al. A novel ultrasound software system for lumbar level identification in obstetric patients. Can J Anesth. 2022;69:1211–9.

Hudgins PA, Fountain AJ, Chapman PR, Shah LM. Difficult lumbar puncture: pitfalls and tips from the trenches. AJNR Am J Neuroradiol. 2017;38:1276–83.

Imbelloni LE, Sakamoto JW, Viana EP, de Aroujo AA, Pottker D, Pistarino MA. Segmental spinal anesthesia: a systematic review. J Anesth Clin Res. 2020;11(6):1000953.

Kachulis B, Tsiouris AJ, Nelson P, Stadnyk I. Dry spinal tap. J Neuroanaesthesiol Crit Care. 2020;8:82–3.

Kotani T, Inoue S, Uemura K, Kawaguchi M. Radiating pain during epidural needle insertion and catheter placement cannot be associated with postoperative persistent paresthesia: a retrospective review. JA Clin Rep. 2021;7:64.

Kurdi MS, Agrawal P, Thakkar P, Arora D, Barde SM, Eswaran K. Recent advancements in regional anaesthesia. Indian J Anaesth. 2023;67:63–70.

le Roux JJ, Wakabayashi K, Jooma Z. Defining the role of thoracic spinal anaesthesia in the twenty-first century: a narrative review. Br J Anaesth. 2023;130(1):e56–65.

Morimoto Y, Ihara Y, Shimamoto Y, Shiramoto H. Use of ultrasound for spinal anesthesia in a super morbidly obese patient. J Clin Anesth. 2017;36:88–9.

Neuraxial Anaesthesia. Available at: https://quizlet.com/201120500/neuraxial-anesthesia-flash-cards/. Last accessed on 28 Apr 2023.

NYSORA. Mechanisms and management of failed spinal anaesthesia; n.d. Available from: https://www.nysora.com/topics/complications/mechanisms-management-failed-spinal-anesthesia/

Oh TT, Ikhsan M, Tan KK, Rehena S, Han N-LR, Sia ATH, Sng BL. A novel approach to neuraxial anesthesia: application of an automated ultrasound spinal landmark identification. BMC Anesthesiol. 2019;19:57.

Parikh KS, Seetharamaiah S. Approach to failed spinal anaesthesia for caesarean section. Indian J Anaesth. 2018;62:691–7.

Prakash N, Kaur U, Singh TK, Dhiraaj S. Allodynia in bilateral lower limbs after epidural catheter insertion. Indian J Anaesth. 2022;66:S177–8.

Ravi PR, Naik S, Joshi MC, Singh S. Real-time ultrasound-guided spinal anaesthesia vs pre-procedural ultrasound-guided spinal anaesthesia in obese patients. Indian J Anaesth. 2021;65:356–61.

Reina MA, Boezaart A, De Andres-Serrano C, Rubio-Haro R, De Andrés J. Microanatomy relevant to intrathecal drug delivery. Methods Mol Biol. 2020;2059:109–20.

Ružman T, Gulam D, HaršanjiDrenjančević I, Venžera-Azenić D, Ružman N, Burazin J. Factors associated with difficult neuraxial blockade. Local Reg Anesth. 2014;7:47–52.

Shih V, Chang SL, Tsai JF, Shih HH. Air-refill phenomenon a simple confirmatory adjunct for loss of resistance technique in labour epidural analgesia. Indian J Anaesth. 2023;67:216–8.

Singh V, Mowar A, Pahade A, Karki G. Sequential combined spinal-epidural anesthesia in a multiple comorbidity patient: an indispensable tool in anesthesiologists' armamentarium. Anesth Essays Res. 2021;15:152–4.

Smitha Y, Naveen Kumar CP. Epidural volume extension technique in high risk obstetric patients-case series. Indian J Anaesth. 2022;66:375–8.

Somani S, Areeruk P, Mok LY, Samy W, Sivakumar RK, Karmakar MK. Dry spinal tap during real-time ultrasound-guided paramedian spinal injection with patient in the lateral decubitus position: a single-centre retrospective study. Eur J Anaesthesiol. 2021;38:259–64.

Subramanian S, Reshma BM, Salim Iqbal M, Harsoor SS. A comprehensive, bed-side scoring system to predict difficult lumbar puncture. J Anaesthesiol Clin Pharmacol. 2023;39:38–44.

Sutagatti JG, Kurdi MS, Bilung PA. Ultrasonographic estimation of skin to sub-arachnoid space depth in the pre-eclamptic Indian parturients and its comparison with physical index based formula – a prospective observational study. Indian J Appl Radiol. 2019;5:135.

Thummala V, Nageswararao L, Swetha D, Sriharitha S, Mounica U. Accidental dural puncture-perioperative management. Indian J Anaesth. 2020;64:425–7.

Vaira P, Camorcia M, Palladino T, Velardo M, Capogna G. Differentiating false loss of resistance from true loss of resistance while performing the epidural block with the CompuFlo® epidural instrument. Anesthesiol Res Pract. 2019;2019:5185901.

Van Zundert A. Difficult subarachnoid anaesthesia prediction and performance. Int J of Reg Anaesth. 2021;2:92–9.

Approach and Troubleshooting in Paediatric Regional Anaesthesia

11

Amrita Banerjee and Ridhima Sharma

Abstract

Regional anaesthesia in paediatric population is the eminent and current highlight to provide pain relief during surgical procedures. It is a fairly recent concept with a steep learning curve since paediatric population has always been on the challenging and demanding end. This chapter not only highlights the methods and techniques for various neuraxial and peripheral nerve blocks in the paediatric population but also accentuates troubleshooting for various complications that can emerge during these procedures. Since the anatomy and physiology of the paediatric group differ from the adult populace, careful tables and references have been contrived for the same. The drug dosages required for each procedure and the toxic dose levels have also been reinforced. This chapter effectively summarizes the contrast between the paediatric and adult populace and how children should not be treated as miniature adults. It also addresses the limitations faced while working with the paediatric cohorts. Not only does this chapter project the landmark techniques for performing the blocks, but it also gives an insight into using the ultrasound for every procedure. It also provides a precise description of the drugs used in a tabulated form for a facile grasping of the concept. It also covers the preoperative and postoperative care of the children. The scope of this chapter thus focuses on a few areas that are rare and taxing.

Keywords

Spinal anaesthesia · Caudal anaesthesia · Epidural · Peripheral nerve blocks · Neonates · Premedication · Discharge criteria · Troubleshooting · Ultrasound

11.1 Spinal Anaesthesia in Paediatric Patients

Spinal anaesthesia in children and especially neonates is the current highlight to provide pain relief during surgical procedures. The administration of spinal anaesthesia in paediatric population is a fairly recent concept compared to spinal anaesthesia administration in adults. This technique was rarely used until Melman reported a case series of infants who were at high risk but underwent successful surgical procedures under spinal anaesthesia. Spinal anaesthesia, especially in pre-terms, who were prone to apnoea of prematurity under general anaesthesia, seemed like a

A. Banerjee (✉)
AIIMS Bilaspur, Bilaspur, Himachal Pradesh, India

R. Sharma
Department of Anaesthesiology and Critical Care, AIIMS, Nagpur, Maharashtra, India

M. K. Prasad, S. J. S. Bajwa (eds.), *Steps to Successful Regional Anesthesia*,
https://doi.org/10.1007/978-981-97-4098-7_11

boon to modern science. Since then, innumerable case series have been reported to be successful and safe under spinal anaesthesia. The main anatomical and physiological differences between adults and paediatric population are enumerated in Table 11.1.

Table 11.1 Anatomical and physiological differences between adults and paediatric population

Adults	Paediatrics	Implication
Conus medullaris ends at L1	Ends at L3	Perform dural puncture below the level of spinal cord to avoid injury
Dural sac ends at S1	Ends at S3	Inadvertent dural puncture is more likely during the performance of a single-puncture caudal block in children if the needle is advanced too far into the epidural space
Sacrum begins more caudad than in infants	Sacrum begins more cephalad than in adults Infants have a small pelvis	Tuffier's line corresponds to L3-L4 interspace in adults and L4-L5 or L5-S1 in infants
CSF volume is 2 mL/kg	CSF volume is 4 mL/kg	Higher local anaesthetic dose requirement in children
CSF is distributed relatively more in the head than in the spinal canal	Distributed more in the spinal canal than in the head Also, state of high cardiac output present	Shorter duration of action of spinal anaesthesia in paediatric population
	Delayed ossification of bones and vertebrae—mostly cartilaginous	Sharp needles can easily traverse them and damage the ossification nuclei—thus compromising further bone and joint development. Thus, bone contact should be avoided during block procedures
Cervical, thoracic, lumbar, and sacrococcygeal spinal curves present	At birth, a single spinal curvature is present Persistent spinal flexibility present Cervical lordosis develops at 3–6 months Lumbar lordosis develops at 8–9 months	Orientation of epidural needles is the same regardless of the intervertebral space
	Fasciae and perineurovascular sheaths are loosely attached to underlying structures	Allows extended spread of local anaesthetics resulting in high-quality nerve blockade
	Epidural fat is very fluid in infants and young children (up to 6–7 years of age)	Allows consistent leakage of local anaesthetics injected within the epidural space—thus large volumes of epidural local anaesthetics (up to 1.25 mL/kg) required to reach desired levels of anaesthesia
	Delayed myelinization of nerve fibres—increased risk of easier intraneural penetration of local anaesthetics	Onset time is shortened, and diluted local anaesthetic is as effective as more concentrated anaesthetic in adults
Sacral vertebrae fused	Lack of fusion of sacral vertebrae	Intervertebral sacral epidural approaches can be performed throughout childhood
Enzymes mature	Enzymatic immaturity	Slower metabolism of local anaesthetics leads to their accumulation
	Low plasma protein content	Increased unbound free fraction of all local anaesthetics—greater danger of systemic toxicity
Sympathetic system matured	Sympathetic immaturity	Haemodynamic stability during neuraxial blocks—fluid loading and use of vasoactive agents are unnecessary

11.1.1 Advantages of Spinal Anaesthesia Over General Anaesthesia in Paediatrics

1. Safer in moribund preterm infants (<60 weeks post-conception) to reduce the incidence of apnea of prematurity postoperatively.
2. Minimal cardio-respiratory imbalances and postoperative nausea and vomiting.
3. Protects against the effects of general anaesthesia on young developing brains (neurobehavioural deficits).
4. More economically sound technique requiring only one drug than general anaesthesia requiring a number of drugs. Spinal anaesthesia is also associated with rapid recovery and shorter hospital stay, thus leading to reduction in cost.
5. No permanent neurological sequelae.
6. Early ambulation and rapid return of appetite.
7. More effective in blunting the neuroendocrine stress and adverse responses to surgery.
8. Preferred technique of choice in children at the risk of developing malignant hyperthermia.
9. Environmentally safe—protects ozone layer against nitrous oxide and inhalational agents.

11.1.2 Indications

The various indications for spinal anaesthesia in children are given in Table 11.2.

11.1.3 Contraindications

The contraindications for spinal anaesthesia in children are mentioned in Table 11.3.

Also consider the surgical site, the anticipated length of the surgery (preferably <90 min), and the surgical position (i.e. spinal, lateral or prone) before administering spinal anaesthesia.

11.1.4 Drug Doses

Local anaesthetics with doses is tabulated in Table 11.4.

11.1.5 Drug Doses Calculation for Spinal Anaesthesia

The spinal anaesthesia drugs and dosage in children are given in Table 11.5.

Table 11.2 Indications for spinal anaesthesia in children

Inguinal hernia repair
Myelomeningocele repair
Lower limb and lower abdominal surgery
Early extubation desired after cardiac surgery—Spinal anaesthesia used for postoperative pain relief instead of opioids
Urologic and orthopaedic procedures

Table 11.3 Contraindications for spinal anaesthesia in children

Absolute contraindications	Relative contraindications
Parental refusal	Non-sedated child in a surgery duration of >60 min
Severe coagulation disorders (haemophilia or DIC)	Anatomical abnormalities of the spine
Severe infection, e.g. septicemia or meningitis	Systemic infection or localized bacterial infection at puncture site
Intracranial tumour with increased intracranial pressure	Coagulopathy
True allergy to local anaesthetics—rare	Degenerative neuromuscular disease
Most are reactions to preservatives such as metabisulfite and methylparaben. Some are symptoms of overdose toxicity	Minimally increased intracranial/intraocular pressure
Certain chemotherapies, e.g. cisplatin (used in hepatoblastoma)—known to induce subclinical neurologic lesions that can be acutely aggravated by a block procedure	Ventriculoperitoneal/ventriculoatrial shunts
Uncorrected hypovolemia	Poorly controlled seizures
Cutaneous or subcutaneous lesions (infection, angioma, tattoo, dystrophic) at the site of puncture	

Table 11.4 Spinal anaesthesia drugs and dosage in children

Local anaesthesia used: Ropivacaine 0.5% (0.5 mg/kg) or 0.5% bupivacaine (0.5–1 mg/kg) in children <10 kg weight
Additives used: 1. "Epinephrine wash" of the syringe rather than a standard dose of epinephrine. Otherwise, epinephrine 5 mg/L or 1/2,00,000 concentration is frequently coadministered with local anaesthetics to decrease plasma peak concentration and prolong the duration of blockade. 2. Clonidine 1 mcg/kg (use a dose of caffeine (10 mg/kg) i/v to prevent potential postoperative apnea, especially if clonidine (2 mcg/kg) is used in the spinal anaesthetic solution). 3. Caudal injection—0.1% bupivacaine. 4. Morphine 10 mcg/kg—only for cardiac surgery to facilitate earlier extubation.

Table 11.5 Spinal anaesthesia drugs and dosage in children

To calculate dose for a single hernia repair in children	
Weight (kg)	Dose (0.5% bupivacaine)
Neonates	0.5–0.8 mg/kg
<5	0.5 mg/kg
5–15	0.4 mg/kg
>15	0.3 mg/kg

11.1.6 Drug Additives and Recommended Doses in Paediatric Regional Anaesthesia Doses

The commonly used additives and recommended doses in paediatric regional anaesthesia are given in Table 11.6.

11.1.7 Preparation

Informed consent must be obtained from the parents/guardians, with adequate documentation of the discussion of risk involved.

In the pre-op area, eutectic mixture of local anaesthetic (EMLA) cream or LMX (lignocaine 4% cream) can be applied to the site of needle insertion, after considering the risk of methemoglobinemia, especially in very small premature infants.

Table 11.6 Commonly used additives and recommended doses in paediatric regional anaesthesia

Additive	Recommended doses	Maximum doses
Morphine (epidural)	30 mcg/kg	50 mcg/kg
Morphine (intrathecal)	10 mcg/kg	20 mcg/kg
Fentanyl (epidural)	1–1.5 mcg/kg	2.5 mcg/kg
Sufentanil (epidural)	0.25–0.5 mcg/kg	0.75 mcg/kg
Clonidine (epidural or along peripheral nerves)	1–1.5 mcg/kg	2 mcg/kg
Ketamine (epidural or occasionally along peripheral nerves) (preservative-free S-ketamine)	0.5 mg/kg	1 mg/kg

The operating room should be pre-warmed before taking the patient inside. Radiant heat lamps, warm blankets, and warm fluids help minimize heat loss in infants. Audio-visual aids may be helpful in distracting older children in whom blocks are performed without sedation.

Standard monitoring equipment (electrocardiogram, pulse oximeter, non-invasive blood pressure cuff) should be applied before performing the procedure.

11.1.8 Supplementing Spinal Anaesthesia

Supplemental intravenous sedation or short period of inhalational general anaesthesia may be required in children undergoing spinal anaesthesia. The disadvantage of using general anaesthesia is that it predisposes preterm infants to apnea and bradycardia. The duration of spinal anaesthesia in infants lasts for about 90 min due to their physiology. Thus, in preterm infants undergoing lower abdominal procedures of less than 90 min duration, spinal block without sedation should be preferred.

Spinal anaesthesia can also be combined with caudal or epidural anaesthesia to prolong the analgesic effect.

11.1.9 Premedication

11.1.9.1 Non-pharmacological Measures to Reduce Anxiety

1. *Music therapy*: Along with combination of music, there should be reduction in noise and bright lights in the operation theatre.
2. *Audio-visual aids*: AV aids like virtual reality aids can help calm the paediatric population, especially in the age group of 2–10 years.
3. *Acupuncture*: In a study conducted by Wang et al., it was shown that children of mothers who were subjected to acupuncture therapy were less anxious than those in the control group.
4. *Preoperative interview*: It is a good psychological intervention.

11.1.9.2 Pharmacological Measures to Reduce Anxiety

- *Benzodiazepines*
  1. *Midazolam:* It is the most used premedicant in the preoperative area. Oral midazolam is shown to be more effective in reducing a child's anxiety than parental presence. Higher doses can cause child to become agitated, restless, and dysphoric. A bitter taste is often associated with oral and nasal administration; thus, mixing it with D-25 is recommended. Another advantage of midazolam is anterograde amnesia. Various routes of administration are tabulated in Table 11.7.
  2. *Diazepam*: It is not a preferred choice in children since immature liver enzymes lead to prolonged half-life of the drug. Oral dose is 0.1–0.3 mg/kg.
  3. *Lorazepam:* The routes of administration are oral, intravenous, or intramuscular. It is metabolized by the liver. Oral or IV dose is 0.05 mg/kg. Dose to reduce preoperative anxiety is 0.025 mg/kg.
- *Ketamine*

  It is a phencyclidine derivative and an N-methyl-D-aspartate (NMDA) receptor antagonist which causes dissociative anaesthesia. It is administered along with antisialogogue to reduce secretions and benzodiazepines to reduce hallucinations and emergence delirium. Duration of action is 8–10 min. Various routes of administration of ketamine are mentioned in Table 11.8.
- *Opioids*
- Fentanyl can be administered by parenteral, transdermal, nasal, and oral routes. Oral dose for sedation is 10–15 mcg/kg; IV and transnasal dose is 1–2 mcg/kg.
- *Non-barbiturate Sedatives*

  Chloral hydrate can be given orally or rectally in a dose of 20–75 mg/kg, up to a maximum of 2 grams. It provides sedation in 30–45 min. It can cause airway obstruction in children with large tonsils.
- *Anticholinergic Drugs*

  These are known for their antisialogogue, vagolytic, and central sedative effects. Various routes of administration of anticholinergic drugs are mentioned in Table 11.9.
- *Alpha-2 Agonists*

  Clonidine causes dose-related sedation at 60–90 min after oral administration (3 mcg/kg) and 50 min after rectal administration. Dexmedetomidine provides sedation, analgesia and anxiolysis without causing respiratory depression. Onset of action occurs in 30–75 min. Various routes of administration

Table 11.7 Midazolam doses and routes of administration

Route of administration of midazolam	Dose (mg/kg)
Intravenous	0.025–0.1
Intramuscular	0.1–0.2
Intranasal	0.2
Rectal	1
Oral	0.25–0.75
Sublingual	0.2

Table 11.8 Ketamine doses and routes of administration

Route of administration of ketamine for sedation	Dose (mg/kg)
Intravenous	0.25–0.5
Intramuscular	1–2
Intranasal	6
Oral	3
Rectal	5

Table 11.9 Doses of anti-cholinergics

Drug	Dose
Atropine	0.01–0.02 mg/kg (IV or IO)
Glycopyrrolate	4 micg/kg (IV or IM)
Scopolamine	0.005–0.010 mg/kg (better sedative and amnestic than atropine)

Table 11.10 Dexmedetomidine doses and routes of administration

Route of administration of dexmedetomidine	Dose (mcg/kg)
Transmucosal Intranasal Sublingual Buccal	1–2
Oral	2.5–4

of alpha-2 agonist are mentioned in Table 11.10.

- *Antihistaminics*
  Oral promethazine (0.25–0.5 mg/kg) is an effective sedative, anticholinergic, antiemetic, and antimotion sickness.
- *Topical Anaesthetics*
  EMLA cream, i.e. eutectic mixture of local anaesthetics (2.5% lidocaine and 2.5% prilocaine) can be used 1 h prior to intravenous catheter insertion. The skin on which it is applied should be intact and it should be covered with an occlusive dressing after application. The drawback is that it causes initial venoconstriction and skin blanching, making cannulation more difficult. Methemoglobinemia may also occur secondary to prilocaine. Maximum dose of EMLA is 1 gram. 4% Lignocaine cream is also available which dilates veins better.

11.1.10 Patient Position

The lateral or sitting position is generally preferred for spinal anaesthesia in children. In lateral position, the patient is brought to the edge of the surgical table and held there firmly by the assistant (Fig. 11.1).

If the patient is in the sitting position, especially in neonates, special care should be taken not to flex the neck of the patient since it can result in airway obstruction. Thus, oxygen monitoring should be done vigilantly to ensure patency and adequacy of the airway.

Using a pacifier in a non-sedated infant, while performing the block, is usually helpful.

11.1.11 Technique

Spinal block should be administered below the level of L3 in infants. Thus, L4-L5 or L5-S1 interface is identified. The area should be cleaned and draped in a sterile manner. Preferably, local anaesthesia should be administered in awake patients.

Since the volume of local anaesthetic needed is small in neonates, it is important to measure the volume corresponding to the hub of the needle and to include this volume, too, in the total dose of local anaesthetic.

An insulin syringe and a short 22 or 25 gauze spinal needle (Quincke) are often used. Spinal needle should be shorter than 50 mm.

The spinal needle is then advanced into the skin, subcutaneous tissue, supraspinous and interspinous ligament, and finally into ligamentum flavum and dura mater.

Since the ligamentum flavum is very thin and soft in children, a distinctive "pop" sound may not be appreciated when the dura is penetrated.

Once there is free flow of CSF from the needle, the drug may be injected into the intrathecal space slowly (@ 0.2 mL/s).

During spinal block, barbotage method is not recommended since it can lead to high spinal block. After giving spinal anaesthesia, the lower limbs of the infant should not be immediately raised up to place the electrocautery return electrode on the back of the infant, since it can lead to total spinal anaesthesia.

In the dawn of the new era, the use of USG for providing spinal anaesthesia has risen. Spinal anaesthesia can be administered by using the median or the paramedian (Fig. 10.12) approach.

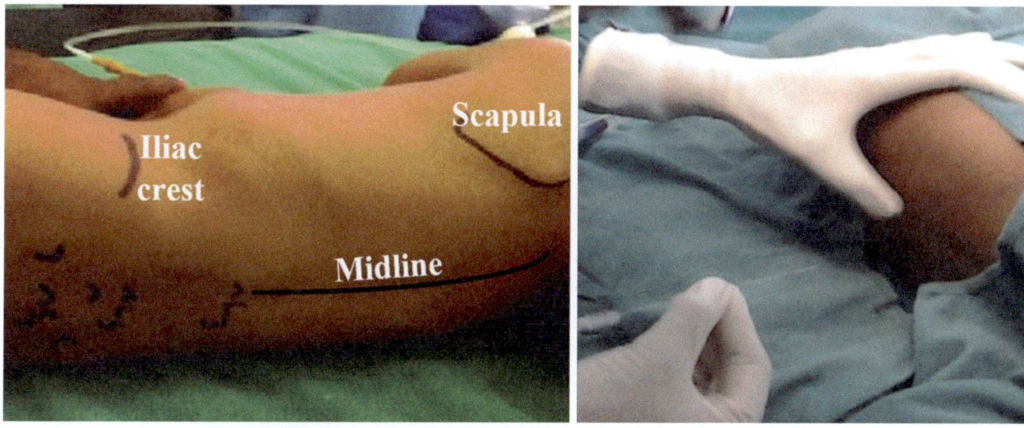

Fig. 11.1 Lateral positioning of children for spinal anaesthesia

USG is especially useful in identifying the subarachnoid space in obese children and in children with malformed vertebrae like those from the VACTERL (vertebral anomalies, anal atresia, cardiac defects, tracheo-oesophageal fistula or oesophageal atresia, renal defects, and limb anomalies) category.

Intraoperative Sedation Choices

- Benzodiazepines like midazolam (IV 0.025–0.1 mg/kg).
- Opioids like fentanyl (IV 1–2 micg/kg).
- Ketamine (IV 0.25–0.5 mg/kg).

Gara Technique (GA with Regional Anaesthesia)

Regional anaesthesia practice in children has brought a paradigmal shift in the way we view our anaesthesia delivering options in children. It previously included only neuraxial techniques, but lately it incorporates advanced peripheral nerve blocks as well. These novel blocks not only provide opioid-sparing analgesia but also minimize invasiveness and risk. These techniques have expanded from single-shot spinal anaesthesia to combined spinal/epidural techniques. Data from large prospective registries suggest that providing regional anaesthesia to children while under general anaesthesia is as safe as in the sedated or awake patient.

11.1.12 Intraoperative Fluid Management

This is done according to Holliday–Segar formula, i.e. 4:2:1 rule, to estimate maintenance hourly fluid requirements (Table 11.11).

11.1.13 Assessing the Block

It is difficult to assess a spinal block in children, especially who are under sedation. In infants, pin-prick or skin pinch or response to a cold stimulus (alcohol swab) may be used to assess the sensory blockade. Ventilator rate and pattern should be observed.

Bromage scale is used in children above 2 years of age to assess the motor blockade (Table 11.12). Below this age, observe the child's response to movement and their response to very gentle palpation of the operative site.

In case of a rapidly rising level of block which mostly features as bradycardia followed by arrest, place the patient in reverse Trendelenburg position.

Table 11.11 Intraoperative maintenance hourly fluid requirements

Weight (kg)	Hourly	Daily
<10	4 mL/kg/h	100 mL/kg/day
10–20	40 mL + 2 mL/kg for every kg >10 kg	1000 mL + 50 mL/kg/day for every kg >10 kg
>20	60 mL + 1 mL/kg for every kg >20 kg	1500 mL + 20 mL/kg/day for every kg >20 kg

Table 11.12 Bromage scale

No block	Free movement of knees and feet is possible
Partial block	Able to only flex knees, but free movement of feet is still possible
Almost complete block	Unable to flex knees, but flexion of feet is still possible
Complete block	Unable to move legs or feet

11.1.14 Recovery and Discharge Criteria

Before shifting the patient to recovery room, ensure the following:

1. Stable vital signs.
2. Intact gag, swallowing and cough reflexes.
3. Adequate respiration.

Discharge criteria should include:

1. Ambulation (appropriate for age).
2. Orientation to time, place, and person (appropriate for age).
3. Tolerance of oral fluids with minimal nausea and vomiting. According to ERAS (early recovery after surgery) guidelines, oral hydration should be started following recovery of the swallowing reflex when the child is calm and conscious.
4. Voiding helps establish degree of residual block and fluid status. Children can be catheterized for long duration surgeries (>2 h).

If residual sensory block is present, give instructions to protect the child from hot, cold, or sharp objects (Table 11.13).

11.1.15 Adverse Effects and Troubleshooting

11.1.16 Precautions/Preventions and Treatment

1. **Bloody tap**: If a bloody tap is encountered during spinal anaesthesia, it is best to remove the needle, flush it with normal saline, and re-insert the spinal needle in a different space.
2. **Sugar nipple**: Sugar-coated nipples can be used to pacify/comfort the infant while the spinal anaesthesia is being performed.
3. **Avoid flexion of head**: While positioning the head of the newborn/infant for giving spinal anaesthesia in sitting position, avoid flexion of the head since it can lead to airway obstruction.

11.1.17 Limitations

Despite several advantages, this technique has its share of limitations as well:

1. Single-shot spinal technique provides only 80–90 min of surgical anaesthesia.
2. Need for sedation and GA in some children for performing the block.
3. *Technical difficulties*: Lack of cooperation makes spinal anaesthesia more challenging in paediatrics. Due to their unique anatomical features, bloody tap is more commonly associated.

Table 11.13 Adverse effects and troubleshooting

Intraoperative	
Adverse effects	**Troubleshooting**
1. Hypotension and bradycardia	Less common in children Preloading and co-loading to increase preload is rarely needed—if required can be done @ 10 mL/kg If bradycardia not resolved, give atropine 0.02 mg/kg iv. If still not resolved, use epinephrine 0.01 mg/kg iv (0.1 mL/kg of 1:10,000 concentration)
2. Local complication of inappropriate needle insertion damaging the nerves and surrounding structures	Use adequate devices and proper technique and ultrasound wherever required
3. Intravenous injection of local anaesthetic causing neurological and cardiovascular complications	Treat via maintaining airway, breathing, and circulation by oxygenation, cardiac massage, and epinephrine (1–2 micg/kg) Administer 20% intralipids (1.5 mL/kg) by iv bolus over 1 minute (can repeat after 5 minutes to maximum 3 doses). Followed by an iv infusion at 15 mL/kg/hr. (maximum cumulative dose up to 10 mL/kg)
Postoperative	
Adverse effects	**Troubleshooting**
1. Post-dural puncture headache (PDPH)	Incidence lower in children Epidural blood patch can be performed with 0.3 mL/kg of blood if headache persists
2. Transient radicular symptoms	Reported in children but transient in nature without long-term adverse effects

4. Paediatric spinal needles are more expensive and may not be freely available.

Conclusion
Spinal anaesthesia in paediatric population is an upcoming and safe technique to practice, especially in preterm neonates who are prone to apnoea of prematurity. It can be safely and judiciously used compared to general anaesthesia and should thus be promoted.

11.2 Caudal Anaesthesia in Paediatric Patients

Epidural analgesia is commonly used in paediatric population for postoperative pain relief and in addition to general anaesthesia. The approach to the epidural space can be at the thoracic, lumbar, or caudal level. In this section, we will be focussing upon caudal epidural anaesthesia.

11.2.1 Definition

Caudal anaesthesia (CA) is epidural anaesthesia of the cauda equina roots in the sacral canal, accessed through the sacral hiatus.

At birth, the sacral plate, which is formed by five sacral vertebrae, is not completely ossified and continues to fuse until approximately 8 years of age (although it may take until 21 years of age). There is a 6% incidence of sacral atresia. The incomplete fusion of the sacral vertebral arch forms the sacral hiatus.

The caudal epidural space can be accessed easily in infants and children through the sacral hiatus. Because of the continuous development of the sacral canal roof, there is considerable variation in the sacral hiatus.

11.2.2 Anatomical and Physiological Implications

Various anatomical and physiological differences between adult and children and their implications are tabulated in Table 11.14.

11.2.3 Advantages of Pain Relief from Epidural Analgesia

1. Early ambulation.
2. Facilitates weaning from ventilators.
3. Reduces time spent in catabolic state.
4. Lowers circulating stress hormone levels.
5. Precise placement of epidural needles for single-injection techniques and catheters for continuous epidural anaesthesia ensures that the dermatomes involved in the surgical procedure are selectively blocked, allowing for lower doses of local anaesthetics to be used and sparing unnecessary block in non-desired regions.

11.2.4 Local Anaesthetics for Caudal Anaesthesia in Children

Bupivacaine, ropivacaine, and levobupivacaine are the most commonly used local anaesthetics for neuraxial anaesthesia in children (Table 11.15). The adjuvants used with local anaesthetics are mentioned in Table 11.16. The volume of drug needed for different surgeries is mentioned in Table 11.17.

11.2.5 Techniques

Caudal Epidural Analgesia: Single-Injection Technique

Choice of Needle

- Short-bevel Tuohy or Crawford needles (5 cm in length) with stylets offer a better tactile sensation when the sacrococcygeal ligament is punctured.
- For children aged 1 year or older, a 22-gauge angiocath is used.
- For children younger than 1 year of age, a 25-gauge needle may be used.
- The use of a styletted needle may reduce the risk of introducing a dermal plug into the caudal space.
- A 23G butterfly needle may also be used in infants to deliver caudal block.
- Some recommend making an entry hole in the skin with a first needle (e.g. 21G hypodermic needle) and then introducing the caudal nee-

Table 11.14 Anatomical and physiological differences

Adults	Children
Conus medullaris – Placed at L1 vertebra	**Conus medullaris** Neonates and infants—placed at L3 vertebra After 1 year of age—placed at L1 vertebra
Sacrum curved and wide	Sacrum is more flat and narrow
Dural sac—ends at S1	**Dural sac** Neonates and infants—ends at S4 Older children—ends at S2 Thus, there is increased risk of accidental dural puncture while placing caudal block in infants
Ultrasound (US) assessment of the neuraxial structures is more challenging due to developed ossification	US assessment is less challenging in younger children because ossification is less developed In infants, the spinal cord fibres, the cerebrospinal fluid (CSF), and the dura mater are easily identified using linear high-frequency US probes
Epidural fat is densely packed	Epidural fat is less densely packed—facilitates the spread of local anaesthesia and helps achieve a quicker block onset
Spinal cord is myelinated	In neonates, spinal cord is still non-myelinated; thus, lower concentrations of local anaesthetics can be effectively used
Lower cardiac output than children	Higher cardiac output—thus, systemic absorption of local anaesthetics occurs faster It leads to shorter duration of block and can also lead to toxic plasma levels

Table 11.15 Comparison between commonly used local anaesthetics

Bupivacaine	Levobupivacaine	Ropivacaine
Maximum safe dose = 2–2.5 mg/kg	Maximum safe dose = 2.5–3 mg/kg	Maximum safe dose = 3–4 mg/kg
Amide group of local anaesthetics	S (−)-isomer of bupivacaine	Long-acting amide local anaesthetic with higher therapeutic index than bupivacaine
Most cardiotoxic among the local anaesthetics. It inhibits cardiac conductivity and contractility and may induce ventricular fibrillation	Less likely to cause myocardial depression and fatal arrhythmias	Decreased incidence of cardiac toxicity
Less neurotoxic than lignocaine but more neurotoxic than levobupivacaine or ropivacaine	Less toxic to the central nervous system than racemic bupivacaine	Less motor block and equivalent analgesia compared to bupivacaine with a decreased incidence of central nervous system toxicity
Intrathecal dose: Neonates = 0.5 mg/kg Older children = 0.3 mg/kg Adults = 0.2 mg/kg	Intrathecal dose = 0.3 mg/kg	Intrathecal dose = 0.5 mg/kg
For single-shot epidural: 0.25% bupivacaine @ 2 mg/kg	For single-shot epidural: 0.25% Levobupivacaine @ 1.5–2 mg/kg	For single-shot epidural: 0.2% Ropivacaine @ 1.5 mg/kg
For continuous epidural infusion: Neonates = 0.2 mg/kg/h of 0.0625% bupivacaine Older children = 0.2–0.4 mg/kg/h of 0.125% bupivacaine	For continuous epidural infusion: (0.125%) Neonates = 0.25 mg/kg/h Older children = 0.25–0.5 mg/kg/h	Infusion (maximum up to 48 h): Neonates = 0.375 mg/kg/h of 0.1% ropivacaine Older children = 0.2–0.4 mg/kg/h of 0.2% ropivacaine
Duration of neonatal epidural infusions should be limited to 48 h in view of cumulative toxicity		Possible vasoconstricting properties—Undergoes slower systemic absorption than bupivacaine This may have clinical implications when a prolonged local anaesthetic infusion is used in children with impaired hepatic function
Single-injection caudal block = 2.5 mg/kg of 0.25% bupivacaine	Single-injection caudal block = 2–2.5 mg/kg of 0.25% levobupivacaine	Single-injection caudal block = 2 mg/kg of 0.2% ropivacaine

Table 11.16 Adjuvants for caudal anaesthesia in children

Epinephrine	Opioids	Clonidine	Ketamine
Most commonly used adjuvant to local anaesthetics	Safe to be used in in-patients with intraoperative and postoperative monitoring	Best non-opioid adjunct	Preservative-free S-ketamine to be used
Concentration of 1:2,00,000 = decreases the absorption rate of local anaesthetic plus serves as a marker for inadvertent intravascular injection	Fentanyl dose: Single-injection caudal anaesthesia = 2 mcg/kg Continuous epidural infusion = 1–2 mcg/mL to 0.1% bupivacaine Caudal morphine = 30–90 mcg/kg	Single-injection caudal block = 1–5 mcg/kg Continuous epidural infusion = 0.1 mcg/kg/h	Dose = 0.25–1 mg/kg

(continued)

Table 11.16 (continued)

Epinephrine	Opioids	Clonidine	Ketamine
	Side effects: (a) Respiratory depression (b) Nausea and vomiting (c) Itching/pruritus (d) Urinary retention	Mechanism of action: Alpha-1 agonist acts by stimulating the descending noradrenergic medullospinal pathways, which inhibits the release of nociceptive neurotransmitters in the dorsal horn of the spinal cord	Side effects: (a) Psychomimetic effects (b) Controversial use in neonates due to study suggesting apoptotic neurodegeneration in the developing brain
		Side effects: (a) Sedation (b) Haemodynamic instability (c) Hypotension (d) Bradycardia (e) Epidural clonidine blunts the ventilatory response to increasing levels of end-tidal carbon dioxide (f) Apnea (rare)	

Table 11.17 Armitage regime for caudal block (0.25% bupivacaine)

Volume (mL/kg)	Dermatomal level	Indication
0.5	Sacral	Circumcision
0.75	Inguinal	Inguinal herniotomy
1	Lower thoracic (T10)	Umbilical herniorrhaphy, orchidopexy
1.25	Mid-thoracic	Repair for trachea-oesophageal fistula

dle into the previously broken skin if a styletted needle is not being used.

- Use of a 22-gauge angiocath—easier to detect intravascular placement and intraosseous placement with this needle. It is not intended to be an epidural caudal catheter. To avoid tissue coring with the angiocath, the needle must be removed before any injection is made.
- Continuous caudal catheters can be inserted using a 20G epidural catheter or 18G angiocath. The dose of LA in them is 0.4 mL/kg of 0.1–0.25% bupivacaine with fentanyl as an additive @ 2–5 mcg/kg. These caudal catheters can be used to prolong analgesic administration in postoperative period.

11.2.5.1 Landmark Approach

- Ensure adequate prevention of heat loss during the procedure. In infants, preventing heat loss with a sterile transparent drape also allows visualization of patient's breathing.
- The patient is placed in a lateral decubitus position with the neck flexed and the knees drawn up to the chest. After proper positioning, the landmarks for caudal epidural block are easily identified in children (Fig. 11.2).
- Initially, the coccyx is identified, and, continuing to palpate in the midline in a cephalad fashion, the sacral cornua can be felt on either side of the midline approximately 1 cm apart. The sacral hiatus is felt as a depression between two bony prominences of the sacral cornua.
- Under sterile conditions, the needle is inserted and advanced into the sacral hiatus at approximately a 70-degree angle to the skin until a

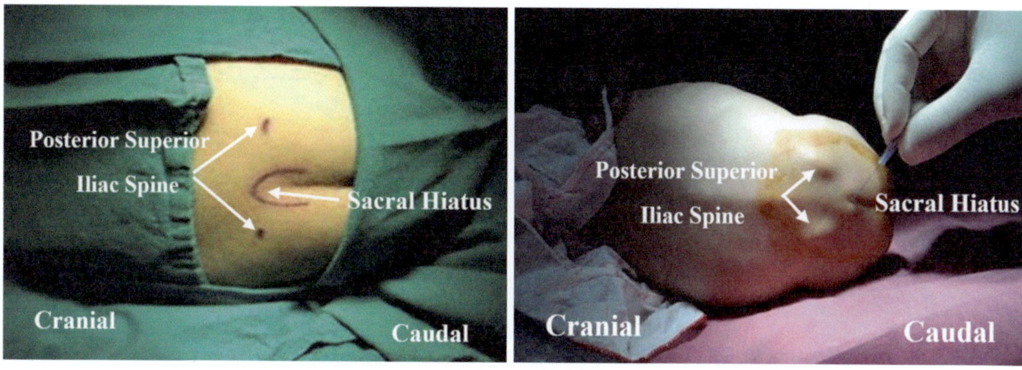

Fig. 11.2 Patient positioning and landmark technique for a caudal block

distinctive "pop" is felt as the sacrococcygeal ligament is punctured.

- After this puncture, the angle of the needle should be reduced to approximately 20–30 degrees, while the needle is advanced 2–4 mm into the caudal canal.
- Any advancement past this point is not recommended because the risk of inadvertent dural puncture increases significantly.

11.2.5.2 Ultrasound (US)-Guided Approach

- The patient is placed in the lateral decubitus position with the knees flexed towards the chest.
- The US machine is placed opposite the operator so that he or she can look over his or her hands towards the screen.
- The patient is prepared, and the US probe is sterilely covered.
- A high-frequency probe is used: A linear hockey-stick probe is used in infants, whereas a probe with a large footprint is preferable in children weighing more than 10 kg, as it allows more intervertebral spaces to be imaged at a time in the sagittal plane.
- The probe is positioned first in a transverse plane at the sacrum level; this is called the short-axis view (SAX). The exact position of the cornua and the sacrococcygeal ligament are defined (Fig. 11.3).
- With the sacrococcygeal ligament in the middle of the image (Fig. 11.3), the probe is then rotated 90 degrees into a midline sagittal position over the lower sacrum, which is called the long-axis view (LAX).
- The sacrococcygeal ligament and the ventral and dorsal layer of the os sacrum, with the caudal epidural space in between, are easily identified (Fig. 11.4).
- After this pre-procedural US assessment of the caudal anatomy, the needle can be introduced into the sacral hiatus with the probe in either axis. If the probe is held in the SAX, the needle insertion will be automatically in the out-of-plane (OOP) approach.
- If the probe is held in the LAX, the needle insertion will then be in the in-plane (IP) approach.
- The needle insertion angle is noted during the scan. The needle may be advanced 2–4 mm into the caudal space, and the stylet is removed. To ensure optimal caudal placement of the needle, a small bolus of saline or local anaesthetic is administered under US guidance with the probe in the midline (LAX).
- The probe is positioned as cephalic as needed to visualize the dural sac in the US screen (Fig. 11.5).
- When the injection starts, we will notice the dura being displaced ventrally, especially in younger children. The spread of local anaesthetic can be monitored by moving the probe cephalic up the spine in the midline or in a paramedian sagittal axis.

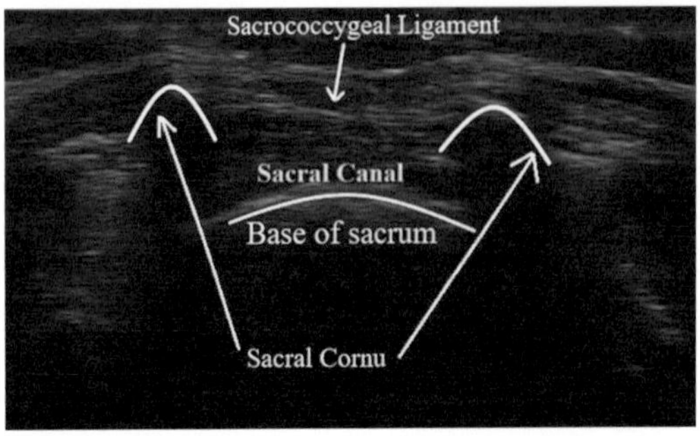

Fig. 11.3 US image in the short-axis view showing the sacral cornua and sacrococcygeal ligament

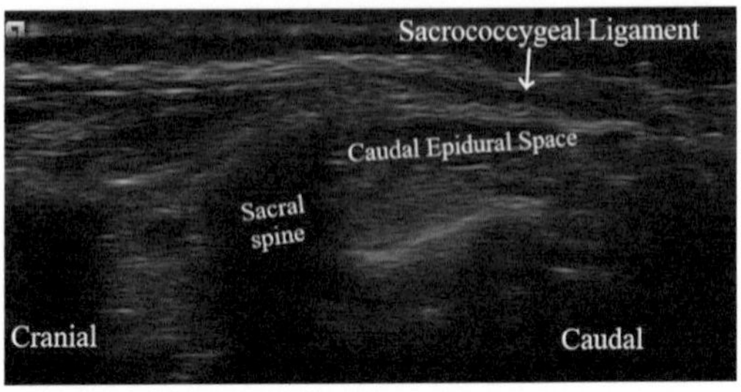

Fig. 11.4 US image in the long-axis view showing the sacrococcygeal ligament and caudal epidural space

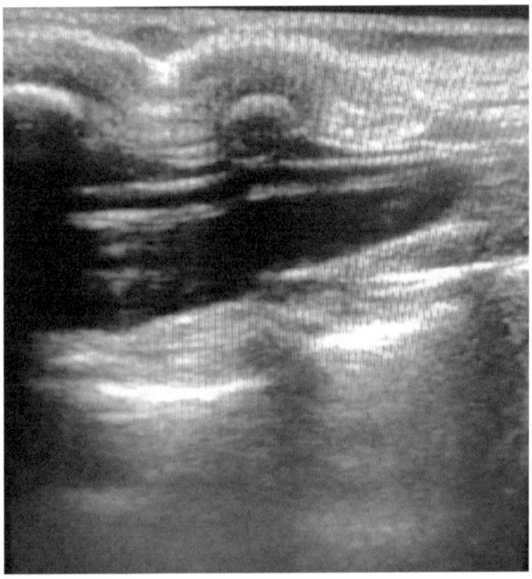

Fig. 11.5 Dural sac visualized before injection in the long-axis view

The same dura movement can be visualized with the probe in the SAX in more cephalic positions.

Confirmation of Correct Local Anaesthetic Distribution

- The classic "pop" felt as the SCM is pierced is usually sought to confirm proper caudal needle placement.
- The absence of subcutaneous bulging and the lack of resistance upon injection are additional signs of correct needle placement and local anaesthetic distribution.
- Aspiration of the needle should be clear of blood and CSF, and a negative response to a test dose of epinephrine should also be used to rule out intravascular placement.
- US has been used to provide real-time needle guidance into the caudal space and to assess the spread of local anaesthetic.

Continuous Caudal Epidural Analgesia

- Continuous caudal epidural analgesia overcomes the limited duration and segmental effect of a single-injection technique.
- Caudal catheters can be advanced to the lumbar or thoracic level.
- Technique for needle insertion:
  - An IV catheter (an 18-gauge angiocatheter for a 20-gauge epidural catheter or a 16-gauge angiocatheter for a 19-gauge epidural catheter).
  - An 18-gauge Crawford or Tuohy needle inserted through the sacrococcygeal membrane.
- The epidural catheter is then advanced carefully from the caudal space to the target level.
- Minor resistance to the passage of the catheter can usually be overcome by simple flexion or extension of the patient's vertebral column and/or by simultaneously injecting normal saline through the catheter.
- It is extremely important to know where the tip of the catheter is finally located: too low a catheter tip level will result in poor analgesia; too high may cause respiratory depression.
- Because catheters do not travel linearly in the epidural space, measuring the length of the catheter against the patient's back does not

accurately determine the targeted surgical level.

- Therefore, the location of the catheter tip should be verified using an objective test (i.e. radiography, nerve stimulation, electrocardiography, or US).

Postoperative Caudal Epidural Infusion for Analgesia

Either bupivacaine 0.125% or ropivacaine 0.1–0.2%, with or without fentanyl 1–2 mcg/mL, is administered at the following rates:

- Age > 3 months: 0.20–0.35 mL/kg/h (< 0.4 mg/kg/h bupivacaine).
- Age < 3 months: 0.1–0.15 mL/kg/h (< 0.2 mg/kg/h bupivacaine).

11.2.6 Complications and Troubleshooting

The complications associated with caudal anaesthesia are tabulated in Table 11.18.

Table 11.18 Complications associated with caudal anaesthesia

Complications	Troubleshooting
Neurologic injury—direct damage to spinal cord causing transient paresthesia or paraplegia or quadriplegia	Keep the patient spontaneously breathing while performing neuraxial block so that pain or paresthesia can be perceived Preprocedural ultrasound scanning of the neuraxial anatomy where available is highly recommended to assess depth to the epidural space
Hypotension—can compromise spinal perfusion	Rare occurrence. Total spinal anaesthesia and/or an intravascular injection needs to be ruled out
Infection—can occur with prolonged use of caudally placed catheters owing to the proximity of the sacral hiatus to the rectum Sacral osteomyelitis can occur	To reduce the risk of contamination by stool and urine, techniques such as catheter tunnelling and fixing the catheter with occlusive dressing in a cephalad direction can be used A strict aseptic technique including the use of a sterile closed-infusion system should also be used Care should be taken to avoid local tissue trauma Daily inspection of the dressing and entry site should be done If the child develops a persistent fever greater than 38 °C of unknown origin, the catheter should be removed and sent for culture
Dural puncture and post-dural puncture headache (PDPH)—occurs when the needle is advanced too far into the sacral canal	Use real-time ultrasound imaging to control needle position Treatment: (a) Bed rest (b) Oral or IV hydration (c) Analgesia (paracetamol, NSAIDs, anti-emetics) (d) Caffeine—not regularly used in paediatric population (e) Epidural blood patch—0.3 mL/kg of autologous blood injected in the awake or mildly sedated patient to detect the appearance of radicular symptoms
Haemodynamic effects and total spinal anaesthesia—significant changes in blood pressure are uncommon in paediatric patients. Therefore, hypotension should raise the suspicion of total spinal anaesthesia and/or an intravascular injection, leading to local anaesthetic toxicity	If total spinal anaesthesia has occurred, provide supportive measures until the effect of the block has dissipated In the event of a life-threatening extension of a total spinal anaesthesia, cerebrospinal lavage may be considered as a last manoeuvre—20–30 mL of CSF can be withdrawn and replaced with 30–40 mL of preservative-free normal saline, Ringer's lactate, or plasmalyte via the epidural catheter
Local anaesthetic systemic toxicity (LAST)—due to accidental intravascular injection into epidural blood vessels	Do careful aspiration and test dosing Avoid usage of sharp-tipped needles Use dilute solutions of local anaesthetics (<0.125% bupivacaine) in continuous epidural infusions

11.3 Epidural Anaesthesia in Paediatric Patients

The paediatric epidural is a widely used technique for providing children with improved analgesia. The various benefits of this technique comprise faster ambulation, effective pain relief, a decrease in stress hormone levels, and early postoperative recovery and discharge. Precise placement of the epidural needle (single injection or continuous anaesthesia) can selectively block the dermatomes involved in the surgical procedure. This circumvents the use of higher doses of local anaesthetics and prevents unnecessary blocking of the unblocked region. Also, due to improvements in ultrasonography, newer methods have supplanted paediatric epidural analgesia (PEA) as being equally effective and safe. However, PEA is still a crucial skill to develop and use.

11.3.1 Anatomy of the Epidural Space

The epidural space surrounds the spinal cord and meninges from the foramen magnum to the sacral hiatus. The ligamentum flava and the vertebral laminae limit it posteriorly. It communicates with the paravertebral space and root sleeve freely. The arachnoid granulations protrusion near the spinal ganglia (dural cuff region) is nearly connected with the subarachnoid space and can be easily transversed by local anaesthetic agents.

At birth, the spinous processes are parallel at all levels to each other due to the single concavity (kyphosis) in the spine. The development of the lumber lordosis occurs when the child starts walking. Therefore, the orientation of the needle is kept perpendicular in all the approaches. Up to the age of 6–8 years, the epidural space in infants and children contains blood vessels, lymphatics, and fat (which is fluid in nature).

The line joining the two iliac crests, also known as the Tuffier's line, crosses the L5-S1 vertebrae (up to 1 year of age) instead of the L4-L5 vertebrae in older children and adults. The elasticity of the ligaments provides better mobility of the vertebral column. Flexion of the spinal cord forward will further expand the epidural space in the lateral position; hence, this position is preferred in children for epidural blocks. The midline approach is widely used, as the ligament flavum is widest in the midline and the risk of inadvertent epidural vessel puncture is low.

11.3.2 Indications and Contraindications

Table 11.19 presents the indications and contraindications of epidural.

11.3.3 Local Anaesthetics for Epidural Anaesthesia in Children

Bupivacaine has mainly been replaced in practice by the more recent local anaesthetic drugs, L-bupivacaine and ropivacaine, because they are safer than bupivacaine. The effectiveness of one agent appears to be no better than another, but ropivacaine infusions may have a greater therapeutic ratio.

11.3.3.1 Dosing of the Drugs

The drug volume depends upon the level of blockade required for the surgery. General estimation of dosing for epidural injection is as follows:

Estimation of dose (general)	0.5–1 mL/kg (maximum 20 mL)
Blockage of a dermatome	0.1 mL/year of age
Lumbar epidural block	Weight × 0.04 mL/dermatome

Table 11.20 presents the standard dosing infusion regimen for paediatric epidural anaesthesia.

Table 11.21 presents the adjuvants for epidural anaesthesia.

Table 11.19 Indications and contraindications of epidural

Indications	Contraindications
Epidural anaesthesia is recommended in all major abdominal, thoracic, retroperitoneal, pelvic surgeries, including scoliosis and pectus excavatum repair	1. Severe coagulation disorders: Haemophilia, acquired (disseminated intravascular coagulation), or therapeutic 2. Septicemia or meningitis 3. Hydrocephaly and intracranial tumoral process 4. Allergy to local anaesthetics 5. Certain chemotherapies (such as with cisplatin) prone to induce subclinical neurologic lesions that can be acutely aggravated by a block procedure 6. Uncorrected hypovolemia 7. Cutaneous or subcutaneous lesions, whatever their nature (infection, angioma, dystrophic or tumoral, tattoo) at the contemplated site of puncture. 8. Parental refusal is a nonmedical absolute contraindication **Relative** 1. Severe malformations of the spine and spinal cord 2. Intraspinal tumours and lesions 3. Tethered cord syndrome 4. History of hydrocephalus 5. Elevated intracranial pressure 6. Unstable epilepsy or reduced intracranial compliance
The intervertebral level depends on the anaesthesiologist experience and patient's age. Lumber approach is mostly used in older children, in contrast to caudal approach in infants and young children	
Thoracic epidural block is a reliable approach in high thoracic dermatome sensory blockade	

Table 11.20 Standard dosing infusion regimen for paediatric epidural anaesthesia

Drug	Initial dose	Infusion	Recurrent dose
Bupivacaine/levobupivacaine	0.25% with 5 μ/mL <20 kg: 8–10 mL/0.1 mL/year >40 kg: Similar to adult	<4 months: 0.2 mg/kg/h (0.15 mL/kg/h of a 0.125% concentration or 0.3 mL/kg/h of a 0.0625%) 4–18 months: 0.25 mg/kg/h (0.2 mL/kg/h of a 0.124% concentration or 0.4 mL/kg/h of a 0.0625%) >18 months: 0.3–0.375 mg/kg/h (0.3 mL/kg/h of a 0.125% solution or 0.6 mL/kg/h of a 0.0625% solution)	0.1–0.3 mL/kg every 6–12 h of a 0.25% or 0.125% concentration
Ropivacaine	0.2% concentration (same dosing as bupivacaine)	0.1%,0.15%, 0.2% Same dosing as bupivacaine	0.1–0.3 mL/kg every 6–12 h of a 0.15% or 0.2% concentration

Table 11.21 Adjuvants for epidural anaesthesia

Drug	Initial dose	Infusion	Recurrent dose
Adjuvants	Fentanyl: 1–2 μg/kg Sufentanil: 0.1–0.6 μg/kg Clonidine: 1–2 μg/kg	Only one adjuvant to be used Morphine: 1–2 μg/mL Fentanyl: 1–2 μg/mL Sufentanil: 0.25–0.5 μg/mL Hydromorphine:1–3 μg/mL Clonidine: 0.3 at 1 μg/mL of solution	Morphine: 25–30 μg/kg every 8 h

11.3.4 Epidural Space Approach Recommendations

The approach to the epidural space depends on the patient's age, site of surgery, and experience of the anaesthesiologists (Table 11.22).

11.3.5 Equipment for the Epidural Block

In the present scenario, there are three sizes of Tuohy needle used for children. Shorter needle is easier to handle, and the small bevels are considered appropriate for the narrow epidural space.

I. 18G Tuohy needle (10 cm)
II. 19G and 20G (5 cm, short) for infants and children weighing less than 10 kg.

11.3.6 Technique

The lumber epidural space is mostly used via the midline approach below the L2-L3 space, representing the lower limit of conus medullaris. After the anaesthesia, child is positioned in the lateral position. Loss of resistance (LOR) technique is used for the confirmation of the epidural space. Medium selection (saline/air) for the LOR is a topic of debate. LOR to air can lead to nerve root compression, higher incidence of inadequate analgesia, venous air embolism, and paraesthesia. In infants, the most dependable is air/preferably CO_2, whereas in children older than 8–10 years, saline is the preferred technique for LOR. The amount of air to be injected for the confirmation of LOR technique is to be limited to 2 mL. The combination of air and saline can be used as the best technique due to improved perception and reduced risk of injecting air, when the epidural space is entered.

The distance from the skin to the epidural space can be calculated with the child's age and size.

Neonate	**1 cm**
Children 10–25 kg	**1 mm/kg**
Children > 25 kg (depth in cm)	**0.8+ (0.05 × weight (kg)**
Depth (cm)	**1 + (0.15 × age in years)**

After the epidural space confirmation, LOR syringe is disconnected from the epidural needle and after negative aspiration of CSF and blood, the local anaesthetic solution is injected either as a single shot or catheter is injected into the epidural space.

The catheter can be threaded from the lumber to the thoracic level, with the bevel of the Tuohy needle directed cephalad. The passage of the catheter should be smooth. A catheter should not be passed against resistance. The catheter should never be withdrawn with the epidural needle in space; otherwise, shearing will occur. In cases of difficult catheter insertion, the entire assembly of the catheter must be removed, i.e. the epidural needle and catheter.

The meniscus test can also be used to confirm epidural catheter placement. The test involves three steps:

Table 11.22 Various epidural approach according to site of surgery

Surgical intervention	Method	Approach
Intervention above umbilicus (thoracic/upper abdomen)	Catheter can be placed for analgesia	Thoracic approach with catheter (experienced anaesthesiologists)
Intervention below umbilicus	Single shot	Lumbar approach in older children Caudal in infants and children <8 years
	Catheter	Lumbar approach Caudal catheters are subjective to the possibility of contamination

1. After negative aspiration for CSF and blood, saline is injected through the filter into the epidural catheter, and the filter is thereby removed.
2. The open end of the catheter is lifted, and the liquid meniscus present in the catheter starts dropping rapidly.
3. The open end of the catheter is lowered, and the liquid meniscus is observed to fill the catheter with clear liquid without any blood.
4. The presence of air in the catheter during backflow confirms its accurate position in the epidural space.

Test Dose

- Local anaesthetic toxicity early symptoms cannot be detected easily in children because of the large number of blocks performed under general anaesthesia or deep sedation.
- Negative aspiration of blood has low sensitivity in predicting intravascular epidural needle or catheter placement.
- A small dose of epinephrine (0.5 g/kg in 0.1 mL/kg of lignocaine) can be used for the test dose.
- A 10-beat increase in heart rate after injection is indicative of intravascular injection.
- Changes in ST segment and T wave amplitude are more sensitive for detecting inadvertent intravenous injection. The recommendation is to inject small aliquots of local anaesthesia and observe the ECG for ST changes.
- The symptoms of inadvertent systemic injection can be delayed for up to 60–90 s after the test dose. Therefore, a period of 90 s' observation is warranted.
- Despite the negative aspiration, the local anaesthetic should be administered in an incremental fashion (0.1–0.2 mL/kg).

11.3.7 Complications

(a) **Neurologic injury**
(b) **Epidural hematoma**
(c) **Infection**
(d) **Dural puncture and post-dural puncture headache**: Use of atraumatic needles for dural puncture (25 or 27G). The diagnosis of PDPH in infants is more difficult because of the infant's inability to localize symptoms. The headache generally resolves after 3–5 days, and non-opioid analgesia or caffeine at 10 mg/kg per 24 h in two to three divided doses may be required. The use of an epidural blood patch is reserved for refractory cases. A blood patch involves aseptic injection of the patient's blood (0.1–0.2 mL/kg) into the epidural space at the level of the dural leak.
(e) **Hemodynamic Effects and Total Spinal Anaesthesia.**
(f) **Local Anaesthetic Systemic Toxicity.**
(g) **Apnoea**: The risk of postoperative apnoea is greatest in premature neonates, ex-premature infants, and those with anaemia.

11.4 Peripheral Nerve Blocks in Paediatrics

11.4.1 Brachial Plexus Block Above the Clavicle

Indications for brachial plexus blocks are to provide anaesthesia and analgesia for surgeries of the upper extremity.

11.4.1.1 Interscalene Approach

The interscalene approach aims to enter the interscalene space at its upper extremity, close to the transverse process of C6.

Position: The child placed in the (dorsal) recumbent position with the arms extended alongside the thorax and head turned (slightly) to the contralateral side.

Puncture site: Located at the projection of Chassaignac tubercle in the interscalene groove, (just posterior to the lateral border of the sternocleidomastoid muscle).

Technique: The needle is inserted at an 80-degree angle (not perpendicularly) to the skin.

Dorsal and slightly caudal aiming towards the clavicle mid-point, primary trunks (instead of roots) of the brachial plexus are located by elicited muscle twitches in the upper arm. Any distal motor twitch and biceps, triceps, or deltoid muscles are adequate. Contraction of the diaphragm indicates phrenic nerve stimulation and anterior placement of the needle tip. Alternatively, trapezius muscle stimulation indicates that needle placement is too posterior.

Muscle twitches in the upper arm are used to detect the primary trunks of the brachial plexus rather than its roots. Biceps, triceps, and/or deltoid muscles, or any distal motor twitch, are sufficient. Phrenic nerve stimulation is suspected with the diaphragmatic contraction and confer anterior needle tip placement. Conversely, trapezius contraction indicates posterior needle placement.

Adverse effects: Ipsilateral phrenic nerve blockade, vascular damage (vertebral.

artery and vein), and accidental cervical epidural and intrathecal penetration.

USG-guided: The probe is placed at the level of the cricoid cartilage in a transverse oblique plane. The trunk and roots are identified as a hypoechoic structure (round to oval) between the scalene anterior and middle muscle. The major vessels and artery (internal jugular vein and carotid) are placed medially and can be easily visualized. The needle is advanced from lateral to medial side of the probe towards the nerves to be targeted.

11.4.1.2 Supraclavicular Brachial Plexus Block

The brachial plexus trunks gather at the lower part of the interscalene space, where they surround the subclavian artery. The trunks are most compact in this area.

Technique Probe (high frequency) placed parallel and against the clavicle in the coronal oblique plane, the brachial plexus (trunk or division) look as a cluster of hypoechoic nodules located lateral, posterior, and superior to the subclavian artery, just above the underlying first rib. Avoid intravascular injection of surrounding vessels (i.e. the suprascapular artery or dorsal scapular artery) by using Doppler (colour). Advance the needle slowly under direct visualization (in-plane approach), from lateral to medial toward the angle made by the first rib and the subclavian artery. Local anaesthetic should reach the angle between the first rib and the subclavian artery.

11.4.2 Brachial Plexus Block Below the Clavicle

Axillary Block

Most commonly used approach to the brachial plexus in the paediatric subset aims to contact terminal nerves of the plexus in the axilla and nerves. The block is easy and safe with high degree of success rate. The surgery involving the forearm and the hand can be easily done under axillary block.

Technique

The child is placed in the supine position with the arm adducted to 90° and supinated. The block can be given both with the help of nerve stimulator and USG. Muscle twitches (with nerve stimulator) are elicited in the forearm and hand. The other way is to visualize the nerve tip close to one of the three cords, mainly the posterior cord and often close to the scapula coracoid process.

Dose of brachial plexus above and below the clavicle	
Bolus	0.3–0.5 mL/kg
Infusion	0.1–0.2 mL/kg/h (infusion)

11.4.3 Recommended Volume of Local Anaesthetics with Nerve Stimulation for Single-Shot Block

11.4.4 Thoracic Wall Blocks

11.4.4.1 PECS 1 and 2 Block

PEC 1 block is an anterior trunk fascial block. It targets medial and lateral pectoral nerves located superficial to the pectoralis minor and deep to the pectoralis major muscle.

PEC 2 block targets intercostal nerves, intercostobrachial nerve, and long thoracic nerve between the pectoralis major and the serratus anterior muscle. Bupivacaine (0.25%) 0.15 mL/kg (max.10 mL) and 0.3 mL/kg (max. 20 mL) can be used in PECS 1 and 2 block, respectively (Table 11.23).

11.4.4.2 Erector Spinae Block

A new interfascial plane block is the erector spinae plane (ESP) block. The vertical parasagittal vertebral plane is traversed by a network of paired muscle bundles and tendons that make up the erector spinae muscle. The dorsal and ventral rami of the thoraco-abdominal spinal neurons are blocked, when drug (local anaesthetic) is deposited along the fascial plane deep to the erector spinae muscle, causing both paravertebral spread and craniocaudal spread (the latter via the costotransverse foramen).

Technique The probe is placed craniocaudally and ESP is visualized covering the transverse processes observed in short axis. The erector spinae muscle is injected ventrally as the needle point is advanced in plane to the transverse processes, and ventral to the erector spinae, local anaesthetic is deposited. The paediatrics literature is currently limited and optimal paediatric dosing regimens are undetermined.

11.4.5 Abdominal Blocks

The abdominal blocks include the transverse abdominis block (TAP), rectus sheath block, and the ilioinguinal/iliohypogastric nerve block.

11.4.5.1 Transverse Abdominis Block (TAP)

Indications: Cholecystectomy, laparoscopic incisions, appendectomy, hernia repair, iliac crest bone graft harvest, and other anterolateral abdominal wall incisions.

Area covered: It blocks the segmental nerves from T9 to T12 and L1.The local anaesthetic is deposited between the transverse abdominal and the internal oblique muscle (abdominal) and provides abdominal wall analgesia.

Technique:

(a) **Landmark-guided**: The triangle of petit consists of a space bounded by the iliac crest, latissimus dorsi, and external oblique muscle is used for landmark-

Table 11.23 Recommended volume of local anaesthetics with nerve stimulation for single-shot block

Block	<10 kg (mL/kg)	11–30 kg	31–60 kg	>60 kg (mL)
Brachial plexus bock above clavicle	1	10 mL + 0.5 mL/kg above 10 kg	20 mL + 0.25 mL/kg above 30 kg	30
Brachial plexus bock above clavicle	0.5	5 mL + 0.25 mL/kg above 10 kg	10 mL + 0.15 mL/kg above 30 kg	15
Any nerve block at elbow	0.2	0.15 mL/kg	0.15 mL	10
Any nerve block at wrist	0.05	0.05 mL/kg	0.05 mL/kg	3–5

guided technique. The two pop sensations include first pop after piercing the external oblique and second pop after internal oblique penetration.

Dose: 0.3–0.4 mL/kg of LA can be used on both the sides.

(b) **USG-guided**: The USG probe is placed on the midaxillary line between the iliac crest and the costal margin, the block is performed in an in-plane method.

Complications

(a) Failure of block.
(b) Liver trauma.
(c) Vessel and bowel puncture.

11.4.5.2 Rectus Sheath Block

Indications: Umbilical or epigastric hernia repair, pyloromyotomy, single port laparoscopic surgery, and other midline incision surgeries (small).

Area covered: Blocks the terminal branches of 9th, 10th, and 11th intercostal nerves.

Technique

(a) **Landmark-guided**: The injection is best performed lateral to the maximal depth of the rectus sheath muscle within a potential space between the rectus abdominis muscle and posterior aspect of the rectus sheath, to assure the blockage of the nerve prior to the origin of the anterior cutaneous nerve.
(b) **USG-guided**: The use of USG is strongly recommended to improve success rate, and to avoid complications, probe (linear) is placed just below the umbilicus to visualize the anterior and posterior rectus sheath and the rectus abdominis muscle. Short bevel is inserted in-plane with the tip directing inside the rectus sheath (near the posterior aspect of the rectus muscle).

Dose*:* 0.1 mL/kg.

11.4.5.3 Ilioinguinal/Iliohypogastric Block

Indications: Hernia repair, orchiopexy, hydrocele surgery.

Area covered: Ipsilateral analgesia in the inguinal region.

Technique.

Landmark-guided: 22G needle (short bevel) is inserted medial and below the anterior superior iliac spine. The medial distance from the ASIS varies depending upon child's size (0.5 cm in infants and 2 cm in the adolescents). The needle is advanced slowly, until the pop of the external oblique muscle aponeurosis.

Dose: 0.4–0.5 mL/kg.

USG-guided: It is more effective than the conventional landmark-guided technique. The needle tip is placed between the ilioinguinal and iliohypogastric nerves. The real-time image helps in visualization of the local anaesthetic spread and thus allows decrease in the drug volume.

11.4.6 Lower Extremity Block

11.4.6.1 Lumbar Plexus Block

The lumbar plexus (LP) is formed by the union of the anterior rami of the first four lumbar nerves (L1–L4) with variable input from the 12th thoracic nerve (T12) and L5.

The LP lies in the psoas compartment in the paravertebral space. The quadratus lumborum muscle forms the posterior border of the lumbar plexus, which is bordered anteriorly by the psoas major muscle and by the psoas compartment in the paravertebral region. It contributes four nerves to the lower extremity, including femoral, lateral cutaneous, obturator, and genitofemoral nerves. The main difference between the children and adult is smaller size of the nerves trunks, which can lead to extensive spread of local anaesthetic. These nerves are less echoic than aponeurosis; this warrants extensive knowledge of anatomy and fascia and nerves relationship.

Indication	Contraindication	Complication
Femoral shaft fracture (femoral and fascia iliaca block)	No specific contraindication to femoral nerve blocks	Direct trauma to the retroperitoneal structure (right kidney mainly)/ intraperitoneal content
Muscle biopsy under femoral and lateral cutaneous nerve block (slight sedation)		Inadvertent spread to neuraxial space (subarachnoid space mainly)
Catheter placement can lead to prolong analgesia in femur surgeries		Nerve impalement and permanent damage

11.4.6.2 Femoral Nerve Block

Indications: Femoral shaft or knee surgeries.

Position: Place the child supine, preferably with the ipsilateral limb slightly abducted. The landmarks are the femoral artery and the inguinal ligament.

Puncture site: Located 0.5–1.0 cm both below the inguinal ligament (not the inguinal crease) and lateral to the femoral artery.

Technique:

(a) **Landmark-guided**: The block needle is inserted posteriorly, either perpendicular to the anterior aspect of the thigh or, especially during the catheter insertion, at a 45-degree angle cephalad, pointing to the umbilicus, until twitches are observed in the quadriceps muscle with neurostimulation use.

(b) **USG-guided**: The probe is placed slightly above and parallel to the inguinal ligament.

11.4.6.3 Sciatic Nerve Block

The sacral plexus is formed by the anterior rami of the L4–L5 nerves and the S1, S2, S3 sacral nerves with variable input from the fourth sacral nerve. The plexus lies on the sacrum surface, anterior to the piriformis muscle. The sacral plexus gives rise to the other two nerves that innervate the posterior cutaneous nerve of the thigh and the sciatic nerve. It is the largest mixed nerve of the body. At the level of popliteal fossa, it divides into common peroneal and posterior tibial nerves. The common nerve continues its descent around the head and neck of the fibula. The terminal branches form the superficial and deep peroneal nerves.

Technique Posterior approach is the most classic approach. This child is positioned in the semi-prone position. The puncture site is mid-distance between the greater trochanter of the femur and the coccyx (caudal extremity). The needle is inserted perpendicularly to the skin (both medial and ventral), pointing towards the ischial tuberosity and twitches are observed in the leg/foot or both.

Indications	Contraindications	Complications
Surgeries on the foot and the leg (saphenous nerve block is often required because this nerve provides (cutaneous) innervation of the medial aspect of the leg)	Sciatic blocks have no specific contraindications	Risk for the compartment syndrome Requires close monitoring and use of diluted solution to avoid motor blockade

11.4.6.4 Obturator Nerve Block

This procedure is performed with the child supine and the thigh slightly abducted and externally rotated (if possible). The landmarks are the groove between the tendon of the long adductor muscle and medial border of the pectineus muscle.

Puncture site: It is in the groove at the level of the greater trochanter of the femur.

With neurostimulation, the needle is inserted following a strict anterior to posterior path until twitches are elicited in the long and short adductor muscles (stimulation of the anterior division branch of the obturator nerve). The needle is further advanced dorsally over 1–2 cm until twitches are elicited in the great adductor (posterior branch).

Dose: 0.1 mL/kg up to a maximum of 5 mL per nerve.

USG-guided: The probe is placed below the pubic tubercle, parallel to the inguinal ligament. The aponeurosis of the sartorius and long and short adductors are easily identified. The anterior branch lies between the long and short adductors, and the posterior branch can be found between the short and great adductors.

11.4.7 Other Nerve Blocks

Penile Block

The penis is innervated by the S2–S4 pudendal nerves that further divide into right and left dorsal nerves of the penis and run beneath the pubic symphysis to travel below the bucks fascia to supply innervation of the penis.

Indications: Circumcision, hypospadias, paraphimosis, and phimosis.

Technique.

Landmark-guided: The penis is pulled downward and puncture site identified at 10 and 2 O clock position, at the base of the penis (below the pubic symphysis). The needle is advanced perpendicularly, until LOR (indicative of piercing the buck's fascia).'The procedure is repeated similarly on the opposite site.

USG-guided: The probe is placed along the shaft in the sagittal plane. The subpubic space is identified, with the deep penile fascia inferiorly and pubic symphysis superiorly.

Depth of insertion: Neonate 0.5 cm; 3 cm in an adolescent.

Dose: 0.1 mL/kg of local anaesthetic.

Contraindication: Epinephrine is contraindicated due to the likelihood of ischemia and necrosis (dorsal artery of penis is an end artery).

11.5 Conclusion

Regional anaesthesia in the paediatric populace is an exigent area that needs to be explored more in order to make this field easier and less challenging. The pain experienced during the surgical procedures needs to be addressed especially in the neonates, and the methods to annihilate them surmised. This chapter adds details to such methods in a meticulous way which is easy to grasp and understand. It provides a comprehensive overview of the differences in anatomy, physiology, the indications and contraindications, the drug dosing, the methods of elucidating the blocks, and the troubleshooting. It focuses on the key aspects required in executing regional anaesthesia in children and also managing the complications if they occur. The details added to each procedure like spinal, epidural, caudal, and peripheral nerve blocks make this chapter the precise synopsis for regional anaesthesia in children. This chapter has been extensively updated to reflect the latest information. The use of not only the landmark techniques but also of the ultrasound in an easy-to-grasp language gives this chapter an extra edge over the others. This chapter thus acts as a comprehensive foundation to regional anaesthesia in the paediatric population in an uncomplicated fashion and categorizes the paediatric population as a separate cohort.

Further Reading

American Society of Anesthesiologists Task Force on Acute Pain Management. Practice guidelines for acute pain management in the perioperative setting: an updated report by the American Society of Anesthesiologists Task Force on acute pain management. Anesthesiology. 2012;116:248–73.

Butterworth JF IV, Mackey DC, Wasnick JD, et al. Morgan & Mikhail's. Clin Anesthesiol. 2017a;5:583–90.

Butterworth JF IV, Mackey DC, Wasnick JD, et al. Morgan & Mikhail's. Clin Anesthesiol. 2017b;5:591–9.

Campbell MF. Caudal anesthesia in children. J Urol. 1933;30:245–50.

Dogliotti AM. Research and clinical observations on spinal anesthesia: with special reference to the peridural technique. Anesth Analg. 1933;12:59–65.

Ecoffey C, Dubousset AM, Samii K. Lumbar and thoracic epidural anesthesia for urologic and upper abdominal surgery in infants and children. Anesthesiology. 1986;65:87–90.

Gupta A, Saha U. J Anaesthesiol Clin Pharmacol. 2014;30(1):10–8.

Hammer GB, Ramamoorthy C, Cao H, et al. Postoperative analgesia after spinal block in infants and children undergoing cardiac surgery. Anesth Analg. 2005;100:1283–8.

Lam DK, Corry GN, Tsui BC. Evidence for the use of ultrasound imaging in pediatric regional anesthesia: a systematic review. Reg Anesth Pain Med. 2016;41:229–41.

Maria BD, Tielens L, Roberts S. NYSORA paediatric epidural and spinal anesthesia and analgesia. 2019.

Miller RD. Miller's anesthesia, vol. 9. Elsevier Health Sciences; 2019a. p. 1189–94.

Miller RD. Miller's anesthesia, vol. 9. Elsevier Health Sciences; 2019b. p. 1195–9.

Motoyama, EK, Davis, Peter J. Smith's anesthesia for infants and children. 2006.

Peutrell JM, Lonnqvist PA. Neuraxial blocks for anaesthesia and analgesia in children. Curr Opin Anaesthesiol. 2003a;16:461–70.

Peutrell JM, Lonnqvist PA. Neuraxial blocks for anaesthesia and analgesia in children. Curr Opin Anaesthesiol. 2003b;16:471–82.

Ruston FG. Epidural anaesthesia in infants and children. Can Anaesth Soc J. 1954;1:37–44.

Ruston FG. Epidural anaesthesia in pediatric surgery. Anesth Analg. 1957;36:76–82.

Ruston FG. Epidural anaesthesia in paediatric surgery: present status in the Hamilton general hospital. Can Anaesth Soc J. 1964;11:12–34.

Schulte-Steinberg O. History. In: Saint-Maurice C, Schulte-Steinberg O, editors. Regional Anaesthesia in children. New York: Appleton & Lange; 1990. p. 13–4.

Short TG. Miller's Anesthesia. In: Anaesthesia and intensive care, 39(6), pp. 1162+. Gale Academic OneFile; 2011, https://go.gale.com/ps/i.do?p=AONE&u=anon~1381e34a&id=GALE|A274409805&v=2.1&it=r&sid=googleScholar&asid=61d0f3a8. Accessed 31 Jan 2023.

Suresh S, Long J, Birmingham PK, et al. Are caudal blocks for pain control safe in children? An analysis of 18,650 caudal blocks from the pediatric regional anesthesia network (PRAN) database. Anesth Analg. 2015;120:151–6.

Tsui BC. Ultrasound imaging for regional anesthesia in infants, children, and adolescents: a review of current literature and its application in the practice of neuraxial blocks. Anesthesiology. 2010;112:719–28.

Neuraxial Labour Analgesia

12

Kanchan Rani and Sukhminder Jit Singh Bajwa

Abstract

Labour pain is described as the most unbearable pain women have ever encountered, with the majority of parturient reporting it as severe or extremely severe. This stressful situation has an adverse effect on maternal and foetal metabolism. The optimal way of evidence-based pain management in labouring mothers is still being debated. Pain relief strategies have traditionally been classified as non-pharmacological, pharmacological, and regional. Inhalational agents, parenteral opioids, and nonopioids are examples of pharmacological techniques. The efficacy of hypnosis, biofeedback, sterile water injection, aromatherapy, and transcutaneous electrical nerve stimulation is unknown due to a lack of robust evidence.

Although many methods for treating pain during labour have been investigated, neuraxial analgesia has been regarded as unrivalled due to its demonstrated efficacy and adaptability with maternal satisfaction.

One of the most frequently used neuraxial labour analgesia is the lumbar epidural. Lumbar epidural analgesia, also known as "mobile epidural" or "walking epidural", aims to produce a selective sensory block from T10 to L1 while preserving motor supply to the lower extremities.

The myths and controversies surrounding neuraxial labour analgesia for the woman and foetus must be dispelled. The proper monitoring of labouring women on neuraxial analgesia by multidisciplinary team is critical. Neuraxial analgesia side effects and complications must be recognised and addressed at the earliest.

Keywords

Analgesia · Labour · Epidural · Combined spinal-epidural

12.1 Introduction

Most labouring women experience excruciating pain during childbirth. They consider birthing pain to be the most extreme suffering they have ever endured, describing it as severe to extremely severe.

Every parturient should have access to some kind of pain management practices and should not be denied pain relief during delivery. It is

K. Rani (✉)
Department of Obstetrics and Gynaecology, Teerthanker Mahaveer Medical College and Research Centre, Moradabad, Uttar Pradesh, India

S. J. S. Bajwa
Department of Anaesthesiology and Critical Care, Gian Sagar Medical College and Hospital, Patiala, Punjab, India

M. K. Prasad, S. J. S. Bajwa (eds.), *Steps to Successful Regional Anesthesia*,
https://doi.org/10.1007/978-981-97-4098-7_12

a woman's entitlement to anticipate pain relief from her obstetrician.

As per ACOG and ASA, "labour results in severe pain for many women. There is no other circumstance where it is considered acceptable for a person to experience untreated severe pain, amenable to safe intervention, while under a physician's care… Maternal request is a sufficient medical indication for pain relief during labour".

12.2 Anatomy of Labour Pain and Analgesia

Labour pain is comprised of both visceral and somatic components.

Pain in first stage of labour arises from uterine contraction and cervical dilatation and is referred to T10-L1 dermatomes. Pain in second stage of labour is caused by distension of perineum by the presenting part, stretch on bladder, urethra, rectum and is referred to lower lumbar and sacral segments (L1-L2 and S2-S4). Pain is carried by A delta and C fibres.

12.3 Method of Labour Analgesia

Conventionally, pain relief methods are classified into non-pharmacological, pharmacological, and regional techniques· (Fig. 12.1).

12.3.1 Non-pharmacological

Massage, deep breathing techniques, acupuncture, hypnosis, transcutaneous electrical nerve stimulation, aromatherapy, acupuncture, and hydrotherapy are all viable options for mild labour pain.

12.3.2 Pharmacological

Pharmacological methods include inhalational agents like entonox, sevoflurane, parenteral opioids like fentanyl, sufentanil, remifentanil, tramadol, pethidine, nalbuphine, and butorphanol, and nonopioids like antihistamines, antispasmodics, sedatives, and nonsteroidal anti-inflammatory drugs (NSAIDs).

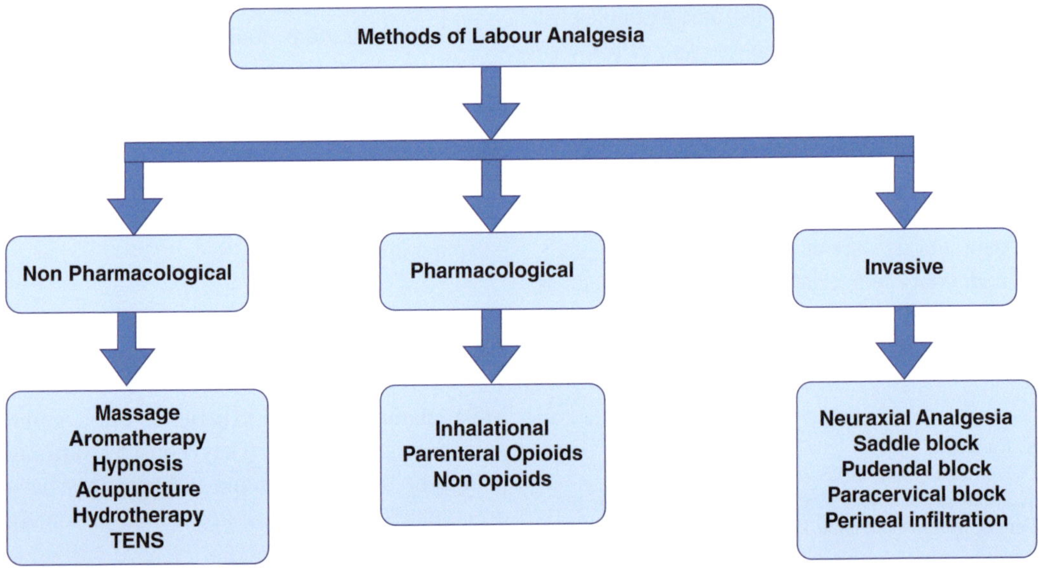

Fig. 12.1 Methods of labour analgesia

12.3.3 Invasive

Among the invasive methods are neuraxial labour analgesia, saddle block, pudendal block, paracervical block, and perineal infiltration.

12.3.3.1 Neuraxial Labour Analgesia

Although many methods have been used by obstetric anaesthesiologists for labour analgesia, neuraxial analgesia has been regarded as unequalled due to its proven efficacy and adaptability with maternal satisfaction. The neuraxial methods are appropriate for both labour analgesia and surgical anaesthesia.

Indications for Neuraxial Labour Analgesia

The primary indications and certain special situations where labour epidurals may be beneficial are tabulated in (Table 12.1).

Contraindication for Neuraxial Labour Analgesia

The contraindication for neuraxial labour analgesia is presented in Table 12.2.

Prerequisite for Neuraxial Labour Analgesia

- Informed consent.
- One to one nursing care should be available for the patient.
- A thorough history and physical examination to identify obstetric and anaesthetic risk factors.

Table 12.1 Indications for neuraxial labour analgesia

Absolute	Maternal request
Relative	Labour augmentation Pre-eclampsia (without severe thrombocytopenia or coagulopathy) High risk for assisted vaginal delivery, e.g., breech or multiple gestation Trial of labour after previous caesarean section Certain cardiac disease Cerebrovascular or respiratory disease High body mass index (BMI) Anticipated difficult airway or other risk factors for general anaesthetic Spinal disorders, e.g., with scoliosis where 'urgent' neuraxial anaesthesia placement may be difficult

Table 12.2 Contraindication for neuraxial labour analgesia

Absolute	Relative
Patient refusal Severe coagulopathy Thrombocytopenia (platelets <75,109/L) LMWH (prophylactic dose within last 12 h, therapeutic dose within 24 h) Hypovolaemia Cardiovascular instability Increased intracranial pressure Local infection Allergy to local anaesthetic drugs	Systemic infection Fixed cardiac output status Certain neurological conditions Previous lumbar spinal surgery Severe anatomical deformity of spine Mild coagulopathy Preexisting central or peripheral neurological condition Unco-operative patient

- All the relevant laboratory investigations should be reviewed properly.
- Examination of the back for any anatomical deformity or any local infection.
- Discussion with obstetrician about obstetric plan.
- Assessment of the foetal heart rate status by CTG for 20 min.
- Assessment of maternal vitals.
- Equipment check (routine and emergency resuscitation drugs and equipment).
- Obtain intravenous access.
- Oral intake of moderate amounts of clear liquid may be allowed, but solid foods should be restricted.
- Antacid prophylaxis every 12 hourly till epidural analgesia is continued.
- Women should be properly instructed on how to use remote dose cord in case of patient-controlled epidural analgesia (PCEA).

Drugs for Neuraxial Labour Analgesia

Once an epidural catheter has been inserted, local anaesthetics, with or without adjuvant medications, are used to provide analgesia. For details of the drugs, kindly refer to Chap. 2 on local anaesthetics.

Techniques of Neuraxial Labour Anaesthesia

Most commonly practised neuraxial labour analgesia is lumbar epidural. There are many alternative neuraxial techniques also (Fig. 12.2).

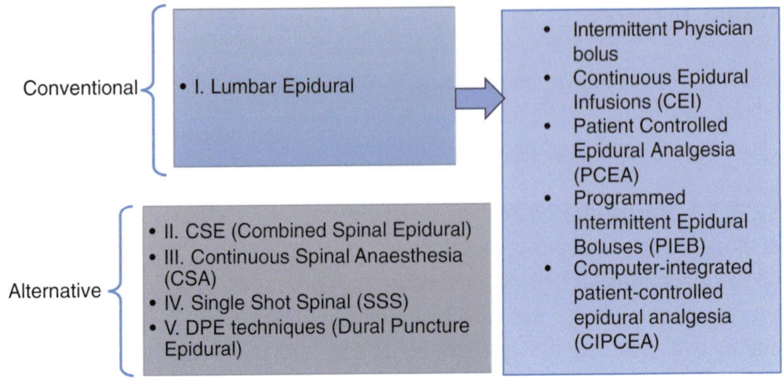

Fig. 12.2 Different neuraxial techniques for neuraxial labour analgesia

The choice of technique usually depends on anaesthetist experience and the clinical scenario.

I. Conventional lumbar epidural or labour epidural.
II. Combined spinal epidural (CSE).
III. Continuous spinal anaesthesia (CSA).
IV. Single-shot spinal (SSS).
V. Dural puncture epidural (DPE) techniques.

I. **Lumbar Epidural**

- Traditional epidural analgesia entails inserting a catheter into the epidural area, administering an initial bolus dosage, and then infusing a local anaesthetic agent with an opioid.
- Lumbar epidurals are popular and safe, providing good analgesia for labouring women.
- Lumbar epidurals can also be used to give anaesthesia for a vaginal delivery or a caesarean section.
- Lumbar epidural analgesia, often known as the "mobile epidural or walking epidural", seeks to generate a selective sensory block from T10 to L1 while sparing the motor supply to the lower limbs (L2-L5).
- Low dose mixture (LDM) labour epidural dosage regimens (e.g., 0.0625–0.125% bupivacaine with 2–4 mcg/ml fentanyl or 0.4 mcg/ml sufentanil) lower the total local anaesthetic dose necessary and motor block experienced, potentially enabling the parturient to be mobile.
- The modern dosing regimens for labour epidural mixture (LDM) produce very less motor block, with no interference with labour progress and minimal maternal and foetal adverse effects.

Low-dose mixture (LDM): 10–15 mL

Bupivacaine (0.0625–0.125%) or ropivacaine 0.08–0.20% or levobupivacaine: 0.05–0.125% with fentanyl (1.5–3 µg/mL) or sufentanil (0.2–0.4 µg/mL).

Epidural Infusion (Low Dose Infusion): 10–15 mL/h

- Bupivacaine 0.0625–0.125% with fentanyl 1.5–3 µg/mL or sufentanil 0.2–0.5 µg/mL. OR
- Ropivacaine 0.08–0.20% with fentanyl 1.5–3 µg/mL or sufentanil 0.2–0.4 µg/mL.

I.1 Regimes for Administering Lumbar Epidural Analgesia

(i) **Intermittent Physician Bolus**

Before the introduction of infusion pumps, epidural analgesia was maintained by intermittent administration of bolus doses of local anaesthetic when analgesia began to wane. When pain returned, analgesia was typically restored with a bolus injection of a local anaesthetic/opioid solution with a lockout period of 10–20 min.

(ii) **Continuous Epidural Infusions (CEI)**

With the introduction of the infusion pump in the early 1980s, the continuous infusion technique became widespread and it reduces the variability of analgesia during labour.

It offers sufficient and smoother analgesia and haemodynamic stability with titrated doses of local anaesthetics and opioid by infusion devices and can be adjusted to individualise analgesia. However, it necessitates higher doses of local anaesthetics, which may impair the ability to bear down during the second stage of labour, leading to a rise in the rate of instrumental deliveries, and many patients require top ups by a clinician or experience unacceptable motor blockage.

(iii) **Patient-Controlled Epidural Analgesia (PCEA)**

This method enables the parturient to control the dose of local anaesthetics based on the severity of pain, improving maternal satisfaction with the psychological benefit of having control over her own pain management. When compared to continuous epidural infusion, there is decreased clinician intervention, the quantity of local anaesthetics and opioid required, and the occurrence of motor block.

Epidural mixture boluses are delivered on demand of patient with a lockout period of 10–20 min. PCEA can be given with or without a baseline infusion. Background infusion decreased the need for anaesthetist-administered supplementary epidural boluses, provided more effective pain control without an increase in the use of local anaesthetics.

(iv) **Programmed Intermittent Epidural Boluses (PIEB)**

It is a comparatively new innovative protocol used for labour analgesia maintenance in which a predetermined amount of epidural mixture is given as a bolus at timed intervals by a drug delivery pump. Instead of background infusion, the hourly total amount of local anaesthetic solution typically used in a CEI is administered as intermittent boluses of LDMs in programmed intermittent epidural bolus (PIEB).

When compared to a CEI, this offers comparable analgesia, higher maternal satisfaction, fewer unscheduled rescue boluses, and lower bupivacaine consumption with less motor blockade.

(v) **Computer-Integrated Patient-Controlled Epidural Analgesia (CIPCEA)**

It is an advanced and innovative epidural analgesia delivery system with a pre-programmed algorithm that analyses the dose of LA and adjusts the basal infusion rate based on the requirement in the previous hour. A computer is connected to PCEA pump. It transforms a continuous infusion pump into a computer-integrated PCEA (CIPCEA), which is more adaptable to the requirements of the parturient. This interactive programme tracks the analgesic requirements over the previous hour and according to the number of demand boluses, it adjusts the amount of its basal infusion.

I.2 Drug Doses in Different Regimens of Lumbar Epidural Analgesia

The drug doses in different regimens of epidural analgesia are provided in Table 12.3.

PCEA Recipes (Patient-Controlled Epidural Analgesia)

The attending anaesthetist has the option of varying PCEA programme settings such as demand bolus, lockout interval, background infusion rate, and hourly maximum dose limits accordingly—maximum 30–35 mL/h (total infusion plus boluses).

I.3 Advantages and Disadvantages of Different Epidural Analgesia Regimens

The advantages and disadvantages of different epidural analgesia regimens are presented in Table 12.4.

Alternative Neuraxial Technique

II. Combined Spinal-Epidural Analgesia (CSEA)

A CSE analgesia incorporates the advantages of continuing labour analgesia with the epidural component with the quick onset of analgesia from the spinal component.

It can be carried out using a needle-through-needle technique or as a single-shot spinal

Table 12.3 Drug doses in different regimens of labour epidural analgesia

Regimen of classic labour epidural	Initial bolus dose	Maintenance with background infusion	Maintenance without background infusion (demand only)	Lockout time (dose interval)
Intermittent physician bolus	10–15 mL LDM	5–8 mL/h LDM Bolus LDM can be given as required[a]	10–15 mL LDM	10–20 min
Continuous epidural infusion (CEI)	LDM 0.0625% bupivacaine with 2 mcg/mL of fentanyl, infusing at 10–12 mL/h			
Patient-controlled epidural analgesia (PCEA)	5–10 mL LDM	5–8 mL/h LDM (background infusion) Bolus dose: 5–8 mL (as required by parturient)	8–12 mL LDM (as required by parturient)	10–20 min
Programmed intermittent epidural boluses (PIEB)	Replace 10–12 mL/h infusion with timed bolus, similar hourly dose, usually with additional PCEA doses Like 6–8 mL Q 30 min, 9–10 mL Q 45 min, 12 mL Q 60 min			

[a]LDM—Low-dose mixture: bupivacaine (0.0625–0.125%) 10–15 mL with fentanyl (1.5–3 μg/mL) or sufentanil (0.2–0.4 μg/mL)

Table 12.4 Advantages and disadvantages of different epidural analgesia regimens

Regimes for administering labour epidural analgesia	Advantages	Disadvantages
Intermittent physician bolus	Improved analgesia in comparison to continuous infusion	Requires frequent provider intervention Pain relief may be interrupted by regression of analgesia between two boluses Can cause blockade of the sacral segments or intense motor blockade or both
Continuous epidural infusions (CEI)	Gives adequate and more uniform analgesia as well as better haemodynamic stability	Requires larger doses of local anaesthetics May impair the ability to bear down during second stage of labor May increase the rate of instrumental deliveries
Patient-controlled epidural analgesia (PCEA)	Improved maternal satisfaction Decreased clinician's intervention Decreased requirement of local anaesthetics and opioid Decreased incidence of motor block [in comparison to CEI]	Requirement of a dedicated infusion pump Proper education of the parturient is required
Programmed intermittent epidural boluses (PIEB)	Higher maternal satisfaction Less need for unscheduled rescue boluses Reduced consumption of LA Less motor blockade (in comparison to CEI)	
PIEB with PCEA	Reduced consumption of LA Less PCEA demand boluses [in comparison to PCEA with standard continuous background infusion]	
Computer-integrated patient-controlled epidural analgesia (CIPCEA)	Significant reduction in the incidence of breakthrough pain without increasing local anaesthetic consumption or incidence of side effects	Requires computer-integrated drug delivery system

followed by the insertion of an epidural catheter as a separate procedure.

There is no difference in inadvertent dural puncture, the frequency of post-dural puncture headache (PDPH), need for rescue analgesia, mode of delivery or maternal satisfaction between CSEs and labour epidurals. Compared to labour epidurals, there is a higher risk of transient hypotension and foetal bradycardia. There is a theoretical risk of using an untested epidural catheter for labour analgesia because of complexity of the procedure.

III. **Continuous Spinal Analgesia (CSA)**

Continuous spinal analgesia (CSA) can be provided by intermittent injection or continuous infusion via intrathecal placement of catheter, similar to the use of an epidural catheter.

Although CSA is most commonly used after an unintentional dural puncture while attempting to place an epidural catheter, some clinician feels that CSA is more dependable than continuous epidural analgesia because of objective verification of catheter placement and LA enters directly to CSF.

Patients with previous spinal surgery, morbid obesity, failure of repeated attempts at epidural catheter placement, or ineffective analgesia with an epidural catheter in situ are very few indications where CSA can be used.

Precaution

CSA has much more safety issues than labour epidural as these catheters are placed in the intrathecal space, several safety concerns arise that are not as serious with epidural catheters.

The pump and the catheter should be properly labelled, and all the staff should be well informed regarding the presence of an intrathecal catheter, exact combination, concentration and doing of drugs.

IV. **Single-Shot Spinal (SSS)**

A single-shot spinal block for labour analgesia can provide instant pain alleviation. However, due to the short duration of action and the high risk of headache when a large-bore needle is used, the use of spinal analgesia is restricted.

Due to the rapid progression of labour, multiparous parturients are likely the best candidates for this procedure. It has been demonstrated that the analgesic effect of a dosage of 2.5 mg bupivacaine and 25 mcg fentanyl can last up to 2 h.

V. **Dural Puncture Epidural (DPE)**

The DPE technique involves a purposeful puncture of the dura with a spinal needle without the administration of intrathecal medication. This technique allows partial confirmation of epidural catheter placement by observing cerebrospinal fluid in the spinal needle placed through the epidural needle.

Although DPE improves analgesia compared to epidurals alone by allowing anaesthetic to flow from the epidural space into the intrathecal space, at present this technique is not in common practice.

Various Indications for Different Neuraxial Analgesia Techniques (Table 12.5)

Table 12.5 Indications for different neuraxial analgesia techniques

Neuraxial analgesia technique	Indications
Conventional lumbar epidural	Maternal request (method of choice for labour analgesia)
Combined spinal epidural analgesia; (CSEA)	For early onset of labour analgesia For immediate pain relief when parturient in advanced labour Morbidly obese patients Patients having difficult spine anatomy Epidural catheter verification for insufficient pain relief
Continuous spinal analgesia (CSA)	Difficulty in placing epidural catheter owing to previous spine surgery or morbid obesity Technique for salvaging after unintentional dural puncture during labour epidural
Single-shot spinal (SSS)	Patients in advanced labour having severe pain In resource-limited setups
Dural puncture epidural analgesia (DPEA)	To enhance the effectiveness of epidural analgesia Indication same as for CSEA

Table 12.6 Dosing of different neuraxial labour analgesia regimes

Neuraxial anaesthesia technique	Loading dose	Maintenance dose with background infusion	Maintenance dose without background infusion	Lockout time
Combined spinal-epidural analgesia (CSEA)	Intrathecal 0.5% B (1–2.5 mg) + F (10–25 μg) or S (2.5–10 μg)	Epidural 5–8 mL/h LDM Bolus*LDM can be given as required	Epidural 5–10 mL LDM	10–20 min
Continuous spinal analgesia (CSA)	Intrathecal 0.5% B (1.75–2.5 mg) +F (15–20 μg) or S (5 μg)	Intrathecal basal infusion B (0.05–0.125%) + F 2–5 μg/ml at 0.5–3 mL/h (titrated to a T8–10 sensory level) or S (2.5–5 μg/h) as required	Intrathecal bolus dose 0.5% B (1.75–2.5 mg) + F (15–20 μg/1–2 h) or S (5 μg SOS)	–
SSS	Local anaesthetic opioid 2.5 mg bupivacaine and 25mcg fentanyl have been shown to last up to 2 h in duration Low-dose Combination (fentanyl 25 μg, bupivacaine 2.5 mg, and morphine 250 μg) in one injection provides up to 4 h of ambulatory pain control			
Epidural (DPE) loading dose	Local anaesthetic opioid 10–15 mL bupivacaine 0.125% Fentanyl 50–100 μg (50 μg probably enough) 10–15 mL ropivacaine and 0.2% sufentanil 10 mg			

Dosing of Different Neuraxial Labour Analgesia Regimes

The local anaesthetic and adjuvant drug dosing are provided in Table 12.6.

Monitoring of Patients on Neuraxial Analgesia

- Assessment by attending anaesthetist should be done during first dose, after 30 min then at regular interval and at call of floor duty nurse.
- Verbal contact should be maintained to women while giving bolus doses.
- Monitoring of maternal heart rate and blood pressure every 5 min for 20 min after initial loading dose or clinician's bolus, then hourly.
- Level of sensory and motor block, pain score, and sedation score should be done 20 min after loading dose or clinician bolus, then hourly.
- Foetal heart rate monitoring.
- For low risk pregnancy: CTG for 30 min after loading dose or clinician bolus, then FHR monitoring every 15 min.
- For high risk pregnancy: Continuous CTG.
- Bladder care: Monitor and encourage regular voiding (at least four hourly, void must be >200 mL/4 h), otherwise insert bladder catheter.
- No further boluses should be given if the woman feels unwell after a bolus or shows symptoms of maternal hypotension or develops sudden marked motor weakness of the legs. The lady should be placed in the left lateral position, and the IV fluid infusion should be increased to provide a 250-mL fluid bolus.
- Labour monitoring should be done as per obstetrics protocol while encouraging patient to change positions at least every 20 min to facilitate foetal descent and rotation.

Troubleshooting

- If visual analogue score (VAS) for pain assessment is <4 on a VAS of 0–10, it means the analgesia is satisfactory and parturient can cope with the pain, whereas if it is >4, evaluate for inadequate block (Fig. 12.3).

  Troubleshooting

  1. Inadequate analgesia: Additional top up.
  2. Unilateral block or missed segment
     - Position patient on unblocked side → if ineffective → withdraw the catheter by 1 cm.

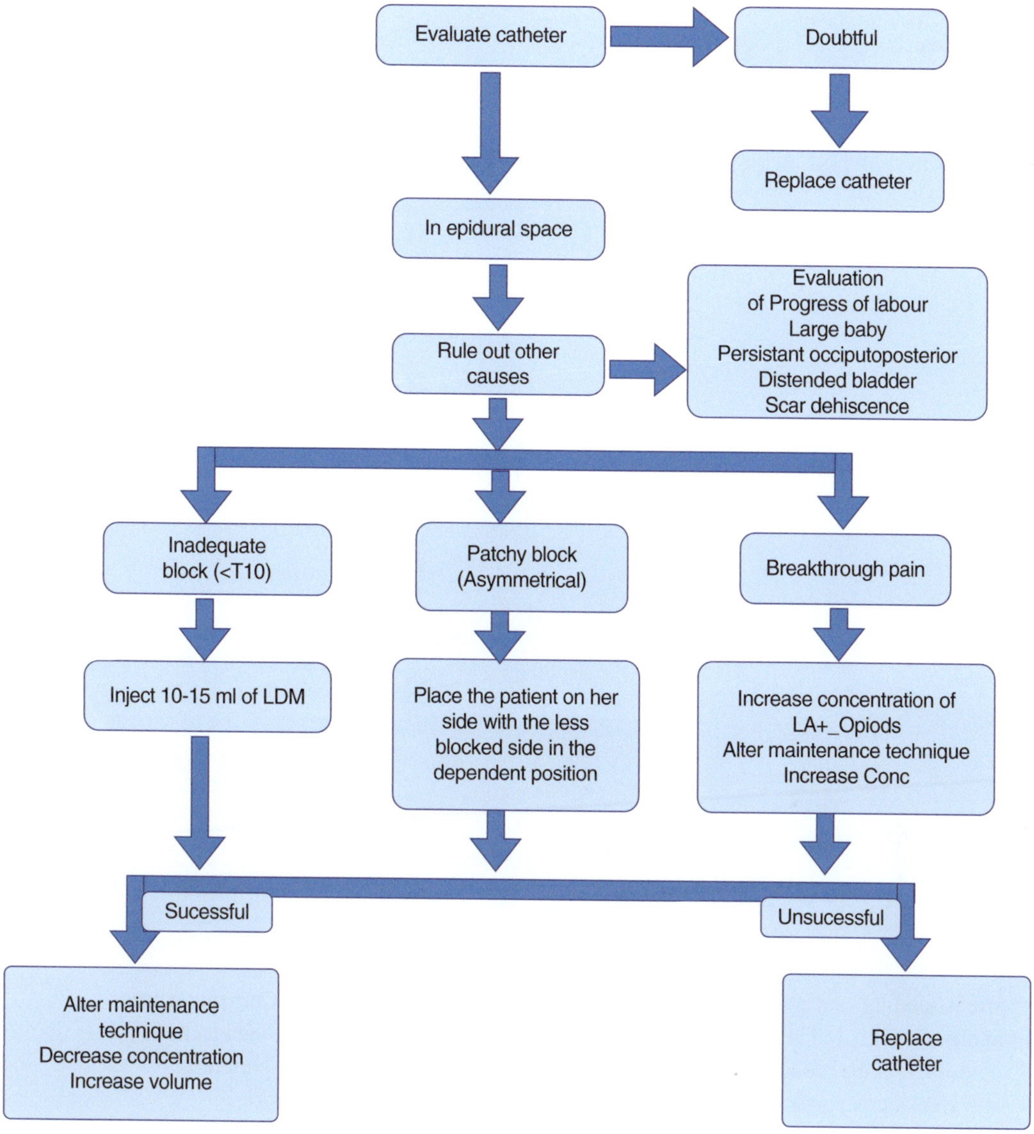

Fig. 12.3 Evaluation of inadequate block

  - Still not effective Reposition the catheter.
- If bloody tap occurs on aspiration of catheter, troubleshooting protocols need to be followed and are mentioned in Fig. 12.4.

Controversies and Concerns

- There is no link between the risk of caesarean birth and neuraxial labour analgesia versus non-neuraxial analgesia.
- There is a higher risk of instrumental vaginal delivery.
- Epidural analgesia prolongs the second stage of labour with no adverse effects on the foetus or neonate.
- The "early vs. late" debate for epidural analgesia has been settled in support of analgesia at the patient's request, independent of cervical examination.
- There is no difference in the incidence of long-term low back pain.

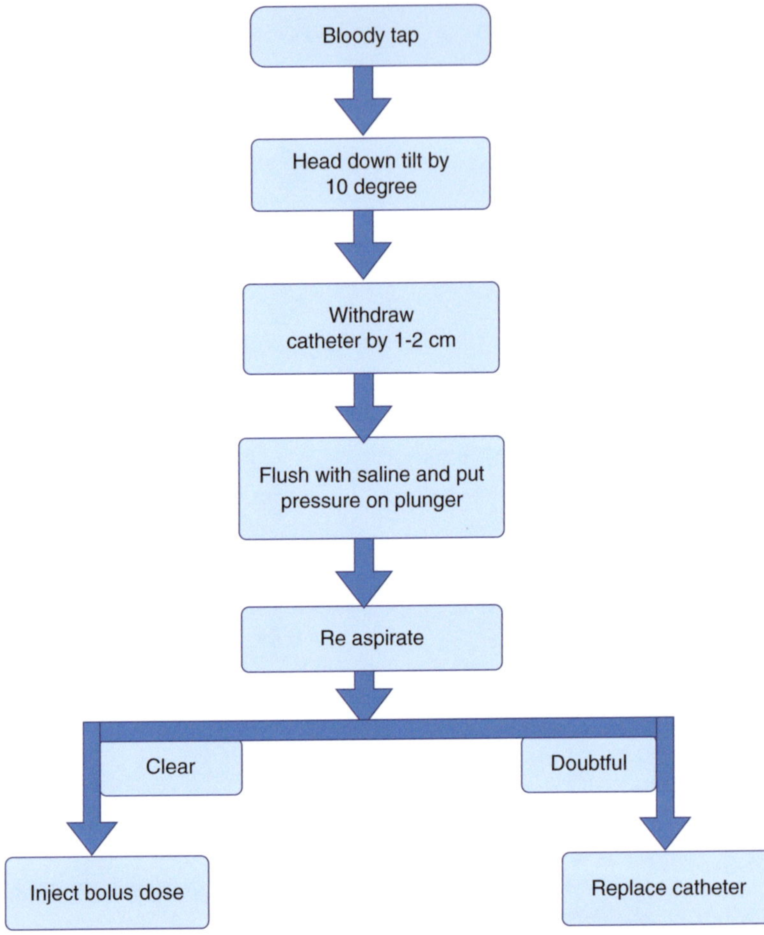

Fig. 12.4 Troubleshooting for bloody tap

- Breastfeeding success and epidural labour analgesia with fentanyl were not affected by epidural fentanyl concentration when analysed at 6 weeks postpartum.
- Epidural analgesia can be used during labour trials for vaginal birth after previous caesarean delivery (VBAC), and sufficient pain relief may encourage more women to try VBAC; epidural analgesia is not anticipated to mask signs of scar rupture.

Side Effects of Neuraxial Analgesia
- Hypotension.
- Uterine tachysystole and foetal bradycardia.
- Pruritus.
- Fever.
- Nausea and vomiting.
- Urinary retention.

Neuraxial Analgesia Complications
- Post-dural puncture headache (PDPH) due to unintentional dural puncture.
- Respiratory depression.
- Local anaesthetic systemic toxicity (see Chap. 2 for details).
- High or total spinal anaesthesia.

12.3.4 Saddle Block

When time or other constraints prevent the use of continuous catheter spinal or epidural anaesthetic techniques in obstetrics, this approach is used (e.g., routine delivery, assisted deliveries like forceps or vacuum, episiotomy or perineal repair, or other obstetric procedures).

12.3.5 Pudendal Nerve Block

Pudendal nerve block is indicated in instrumental vaginal delivery or labour analgesia in second stage when epidural analgesia is contraindicated. See Chap. 13 for details.

12.3.6 Paracervical Block

In the first stage of labour, a paracervical block (an injection of local anaesthetic into the cervix) is used to alleviate the labour pains in active phase of labour when no safer alternative is available. It is not used routinely.

Further Reading

American College of Obstetricians and Gynecologists' Committee on Practice Bulletins—Obstetrics. ACOG practice bulletin no. 209: obstetric analgesia and anesthesia. Obstet Gynecol. 2019;123(3):e208–25.

Anim-Somuah M, Smyth RM, Cyna AM, Cuthbert A. Epidural versus non-epidural or no analgesia for pain management in labour. Cochrane Database Syst Rev. 2018;5(5):CD000331.

Ashagrie HE, Fentie DY, Kassahun HG. A review article on epidural analgesia for labor pain management: a systematic review. Int J Surg Open. 2020;24:100–4.

Auckland District Health Board. Epidural-Analgesia-in-labour-management-and-care. Available from: https://www.nationalwomenshealth.adhb.govt.nz/assets/Womens-health/Documents/Policies-and-guidelines/Epidural-Analgesia-in-Labour-Management-and-Care.pdf. Accessed 01 Apr 2023.

Bauchat J, Wong CA. Neuraxial labor analgesia and effect on labor. In: Santos AC, Epstein JN, Chaudhuri K, editors. Obstetric anesthesia. McGraw Hill; 2015.

Bhagat K, Daftary SN. Pain relief in labour: an indian perspective. Available from: https://icogonline.org/wp-content/uploads/pdf/gcpr/pain-relief-in-labour.pdf. Accessed 1 Apr. 2023.

Bilić N, Djaković I, Kličan-Jaić K, Rudman SS, Ivanec Ž. Epidural analgesia in labor – controversies. Acta Clin Croat. 2015 Sep;54(3):330–6.

Chestnut DH, Wong CA, Tsen LC, Ngan Kee WD, Beilin Y, Mhyre JM, et al., editors. Chestnut's obstetric anesthesia: principles and practice. 5th ed. Elsevier Saunders: Philadelphia; 2014.

George RB, Allen TK, Habib AS. Intermittent epidural bolus compared with continuous epidural infusions for labor analgesia: a systematic review and meta-analysis. Anesth Analg. 2012;116:123–44.

Grigg PWSaddle Block Anesthesia. Available at: https://basicmedicalkey.com/saddle-block-anesthesia/ BasicmedicalKey. Assessed on 03 Apr 2023.

Gupta S, Partani S. Neuraxial techniques of labour analgesia. Indian J Anaesth. 2018;62(9):658–66.

Halliday L, Nelson SM, Kearns RJ. Epidural analgesia in labor: a narrative review. Int J Gynaecol Obstet. 2022;159(2):356–64.

Jones L, Othman M, Dowswell T, et al. Pain management for women in labour: an overview of systematic reviews. Cochrane Database Syst Rev. 2012;3:CD009234.

Kingsley C, McGlennan A, Browni J, Gill A The labour epidural: the basics. World Federation of Society of Anaesthesiologist. Obstetric Anaesthesia Tutorial 365. https://resources.wfsahq.org/wp-content/uploads/365_english.pdf. Accessed 01 Apr 2023.

Kocarev M, Khalid F, Khatoon F, Fernando R. Neuraxial labor analgesia: a focused narrative review of the 2017 literature. Curr Opin Anaesthesiol. 2018;31(3):251–7.

Lam KK, Leung MKM, Irwin MG. Labour analgesia: update and literature review. Hong Kong Med J. 2020;26(5):412–20.

Leo S, Ocampo CE, Lim Y, Sia AT. A randomized comparison of automated intermittent mandatory boluses with a basal infusion in combination with patient-controlled epidural analgesia for labor and delivery. Int J Obstet Anesth. 2010;19:357–64.

Narayanappa A, Gurulingaswamy S, Prabhakaraiah U, Kempegowda K, Hanumantharayappa NB. Practice of labor analgesia among anesthesiologists across India: cross-sectional study. Anesth Essays Res. 2018;12(3):651–6.

Novikova N, Cluver C. Local anaesthetic nerve block for pain management in labour. Cochrane Database Syst Rev. 2012;4:CD009200.

Obstetrics Anaesthetists Association. Available from: https://www.oaa-anaes.ac.uk/assets/_managed/editor/File/Guidelines/epidural%20for%20labour/Painrelief_for_labour_Swales_Southampton.pdf. Accessed 1 Apr 2023.

Onuoha OC. Epidural analgesia for labor: continuous infusion versus programmed intermittent bolus. Anesthesiol Clin. 2017;35:1–4.

Othman M, Jones L, Neilson JP. Non-opioid drugs for pain management in labour. Cochrane Database Syst Rev. 2012;7:CD009223.

Pandya ST. Labour analgesia: recent advances. Indian J Anaesth. 2010;54(5):400–8.

Shatil B, Smiley R. Neuraxial analgesia for labour. BJA Educ. 2020;20(3):96–102.

Sng BL, Sia ATH. Maintenance of epidural labour analgesia: the old, the new and the future. Best Pract Res Clin Anaesthesiol. 2017;31(1):15–22.

Ullman R, Smith LA, Burns E, Mori R, Dowswell T. Parenteral opioids for maternal pain relief in labour. Cochrane Database Syst Rev. 2010;9:CD007396.

University Hospital Wishaw Women's Services Directorate. Available from: https://nhslguidelines.scot.nhs.uk/media/1851/fetal-heart-rate-monitoring-in-labour-v2-june-2021-281021.pdf. Assessed on 1 Apr 2023.

Van de Velde M, Teunkens A, Hanssens M, Vandermeersch E, Verhaeghe J. Intrathecal sufentanil and fetal heart rate abnormalities: a double-blind, double placebo-controlled trial comparing two forms of combined spinal epidural analgesia with epidural analgesia in labor. Anesth Analg. 2004;98(4):1153–9.

Waldum ÅH, Lukasse M, Staff AC, Falk RS, Sørbye IK, Jacobsen AF. Intrapartum pudendal nerve block analgesia and childbirth experience in primiparous women with vaginal birth: a cohort study. Birth. 2023;50(1):182–91.

Wong CA. Advances in labor analgesia. Int J Women's Health. 2010;1:129–54.

Yeo ST, Holdcroft A, Yentis SM, Stewart A. Analgesia with sevoflurane during labour: determination of the optimum concentration. Br J Anaesth. 2007;98(1):105–9.

Regional Nerve Blocks for Minor Obstetrics and Gynaecological Procedures

13

Kanchan Rani and Mukesh Kumar Prasad

Abstract

In minor obstetrical and gynaecological procedures such as hysteroscopy, cervical ablation or excision, intrauterine device placement, dilatation and evacuation, perineal repair, part of labour analgesia, and in certain pain conditions such as pudendal neuralgia, vaginismus, anorectal pain, and genital pain, regional anaesthesia has a number of advantages over general anaesthesia. In addition to avoiding systemic drug side effects and airway manipulation, regional anaesthesia promotes quicker healing, better post-operative pain relief, and early hospital discharge. Pudendal nerve blocks and paracervical blocks are commonly performed for minor obstetrical and gynaecological procedures. Blocks can be performed by gynaecologists in outpatient operating rooms using landmark, PNS, or ultrasound guidance.

K. Rani (✉)
Department of Obstetrics and Gynaecology, Teerthanker Mahaveer Medical College and Research Centre, Moradabad, Uttar Pradesh, India

M. K. Prasad
Department of Anaesthesiology, Teerthanker Mahaveer Medical College and Research Centre, Moradabad, Uttar Pradesh, India
e-mail: mukeshkumar2002@gmail.com

Keywords

Pudendal nerve · Pudendal block · Paracervical block · Local anaesthesia · Minor gynaecological surgery

13.1 Pudendal Nerve Block

13.1.1 Introduction

- The sensory and motor supply to the perineum and external genitalia is primarily controlled by the mixed pudendal nerve (S2-S4) in both sexes.
- The nerve is bilateral, with branches emanating from the left and right pudendal nerves that innervate the rectal canal, anus, perineum, and external genitalia.
- A local anaesthetic injection near the trunk of the pudendal nerve at the level of the ischial spine causes analgesia in the lower vagina, posterior perineum, and vulva.

A pudendal nerve block does not totally remove sensation in the anterior part of the perineum because branches of the ilioinguinal and genitofemoral nerves supply that area. Because pudendal block does not affect the cervix or upper vagina, it is also ineffective in relieving pain caused by uterine manipulation.

M. K. Prasad, S. J. S. Bajwa (eds.), *Steps to Successful Regional Anesthesia*,
https://doi.org/10.1007/978-981-97-4098-7_13

13.1.2 Anatomy

The pudendal nerve anatomy is mentioned in Table 13.1.

13.1.3 Indications

The indications for pudendal nerve block are given in Table 13.2.

13.1.4 Contraindications

The contraindications for pudendal nerve block are given in Table 13.3.

13.1.5 Preparations

The preblock preparations for pudendal nerve block are given in Table 13.4.

13.1.6 Block Approaches

- A pudendal nerve block aims to block the nerve where it enters the lesser sciatic foramen, which is 1 cm inferior and medial to the sacrospinous ligament's attachment to the ischial spine.
- The block is usually bilateral or may be unilateral.
- The syringe is not attached until the needle has reached its final position.

Table 13.1 Pudendal nerve anatomy (Fig. 13.1)

Roots	Originates from the anterior rami of the S2, S3, and S4 spinal nerves of sacral plexus			
Course	Begins in the pelvic cavity and is situated next to the lateral wall of the pelvic cavity Exits the pelvis via the greater sciatic foramen inferior to the piriformis muscle and bends around the posterior aspect of the sacrospinous ligament before entering the perineum via the lesser sciatic foramen After exiting the lesser sciatic foramen and entering the perineum, the nerve passes through the pudendal (Alcock's) canal, a sheath of connective tissue on the medial wall of the obturator internus muscle The pudendal nerve is proximal to the ischial spine in the gluteal region, where it is the target of a pudendal nerve block Throughout most of its path, the nerve is closely associated with the branches of the internal pudendal artery and vein			
Branches		**Dorsal nerve of the penis (males) or clitoris (females)**	**Perineal nerve (superficial and deep branch)**	**Inferior rectal (anal) nerve**
Innervations/ actions [30% autonomic and 70% somatic (50% sensory and 20% motor)]	Motor	Muscles involved in penile and clitoral erection and ejaculation in males	Superficial and deep perineal muscle, bulbospongiosus, ischiocavernosus, urethral sphincter, anterior part of external anal sphincter, and some part of levator ani	Levator ani muscle External anal sphincter
	Sensory	Erectile tissue of corpus cavernosum and crus of penis/ clitoris Skin over dorsolateral aspect of foreskin, glans, and penis/ clitoris	Lower third of vagina and urethra Posterior portion of perineal skin and scrotum/ labia majora and minora	Anal circumference skin Caudal third of rectum Posterior vulva
	Autonomic	Erection initiation and maintenance (parasympathetic)	Conscious awareness of need to urinate	Conscious awareness of need to defecate

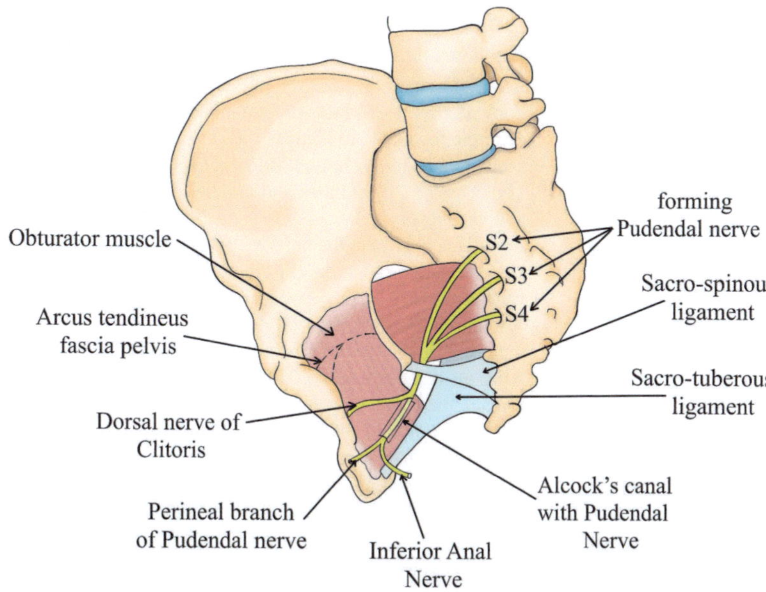

Fig. 13.1 Pudendal nerve anatomy

Table 13.2 Indications for pudendal nerve block

Operative/acute pain	Chronic pain (diagnosis and treatment)
Operative vaginal delivery Outlet instrument delivery (obstetrics forceps) Perineal repair Labour analgesic for the second stage of labour when neuraxial anaesthesia is contraindicated Procedure on lower vagina or posterior perineum	Pudendal neuralgia Vaginismus Anorectal pain Genital pain Proctalgia fugax

Table 13.3 Contraindications for pudendal nerve block

Absolute	Relative
Allergy to local anaesthetic Skin and soft tissue infections at the injection site	Uncorrected coagulopathies Prior surgery in the area with changed local anatomy

Table 13.4 Preblock preparations for pudendal nerve block

Pre-requisites	Equipment/materials required
Informed consent NPO status Optimal sedation if necessary Emergency, resuscitation drugs, and equipment Secure IV access Monitoring (HR, NIBP, Spo2, ECG, RR, etc.) and oxygen supply Site and side of block should be marked and confirmed	Sterile towels 10–20 mL syringes with local anaesthetic Sterile gloves, marking pen, and surface electrode One 1.5 in., 25-gauge needle for skin infiltration A 5-cm long, 21–22 gauge short-bevel, insulated stimulating needle Injection pressure monitor Low frequency curvilinear (2-5 MHz) probe, sterile sleeve, and gel Local anaesthetic

13.1.6.1 Landmark/PNS-Guided Approach

The Transvaginal Approach

- This approach is common for obstetric and gynaecological procedures. Usually, 10 mL is used each side, but this varies.

The transvaginal approach to pudendal nerve block is mentioned in Table 13.5.

The Transperineal Approach

This approach is used for

Table 13.5 The transvaginal approach to pudendal nerve block

Position	Lithotomy position
Landmark technique, POE, and end point (Fig. 13.2)	After all aseptic preparation, palpate the posterolateral vaginal sidewall and identify bony protrusion (ischial spine) that differ from the rest of the sidewall (**Tip**: If the examiner is unable to identify the ischial spines, palpate the firm band of the sacrospinous ligament and follow it laterally from the sacrum to the ischial spine) The operator's right index and middle fingers are used to palpate the right ischial spine and vice versa Introduce and direct the needle guide under fingers to reach ischial spine Needle guide is positioned 1 cm medial and inferior to the ischial spine, against the vaginal mucosa on the sacrospinous ligament The spinal needle is inserted into needle guide and advanced through the vaginal mucosa into the sacrospinous ligament, a distance of about 1 cm After negative aspiration, 3 mL of local anaesthetic is injected into the ligament Finally, the needle is gently advanced until resistance caused by the ligament is gone. The needle should now be inserted into the loose areolar tissue behind the ligament, which contains the pudendal nerve The remaining 7 mL of anaesthetic is injected after negative aspiration (**Tip**: The pudendal and inferior gluteal vessels lie adjacent to the pudendal nerve so any positive aspiration indirectly confirms the approximate position of nerve and drug can be deposited after repositioning the needle) Same procedure is repeated for the other side
Needle	A 10 cm spinal needle with needle guide
End point	Loss of anal wink reflex
Drug dosage	10 mL of local anaesthetic (individual or in combination) Surgical anaesthesia: 0.5–0.75% ropivacaine, 0.25–0.5% bupivacaine,0.25–0.5% levobupivacaine, 1–2% lidocaine with or without epinephrine Analgesia: 0.2–0.375% ropivacaine, 0.125–0.25% bupivacaine, 0.125–0.25% levobupivacaine,0.5%–1% lidocaine with or without epinephrine)

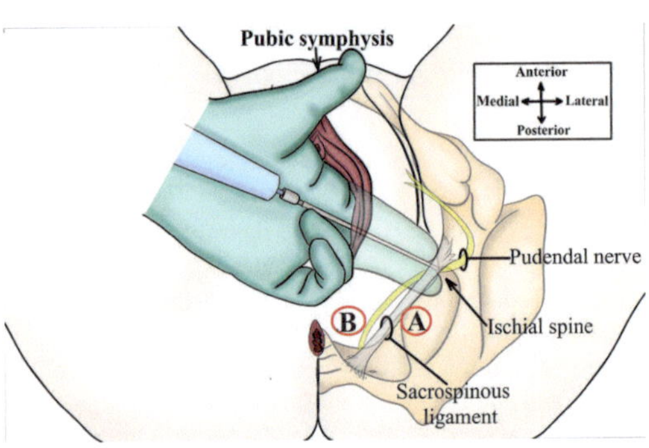

Fig. 13.2 Landmark-guided pudendal nerve block (transvaginal approach), (**a**) POE for the transperineal approach to pudendal nerve block (**b**) POE for the perirectal approach to pudendal nerve block)

- Anorectal and urological procedures, as well as pudendal neuralgia in men.
- The descent of the presenting part may block the vaginal route for the guiding finger, which is the primary indication for the transperineal approach.
- It is preferable to use ultrasound imaging guidance for this approach.

  The transperineal approach to pudendal nerve block is given in Table 13.6.

Perirectal Approach

- Most commonly used for anorectal procedure and pudendal neuralgia.

  The perirectal approach to pudendal nerve block is given in Table 13.7.

13.1.6.2 Ultrasound-Guided Pudendal Nerve Block

- Ultrasound imaging enables the needle pathway to the target to be guided more precisely while avoiding any damage to the nearby structures.

Anterior Approach

It was first reported by Parras and Blanco in 2013.

Table 13.6 The transperineal approach to pudendal nerve block

Position	Lithotomy position
Landmark technique and POE (Fig. 13.2)	After all aseptic preparation, palpate the ischial spine by inserting index finger into vagina or rectum The skin entry point is 2.5 cm posteromedial to the ischial tuberosity, overlying the ischiorectal fossa which is identified by palpation or under ultrasound guidance The needle is advanced lateral to the clinician's finger in the posterolateral direction until it reaches the ischial spine Needle is positioned 1 cm medial and inferior to the ischial spine through the sacrospinous ligament After negative aspiration, 3 mL of local anaesthetic is injected into the ligament Finally, the needle is gently advanced until loss of resistance is encountered marking complete penetration of the ligament The needle should now be inserted into the loose areolar tissue behind the ligament, which contains the pudendal nerve The remaining 7 mL of anaesthetic is injected after negative aspiration Same procedure is repeated for the other side
Needle	A 10 cm spinal needle
End point	Loss of anal wink reflex or pinprick sensory test in the anogenital area
Drug dosage	Same as in transvaginal approach

Table 13.7 The perirectal approach to pudendal nerve block

Position	Recumbent position
Landmark technique, POE, and end point (Fig. 13.2)	After all aseptic preparation, palpate the ischial spine by inserting index finger into the rectum (or vagina) The needle is inserted lateral to rectum and advanced lateral to the clinician's finger in the posterolateral direction until it reaches the ischial spine Needle is positioned 1 cm medial and inferior to the ischial spine through the sacrospinous ligament After negative aspiration, 3 mL of local anaesthetic is injected into the ligament (optional) Finally, the needle is gently advanced until loss of resistance is encountered marking complete penetration of the ligament The needle should now be inserted into the loose areolar tissue behind the ligament, which contains the pudendal nerve The local anaesthetic is injected after negative aspiration Same procedure is repeated for the other side
Needle	A 10 cm spinal needle or insulated needle
PNS stimulation	Current intensity started at 1.5 mA (2 Hz, 0.1–0.3 ms) and decreased to 0.4–0.5 mA (can be used)
End point	Maximal anal sphincteric tone if nerve stimulation is used or loss of anal wink reflex or pinprick sensory test in the anogenital area
Drug dosage	Same as in transvaginal approach

USG-guided anterior approach for pudendal nerve block is mentioned in Table 13.8.

Posterior/Transgluteal Approach

USG-guided posterior/transgluteal approach for pudendal nerve block is mentioned in Table 13.9.

13.1.7 Efficacy

- Analgesia starts within 5 min, elicited by pinching the lower vagina and posterior vulva.
- Maximum effects occur after 10–20 min and lasts for 30–60 min.

13.1.8 Troubleshooting

- The most common reason for block failure is not allowing enough time for the anaesthetic to take effect.
- In case of unilateral block, additional 5 mL of LA is injected into the unanesthetized side.

Table 13.8 USG-guided pudendal nerve block (anterior approach)

Position	Lithotomy position
Landmark (Fig. 13.3a, b)	After skin asepsis, sterile transducer preparation, and required sedation, the linear US transducer (10–15 MHz) is kept lateral to the vulvar/scrotal junction with the rectum, in an oblique sagittal or transverse position Identify the ischiopubic ramus of the ischial tuberosity on lateral side of transducer Identify the small hyperechoic structures of approximately 3 mm in diameter as pudendal nerve (Tips: Since nerve diameter is very small, it is difficult to identify it. Switching on colour Doppler helps in identifying internal pudendal artery which helps in identifying pudendal nerve simultaneously)
POE	Needle is inserted either in-plane from medial side of probe or out-of-plane (Fig. 13.3a, b)
Needle	Blunt 22G, 50 mm neurostimulation needle inserted in-plane or out-of-plane towards the target
PNS stimulation	Current intensity started at 1.5 mA (2 Hz, 0.1–0.3 ms) and decreased to 0.4–0.5 mA
End point	The contraction of the anal sphincter or of the peripheral perineal structures in proximity to the neural structure (tips: Since pudendal nerve is smaller in size and is mixed nerve with lower percentage of motor fibres so neurostimulation may not be 100% reliable. In the absence of neurostimulation, drug is deposited around internal pudendal artery after negative aspiration)
Drug dosage	Same as in transvaginal approach

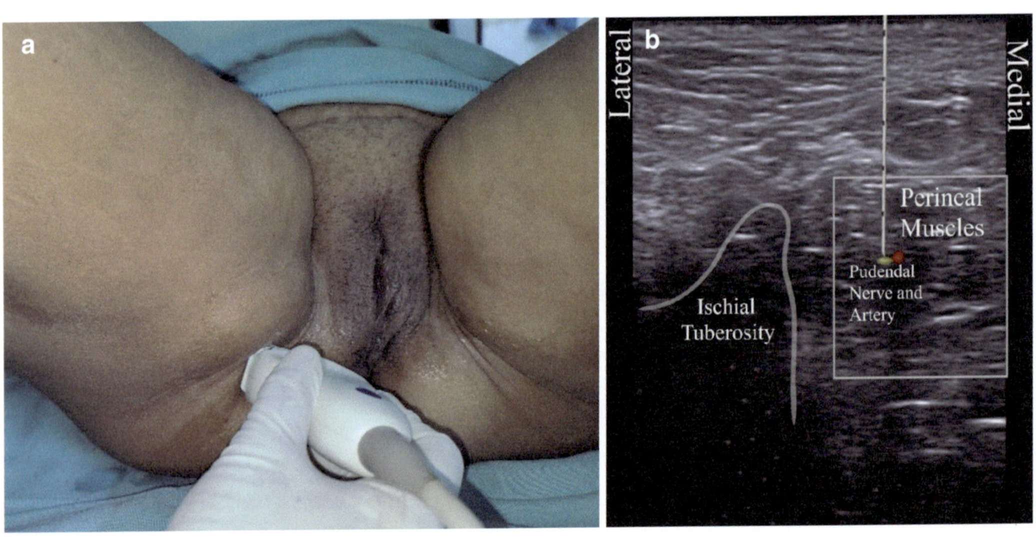

Fig. 13.3 (**a**) Probe position for pudendal nerve block. (**b**) Ultrasound image showing pudendal nerve and vessels

Table 13.9 USG-guided pudendal nerve block (posterior/transgluteal approach)

Position	Prone position or lateral decubitus position
Landmark (Fig. 13.4a)	After skin asepsis, sterile transducer preparation, and required sedation, the curvilinear US transducer (2–5 MHz) is kept transversally, starting scan from PSIS towards caudal and lateral direction **At PSIS level** (Fig. 13.4a–c) – Iliac crest with 3 layers of gluteus seen (maximus, medius, and minimus posterior to anterior) **At sciatic notch** (Fig. 13.4a,d,e) – Ischium appears as curved structure as it forms posterior wall of acetabulum – Identify two muscles: Gluteus maximus posterior and piriformis anterior – Sciatic nerve and inferior gluteal artery are seen anterior/deep to piriformis **At level of ischial spine** (Fig. 13.4a,f,g) – Ischium spine becomes straight and hyperechoic – Sacrospinous ligament appears as hyperechoic line medial to ischium (SSL does not cast an anechoic structure as compared to bone) – Piriformis disappears – Internal pudendal artery can be identified on medial portion of ischial spine – The pudendal nerve will lie medial to the pudendal artery at this level between sacrospinous and sacrotuberous ligaments
POE	Needle is inserted from medial side of probe (Tip: Needle can be inserted from lateral side of probe when probe scanning starts from midpoint of greater trochanter and the posterior superior iliac spine identifying continuous hyperechoic line of iliac bone and then parallel and caudal to lesser sciatic notch where pudendal nerve and vessels can be seen)
Needle	10–15 cm needle inserted in in-plane technique from medial to lateral direction
End point	Needle tip between sacrotuberous and sacrospinous ligament with adequate local anaesthetic spread within the interligamentous plane
Drug dosage	Same as in transvaginal approach

- The pudendal block has no effect on pain in the anterior perineum, upper vagina, or cervix, and subcutaneous infiltration of LA is needed in these areas.

13.1.9 Complications

Although complications are uncommon, potential complications include:

- **Hematoma**
- **Infection:** A localized infection can spread into the retro-psoas space, gluteal muscle, or hip joint less frequently.
- **Nerve injury:** Ischial region paresthesias or sacral neuropathy can occur.
- Urinary or faecal incontinence and numbness in the pudendal nerve area.
- **Systemic toxicity:** Intravenous administration can cause local anaesthetic systemic toxicity (LAST).
- **Neonatal anaesthetic toxicity:** Neonatal anaesthetic toxicity after maternal pudendal block is extremely rare. Neonatal lidocaine intoxication can lead to transient hypotonia, apnea, seizures, mydriasis, cyanosis, and the need for mechanical ventilation.

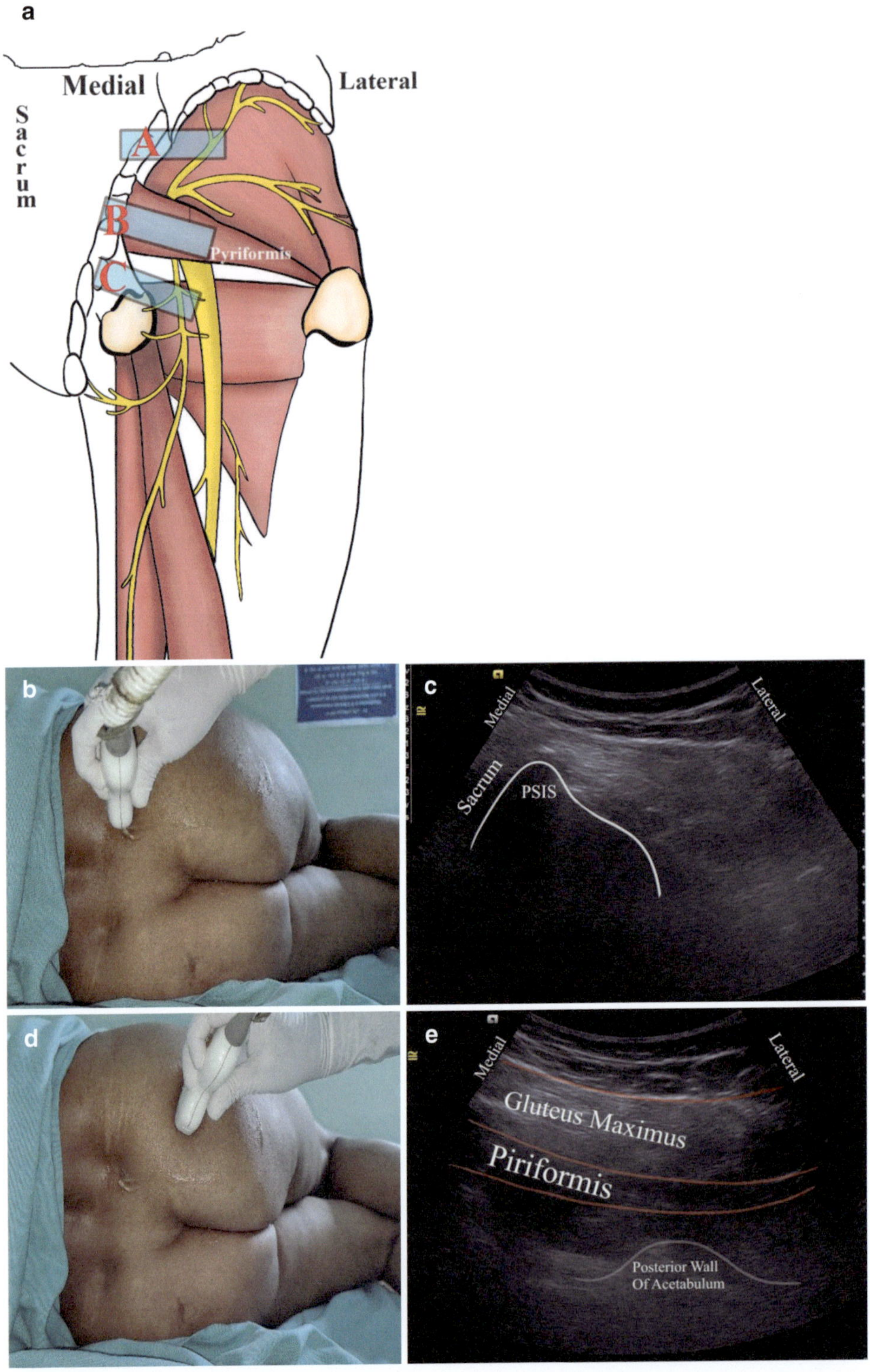

Fig. 13.4 (**a**) Schematic representation and different probe positions during USG-guided pudendal nerve block. (**b**) Probe position (A) at PSIS level. (**c**) USG image at PSIS level (A). (**d**) Probe position (B) at sciatic notch. (**e**) Probe position and USG image at sciatic notch (B). (**f**) Probe position (C) at ischial spine. (**g**) USG image at ischial spine(C)

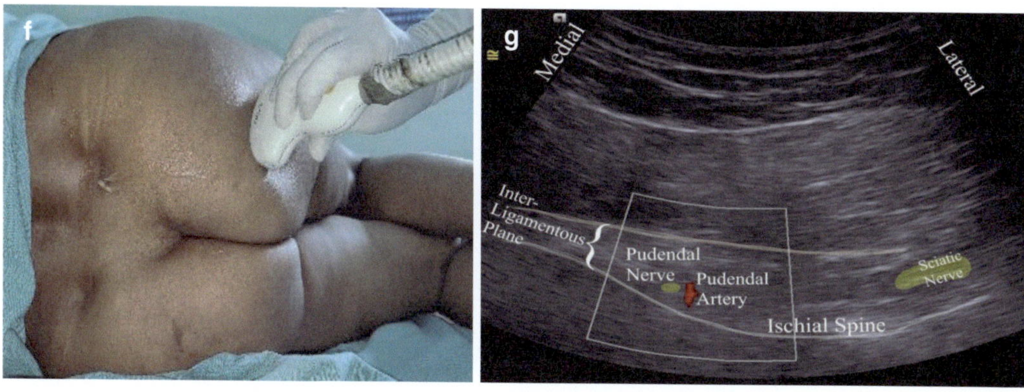

Fig. 13.4 (continued)

13.2 Paracervical Block

13.2.1 Introduction

- Paracervical block is most frequently used to provide analgesia during gynaecologic procedures involving cervical dilation or manipulation.
- It prevents pain transmission via sympathetic, parasympathetic, and visceral sensory fibres before they enter the uterus at the internal os. Motor pathway and perineal sensation remain intact.

13.2.2 Anatomy

- The uterovaginal (or Frankenhäuser) plexus, which is made up of fibres from the inferior hypogastric (pelvic) plexus (T10-L1) and sacral nerve roots, innervates the upper vagina, cervix, and lower uterus (S1-S4).
- It is located just lateral to the cervix and uterus.

13.2.3 Indications

The indications for paracervical nerve block are given in Table 13.10.

13.2.4 Preparations

The preblock preparations for paracervical nerve block are mentioned in Table 13.11.

13.2.5 Local Anaesthetics Choice

- **For gynaecological procedures:** LA with vasoconstrictor is preferred.
- 1% lidocaine and 0.5% ropivacaine are most commonly used with epinephrine (1:200,000 or 5 mcg/mL) or vasopressin (3–5 units in 10–20 mL of LA). However, these adjuvants should be used cautiously in hypertensive patients and coronary artery disease with heart diseases.

Table 13.10 Indications for paracervical nerve block

Gynaecologic procedures	Obstetric procedure
Hysteroscopy Cervical ablation or excision Intrauterine device placement	Manual vacuum aspiration (MVA) Dilatation and evacuation Labour pain management when there is not a safer alternative available during the active phase of labour

Table 13.11 Preblock preparations for paracervical nerve block

Pre-requisites	Equipment/materials required
Informed consent Emergency, resuscitation drugs and equipment Secure IV access Monitoring (HR, NIBP, Spo2, ECG, RR, etc.) and oxygen supply	10–20 mL syringes with local anaesthetic Sterile gloves A 23G 8–10 cm needle Local anaesthetic

- Various doses were used ranging from 50 mg to 200 mg. Typically, 100–200 mg is used.
- **For obstetric procedures:** LA without vasoconstrictor is preferred.
- Amide-type anaesthetics is preferable in obstetrics patients as only small amounts of non-metabolized drug reach the foetus.
- Bupivacaine may be avoided due to its association with foetal death and cardiac toxicity in healthy adults.

13.2.6 Paracervical Block for Gynaecological and Minor Obstetrics Procedure

13.2.6.1 Block Approach

Landmark-guided paracervical block is given in Table 13.12.

13.2.6.2 Efficacy of Block

- Onset of analgesia occurs within minutes of injection which decreases with increased concentrations.
- It is recommended to wait for 3–4 min following the injection.

13.2.6.3 Tips

- With longer injection cannula (80 mm), it is easier to reach the sacrouterine ligaments and causes less discomfort to patient.

Table 13.12 Landmark-guided paracervical block

Position	Lithotomy position
Landmark technique and POE (Fig. 13.5)	After all aseptic preparation of cervix and vaginal vault, vaginal speculum and tenaculum are used for optimal exposure Commonly LA is injected either at two-point (at **4 and 8 o'clock**) or four-point (at **2, 4, 8, and 10 o'clock**) into the cervicovaginal junction
Needle	A 23G 8–10 cm needle
End point	LA is injected at least 1 cm into the cervical stroma at the cervicovaginal junction
Drug dosage	Regardless of the number of injection sites, 10–20 mL of LA is used

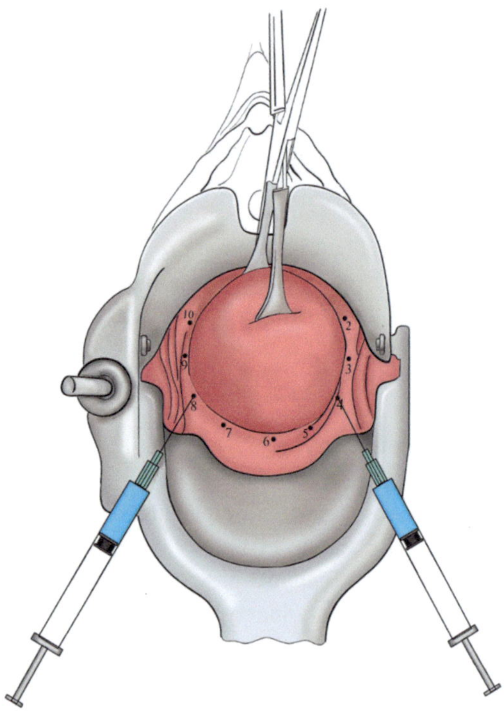

Fig. 13.5 Paracervical block at 4 and 8 O′ clock position)

- Deeper injections (2–3 cm) provide better analgesia.
- Always aspirate prior to infiltration.

- Reposition of needle in case of intravascular placement of needle.
- If there is excessive resistance, withdraw the needle for a few millimetres and reposition it.
- The two-point technique seems equally effective to four-point technique.

13.2.6.4 Complications

Paracervical block complications are uncommon

- Bleeding from the puncture site.
- Hematoma formation.
- Infection.
- Local anaesthetic systemic toxicity (LAST) due to intravascular injection.
- Drowsiness and ringing in the ears, confusion, seizure, coma, and ventricular arrhythmia can occur.
- Vasovagal syncope: Ineffective paracervical block can result in vasovagal syncope.

13.2.6.5 Paracervical Block for Labour Analgesia

- Paracervical block can be used to reduce the pain associated with cervical dilation during the active phase of labour when no safer alternative is available.
- It is administered only during active labour, when cervical dilatation is between 4 and 8 cm. If administered before 4 cm, there is possible risk of overdosing because of repeated administrations.
- It is not recommended beyond 8 cm of dilatation due to increased procedural complexity, decreased efficacy, and a greater potential for foetal bradycardia induction.

Further Reading

Anderson D. Pudendal nerve block for vaginal birth. J Midwife Women's Health. 2014;59(6):651–9.

Dokken K, Fairley P. Sodium channel blocker toxicity. In: StatPearls [Internet]. Treasure Island (FL): StatPearls Publishing; 2023.

Ghanavatian S, Leslie SW, Derian A. Pudendal nerve block. In: StatPearls [Internet]. Treasure Island (FL): StatPearls Publishing; 2023.

Hoffman BL, Schorge JO, Bradshaw KD, et al. Intraoperative considerations. In: Williams gynecology. 3rd ed. McGraw Hill Education; 2016. p. 842.

https://www.ipas.org/clinical-update/english/pain-management/paracervical-block. Last reviewed: January 26, 2022.

Kapp N, Lohr PA. Modern methods to induce abortion: safety, efficacy and choice. Best Pract Res Clin Obstet Gynaecol. 2020;63:37–44.

Kaur J, Leslie SW, Singh P. Pudendal nerve entrapment syndrome. In: StatPearls [Internet]. Treasure Island (FL): StatPearls Publishing; 2023.

Kim S, Song SG, Paek OJ, Lee HJ, Park DH, Lee JK. Nerve-stimulator-guided pudendal nerve block by pararectal approach. Color Dis. 2012;14(5):611–5.

Kinter KJ, Newton BW. Anatomy, abdomen and pelvis, pudendal nerve. In: StatPearls [Internet]. Treasure Island (FL): StatPearls Publishing; 2023.

NCBI Bookshelf. A service of the national library of medicine, National Institutes of Health. StatPearls [Internet]. Treasure Island (FL): StatPearls Publishing; 2022.

Neal JM, et al. ASRA practice advisory on local anesthetic systemic toxicity. Reg Anesth Pain Med. 2010;35(2):152–61.

Neis F, Wallwiener D, Henes M, Krämer B, Brucker S. Opinion paper: gynecological surgery in local anesthesia? Arch Gynecol Obstet. 2022;306(4):1063–8.

Novikova N, Cluver C. Local anaesthetic nerve block for pain management in labour. Cochrane Database Syst Rev. 2012;2012(4):CD009200.

Renner RM, Jensen JT, Nichols MD, Edelman AB. Pain control in first-trimester surgical abortion: a systematic review of randomized controlled trials. Contraception. 2010;81(5):372–88.

Rojas-Gómez MF, et al. Regional anesthesia guided by ultrasound in the pudendal nerve territory. Col J Anesthesiol. 2017;45(3):200–9.

Tangsiriwatthana T, Sangkomkamhang US, Lumbiganon P, Laopaiboon M. Paracervical local anaesthesia for cervical dilatation and uterine intervention. Cochrane Database Syst Rev. 2013;30(9):CD005056.

Wolman I. Berek and Novak's gynecology 15th edition. J Obstet Gynecol India. 2014;64(2):150–1.

Re-emerging Techniques in Anaesthesia

14

Harkomal Kaur and Mukesh Kumar Prasad

Abstract

With modern medical infrastructure increasing the safety of surgical procedures, many anaesthesia techniques have been brought to mainstream practice from the archives. Most notable of these are segmental spinal anaesthesia and Bier block or intravenous regional anaesthesia. In the past, these techniques were not favoured due to increased side effects, meagre monitoring and safer alternatives. In the light of new research and advent of modern monitoring devices, these devices are re-emerging as acceptable alternatives to the existing techniques. Segmental spinal anaesthesia or thoracic spinal anaesthesia can be highly beneficial in patients in whom general anaesthesia is contraindicated. Likewise, Bier block can be utilised in emergency settings when and where situations might not be favourable for immediate general anaesthesia. Another such procedure that has gained its foothold in the cosmetic dermatosurgical procedures is tumescent anaesthesia. It has found application beyond fat removing surgeries and is now used for various other outpatient dermatological procedures including hair transplants. These techniques need to be included in the present-day curriculum to explore their use beyond what they were originally meant for.

Keywords

Bier block · WALANT · Tumescent · Segmental spinal

14.1 Introduction

Advances in modern anaesthesia and increased safety due to monitoring have brought many unorthodox and dated techniques into the forefront. These techniques provide an alternative to the mainstream general and regional anaesthesia and provide a safer alternative in the patients who have increased risk pertaining the routine modes of anaesthesia. The most noteworthy of these techniques are intravenous regional anaesthesia (IVRA), tumescent anaesthesia and segmental spinal anaesthesia. In this chapter, we discuss the techniques with their new found applications and advantages in modern anaesthesia practice.

H. Kaur (✉)
Department of Anaesthesiology, Nalanda Medical College and Hospital, Patna, Bihar, India

M. K. Prasad
Department of Anaesthesiology, Teerthanker Mahaveer Medical College and Research Centre, Moradabad, Uttar Pradesh, India
e-mail: mukeshkumar2002@gmail.com

M. K. Prasad, S. J. S. Bajwa (eds.), *Steps to Successful Regional Anesthesia*,
https://doi.org/10.1007/978-981-97-4098-7_14

14.2 Bier Block

German surgeon, August Bier introduced intravenous regional anaesthesia or Bier block in 1908. The simplicity of this block, the minimal learning curve and safety under monitored settings have made this technique relevant in a number of surgical and pain management procedures.

14.2.1 Mechanism of Action

In Bier block, the local anaesthetic is given into the vein directly in the upper or lower extremity after exsanguinating the area involved by means of a tourniquet. The mechanism of action is by two routes:

(a) **Direct anaesthesia** or peripheral infiltration block due to the nerves directly immersed in the local anaesthetic.
(b) **Indirect anaesthesia** or conduction block caused due to infiltration of the local anaesthetic into the substance of nerves via the vasa vasorum.

14.2.2 Indications

- Brief surgical procedures of the extremities lasting less than 1 h.
- Upper limb: Dupuytren contracture release, carpal tunnel release, ganglionectomy, reduction of fractures distal in position.
- Lower limb surgeries: Excision of mass, digital nerve repair, foot or ankle surgeries less than 45 min in duration.

14.2.3 Contraindications

- Crush injury
- Inability to locate or maintain a peripheral line
- Allergy to local anaesthetic
- Compound fractures
- Cellulitis or local skin infection
- Previous arteriovenous shunt
- Surgery longer than 1 h
- Peripheral vascular disease
- Sickle cell disease

14.2.4 Technique

Equipment Required

- Standard ASA monitors and resuscitation equipment
- 20 or 22 gauge intravenous cannula
- Two pneumatic tourniquets of appropriate size
- Esmarch bandage (60 cm long and 10 cm wide)
- 30 or 50 mL syringe
- Adhesive tapes
- Appropriate local anaesthetic in adequate concentration

14.2.4.1 Upper Extremity Bier Block

1. Intravenous catheter is secured into a peripheral vein as distally as possible. The preferred veins are the veins in the dorsum of the hand.
2. The double pneumatic tourniquet is placed around the biceps area with the proximal cuff higher on the upper arm (Fig. 14.1).
3. Elevate the entire arm to passively exsanguinate the arm. Drape the Esmarch bandage from the fingertips of the hand till the distal cuff.
4. Inflate the proximal pneumatic cuff 50–100 mmHg above the systolic blood pressure. The axillary artery is occluded digitally beforehand (Fig. 14.2).
5. Remove the Esmarch bandage after the cuff inflation and inject 30–50 mL of 0.5% lignocaine into the indwelling intravenous catheter (Fig. 14.3).
6. The intravenous cannula is withdrawn and pressure applied using sterile gauge.

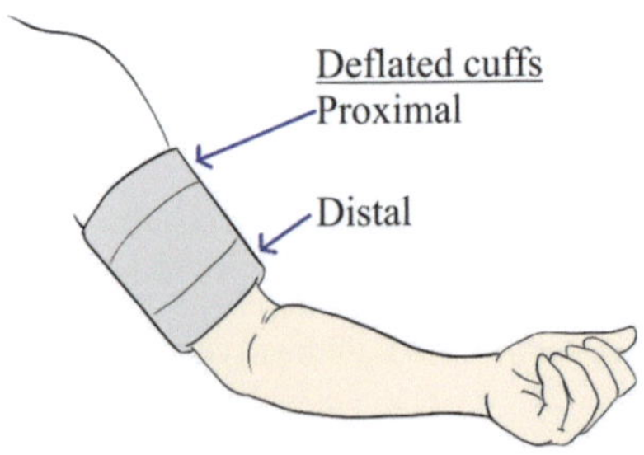

Fig. 14.1 Proximal and distal cuff

7. After 25–30 min of onset of analgesia or when the patient complains of the tourniquet pain, the distal cuff is inflated and the proximal cuff is released (Figs. 14.4 and 14.5).

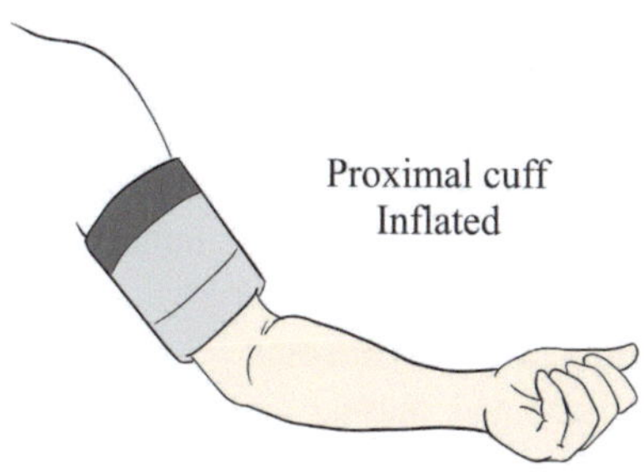

Fig. 14.2 Inflated proximal cuff

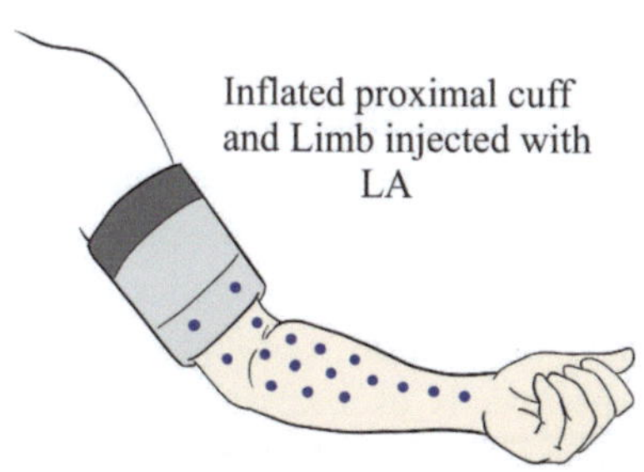

Fig. 14.3 Inflated proximal cuff with LA injected

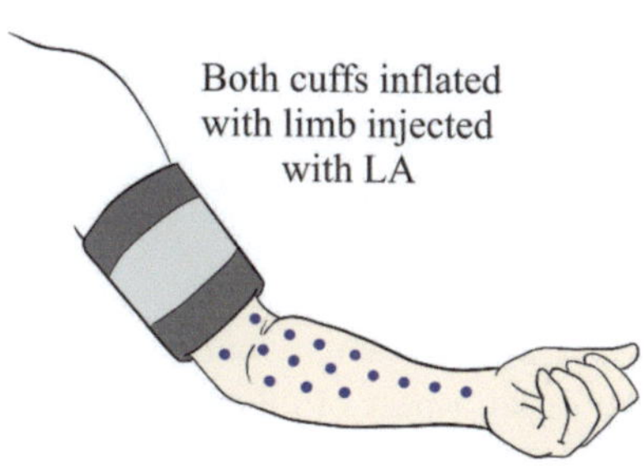

Fig. 14.4 Both cuffs inflated with LA injected

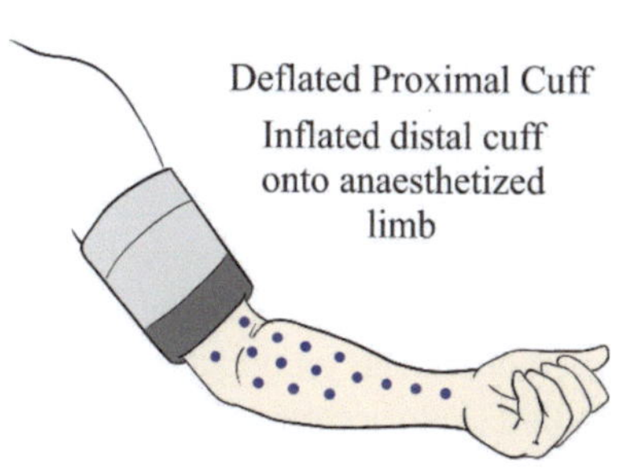

Fig. 14.5 Inflated distal cuff with LA injected

14.2.4.2 Lower Extremity Block

The only difference in the lower extremity block is that the larger venous compartment requires larger volume of dose, i.e. 100 mL versus 50 mL.

14.2.4.3 Drugs Used

Local Anaesthetics

- Lignocaine HCl 0.5%
  - Most common
  - Onset in 4–5 min
  - Termination of anaesthesia after tourniquet deflation: 5–6 min
  - Maximum dosage: 3 mg/kg
- Prilocaine 0.5% with maximum dosage up to 3–4 mg/kg
- Ropivacaine 0.3% or 1.2 mg/kg
- Bupivacaine 0.25%

Adjuvants to Local Anaesthesia in IVRA

Various adjuvants have been used to enhance the analgesia, improve the sensory and motor outcomes as enumerated below.

1. **Alpha-2 agonists**: Clonidine and dexmedetomidine both have been successfully added to the local anaesthetic solution for IVRA. Clonidine in a dose of 2 micrograms/kg decreases tourniquet pain. However, no significant effect on the onset or duration of the sensory or motor block has been seen. Dexmedetomidine, however, significantly decreases the sensory onset and prolongs the duration of analgesia in a dose of 0.5micrograms/kg. This effect can be attributed to the fact that dexmedetomidine is more selective towards alpha-adrenoreceptors.
2. **Opioids:** Addition of opioids like fentanyl and tramadol has been found beneficial in decreasing the tourniquet pain and in lowering the concentration of local anaesthetic preventing its potential toxicity.
3. **Muscle relaxants:** Atracurium has been successfully added in a dosage of 2 mg to the IVRA solution. It has been shown to provide muscle relaxation and easier reduction of fractures in hand and forearm surgeries.
4. **Neostigmine:** Neostigmine (0.5–1 mg) has shown analgesic properties when added with IVRA.

5. **Nonsteroidal anti-inflammatory analgesics**: NSAIDs such as ketorolac (0.3 mg/kg) and tenoxicam have provided better analgesic outcomes when combined with 0.5% lignocaine.
6. **Nitroglycerine:** The ability of NTG to modulate pain in the central and peripheral nervous system is due to increase in the intracellular cyclic GMP that may aid in shortening the onset of anaesthesia. Its vasodilatory properties may also contribute to the increased uptake of local anaesthetic.
7. **Corticosteroids:** Steroid IVRA has been used in complex regional pain syndrome type I. Methylprednisolone 40 mg is added to 40 mL of 0.5% lignocaine to achieve the desired effect.
8. **Sympatholytic drugs**: Intravenous regional administration of guanethidine and reserpine inhibits sympathetic activity in the isolated area. This effect has been utilised in the treatment of reflex sympathetic dystrophy, rheumatoid arthritis, frostbite and CRPS. Guanethidine may produce hypotension and is to be used carefully in patients susceptible to angina.

Deflation of Tourniquet

The tourniquet is not deflated before 30 min even when the surgery ends before that time as a rule. The distal tourniquet is clamped off and patient is monitored in the PACU till 30 min are completed. Following which the tourniquet is deflated in a cyclical manner to avoid any systemic toxicity of the drugs. The patient must be monitored for at least 15 min following tourniquet declamping.

Cyclical Tourniquet Deflation Technique

The cuff is deflated and immediately reinflated, and the signs of any systemic toxicity are observed. If no signs of systemic toxicity occur after 1 min, the cuff is deflated and again reinflated for 1–2 min. If no signs of systemic local anaesthetic toxicity occur, the cuff is deflated and removed from the extremity.

14.2.4.4 Complications

Drug Related

- Systemic toxicity of local anaesthetics
- Methemoglobinemia with use of prilocaine
- Adjuvant related

Tourniquet Related

- **Tourniquet pain**
- **Nerve injury:** Injury to median, ulnar and radial nerve due to direct compression by the tourniquet
- **Compartment syndrome**
- Capillary and muscle damage due to tissue acidosis

14.2.4.5 Recent Modifications and Applications

Modified Forearm Bier Block

The single forearm tourniquet procedure or MFBB was introduced as an effective method for short forearm and hand surgeries. The major advantage of forearm tourniquet technique is decreased toxicity of local anaesthetic as lower volumes are required. MFBB was earlier not favoured due to assumption that local anaesthetic toxicity may occur through the intraosseous vasculature. However, over a period of time, studies have ruled out the risk as minimal and have suggested it to be a safe alternative to the conventional technique.

Technique

In this procedure, a single tourniquet is applied over the distal aspect of elbow as per standard tourniquet recommendations. Intravenous local anaesthetic is then injected into the vein.

The most commonly used local anaesthetic is 0.5%lignocaine in a dosage of 1.5 mg/kg. The maximum volume used is up to 25 mL which is almost half of the conventional volume.

Tourniquet time: The tourniquet can be removed immediately after the surgery due to low volume of local anaesthetic and hence no fear of toxicity. The average tourniquet time has been found to be 11 min according to recent studies.

Advantages Over Bier block

- Lesser tourniquet pain leading to decreased requirement of sedation
- Decreased risk of local anaesthetic toxicity
- Lesser tourniquet time

14.2.5 Wide Awake Local Anaesthesia No Tourniquet (WALANT) Hand Surgery

A newer addition to the spectrum of local aesthetic blocks is the WALANT hand surgery technique that requires no sedation or tourniquet and is indicated for short-hand and distal forearm surgeries. This technique was introduced by Canadian plastic surgeon Dr. Lalonde in 2005.

14.2.5.1 Indications

- Hand surgery in patients with comorbidities who are at higher risk of general anaesthesia.
- Patient with contraindications to tourniquet like ESRD with AV fistula.
- Short outpatient minor procedures for ambulatory surgery.

14.2.5.2 Contraindications

Absolute

- Lack of consent
- Uncooperative patient

Relative

- Hypercoagulable state
- Lidocaine hypersensitivity
- Infection
- Anxious
- Peripheral vascular disease
- Polytrauma

14.2.5.3 Technique

This technique requires mixing an amide local aesthetic with epinephrine for haemostasis. The analgesic haemostat mixture comprises 1% lignocaine with 1:100.00 epinephrine with 8.4% sodium bicarbonate (1 mL in per 10 mL of lignocaine epinephrine solution} optionally.

The solution is administered approximately 30 min prior to incision. Phentolamine 1gm in 10 mL of 0.9% normal saline may be needed if epinephrine reversal is required.

The infiltrations done are as follows:

- **Carpal tunnel release:** Administer a 10 mL injection located 5 mm above the wrist crease and 5 mm towards the ulnar side of the median nerve. Additionally, inject another 10 mL deeply at the site of the incision.
- **Dupuytren's contracture:** Inject 10 mL into the palm, followed by 2 mL into the proximal phalanx and 2 mL into the middle phalanx.
- **Trigger finger:** Inject 4 mL into the subcutaneous tissue located just beneath the incision site. Be cautious to avoid injecting into the sheath.
- **ORIF distal radius:** Inject 5 mL into the area of the distal radius fracture. Administer 10 mL into either the volar or dorsal region of the distal radius. Utilise a more concentrated solution of 1% lidocaine–epinephrine at a ratio of 1:40,000 due to the need for increased haemostasis during the procedure. In the case of volar plating, inject 5 mL into the pronator quadratus. For dorsal plating, inject 5 mL underneath the extensor retinaculum.
- **Finger sensory block:** Inject 2 mL into either the dorsal or volar side of the proximal phalanx, positioned distal to the crease between the finger and palm.
- **Metacarpal fractures:** Administer a total of 40 mL around the circumference of the metacarpal bone.

14.2.5.4 Advantages

- This procedure can be done on an outpatient basis.
- Short, easy to administer, suitable for ambulatory surgery.
- Prevent stiffness and adhesion formation as patient participation and mobilisation start very early.

14.2.5.5 Complications

- Vasovagal response
- Anxiety

Rare complications are:

- Inadequate anaesthesia needing lignocaine supplementation
- Epinephrine-induced cardiac ischemia
- Seizures and altered mentation
- Bupivacaine-induced cardiotoxicity

14.3 Tumescent Anaesthesia

The word tumescent translates to swollen or firm or tense. In tumescent (local) anaesthesia (TLA/TA), dilute local anaesthetic is infiltrated into the subcutaneous tissue till it becomes tense providing a painless and relatively bloodless plane for the surgical procedure. Its application was earlier limited to liposuction alone, but it has now found acceptance in varied surgical procedures, such as plastic surgery and dermatosurgical. Its advantages include prolonged anaesthesia extending into postoperative period, decreased blood loss due to vasoconstriction by adrenaline and its relative safety in monitored care.

14.3.1 Indications

Various indications for tumescent anaesthesia are mentioned in Table 14.1.

Table 14.1 Indications for tumescent anaesthesia

Plastic surgery	**Surgical indications**
Liposuction	Endovenous laser therapy for varicose veins
Anaesthesia for post-burn contractures and scars	Mastectomy with axillary lymph node dissection
Breast surgeries for augmentation, reduction	Post-burn contracture release in adult as well paediatric patients
Dermatosurgical indications:	Tumescent technique for inguinal hernia repair
Hair transplant	**Acute pain management**
Face laser resurfacing	Post-herpetic neuralgia
Dermabrasions	
Vitiligo surgery	
Anaesthesia for zoster dermatitis	
Axillary hyperhidrosis	

14.3.2 Procedure:

14.3.2.1 Klein's Solution or Standard Tumescent Solution.

This solution is prepared by adding 50 mL 1% lignocaine with 1 mL of 1:1000 adrenaline to 1 litre of saline. This mixture contains 0.05% lignocaine with 1:1000000 adrenaline. To alkalise the solution, 10 milliequivalents of $NaHCO_3$ are added to avoid the stinging during infiltration. Addition of sodium bicarbonate also increases the percentage of nonionised local anaesthetic, facilitating the transition into the cellular bodies.

14.3.2.2 Pharmacological Considerations

The most commonly used drug is lignocaine hydrochloride. Although the maximum recommended dose of lignocaine with adrenaline is 7 mg/kg, in tumescent anaesthesia doses as high as 35–55 mg/kg can be used.

The above-mentioned concentration is safe because:

- Tumescent lignocaine is absorbed slowly from the subcutaneous tissue like a depot formulation leading to delayed peak levels of drug concentration and rapid hepatic clearance.
- In liposuction procedures, about 30% of the lignocaine is sucked out with the fat.
- High dilution leads to insufficient gradient for absorption.
- Epinephrine-induced vasoconstriction leads to decreased absorption.
- The dose of epinephrine is 0.07 mg/kg. As epinephrine is unstable in alkalised lignocaine solution leading to decrease in its concentration, it should be mixed fresh on the day of surgery.

14.3.3 Anaesthetic Applications of TLA Beyond Liposuction

Tumescent (local) anaesthesia was originally used solely for liposuction. With evolving medical infrastructure and need for minimally invasive and ambulatory surgical procedures, it has found its place beyond what it was originally proposed for. The various applications include:

1. **TLA For Endovascular Thermal/Laser Ablation of Varicose Veins (EVLT)**

   The use of TLA for end-vascular laser ablation is well accepted by the patients as well as the surgeons. In EVLT, the tumescent solution is injected circumferentially around the vein using ultrasound guidance.

   It provides analgesia and prevents thermal energy induced tissue damage. In addition, it also provides perivenous compression of the vein providing better contact between the vein and laser.

   Volume of Tumescent Anaesthesia Used

   10 mL of tumescent solution is used per centimetre of the vein. The average volume reported has been 250–665 mL with lignocaine dose in the range of 3–10 mg/kg.

   Complications

   In EVLT, the solution is injected around the vascular space as compared to avascular spaces in liposuction. Hence, the risk of systemic absorption of epinephrine is increased. Thus, epinephrine can be omitted from the solution which can lead to earlier peak concentrations of the local anaesthetic.

2. **Breast Surgery**

   The use of tumescent anaesthesia has expanded its use to aesthetic procedures of the breast and mastectomy. Mastectomy under TLA was first performed by Worland in 1996. It not only provides pain-free and bloodless surgical area, but also hydrodissection of the anatomical plane provides assistance to the surgical procedure. Along with this, epinephrine in the tumescent solution provides vasoconstriction, and the volume of the fluid provides the tamponade effect offering desired homeostasis.

   Tumescent Cocktail for Breast Surgery

   The volume of the infiltrate is calculated using the estimated breast volume as per the equation: breast volume = 0.973 × (breast circumference/6.28). Twice the amount of volume calculated is taken for infiltration. Lignocaine 2% up to a dosage of 35 mg/kg or bupivacaine 0.5% up to a maximum of 9.5 mg/kg can be used.

   The infiltration is done using a 5 mm liposuction needle at the surgical site till the tissue becomes tense. Additional infiltration in the subdermal planes is done to block the infra clavicular nerves in the caudal aspect of the clavicle, for the lateral cutaneous branches of intercostal nerves in the mid-axillary line, along the sternum for intercostal nerves and retromammary plane for nerves of pectoral fascia.

   Advantages

   - Elderly and multimorbid patients of ASA III or IV can benefit from these where the risk of general anaesthesia is high.
   - Analgesia extends in the postoperative period avoiding opioids.
   - Ambulatory aesthetic procedures for breast can be done without risking the complications of general anaesthesia.

   Complications

   - Local anaesthetic systemic toxicity.
   - Skin flap necrosis can occur due to the vasoconstrictive effect of epinephrine and the compressing effect of volume of the solution.

3. **Cardiothoracic Surgical Procedures**

   Successful placement of subcutaneous implantable cardioverter defibrillator device has been reported using tumescent anaesthesia technique. This provides an alternative pain-free method in otherwise high-risk cardiac patients. TLA has shown excellent patient satisfaction and acceptability.

4. **Inguinal Hernia Repair**

   Although inguinal hernia surgery has been performed under local anaesthesia alone, tumescent anaesthesia provides better operating conditions, lesser risk of toxicity of local anaesthetic, early ambulation and no risk of injury to the femoral nerve as reported by some studies. The tumescent solution of 1% lignocaine with 0.5% bupivacaine and epinephrine has been utilised in a step-by-step infiltration techniques.

The tumescent solution infiltration is done in the subcutaneous tissue first, then after the exposure of external oblique fascia. Additional nerve block is given using 10 mL of 1% lignocaine along with 0.2% bupivacaine to block the nerve at the root of spermatic cord.

Tumescent TAPP

Laparoscopic transabdominal preperitoneal inguinal hernia repair using tumescent solution of lignocaine along with carbon dioxide gas has also been reported with favourable outcomes.

5. **Surgical Treatment of Burns and Post-Burn Sequelae**

   Post-burn contractures especially around the neck can present anaesthesiologists with difficult airway situation. In such cases, tumescent solution infiltration can be done while the patient is awake or with minimal sedation without compromising the airway.

   TLA in conjunction with general anaesthesia has also proved beneficial in paediatric population for surgical treatment of burns and post-burn sequelae as it provides excellent postoperative analgesia over wide areas.

6. **Post-Herpetic Neuralgia**

   The use of tumescent anaesthesia has also been explored in the acute management of herpetic neuralgia in addition to corticosteroids. Use of 0.05% lignocaine along with steroids injected into the dermatomal area of pain has provided promising results.

14.3.4 Complications of Tumescent Anaesthesia

1. **Local Anaesthetic Systemic Toxicity (LAST)**

   Due to the large volume of the drug used over a wide area, intravascular spread of the local anaesthetic can lead to local anaesthetic systemic toxicity. It presents as neurological, cardiac symptoms and can even lead to cardiac arrest. The incidence of LAST is higher in patients with impaired hepatic function, intake of enzyme inhibitor drugs.

   To prevent local anaesthetic related complications, following considerations must be followed:

   - Detailed history and examination to rule out any systemic disease and enzyme inducers or inhibitors medications must be taken before the procedure.
   - Maximum allowable doses of local anaesthetic must be calculated in mg/kg before preparing the solution.
   - Any additional administration of local anaesthetic for at least 12–18 h after the procedure must be proceeded with great caution.

14.4 Segmental Thoracic Spinal Anaesthesia

Segmental spinal anaesthesia refers to subarachnoid puncture at high thoracic levels as close as possible to the operative field in low dose in order to limit the effect of anaesthesia to the desired dermatome. The concept was introduced in 1934 when the first thoracic spinal anaesthesia was given, but this method could not gain much acceptance as anaesthesiologists feared injuring the spinal cord by performing spinal anaesthesia above the termination of conus medullaris. Thoracic spinal anaesthesia has been successfully administered for various surgeries, including laparoscopic cholecystectomies, breast cancer lumpectomies and abdominal cancer surgery and has been demonstrated to be effective and safe.

14.4.1 Anatomy

The thoracic part of the vertebral canal is the most complex and distinct part of the spine. The morphology of the thoracic vertebrae resembles the cervical vertebrae at the upper end (T1–T4) and the lumbar vertebrae at the lower end (T9–T12). The vertebrae from T1 to T4 have vertically oriented articular processes and spinous processes that project directly posteriorly. The lower thoracic vertebrae from T9 to T12 have broad and flat spinous processes that project directly posteriorly. However, the middle thoracic vertebrae, i.e. T5–T8 have spinous processes that project posteriorly at an extreme acute angle. The inferior border of the spinous processes in middle thoracic vertebrae almost overlies the lamina of the vertebrae below. The transverse processes of the thoracic vertebrae articulate with the corresponding ribs. The transition between L1 and T12 can be used in counting up technique to find the intervertebral space. The laminar spaces in the thoracic vertebrae are narrower than the lumbar vertebrae.

The magnetic resonance imaging (MRI) studies of the spine by Imbelloni LE et al. have revealed that the posterior depth of the subarachnoid space in the mid-thoracic region is greater than the lumbar and upper thoracic level. On measuring the space between the dura mater and the spinal cord in MRI studies, it was found to be 5.19 mm at T5, 5.88 mm at T10 (Fig. 14.6). It was also observed that cauda equina and dura mater touch more anteriorly in the thoracic region as compared to posteriorly in the lumbar region, thus increasing the safety of thoracic spinal anaesthesia.

In addition, upon studying the consequences of accidental dural puncture in the thoracic epidural anaesthesia, it was found that the incidence of neurological complications was low. This can be explained by the deeper subarachnoid space at the thoracic level. Also, the cauda equina is closer to the spinal cord anteriorly in the thoracic region in contrast to the lumbar region where it touches it posteriorly, thus increasing the safety of regional anaesthesia in the mid-thoracic region.

14.4.2 Indications

- Patients with high risk of mortality and morbidity under general anaesthesia.
- Patients with decreased physiological reserves, comorbidities.
- Patients in which conventional lumbar spinal anaesthesia cannot be performed

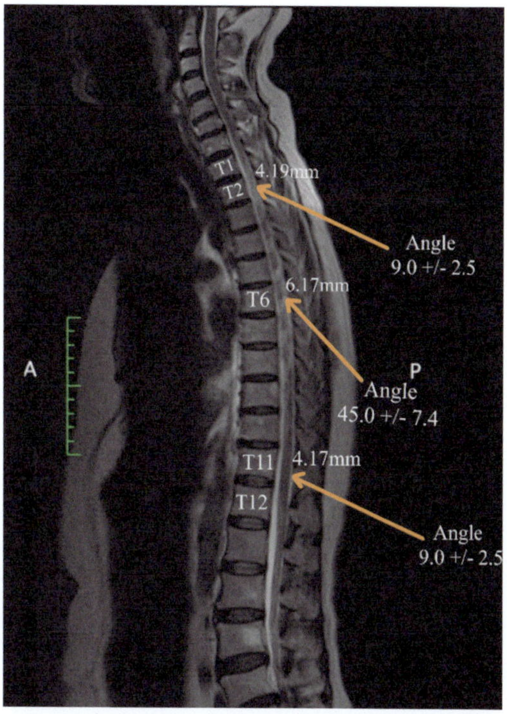

Fig. 14.6 Magnetic resonance imaging of the spinal column, distance of the dura mater to the spinal cord and angle relative to the tangent at the insertion point on the skin at T2, T5 and T10 level

- Patients with poor pulmonary function as an alternate to general anaesthesia.

A variety of surgeries have been performed under segmental thoracic spinal anaesthesia including the breast surgery, laparoscopic cholecystectomy, abdominal surgeries and cardiothoracic surgery.

14.4.3 Contraindications

Table 14.2 Contraindications for segmental thoracic spinal anaesthesia.

14.4.4 Procedure

14.4.4.1 Preparation

A thorough pre-anaesthetic check-up with general and systemic examination along with the

Table 14.2 Contraindications for segmental thoracic spinal anaesthesia

Absolute contraindications	Relative contraindications
Patient refusal Infection at the site of procedure Elevated intracranial pressure Allergy to the drug being used	Pre-existing neurological damage Hypovolemia Septicemia Coagulopathy Fixed cardiac output diseases. Cardiac conditions like left ventricular outflow obstruction

physical examination of the spine for scoliosis, previous surgery and infection at the local site must be made. Airway assessment should be done along with the routine and specific investigations. An informed consent must be taken before the surgery.

In the operating room, intravenous access is secured and standard monitoring is applied and baseline vitals are assessed.

14.4.4.2 Position

Thoracic spinal anaesthesia can be administered in both sitting and left decubitus position. However, sitting position is preferred as it avoids potential rotation of the spine. The patient is asked to flex the neck and push the back backwards to open up the intervertebral spaces.

Palpation of the intervertebral spaces can be done by palpating the T7 spine at the inferior angle of scapula and the 12th rib margin.

The thoracic vertebrae articulate with the corresponding rib, and the intervertebral space can be palpated by counting up.

It is recommended that an experienced anaesthesiologist must administer the spinal anaesthesia under all aseptic precautions.

14.4.4.3 Approach

Both midline and paramedian approaches to the subarachnoid space can be used. The paramedic approach is preferred in the mid-thoracic region as the midline approach requires acute upward angulation of the spinal needle. Forty-five to 60 degrees of angulation of the needle is required for puncturing at the thoracic level. This position increases the distance to a point that allows needle advancement without touching the cord. The midline approach is suitable for the lower thoracic intervertebral spaces.

14.4.4.4 Choice of Spinal Needle

A cutting needle is preferred over pencil tip as the orifice of the pencil point needle is 1.7 mm away from the tip which may increase the chances of neurological complications.

Alternately, a combined spinal epidural kit can be used to first identify the epidural space and then advancing the spinal needle to avoid any neurological damage.

14.4.4.5 Local Anaesthetic

In the beginning, hypobaric solutions were used. In recent times, both isobaric and hyperbaric local aesthetics have been used.

Hyperbaric local anaesthetics provide denser sensory block as they tend to have a greater effect on the posterior roots, while the opposite is true for the isobaric local anaesthetics.

The doses for different dermatome level are given in Fig 14.7.

Adjuvants

Addition of adjuvants to the local anaesthetics can decrease the dose of the local anaesthetic and provides prolonged analgesia. Various practised and potential adjuvants are enumerated below:

- **Opioids**: Opioids are the most extensively used adjuvants for local anaesthetics in central neuraxial blocks. They cause hyperpolarisation of the afferent sensory neurons via the G protein coupled receptor mechanism. This enhances the anti-nociceptive ability of the local anaesthetic, providing prolonged sensory block. However, the use of opioids intrathecally is associated with adverse effects such as pruritus, respiratory failure, nausea and vomiting. These adverse effects are dose-dependent and reversible with antagonists.

  - **Morphine**: Preservative-free morphine has been used in thoracic epidural in the dose of 1–5 mg and provides improved

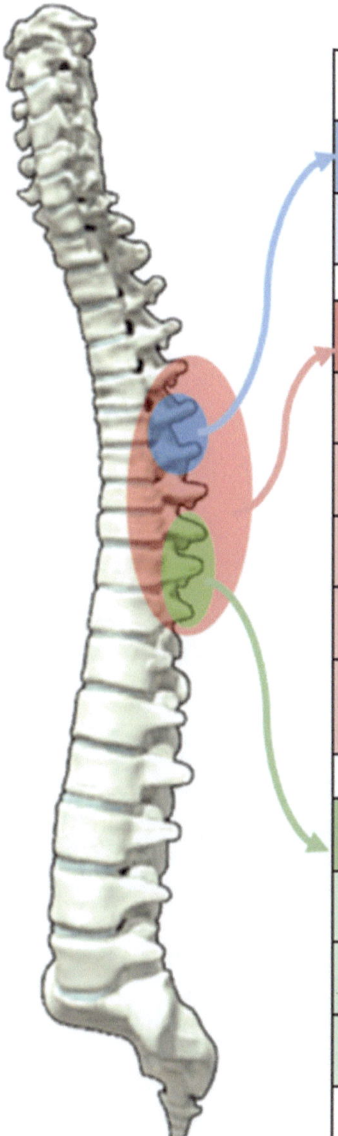

Surgical procedure	Needle insertion level	LA volume range	Sensory level
Thoracic surgery: T5-T6			
Breast surgery	T5-T6	1.1-1.4 ml	T1-T12
Upper Abdominal Surgery: T4-T11			
Laparoscopic cholecystectomy	T8-T11	1.5-2.5 ml	T2-L5
Gastrostomy	T8-T9	1 ml	T3-T12
Gastrostomy	T6-T8	0.9-1.2 ml	T4
Colon resection	T4-T5	1.7 ml	T3-L5
Laparotomy for other abdominal malignancies	T9-T10	2 ml	T2-L3
Lower Abdominal Surgery: T8-T11			
Caesarean delivery	T8-T9	1.4 ml	T4-L2
Cystectomy	T10-T11	1 ml	T6-L2
Nephrectomy	T10-T11	1.3-2 ml	T3-T12
LA: local anaesthetic			

Fig. 14.7 Level of thoracic spinal needle puncture and volume of local anaesthetics

cephalic spread. Intrathecally, it has been used in doses of 100 micrograms or less and has provided better analgesic conditions especially in elderly. In context of thoracic segmental spinal anaesthesia, the dose must be adjusted according to the site of injection.

- **Fentanyl**: fentanyl has been most commonly used in segmental spinal anaesthesia, especially in laparoscopic cholecystectomies. It is usually used in a dosage of 10–25 micrograms intrathecally and has a favourable adverse reaction profile as compared to morphine.
- Others: Other opioids like sufentanil, hydrocodone and buprenorphine have been used in neuraxial blocks with improved efficacy.

- **Midazolam**: The use of preservative-free midazolam has been reported in various case studies of segmental spinal anaesthesia. It provides analgesia by suppressing the spinal sensory functions and acts on GABAergic and opioid receptors. It also acts upon the benzodiazepine receptors in the spinal cord. The intrathecal dose of midazolam is 1–2.5 mg, and this dose has been shown to prolong the sensory effect of local anaesthetic without significant adverse effects.
- **Alpha-2 adrenoreceptor antagonists**: Clonidine and dexmedetomidine have been used in lumbar neuraxial anaesthesia with proven efficacy and safety.
  - **Clonidine:** Intrathecal clonidine can provide increased segmental spread and prolonged duration of analgesia. The intrathecal effect of clonidine has been attributed to its action on the post-junctional alpha-2 receptors in the dorsal horn of spinal cord and the blockage of sympathetic outflow. The recommended dose is 15–40 micrograms and must be adjusted as per the site and keeping in mind the adverse effects like sedation, bradycardia and hypotension that can be deleterious in multimorbid and elderly patients.
  - **Dexmedetomidine:** Addition of dexmedetomidine in a dosage of 1–5micrograms has been found to be more effective in increasing the duration of postoperative analgesia with decreased incidence of hypotension.
- **Ketamine:** Preservative-free ketamine has been found to have analgesic effect when administered intrathecally via the NMDA receptors, cholinergic and 5-hydroxytryptamine receptors. It shortens the onset of sensory and motor block and decreases the duration of the motor block, making it an effective additive in ambulatory surgery. There have been case reports of its use in continuous segmental spinal anaesthesia in a dose of 0.25 mg /kg along with midazolam 0.03 micrograms/kg where it has been shown to be superior to the traditional opioid adjuvants. However, dose-dependent psychomimetic sequelae, drowsiness and nausea can be a limiting factor in its extensive use in higher doses.
- **Steroids**: Intrathecal dexamethasone in the dose of 8 mg has been found to increase the duration of sensory block without significant adverse effects.

14.4.5 Advantages of Thoracic Spinal Anaesthesia

- Thoracic spinal anaesthesia provides better haemodynamic stability as compared to spinal anaesthesia as the sympathetic block is restricted to the dermatome involved.
- As the nerve roots in the thoracic region are thinner and the cerebrospinal fluid volume is also low, lesser volume of drug is required.
- Early ambulation as minimal lower limb motor involvement is seen.
- Over general anaesthesia, it provides:
  - Better intraoperative pain control extending to the postoperative period.
  - Lesser postoperative nausea and vomiting.
  - Early ambulation.
  - Lesser respiratory complications.
  - Reduced cost.
  - Low incidence of deep vein thrombosis.
  - Less airway complications.
  - Decreased neuroendocrine stress response.
  - Protection against thromboembolic events (Table 14.3).

The major concern with high thoracic spinal anaesthesia is ventilatory compromise due to the higher level of block. However, it is to be noted that the active inspiratory muscle is diaphragm, which is innervated by the cervical nerves and expiration is a passive process. Thus, the inspiratory capacity is not significantly decreased. However, the ability of forced expiration and cough is decreased due to the inhibition of nerves innervating the upper anterior abdominal wall.

Table 14.3 Complications

The complications with TSSA are the same as with lumbar spinal anaesthesia.
Direct needle trauma
Infection (abscess, meningitis)
Vertebral canal hematoma
Spinal cord ischemia
Arachnoiditis
Post-dural puncture headache
Hypotension
Nausea/vomiting (typically caused by hypotension)
Bradycardia
Paresthesia
Transient mild hearing impairment
Backache
Urinary retention
TNS
Total spinal anaesthesia
Cardiovascular collapse
Death

In present times, improved drug formulations, sophisticated medical equipment and monitoring have refreshened the possibilities of older techniques to be re-introduced into the routine anaesthetic practice.

Further Reading

Caruselli M, Michel F. Thoracic spinal anesthesia: an interesting alternative to general anesthesia. Minerva Anestesiol. 2020;86(3):244–6.

Chiao A, et al. Single-cuff forearm tourniquet in intravenous regional anaesthesia results in less pain and fewer sedation requirements than upper arm tourniquet. Br J Anaesth. 2013;111(2):271–5.

Chyung JW, et al. Tumescent local anesthetic technique for inguinal hernia repairs. Ann Surg Treat Res. 2014;87(6):325–30.

Dekoninck V, Hoydonckx Y, Van de Velde M, Ory JP, Dubois J, Jamaer L, Jalil H, Stessel B. The analgesic efficacy of intravenous regional anesthesia with a forearm versus conventional upper arm tourniquet: a systematic review. BMC Anesthesiol. 2018;18(1):86.

Elakany MH, Abdelhamid SA. Segmental thoracic spinal has advantages over general anesthesia for breast cancer surgery. Anesth Essays Res. 2013;7(3):390–5.

Ellakany MH. Thoracic spinal anesthesia is safe for patients undergoing abdominal cancer surgery. Anesth Essays Res. 2014;8(2):223–8.

Fish MJ, Bamberger HB. Wide-awake local anesthesia no tourniquet (WALANT) hand surgery. In: StatPearls [Internet]. Treasure Island (FL): StatPearls Publishing; 2023. Available from: https://www.ncbi.nlm.nih.gov/books/NBK570646

Ghaderi K, Rahmani K, Rahmanpanah N, Shami S, Zahedi F, Nasseri K. Comparison of lidocaine-dexmedetomidine and lidocaine-saline on the characteristics of the modified forearm bier block: a clinical trial. J Anaesthesiol Clin Pharmacol. 2021;37:610–5.

Gunes T, et al. Less painful tumescent solution for patients undergoing endovenous laser ablation of the saphenous vein. Ann Vasc Surg. 2015;29(6):1123–7.

Hadzic A. Hadzic's peripheral nerve blocks and anatomy for ultrasound -guided regional Anaesthesia. 2nd ed. China: McGraw-Hill; 2004.

Haghighi M, et al. A comparison between single and double tourniquet technique in distal upper limb orthopedic surgeries with intravenous regional anesthesia. Arch Bone Jt Surg. 2018;6(1):63–70.

Huang YC, et al. WALANT for distal radius fracture: open reduction with plating fixation via wide-awake local anesthesia with no tourniquet. J Orthop Surg Res. 2018;13(1):195.

Hudson AJ, Whittaker DR, Szpisjak DF, Lenart MJ, Bailey MM. Tumescent technique without epinephrine for endovenous laser therapy and serum lidocaine concentration. J Vasc Surg Venous Lymphat Disord. 2015;3:48–53.

Imbelloni LE, Sakamoto JW, Viana EP, de Aroujo AA, Pottker D, de Pistarino MA. Segmental spinal anesthesia: a systematic review. J Anesth Clin Res. 2020;11:953.

Kalagac Fabris L, Biberić M, Zrna S. New concept of fusion technics in regional anesthesia. Acta Clin Croat. 2022;61(Suppl 2):135–44.

Kendler M, Simon JC, Wetzig T. Local anesthesia with lidocaine and prilocaine, using the tumescent technique, for the radiofrequency ablation of lower extremity varicose veins. Int J Dermatol. 2013;52:739e44.

Khater A, Mazy A, Gad M, Taha Abd Eldayem O, Hegazy M. Tumescent mastectomy: the current indications and operative tips and tricks. Breast Cancer (Dove Med Press). 2017;9:237–43.

Klein JA. Anesthesia for liposuction in dermatologic surgery. J Dermatol Surg Oncol. 1988;14:1124–32.

Klein JA. Tumescent technique for regional anesthesia permits lidocaine doses of 35 mg/kg for liposuction. J Dermatol Surg Oncol. 1990;16:248–63.

Kurdi MS, Agrawal P, Thakkar P, Arora D, Barde SM, Kala E. Recent advancements in regional anaesthesia. Indian J Anaesth. 2023;67(1):63–70.

le Roux JJ, Wakabayashi K, Jooma Z. Defining the role of thoracic spinal anaesthesia in the twenty-first century: a narrative review. Br J Anaesth. 2023;130(1):e56–65.

Löser B, Petzoldt M, Löser A, Bacon DR, Goerig M. Intravenous regional anesthesia: a historical overview and clinical review. J Anesth Hist. 2019;5(3):99–108.

Neal JM, Mulroy MF, Weinberg GL. American Society of Regional Anesthesia and Pain Medicine American Society of Regional Anesthesia and Pain Medicine checklist for managing local anesthetic systemic toxicity: 2012 version. Reg Anesth Pain Med. 2012;37(1):16–8.

Novoa JC. Tumescent anesthetic breast surgery (TABS): breast augmentation surgery in an office-based surgical center. In: Mugea TT, Shiffman MA, editors. Aesthetic surgery of the breast. Berlin/Heidelberg: Springer; 2015. p. 107–19.

Prasad MK, Puneet P, Rani K, Shree D. Severe post-burn neck contracture release and skin graft harvest using tumescent local anaesthesia as the sole anesthetic technique. J Anesth. 2012;26(1):97–9.

Romero J, et al. Tumescent local anesthesia for subcutaneous implantable cardioverter-defibrillator implantation: an alternative for general anesthesia. Heart Rhythm Case Rep. 2021;7(5):286–91.

Shatri G, Singh A. Thoracic segmental spinal anesthesia. In: StatPearls [Internet]. Treasure Island (FL): StatPearls Publishing; 2023. Available from: https://www.ncbi.nlm.nih.gov/books/NBK572087/

Spannella F, et al. Thoracic continuous spinal anesthesia for high-risk comorbid older patients undergoing major abdominal surgery: one-year experience of an Italian geriatric hospital. Minerva Anestesiol. 2020;86:261–9.

Swain A, Nag DS, Sahu S, Samaddar DP. Adjuvants to local anesthetics: current understanding and future trends. World J Clin Cases. 2017;5(8):307–23.

Uttamani RR, Venkataram A, Venkataram J, Mysore V. Tumescent anesthesia for dermatosurgical procedures other than liposuction. J Cutan Aesthet Surg. 2020;13(4):275–82.

Vaughn N, Rajan N, Darowish M. Intravenous regional anesthesia using a forearm tourniquet: a safe and effective technique for outpatient hand procedures. Hand (N Y). 2020;15(3):353–9.

Vincenzi P, et al. Continuous thoracic spinal anesthesia with local anesthetic plus midazolam and ketamine is superior to local anesthetic plus fentanyl in major abdominal surgery. Surg Open Sci. 2020;2(4):5–11.

Vincenzi P, et al. Opioid-free segmental thoracic spinal anesthesia with intrathecal sedation for breast and axillary surgery: report of four cases. Local Reg Anesth. 2022;15:23–9.

Volkmar AJ, et al. Safety and efficacy of forearm tourniquet compared to upper arm tourniquet for local intravenous regional anesthesia in hand surgery: a randomized clinical trial. Iowa Orthop J. 2021;41(1):177–81.

Tourniquet and Its Concerns in Anaesthesia

15

Aditi Khare and Mukesh Kumar Prasad

Abstract

Tourniquets are compressive devices routinely used for occluding blood flow during limb surgeries. They have their advantages of bloodless surgical field and decreased intraoperative blood loss but are also associated with physiological changes which become intolerable, especially in cardiac compromised patients. The various complications associated with tourniquet use have been taken care of by various modifications. The surgical and anaesthesiologist team must be well aware of the proper functioning and use of tourniquet to avoid any complications pertaining to it.

Keywords

Tourniquet · Complication · Occlusion pressure · Cuff

A. Khare
Department of Anaesthesiology, Global Hospital, Gwalior, India

M. K. Prasad (✉)
Department of Anaesthesiology, Teerthanker Mahaveer Medical College and Research Centre, Moradabad, India
e-mail: mukeshkumar2002@gmail.com

15.1 Introduction

- A tourniquet is a constricting or compressing device that is used to control venous and arterial circulation to an extremity for a finite period of time. Tourniquet is coined by Jean-Louis Petit (Fig. 15.1).
- Tourniquets are of several types and have several applications, currently most frequently used in the peri-operative period.
- The use of tourniquet is a common practice in orthopaedic surgeries, since they enable minimization of blood loss during limb surgeries and ensure better visibility for the surgeon by enabling a bloodless field.

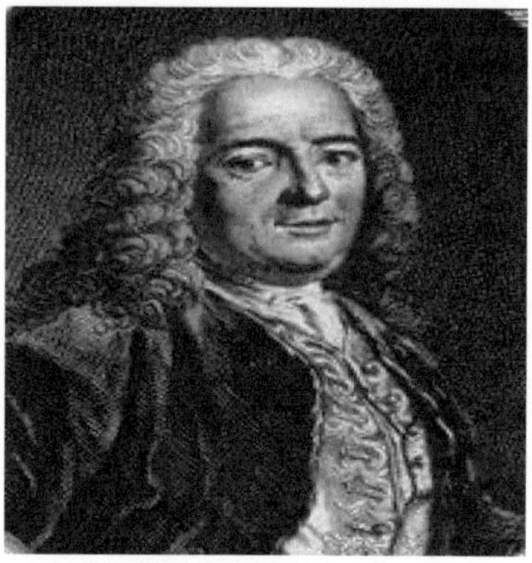

Jean Louis Petit - coined the term "Tourniquet"

Fig. 15.1 Jean-Louis Petit

M. K. Prasad, S. J. S. Bajwa (eds.), *Steps to Successful Regional Anesthesia*,
https://doi.org/10.1007/978-981-97-4098-7_15

- Its use is associated with certain physiological changes as well as complications; hence, it is important to know in detail about its parts, specifications, indications, and contraindications.

15.2 Types of Tourniquet

Tourniquets have evolved over time. They are also used in multiple areas; thus, they have been designed to suit needs of the treating physician. The different types of tourniquet described are as follows (Figs. 15.2, 15.3, and 15.4).

15.3 Physiological Effects and Complications

Tourniquet application has physiological effects on the body, which may turn into complications. The complications may be divided into local and systemic as described in Fig. 15.5 and Tables 15.1 and 15.2.

15.4 Selection of Tourniquet

Selection of tourniquet must be individualized. The following criteria can be used for choosing the appropriate tourniquet:

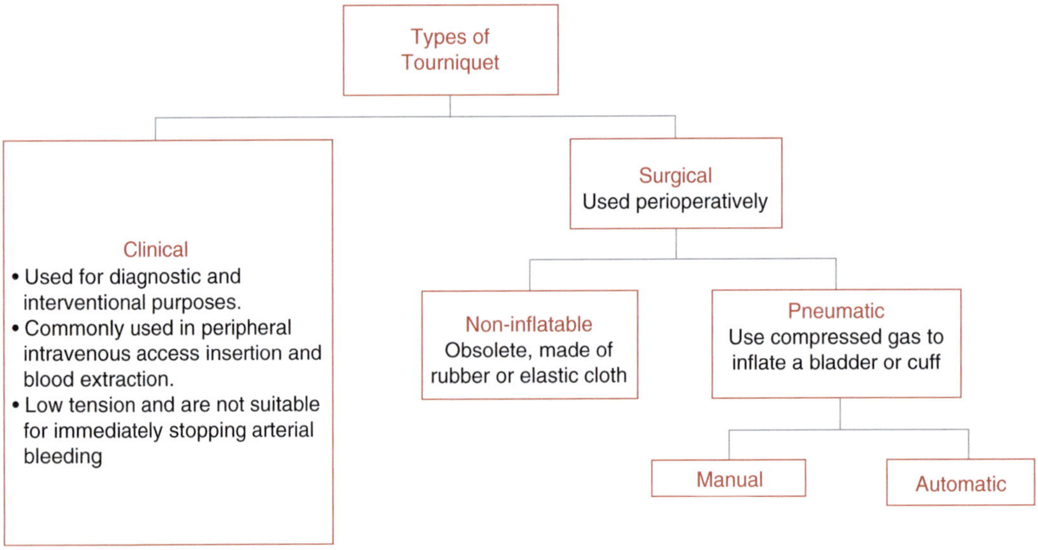

Fig. 15.2 Types of tourniquet

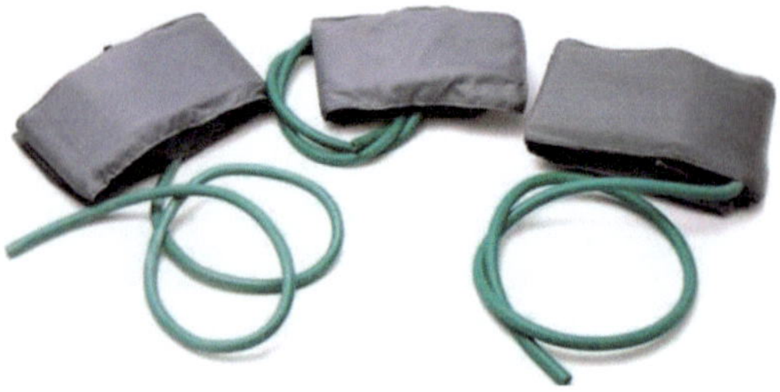

Fig. 15.3 Pneumatic tourniquet

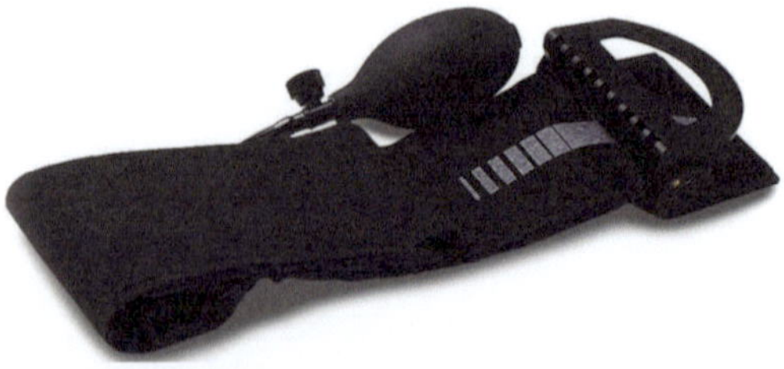

Fig. 15.4 Manual pneumatic tourniquet

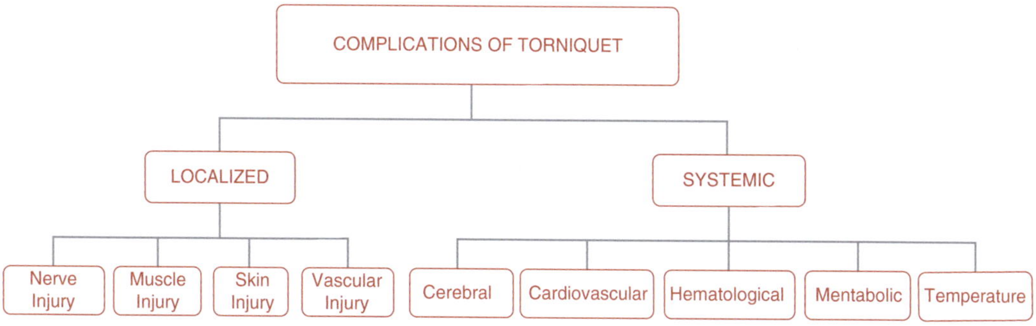

Fig. 15.5 Complications of tourniquet

Table 15.1 Effects and systemic complications of tourniquet application

Cardiovascular system	*On tourniquet inflation*: Limb exsanguination and tourniquet inflation ⟶ increase blood volume and SVR ⟶ increase in central venous pressure Effects can be detrimental in patients with poor cardiac function Heart rate and systolic and diastolic pressures may increase after 30–60 min of tourniquet inflation due to ischaemia and tourniquet pain This persists until tourniquet deflationPoor response to analgesic drugs or increasing depth of anaesthesia *On tourniquet deflation*: Sudden drop in CVP and MAP Due to a combination of a shift in blood volume back into the limb and washout of metabolites from the ischemic limb into the systemic circulation More marked with the simultaneous use of tourniquets on both lower limbs
Respiratory system	Increase in $EtCO_2$ as a result of efflux of hypercapnic venous blood and metabolites into the systemic circulation. Greater with the lower limb tourniquet, increased muscle bulk. Peaks at 1–3 min, returns to baseline at 10–13 min in a spontaneously breathing patient, minute volume needs to be increased in mechanically ventilated patients.
Central nervous system	Tourniquet deflation ⟶ increase in $EtCO_2$ ⟶ increased cerebral blood flow. Patients with reduced intracranial compliance are at risk. Normocapnia can prevent this during tourniquet deflation.
Haematological system	Coagulability and fibrinolysis are both affected. Tourniquet application, pain from surgery ⟶ tissue damage and catecholamines release ⟶ increased platelet aggregation and stimulation of coagulation factors. Deflation of the tourniquet ⟶ release of tissue plasminogen activator, activating the anti-thrombin III, thrombomodulin-protein C anticoagulant system ⟶ increased fibrinolytic activity ⟶ post-tourniquet bleeding. Increased fibrinolysis maximal at 15 min and returns to baseline within 30 min of tourniquet release.
Metabolic changes	Local changes in ischemic limb Increased lactic acid, $PaCO_2$ and K. Decreased PaO_2 and pH. Toxic metabolites ⟶ enter general circulation ⟶ systemic metabolic changes. The degree of these changes correlates with the duration of ischaemia, which are fully reversed within 30 min of tourniquet deflation. Metabolic changes are more pronounced with bilateral tourniquets.
Temperature changes	Core body temperature increases after tourniquet application as the available surface area for heat loss decreases, thereby causing lesser heat transfer from central to the peripheral compartment. Deflation leads to a transient fall in core temperature due to the redistribution of body heat and hypothermic blood from the ischemic limb. Maintenance of normothermia during surgery reduces this decline.

Table 15.2 Localized complications of tourniquet application

Nerve injury	Paresthesia or paralysis. Maximum at proximal and distal edges of cuff. More common in upper limbs. Radial nerve > ulnar nerve > median nerve. Common peroneal nerve most common in lower limb. Due to compression and ischaemia.
Muscle injury	Due to ischaemia and mechanical deformation. This can cause metabolic and microvascular changes. Intracellular CPR, glycogen, O2, ATP exhaust by 3 h. Free radical.
Skin injury	Cutaneous abrasions, pressure, necrosis, blister. Increased risk in paediatric, obese, elderly, peripheral vascular disease.
Vascular injury	Increased risk in paediatric, elderly, peripheral vascular disease, obese

15.4.1 Cuff length and cuff width
15.4.2 Cuff location
15.4.3 Cuff shape
15.4.4 Single- versus dual-bladder design
15.4.5 Disposable versus reusable cuffs.

15.4.1 Cuff Length and Cuff Width

Cuff length and width of tourniquet (Table 15.3).

15.4.2 Cuff Location

Cuffs should be selected on the basis of location of cuff: arms, thighs, or legs.

Tourniquets should be positioned at the point of maximum circumference of the limb.

15.4.3 Cuff Shape

Cuff shape may be cylindrical or conical depending upon the contour of the limb (Cuff shape: Fig. 15.6a Conical contour; Fig. 15.6b Cylindrical cuff).

Table 15.3 Cuff length and width

Length	Cuff overlap at least three inches but not >6 inches
	Excessive overlap causes increased pressure, wrinkling of underlying soft tissue
	Underlap results in ineffective tourniquet inflation and inadequate constriction of the limb
Width	Should be wider than half the limb's diameter
	Wider cuffs disperse pressure over a greater surface area and thus may be lower pressure
	This reduces the risk of injury

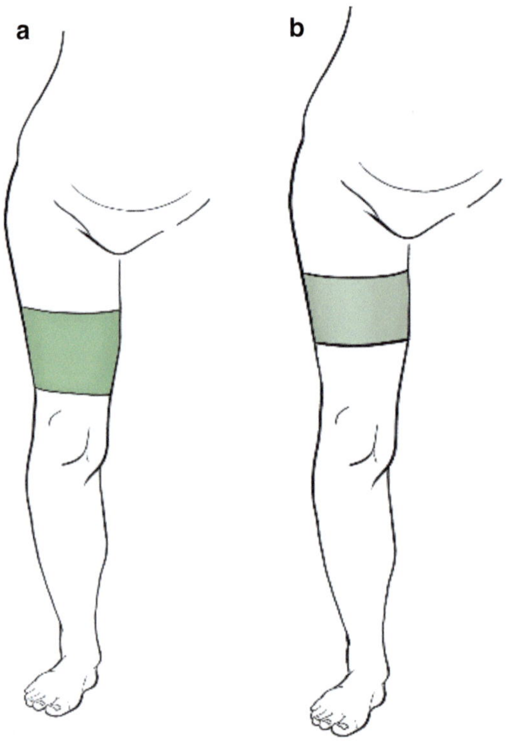

Fig. 15.6 (**a**) Conical cuff. (**b**) Cylindrical cuff

15.4.4 Single- Versus Dual-Bladder Design

Dual-bladder cuffs are useful in surgeries requiring longer duration of tourniquet inflation. These prevent local ischaemia of the skin and structures underlying the tourniquet.

15.4.5 Disposable Versus Reusable Cuffs

This choice is dictated by cost-effectivity, patient condition, and other factors.

15.5 Contraindications

- Severe peripheral vascular disease.
- Sickle cell disease.
  - In sickle cell disease, sickling is precipitated by circulatory stasis, acidosis, and hypoxemia, all of which happen during the use of a tourniquet.
  - With proper necessary precautions, tourniquets can be used safely in most patients with sickle cell disease.
- Severe crush injury.
- Diabetic neuropathic patients.
- Patients with history of deep vein thrombosis and pulmonary embolism.
- Limbs with severe infection.
- Patients with poor cardiac reserve.
- Traumatized limbs.
- Reynaud's disease.

15.6 Tourniquet Usage (Table 15.4)

Table 15.4 Tourniquet usage

Tourniquet cuff pressure	The pressure to which a tourniquet cuff is inflated. It depends on variables: age, skin, blood pressure, shape and size of the extremity, dimensions of the cuff. Should be kept to a minimum. Approximately 200–300 mmHg for adults.
Limb occlusion pressure (LOP)	Defined as the minimum pressure required to stop the flow of arterial blood into the limb distal to the cuff. Determined by gradually increasing tourniquet pressure until distal blood flow is interrupted. Safety margins are recommended for different LOP so as to ensure obliteration of arterial blood flow. This value is to be added to the LOP value to determine the pressure at which the cuff should be inflated: 40 mmHg for LOP <130 mmHg 60 mmHg for LOP 131–190 mmHg 80 mmHg for LOP >190 mmHg. Add 50 mmHg for paediatric patients
Inflation or occlusion time	Time duration for which tourniquet is inflated. Should be minimum. Varies with the patient's age, physical status, and vascular supply to the extremity. Safe time limit: 1–3 h. In case of prolonged surgery, if the anticipated duration is >2.5 h after 2 h of surgery, a 10-min deflation interval is exercised then and at subsequent 1 hour intervals. Paediatric patients inflation time should be <75 min.

Pre-application Precautions

- Check pressure source, cuff, regulator, tubing, and connectors.
- The cuff should not directly overlie bony prominences, and the edge of the tourniquet should be at least 2 cm distal to the head of fibula and 2 cm proximal to the malleoli for calf cuffs.
- The cuff should overlap at least 3 inches, but not more than 6 inches as it may cause generation of high pressures.
- The limb should be exsanguinated by elevating and using an Esmarch bandage or tourniquet Exsanguinators for emptying the blood vessels from the distal end to the proximal end prior to tourniquet inflation.
- Advantages include a clear operating field, reduction in overall blood loss, and reduction in the risk of microemboli at the time of release.

Methods to Lower Effective Cuff Pressure

1. *Double tourniquet technique.*

   Two tourniquets are used and inflated alternately to change the point of compression.

2. *Tourniquet inflation based on limb occlusion pressure.*
   The limb occlusion pressure is determined and cuff is inflated accordingly.
3. *Use of devices to detect absence of arterial pulse.*
   Doppler technique and pulse oximetry to confirm the absence of the arterial pulse to determine the minimum inflation pressure.
4. *Cuff pressure synchronization with systolic blood pressure.*
5. *Controlled hypotension.*
   To decrease direct cuff pressure against the tissue. However, risk of ischaemia is persistent.

Safe Use of Tourniquet

The following are rules for the safe use of tourniquet in order to decrease the complication rate (Table 15.5).

Table 15.5 Rules for the safe use of tourniquet

Pre-requisite	Apply only to a healthy limb or with caution to an unhealthy limb like peripheral vascular disease
Tourniquet measurement	According to patient's physique, size is determined, generally for arm 10 cm and leg 15 cm or wider in large legs/arms
Application area	Upper/mid arm; mid/upper thigh
Pressure	50–100 mmHg above systolic for the arm; double systolic for the thigh
Maximum pressure	Arm 200–250 mmHg, leg 250–350 mmHg
Maximum time	Arms 1.5 h; legs 2 h (10 mininterval if to continue)
Preventive measure	Padding to be done using at least two layers of orthopaedic wool Large cuffs are recommended for larger limbs instead of increasing pressure Avoid high temperatures Keep the tissue moist
Maintenance	Calibrate weekly (minimum) against mercury manometer; 3 monthly maintenance is required

15.7 Specific Complications of Tourniquet

15.7.1 Tourniquet Pain

Tourniquet pain is described as a poorly localized, dull, tight, aching sensation at the site of tourniquet application.

Mechanism

- The A-delta fibres at the site of tourniquet application are blocked by mechanical compression after about 30 minor tourniquet inflation, whereas the C fibres keep functioning.
- Tourniquet compression leads to release of prostaglandins by the injured cells, which in turn increases pain perception by stimulation of pain receptors.
- Also, limb ischaemia causes central sensitisation via NMDA receptor activation due to repeated nociceptive afferent input from the affected limb.

Presentation

- Under regional anaesthesia, it may manifest as pain sometime after inflation of tourniquet.
- During general anaesthesia, it presents as increase in heart rate and mean arterial pressure.
- It is more common under general anaesthesia and occurs most often during lower limb surgeries.

Anaesthetic Implications

- Tourniquet pain has important impacts on anaesthesia.
- Tourniquet pain can be severe and can cause discomfort to the patient.
- Presence of tourniquet pain may result in the requirement to change the plan of anaesthesia to general anaesthesia.
- The only definitive treatment is tourniquet deflation.

Management of Tourniquet Pain

There are various methods used for management of tourniquet pain (Fig. 15.7).

15.7.2 Tourniquet Syndrome

- A series of physiological and pathological changes that occur after deflation of tourniquet.
- Deflation leads to
  - Decrease in mean arterial BP due to the release of metabolites from the ischemic limb into the circulation and the decrease in peripheral vascular resistance.
  - Transient increase in EtCO2.
  - Decrease in temperature.
  - Decrease in central venous pO2.
- Reperfusion syndrome is caused by the re-establishment of blood flow following deflation of tourniquet and can induce a paradoxical extension of ischemic damage mediated by free radicals (Fig. 15.8).

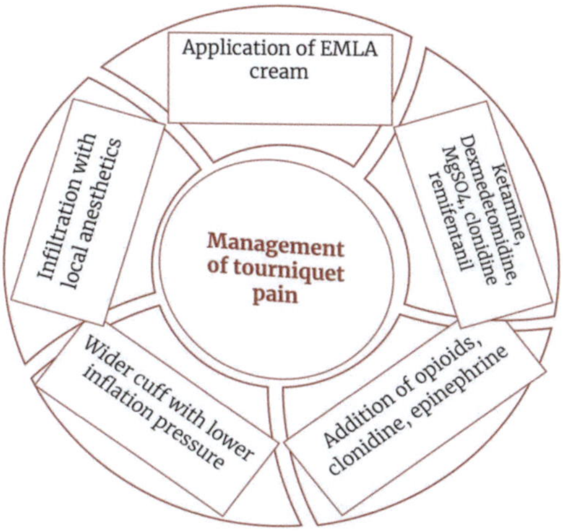

Fig. 15.7 Management of tourniquet pain

Treatment

(a) Hydrogen Sulfide: H_2S affects various metabolic signalling pathways (particularly Akt), mitochondrial integrity and ETC activity, apoptosis, and cell survival.
(b) b. L-arginine: Pre-treatment with individual monoclonal antibodies may limit the ischaemia reperfusion injury.

15.7.3 Post-tourniquet Syndrome

- Prolonged postoperative swelling of the extremity after use of tourniquet.
- May occur after 1–6 weeks.
- Swelling caused by return of blood to the extremity and post-ischemic reactive hyperaemia.
- Characterized by oedema, stiffness, pallor, weakness without paralysis, numbness.
- Occurs in long duration of tourniquet application.
- Also may occur where cuff pressure is sufficient to obliterate arterial flow while

Fig. 15.8 Reperfusion injury after tourniquet deflation

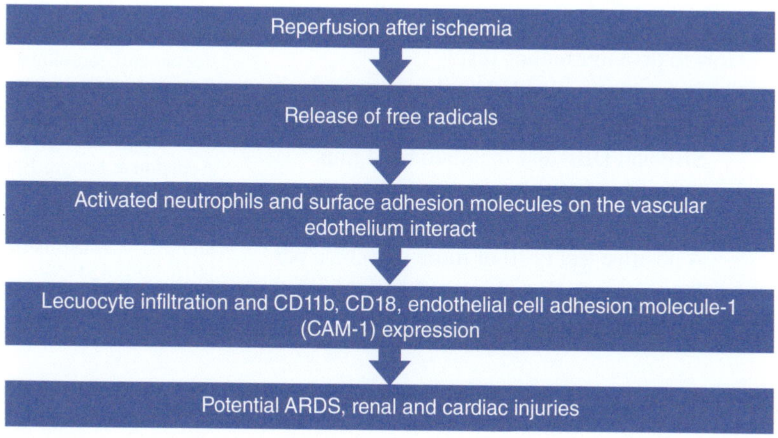

insufficient to allow venous drainage. This may especially be seen in elderly patients, where the calcification of major arteries makes them non-compliant to tourniquet pressure.

15.8 Other Uses of Tourniquet

15.8.1 IV Regional Anaesthesia (Bier's block)
15.8.2 Tourniquet Test
15.8.3 Pneumatic Compression Devices
15.8.4 Phlebotomy and Blood Collection
15.8.5 Military Anti-shock Trousers (MAST).

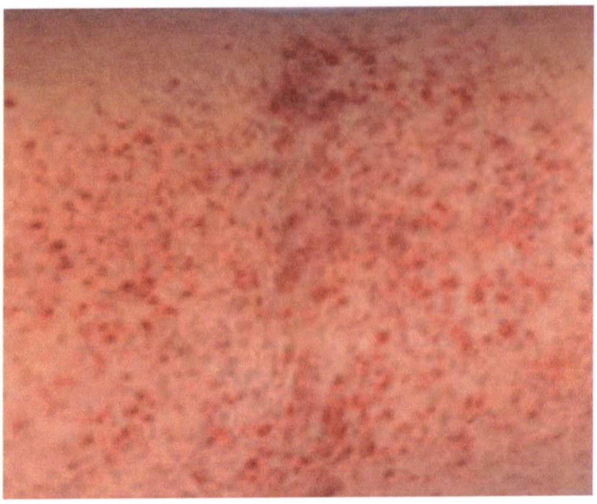

Fig. 15.9 Positive petechiae test

15.8.1 IV Regional Anaesthesia (Bier's Block)

- It is a technique of IV regional anaesthesia and can be used for upper extremity as well as lower extremity procedures.
- Advantages:
  - Ease of administration.
  - Rapid onset.
  - Rapid recovery.
  - Muscle relaxation.
  - Controllable and predictable duration of anaesthesia.

15.8.2 Tourniquet Test

- The tourniquet test has been used for assessment of dengue.
  It is a marker of capillary fragility.
- How to do a tourniquet Test?
  1. Record the patient's blood pressure.
  2. Inflate the cuff to a point midway between SBP and DBP and maintain for 2 min.
  3. Reduce and wait 2 min.
  4. Count petechiae below antecubital fossa.
  5. A positive test is 10 or more petechiae per 1 square inch (Fig. 15.9).

15.8.3 Pneumatic Compression Devices

They are a modified form of tourniquet which can be applied on lower extremities as prophylaxis against deep venous thrombosis.

15.7.4 *Phlebotomy and Blood Collection*
15.7.5 *Military Anti-shock Trousers (MAST).*

Further Reading

AORN Recommended Practices Committee. Recommended practices for the use of the pneumatic tourniquet in the perioperative practice settings. AORN J. 2007;86:640–55.

Clinical assessment [Internet]. cdc.gov. [cited 2023 Feb 4]. https://www.cdc.gov/dengue/training/cme/ccm/page73112.html

Dreyfuss UY, Smith RJ. Sensory changes with prolonged double-cuff tourniquet time in hand surgery. J Hand Surg Am. 1988;13:736–40. Noor-din S, McEwen JA, Kragh JF Jr, Eisen A, Masri BA. Surgical

Groah. Perioperative nursing, vol. 304. 3rd ed. Stamford: Appleton & Lange; 1996.

Kumar K, Railton C, Tawfic Q. Tourniquet application during anesthesia: "what we need to know?". J Anaesthesiol Clin Pharmacol [Internet]. 2016;32(4):424–30.

Kutty S, McElwain JP. Padding under tourniquets in tourniquet controlled surgery: Bruner's ten rules revisited. Injury. 2002;33:75.

Noordin S, McEwen JA, Kragh JF Jr, Eisen A, Masri BA. Surgical tourniquets in orthopaedics. J Bone Joint Surg Am. 2009;91:2958–67.

Oragui E, Parsons A, White T, Longo UG, Khan WS. Tourniquet use in upper limb surgery. Hand. 2011;6:165–73.

Sato J, Ishii Y, Noguchi H, Takeda M. Safety and efficacy of a new tourniquet system. BMC Surg. 2012; 12:17.

Sharma JP, Salhotra R. Tourniquets in orthopedic surgery. Indian J Orthop [Internet]. 2012;46(4):377–83.

Tredwell SJ, Wilmink M, Inkpen K, McEwen JA. Pediatric tourniquets: analysis of cuff and limb interface, current practice, and guidelines for use. J Pediatr Orthop. 2001;21:671–6.

Tuncali B, Karci A, Bacakoglu AK, Tuncali BE, Ekin A. Controlled hypotension and minimal inflation pressure: a new approach for pneumatic tourniquet application in upper limb surgery. Anesth Analg. 2003;97:1529–32.

Wakai A, Wang JH, Winter DC, Street JT, O'Sullivan RG, Redmond HP. Tourniquet induced systemic inflammatory response in extremity surgery. J Trauma 2001;51:922–6. Yamazaki T, Seko Y, Tamatani T, Miyasaka M, Yazaki Y. Expression of intracellular adhesion molecule-1 in rat with ischemia/reperfusion and limitation of infarct size by treatment with antibodies against cell adhesion molecules. Am J Pathol 1993;143:410–8.

Regional Anaesthesia and Coagulation Disorder

16

Sonali Gupta and Rohit Hanmanta Bhandari

Abstract

Regional anaesthesia has truly reached its pinnacle with the introduction of newer and safer modalities. However, it is not without its share of drawbacks and shortcomings. A steady rise in the incidence of thromboembolism and a large pool of patients on antithrombotic medications pose serious safety concerns in patients receiving regional anaesthesia. Individuals with hereditary disorders of coagulation constitute a far smaller proportion, but due to the scarcity of large data points and literature, there is no consensus about the safety of regional anaesthesia in this subset of patients. Given that haemorrhagic complications like vertebral canal haematoma in these patients may be catastrophic and debilitating, it becomes essential to be well-versed with the specific concerns and necessary amendments that may be crucial to individualize the administration of regional anaesthesia in these patients. There is no inviolable approach, and therefore, all cases should be evaluated meticulously and risk stratified individually. Thorough risk–benefit analysis forms the cornerstone of management. However, this chapter aims to provide practical problem-solving scenarios and clear direction not only for anaesthesiology trainees but also for practising anaesthesiologists.

Keywords

Coagulation disorders · Coagulopathy · Regional anaesthesia · Vertebral canal haematoma

16.1 Introduction

Regional anaesthesia (RA) is associated with fewer complications, a shorter length of stay, and reduced number of ICU admissions in patients undergoing lower limb surgery. With the introduction of safer drugs and use of ultrasound guidance to administer regional anaesthesia, there has been an increase in its use as a standalone modality or in conjunction with general anaesthesia to provide anaesthesia as well as analgesia for diverse procedures. The most dreaded complication associated with the use of RA is bleeding into the vertebral canal which can lead to nerve compression and subsequent neurodeficit. As we encounter more patients with coagulation abnormalities, either because of pharmacotherapy or due to disease processes, the risk of bleeding complications becomes a significant patient safety hazard. When administering regional anaesthesia to such patients, the anaesthetist must weigh the risks vs benefits and decide if technique should be altered or abandoned altogether.

S. Gupta (✉) · R. H. Bhandari
North Middlesex University Hospital, London, UK

M. K. Prasad, S. J. S. Bajwa (eds.), *Steps to Successful Regional Anesthesia*,
https://doi.org/10.1007/978-981-97-4098-7_16

16.2 The Coagulation Pathway

It is a critical component of haemostasis, the process that prevents excessive bleeding. It can be summarized as follows:

1. **Vasoconstriction**: When a blood vessel is injured, it constricts (narrows) to reduce blood flow and minimize bleeding.
2. **Primary Haemostasis**: Platelets are recruited to the site of injury, where they adhere to exposed collagen and become activated. This activation causes them to change shape and release chemical signals that further activate platelets.
3. **Secondary Haemostasis**: This consists of two main pathways: the intrinsic and extrinsic pathways.
   (a) Intrinsic Pathway: This pathway is initiated within the bloodstream. It involves a cascade of clotting factors (Factors XII, XI, IX, and VIII) that ultimately lead to the activation of Factor X.
   (b) Extrinsic Pathway: This pathway is initiated by external factors, such as tissue injury. Tissue factor (Factor III) combines with Factor VII to activate Factor X.
4. **Common Pathway**: Factor X, activated in both the intrinsic and extrinsic pathways, leads to the formation of prothrombinase. Prothrombinase converts prothrombin (Factor II) into thrombin (Factor IIa).
5. **Thrombin**: Thrombin is a key enzyme that plays a central role in coagulation. It converts soluble fibrinogen into insoluble fibrin strands, forming a mesh that traps blood cells to create a stable blood clot.
6. **Fibrinolysis**: After the clot has served its purpose, plasmin breaks down the fibrin strands, leading to clot dissolution.

Overall, the coagulation pathway is a highly regulated and intricate process that balances the need to stop bleeding with the risk of excessive clotting. Dysregulation in this pathway can lead to bleeding disorders or thrombotic disorders.

16.3 Coagulation Test

The choice of coagulation tests depends on the clinical context and the specific aspects of coagulation that need to be evaluated.

1. **Prothrombin Time (PT):** This test measures the time it takes for blood to clot through the extrinsic and common pathways. It is often used to monitor warfarin (Coumadin) therapy and assess the extrinsic pathway.
2. **International Normalized Ratio (INR):** INR is calculated based on the PT result and is used primarily to monitor the effectiveness of warfarin therapy, ensuring that the clotting time remains within a target range.
3. **Activated Partial Thromboplastin Time (aPTT):** The aPTT test evaluates the intrinsic and common pathways of coagulation. It is used to monitor heparin therapy and assess various clotting factor deficiencies.
4. **Thrombin Time (TT)**: This test measures the time it takes for fibrinogen to be converted into fibrin by thrombin. It is primarily used to evaluate disorders related to fibrinogen levels.
5. **D-Dimer**: Elevated levels of D-dimer in the blood can indicate the presence of an abnormal blood clot or the breakdown of a clot. It is often used in the diagnosis of conditions like deep vein thrombosis (DVT) and pulmonary embolism (PE).
6. **Platelet Count**: A simple blood test that measures the number of platelets in the bloodstream. Abnormal platelet counts can indicate bleeding or clotting disorders.
7. **Bleeding Time**: Although less commonly used today, this test measures the time it takes for a small skin incision to stop bleeding. It assesses platelet function and vessel wall integrity.
8. **Fibrinogen Assay**: Measures the level of fibrinogen in the blood, which is important for blood clot formation. Abnormal levels can indicate bleeding or clotting disorders.
9. **Factor Assays**: These tests measure the activity of specific clotting factors, such as Factor VIII for haemophilia A or Factor IX for haemophilia B.

10. **Thromboelastography (TEG) and Rotational Thromboelastometry (ROTEM)**: These are more advanced tests that provide a dynamic assessment of the entire coagulation process, offering information about clot formation, strength, and breakdown.

In this chapter, we aim to discuss a variety of conditions and drugs that may result in coagulopathy and how it changes the conduct of regional anaesthesia. We shall also cover the guidelines in place for management of such patients.

16.4 General Considerations and Risks Associated with Administering Regional Anaesthesia in Coagulopathic Patient

16.4.1 Risks Associated with Administering Regional Anaesthesia in Coagulopathic Patient

The most frightful but rare complication one can imagine in coagulopathic patients post-neuraxial anaesthesia would be vertebral canal haematoma (VCH), defined as symptomatic bleeding within the spinal neuraxis, and can lead to paraplegia if not addressed promptly. Permanent neurological complications following peripheral nerve blocks (PNBs) may result in seriously incapacitating consequences. The actual incidence of neurologic dysfunction post central neural blockade resulting from haemorrhagic complications is unknown. However, it was reported to be 0.85 per 100,000 (95% CI 0–1.8 per 100,000) in the third National Audit Project (NAP3). It also identified epidural catheter removal as the time of greatest risk for epidural haematoma development.

Published reports of significant haemorrhagic complications from peripheral nerve and plexus blocks suggest the harm is mainly derived from spinal haematoma, exsanguination, compression of surrounding structures leading to airway obstruction, major blood vessel occlusion, or tissue ischaemia. Relative risk varies and increases from superficial to deep blocks as outlined in Table 16.1. Management of bleeding complications in deep peripheral nerve blocks and central neuraxial blocks (CNB) is difficult as compared to superficial nerve blocks due to the site and non-compressibility. Invasive intervention may be required in some cases.

Experienced and well-trained clinicians may be able to reduce the incidence of vascular puncture, and procedures such as supraclavicular blocks can be performed safely under ultrasound guidance.

Table 16.1 Relative risk associated with individual regional anaesthetic techniques in coagulopathic patient

Low risk → → → → → **High risk**

Superficial blocks	**Perivascular blocks**	**Deep blocks**	**Neuraxial and paravertebral blocks**
– Forearm – Knee – Ankle – Superficial cervical plexus – Wrist – Digital – Bier's block **Fascial blocks** – Ilioinguinal – Iliohypogastric – Transversus abdominis plane	Popliteal / sciatic – Femoral nerve – Intercostal nerve – Interscalene – Axillary	– Coeliac plexus – Stellate ganglion – Proximal sciatic – Obturator – Infraclavicular – Supraclavicular	– Epidural with catheter (highest risk) – Single-shot epidural – Spinal – Paravertebral – Lumbar sympathectomy – Deep cervical plexus

16.4.2 Considerations for Neuraxial Block in Obstetric Patient

Population group which is most likely to receive neuraxial block as an exclusive modality of anaesthesia is the parturient. Not only do they differ in their physiology, but they may also present with conditions that alter the haemostatic mechanism. In general, pregnancy is a procoagulant state. The concentration of all clotting factors rises except Factors II, V, XI, and XIII. This continues for up to 7 days postpartum with an increased risk of thrombotic complications and returns to baseline by 2 weeks postpartum. In the obstetric population, the overall estimated risk of epidural or spinal haematoma following neuraxial anaesthesia is 1:168,000.

Platelet abnormalities are the most common haematological disorder during pregnancy and are most often caused by hypertensive disorders such as preeclampsia, gestational thrombocytopenia, or idiopathic thrombocytopenic purpura. Conventionally, spinal/epidural blocks were considered safe if the platelet count was above 70,000–100,000/cumm. This recommendation has been questioned mainly because thrombocytopenia during pregnancy often occurs with qualitative defects as well, and neuraxial anaesthesia is safer than general anaesthesia for the parturient. Each case must be assessed individually, weighing the risks and benefits.

Another condition seen exclusively during pregnancy is the *acute fatty liver of pregnancy*. It affects almost 1 in 5000–10,000 pregnancies. A potentially fatal obstetric complication is characterized by acute hepatic failure due to fatty liver infiltration. Coagulopathy, electrolyte abnormalities, and multisystem organ dysfunction are among the consequences. If the INR is less than 1.5, neuraxial puncture is considered safe in these patients.

Sepsis and coagulation abnormalities are highly likely to occur following *intrauterine foetal death* (IUFD). In 3% of patients with uncomplicated intrauterine foetal death and 13% of patients with placental detachment or uterine perforation, coagulation abnormalities are present.

Rarely, obstetric patients may have concomitant *inherited coagulation disorders* such as von Willebrand disease, haemophilia A and B, protein C and S deficiency, antithrombin III deficiency, Factor V Leiden mutation, and antiphospholipid antibody syndrome.

Any one of the following three factors can result in nerve injuries caused by regional anaesthetic procedures: trauma to the nerve; chemical damage; or a compression injury. An epidural abscess or spinal hematoma can cause compression injuries. Up to 50% of hematomas occur during epidural catheter removal.

In summary, the following scenarios represent a very high risk of developing VCH with consequent cord compression and permanent impairment after a regional anaesthetic procedure:

1. Platelets less than 75,000 or abnormal coagulation tests in pre-eclamptic patient or HELLP syndrome.
2. Platelets less than 20,000 in idiopathic thrombocytopaenia.
3. Therapeutic dose of LMWH less than 6 h before puncture.
4. aPTTr above normal range in a patient on UFH infusion,
5. INR > 2 in a patient on Warfarin.
6. With abruption or overt sepsis in patients with IUFD.

16.5 Disorders of Coagulation

To discuss coagulation abnormalities and the underlying pathophysiology is beyond the scope of this chapter. In brief, bleeding disorders can be classified as in Fig. 16.1.

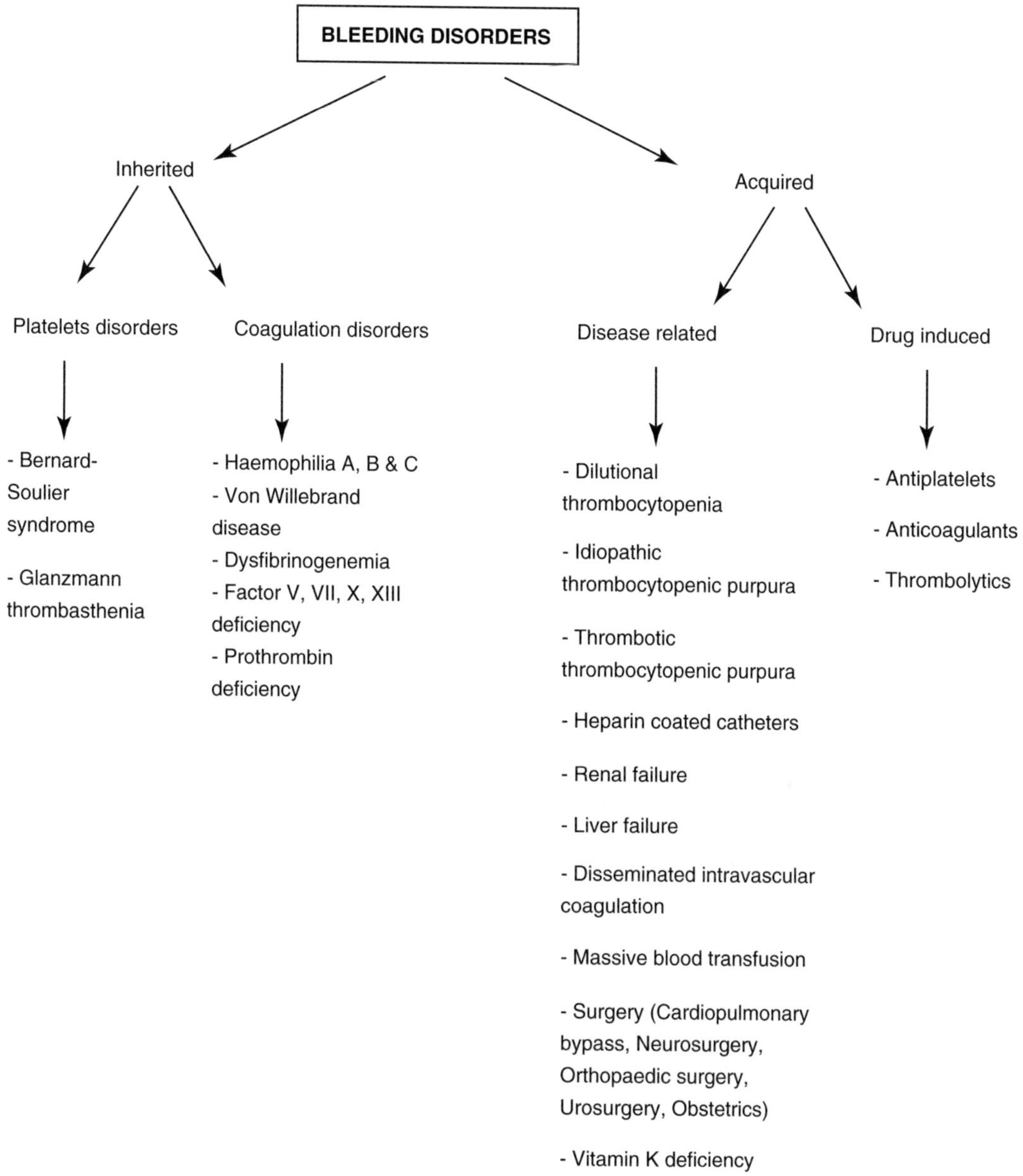

Fig. 16.1 Classification of bleeding disorders

16.6 Approach and Troubleshooting in Patients with Coagulation Abnormalities

16.6.1 Inherited Disorders of Coagulation

Commonly encountered inherited coagulopathies in clinical practice mainly comprise of Von Willebrand's disease (vWD) and haemophilia. The clinical picture can range from asymptomatic to those with severe bleeding tendencies.

vWD is caused by either a quantitative (Type 1 and 3) or a qualitative (Type 2) defect in Von Willebrand factor (vWF), with Type 1 being mild and Type 3 being the most severe. We do not recommend use of regional anaesthesia in Type 2 and 3 vWD. Peripheral nerve blocks under ultrasound guidance in Type 1 vWD can be considered provided that vWF:RCo level (vWF:ristocetin cofactor level) is maintained at about 100 IU/dL perioperatively and > 50 IU/dL in the immediate postoperative period. The Factor VIII (FVIII) plasma concentration should be above 100 IU/dL and sustained above 50 IU/dL in the postoperative period. Desmopressin (DDAVP), FVIII/vWF concentrate, and tranexamic acid can be used to reduce risk of bleeding, if required. DDAVP is administered subcutaneously or intravenously at a dose of 0.3 μg/kg administered 90 min before the procedure. Patients not responsive to DDAVP are candidates for FVIII and/or VWF replacement therapy. Tranexamic acid should be administered at a dose of 10–15 mg/kg intravenously 3–4 times a day. Due to the paucity of large randomized controlled trials, we cannot conclude safety of neuraxial puncture in vWD even though there are case reports of neuraxial anaesthesia in parturient with vWD without bleeding complications. vWF activity level of 0.50–1.50 IU/mL is advised to allow neuraxial anaesthesia in parturient. To conclude, the authors do not recommend performing neuraxial puncture in patients with vWD and appropriate expert haematology opinion should be sought before elective peripheral nerve blocks in Type 1 vWD patients.

Haemophilia is a rare X-linked congenital bleeding disorder characterized by a deficiency of coagulation FVIII, called haemophilia A, or factor IX (FIX), called haemophilia B. Haemophilia A is about four times more common than haemophilia B. A definitive haemophilia diagnosis is based on a factor assay to demonstrate deficiency of FVIII or FIX in a patient presenting with history of easy bruising or spontaneous bleeding. The normal value is 0.5–1.5 IU/mL or 50–150%. World Federation of Hemophilia (WFH) recommends that epidural in carriers of haemophilia is not contraindicated if the coagulation screen is normal and the relevant factor level is above 50 IU/dL or raised to above 50 IU/dL by prophylactic treatment. In the absence of an inhibitor, each IU of plasma derived or recombinant FVIII and FIX per kilogram of body weight infused intravenously 30–60 min before the procedure will raise the plasma level by approximately 2 IU/dL and 1 IU/dL, respectively. For patients with haemophilia undergoing surgery, the WFH advises against CNB. If required, it should be performed only under adequate clotting factor coverage as the safety of neuraxial procedures has not been established in patients with haemophilia.

Key Points
- Obtain a preoperative clotting screen and specific factor assay as required.
- Avoid CNB in all patients with either vWD or haemophilia.
- Safety of labour epidural in asymptomatic carrier of haemophilia is unclear.
- Peripheral nerve block in Type 1 vWD after careful consideration of risk and benefits.

16.6.2 Disease-Related Coagulopathy

Frequently, anaesthesiologists come across patients who may need regional anaesthesia and have concomitant disease that may affect the coagulation system. Common causes include trauma, massive transfusion, renal and/or hepatic dysfunction, disseminated intravascular coagulopathy (DIC), and sepsis.

Severe *sepsis* is associated with a procoagulant state and is usually anticoagulated for deep vein thromboprophylaxis. Consumptive coagulopathy may develop in septic shock. Severe sepsis remains a relative contraindication to central neuraxial anaesthesia due to the presumed increased incidence of epidural abscess, meningitis, and potential coagulopathy.

Haemorrhagic diathesis associated with *uraemia* is primarily due to platelet dysfunction. These patients may also be on regular dialysis and have residual anticoagulation after heparin administration. Heparin should be adequately reversed if regional anaesthesia is performed. In acute scenario, DDAVP has been used to control bleeding, but it cannot be used as a substitute for providing adequate cover in CNB.

Liver is the primary site for synthesis of coagulation factors except Factor VIII. *Liver failure* is associated with haemostatic abnormality and there may be associated thrombocytopenia and abnormal platelet function as well due to associated hypersplenism. Patients with liver failure represent a high-risk group for general anaesthesia. When regional anaesthesia is considered an alternative, coagulopathy should be evaluated and corrected.

The coagulopathy in *trauma* occurs because of tissue trauma, shock, haemodilution, hypothermia, acidosis, and inflammation. When there is a massive transfusion, major trauma is frequently associated with dilutional and consumption coagulopathy. This coagulopathy is a dynamic situation and evaluation of coagulation status should be made when haemorrhage is controlled, and the patient is haemodynamically stable. Viscoelastic haemostatic assays have been used regularly in many trauma units, but there is no clear cost-effective benefit established over conventional tests of coagulation.

Disseminated intravascular coagulopathy is the pathological systemic intravascular activation of coagulation mechanisms in response to a disease process leading to a consumptive coagulopathy. Safe conduct of CNB cannot be established in such cases and alternative anaesthetic techniques should be explored. Peripheral nerve blocks, if considered, should be performed by expert operator at compressible sites and under ultrasound guidance.

Key Points

- Obtain full coagulation screen.
- Consider underlying pathology.
- Ensure adequate blood and blood products are available.
- Functional platelet dysfunction may be helped by administering DDAVP.
- RA is especially high risk in DIC due to alternating prothrombotic and coagulopathic state.

16.6.3 Clinical Case Scenario

A 27-year-old primigravida at 36 weeks of gestation presented with HELLP syndrome to the maternity unit. She had a HR 96/min and BP 158/90 mmHg. Her investigations were as follows: Hb 10.8 g/dL, WBC 15,600/cumm, platelets 84,000, INR 1.5, aPTT 38, bilirubin 1.8, AST 210, ALT 250, ALP 280, and creatinine 1.2 mg/dL. Decision was taken to perform a caesarean section to terminate the pregnancy.

Key Issues

- Coagulopathy secondary to HELLP syndrome.
- Time-sensitive surgery.

The anaesthetist decided to avoid spinal anaesthesia in view of the deranged coagulation profile and decided to go ahead with general anaesthesia. He also planned for a bilateral TAP block under ultrasound guidance for postop pain relief.

Discussion

- Coagulopathy is a relative contraindication for RA. The risks and benefits should be weighed, and a plan should be formed after discussion with the surgeon and the patient.
- Ensure availability of blood and blood products.
- Risk of bleeding after RA varies with the specific technique and proximity to vascular structures. There is a low risk of bleeding after plane blocks like TAP block.
- Use of ultrasound can further reduce the risk as the path of needle can be visualized and any vascular structures can be avoided.
- Some anaesthetists may argue that a single-shot spinal anaesthetic can be performed under FFP cover. However, it is important to note that HELLP syndrome involves rapidly changing coagulation issues, making it advisable to avoid neuraxial block procedures in such patients.

16.6.4 Drug-Induced Coagulopathy

Several classes of antiplatelets and anticoagulants are in clinical use, and their implications for performance of neuraxial puncture vary substantially. A brief classification of these is shown in Figs. 16.2 and 16.3.

The American Society of Regional Anesthesia (ASRA) guidelines are considered to be the industry standard for conduct of regional anaesthesia in patients with drug-induced coagulopathy. It provides recommendations primarily for CNB and states that same precautions should be taken for those undergoing peri-neuraxial, deep plexus, or deep peripheral block. Careful consideration of vascularity and compressibility of the anatomical site and the potential consequences of bleeding at that site should be made for superficial plexus and peripheral nerve blocks. The European Society of Regional Anaesthesia & Pain Therapy also provides recommendations

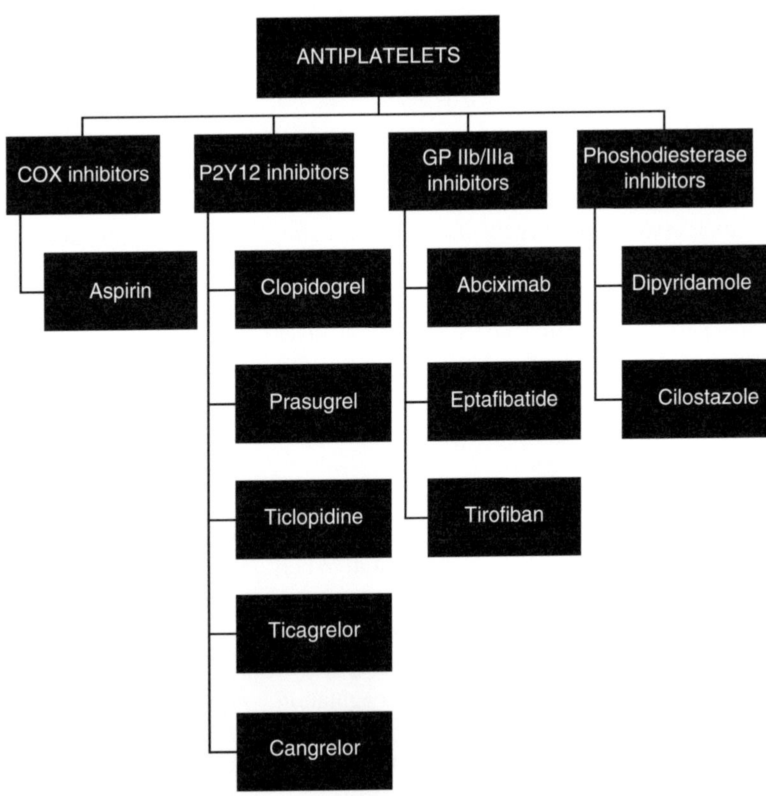

Fig. 16.2 Classification of antiplatelet drugs

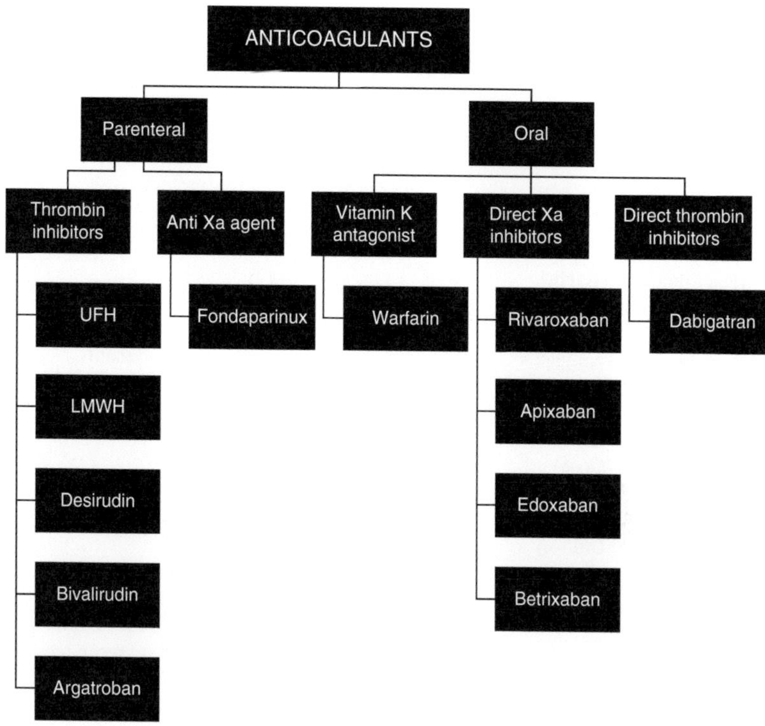

Fig. 16.3 Classification of anticoagulant drugs

along similar line. Furthermore, they state that a parturient on anticoagulants is to be managed same as a non-pregnant patient. Table 16.2 summarizes the guidelines in a concise and easy to use manner.

In case the patient is on long-term anticoagulation, a plan for bridging therapy should be made in consultation with haematologist. For understanding of the readers, Table 16.3 outlines bridging therapy for different agents in a nutshell, but clinical scenarios are often not as straightforward and hence expert haematology opinion is paramount.

The ASRA guidelines are applicable to patients presenting for elective as well as emergency surgeries. In case urgent reversal of anticoagulation is required, drug specific agents can be used. A brief summary is provided in Table 16.4.

Societal recommendations for safe neuraxial puncture recommend a platelet count >1,00,000/cumm and INR < 1.4. It is important to understand that coagulopathy is a relative contraindication for neuraxial anaesthesia. Careful consideration should be given to the risks and benefits of regional vs general anaesthesia, availability of equipment/services to manage bleeding complications, and patient preference.

Key Points

- Consider suitability of regional anaesthesia based on the antiplatelet/anticoagulant patient is on.
- Check coagulation status prior to performing the procedure.
- Ensure appropriate time has passed before performing the procedure.
- In case of emergency, consider use of reversal agents for specific drugs, if available.
- Follow same guidelines for deep plexus block as those for CNB.
- Same guidelines apply for obstetric patient as well.

Table 16.2 Guidelines for administering regional anaesthesia to patients on drugs interfering with haemostasis

Drug	Interval between last dose and neuraxial puncture/catheter removal	Restart anticoagulation after neuraxial puncture/catheter removal	Comments
Fibrinolytics and thrombolytics (t-PA, STK)	Contraindicated	–	Not recommended to perform spinal or epidural anaesthetics except in highly unusual circumstances
Unfractionated heparin – IV infusion Subcutaneous – Low dose prophylaxis (<15,000 U/day) – High dose prophylaxis (>15,000 U/day or > 5000 U/dose) – Therapeutic (> 20,000 U/day or > 10,000 U/dose)	4–6 h 4–6 h 12 h 24 h	1 h 1 h Assess risk vs benefit Assess risk vs benefit	– Assess platelet function prior to neuraxial puncture/catheter removal if patient has received UFH > 4 days – Monitor with aPTT, Anti-Xa, ACT
Low molecular weight heparin – Prophylactic – Therapeutic (enoxaparin 1 mg/kg every 12 h, enoxaparin 1.5 mg/kg daily, dalteparin 120 U/kg every 12 h, dalteparin 200 U/kg daily, or tinzaparin 175 U/kg daily)	12 h 24 h	– First postop dose given 12 h after neuraxial puncture for patient receiving prophylactic dose – Therapeutic-dose LMWH may be resumed 24 h after non-high-bleeding risk surgery and 48–72 h after high bleeding risk surgery – Wait for 4 h after catheter removal before giving therapeutic/prophylactic LMWH	– Not recommended to concomitantly use medications affecting haemostasis, such as antiplatelet drugs, standard heparin, or dextran, regardless of LMWH dosing regimen when there is an indwelling neuraxial catheter – Delay LMWH 24 h postoperatively after a traumatic puncture – Do not use therapeutic dosing with catheter in place
Anti-Xa agents – IV (fondaparinux) Oral – Rivaroxaban – Apixaban – Edoxaban – Betrixaban	– 72 h 72 h 72 h 72 h	6 h 6 h 6 h 6 h 6 h	– Do not maintain neuraxial catheters with anti-Xa agents – Do not perform neuraxial blocks in patients with a CrCl of less than 30 mL/min – In case of unanticipated administration with indwelling catheter, wait for 30 h before removing catheter with rivaroxaban, apixaban, and edoxaban. Wait for 72 h with betrixaban

(continued)

Table 16.2 (continued)

Drug	Interval between last dose and neuraxial puncture/catheter removal	Restart anticoagulation after neuraxial puncture/catheter removal	Comments
Direct thrombin inhibitors – Parenteral (desirudin, bivalirudin, and argatroban) – Oral (dabigatran)	Contraindicated – CrCl <30 mL/minute: Avoid neuraxial puncture – CrCl 30–49 mL/minute: 120 h – CrCl 50–79 mL/minute: 96 h – CrCl ≥80 mL/minute: 72 h – Renal function unknown: 120 h	6 h	– With unanticipated administration with indwelling catheter, we suggest that dabigatran dosing be held for 34–36 h – May be reversed with idarucizumab if necessary
Vitamin K antagonist (warfarin)	5 days		– Reversal for urgent surgery/procedure, consider 2.5–5 mg oral or IV vitamin K; for immediate reversal, consider PCCs, fresh frozen plasma – Patients at high risk of thromboembolism, bridge with therapeutic SC LMWH (preferred) or IV UFH preoperatively
Antiplatelets NSAIDs Platelet P_2Y_{12} receptor blockers – Clopidogrel – Prasugrel – Ticlopidine – Ticagrelor – Cangrelor GpIIb/IIIa inhibitors – Abciximab – Eptifibatide – Tirofiban Phosphodiesterase (PDE) inhibitors – Cilostazol – Dipyridamole Aspirin	No contraindication to neuraxial puncture with concomitant use of NSAIDs 5–7 days 7–10 days 10 days 5–7 days 3 h 24–48 h 4–8 h 4–8 h 2 days 24 h May continue dosage	– Therapy may be resumed immediately after needle placement/catheter removal, provided a loading dose of the drugs is not administered. If a loading dose is administered, wait for 6 h (2C) 8 h 6 h 6 h	– Do not maintain neuraxial catheters with prasugrel, ticagrelor, or cangrelor – Contraindicated for 4 weeks after surgery; monitor neurologic status if given after neuraxial technique for GpIIb/IIIa inhibitors – Remove catheter ≥6 h prior to first postoperative dose for PDE inhibitors

Table 16.3 Overview of bridging therapy

Days	Vitamin K antagonist (VKA)	Direct oral anticoagulants	Antiplatelets
−7			Stop prasugrel
−6			
−5	STOP		Stop clopidogrel
−4	Consider bridging in specific cases		
−3		Stop with impaired kidney/liver function	Stop ticagrelor
−2		STOP	
−1		No bridging	
Surgery			
+1	Start UFH/LMWH Restart VKA with low bleeding risk	Restart VKA with low bleeding risk	Restart P2Y12 inhibitors
+2	Restart VKA with high bleeding risk	Restart VKA with high bleeding risk	

Table 16.4 Options for reversal of drug-induced anticoagulation

Anticoagulant	Possible reversal agents	Options for lab monitoring
Unfractionated heparin	Protamine sulphate	APTT or anti-FXA levels
Low molecular weight heparin	Protamine sulphate (partial neutralization)	Anti-FXA levels
Fondaparinux	None	Anti-FXA levels
Argatroban	None	APTT
Bivalirudin	None	APTT
Warfarin (vitamin K antagonists)	Vitamin K PCC FFP	International normalized ratio (INR)
Dabigatran[a]	Idarucizumab	Thrombin time[b] Dilute thrombin time Ecarin clotting time Ecarin chromogenic assay
Apixaban and rivaroxaban[c]	Andexanet alfa[d] PCC aPCC	Chromogenic anti-FXa assay calibrated against apixaban or rivaroxaban[b]
Edoxaban[c]	PCC aPCC	Chromogenic anti-FXa assay calibrated against edoxaban[b]

However, if there is concern about therapeutic medication levels or desire to monitor drug levels before or after reversal, then these assays may be utilized

Abbreviations: *FFP* fresh frozen plasma, *PCC* prothrombin complex concentrate, *aPCC* activated prothrombin complex concentrate, *APTT* activated partial thromboplastin time

[a]Could consider haemodialysis or activated charcoal for reversal of medication

[b]Not required for use and regular monitoring of anticoagulant

[c]Could consider activated charcoal for reversal of medication

[d]Not approved for reversal in the preoperative setting

16.7 Management of VCH

In the rare event of VCH, early identification and appropriate management are critical.

Usual symptoms of VCH include *acute axial back pain* radiating to corresponding dermatome with or without focal neurologic deficit with signs of nerve root or spinal cord compression within 24–48 h after a neuraxial puncture. Pain is typically exacerbated by percussion over the spine and by increased intraspinal pressure caused by coughing, sneezing, or straining.

Associated symptoms may include numbness, weakness, and urinary or faecal incontinence.

- Any new onset neurological deficit like paraesthesia (numbness/tingling), weakness, unexplained excessive pain following a PNB or effect of the block lasting longer than expected (>48 h after single injection) can be suggestive of hematoma around the nerve.
- It is paramount to rule out any pre-existing neurological symptoms.
- In case the post-op neurodeficit is not consistent with pre-op neurodeficit, then a detailed examination should be carried out including a check for distal pulsations. Special attention should be paid to tight plasters/casts and splints. Consider gentle limb repositioning to relieve pressure over nerves that run a superficial course.
- Discontinue epidural infusion if neurologic deficit is evident, with the catheter left in place, to rule out any contribution from the local anaesthetic.
- Consider an urgent lesion if there is motor deficit and/or progressively worsening symptoms.
- Urgent ultrasound/magnetic resonance imaging (MRI) may be warranted.
- Surgical management is usually required in urgent cases.
- Favourable neurologic recovery can occur if surgery and decompression are performed within 36 h of a complete motor deficit and within 48 h of a partial deficit.
- There are multiple case reports of conservative management and follow-up in non-urgent cases or those with minor deficits.
- Prognosis for neurologic recovery primarily depends on the patient's preoperative neurologic status and duration of neurologic dysfunction.
- The authors recommend neurosurgical consultation when in doubt, considering time-sensitive deterioration.

16.8 Summary

Management of patients with coagulopathy could be challenging even with latest diagnostic modalities. There is no established consensus when it comes to patients with inherited bleeding disorders. Adequate haemostasis before and after puncture and during catheter removal is necessary for safe conduct of regional anaesthesia. Inherited and acquired bleeding disorders and concomitant use of anticoagulant medications deserve special consideration due to the devastating outcome following VCH. Patients should be well counselled regarding the risks associated with the specific anaesthetic procedure with respect to deranged coagulation. If the risk of thromboembolism is high, it may be appropriate to take antithrombotic drugs during the perioperative period. All possible avenues should be explored to minimize the risk of haematoma, and if deemed unfit, general anaesthesia should be administered.

Further Reading

Ashken T, West S. Regional anaesthesia in patients at risk of bleeding. BJA Educ. 2021;21(3):84.

Bauer ME, Arendt K, Beilin Y, Gernsheimer T, Perez Botero J, James AH, et al. The society for obstetric anesthesia and perinatology interdisciplinary consensus statement on neuraxial procedures in obstetric patients with thrombocytopenia. Anesth Analg. 2021;132(6):1531–44.

Bhatia P, Chhabra S. Physiological and anatomical changes of pregnancy: implications for anaesthesia. Indian J Anaesth. 2018;62(9):651.

Butwick AJ, Carvalho B. Neuraxial anesthesia for cesarean delivery in a parturient with type 1 von Willebrand disease and scoliosis. J Clin Anesth. 2007;19(3):230–3.

Castaman G, Goodeve A, Eikenboom J. Principles of care for the diagnosis and treatment of von Willebrand disease. Haematologica. 2013;98(5):667.

Cata JP, Hanna A, Tetzlaff JE, Bishai A, Barsoum S. Spinal anesthesia for a cesarean delivery in a woman with type-2 M von Willebrand disease: case report and mini-review. Int J Obstet Anesth. 2009;18(3):276–9.

Connell NT, Flood VH, Brignardello-Petersen R, Abdul-Kadir R, Arapshian A, Couper S, et al. ASH ISTH NHF WFH 2021 guidelines on the management of von Willebrand disease. Blood Adv. 2021;5(1):301–25.

Faculty of Pain Medicine. Best practice in the management of epidural analgesia in the hospital setting [Internet]. FPM; 2020. Available from: https://fpm.ac.uk/media/2576

Horlocker TT, Vandermeulen E, Kopp SL, Gogarten W, Leffert LR, Benzon HT. Regional anesthesia in the patient receiving antithrombotic or thrombolytic therapy: American Society of Regional Anesthesia and Pain Medicine evidence-based guidelines. Obstet Anesth Dig. 2019;39(1):28–9.

Katz D, Beilin Y. Disorders of coagulation in pregnancy. Br J Anaesth. 2015;115(suppl_2):ii75–88.

Kietaibl S, Ferrandis R, Godier A, Llau J, Lobo C, Macfarlane AJ, et al. Regional anaesthesia in patients on antithrombotic drugs: joint ESAIC/ESRA guidelines. Eur J Anaesthesiol. 2022;39(2):100–32.

Maronge L, Bogod D. Complications in obstetric anaesthesia. Anaesthesia. 2018;73:61–6.

Membership of the Working Party, Harrop-Griffiths W, Cook T, Gill H, Hill D, Ingram M, Makris M, et al. Regional anaesthesia and patients with abnormalities of coagulation: the Association of Anaesthetists of Great Britain & Ireland the obstetric Anaesthetists' association regional Anaesthesia UK. Anaesthesia. 2013;68(9):966–72.

Moster M, Bolliger D. Perioperative guidelines on antiplatelet and anticoagulant agents: 2022 update. Curr Anesthesiol Rep. 2022;12:286–96. https://doi.org/10.1007/s40140-021-00511-z.

O'Flaherty D, McCartney CJL, Ng SC. Nerve injury after peripheral nerve blockade – current understanding and guidelines. BJA Educ. 2018;18(12):384–90.

Palta S, Saroa R, Palta A. Overview of the coagulation system. Indian J Anaesth. 2014;58(5):515.

Peterson W, Tse B, Martin R, Fralick M, Sholzberg M. Evaluating hemostatic thresholds for neuraxial anesthesia in adults with hemorrhagic disorders and tendencies: a scoping review. Res Pract Thromb Haemos. 2021;5(4):e12491.

Ruppen W, Derry S, McQuay H, Moore RA. Incidence of epidural hematoma, infection, and neurologic injury in obstetric patients with epidural analgesia/anesthesia. J Am Soc Anesthesiol. 2006;105(2):394–9.

Shah UJ, Narayanan M, Graham SJ. Anaesthetic considerations in patients with inherited disorders of coagulation. Continu Educ Anaesth Crit Care Pain. 2015;15(1):26–31.

Sridharan M. Anticoagulant reversal- patient blood management resources. International Society of Blood Transfusion. https://www.isbtweb.org/isbt-working-parties/clinical-transfusion/resources/patient-blood-management-resources/16-anticoagulant-reversal.html#:~:text=Parenteral%20anticoagulants%20have%20a%20short,plasma%2C%20or%20prothrombin%20complex%20concentrate.

Srivastava A, Santagostino E, Dougall A, Kitchen S, Sutherland M, Pipe SW, et al. WFH guidelines for the management of hemophilia. Haemophilia. 2020;26:1–58.

Yoon HJ. Coagulation abnormalities and bleeding in pregnancy: an anaesthesiologist's perspective. Anesth Pain Med. 2019;14(4):371–9.

Sympathetic Nerve Blocks

17

Shailendra Kumar, Dhruv Jain,
and Sana Yasmin Hussain

Abstract

Sympathetic nervous system is organized at various levels in the body innervating organs and multiple structures. Visceral organs are supplied by sympathetic plexus like celiac plexus, hypogastric plexus, and ganglion impar. Upper limb and head are supplied by stellate ganglion, while lower limb is supplied by lumbar sympathetic chain. Blocks of these fibres can alleviate pain conditions and other conditions associated with sympathetic activity. Cancer pain is now commonly treated with visceral sympathetic plexus blocks with reasonable success, improving the quality of life in these patients. Chronic regional pain syndrome and peripheral vascular diseases can be effectively managed with stellate or lumbar sympathetic blocks. Proper understanding of anatomy and steps for conduct of these minimally invasive percutaneous interventions is required for precise placement of blocks. Use of fluoroscopy and ultrasound helps in improving efficacy of these blocks by improving success rate and minimizing complications. Long-lasting relief can be provided by destruction of these sympathetic plexus with chemical neurolysis or radiofrequency ablation.

Keywords

Sympathetic nerve blocks · regional anaesthesia · interventional ultrasound · fluoroscopy, chronic pain

17.1 Introduction

Sympathetic nerve blocks are used to treat a wide variety of conditions like sympathetically mediated pain, visceral pain, vascular disorders, and neuropathic pain. Commonly used interventions include stellate ganglion, lumbar sympathetic, and abdominal sympathetic blocks. The block performed can be diagnostic to estimate the response and is performed with local anaesthetic. Therapeutic blocks involve destruction of sympathetic neurons with neurolytic agents like alcohol, phenol, or radiofrequency ablation and provide more sustained pain relief. Understanding the anatomy of the sympathetic chain and transmission of pain signals is important for successful block interventions for acute and chronic pain management.

S. Kumar · D. Jain · S. Y. Hussain (✉)
Department of Anaesthesiology, Pain Medicine and Critical Care, AIIMS, New Delhi, India

M. K. Prasad, S. J. S. Bajwa (eds.), *Steps to Successful Regional Anesthesia*,
https://doi.org/10.1007/978-981-97-4098-7_17

17.2 Abdominal Sympathetic Blocks

They are indicated in the presence of visceral pain of abdomen and pelvic organs. Malignancy or other chronic conditions involving these organs can result in significant pain. Blockade of sympathetic ganglion innervating these organs reduces the pain and the need for analgesics. The visceral afferent pain fibres of the abdomen travel along the sympathetic fibres, with cell bodies located in dorsal root ganglion. The second-order neurons then ascend via the spinothalamic tract. Blockade of sympathetic ganglia thus blocks the visceral afferents resulting in pain relief. The commonly performed sympathetic ganglion blocks for abdominal pain include:

1. *Celiac plexus block*: Liver, pancreas, gall bladder, stomach, small intestine, colon.
2. *Superior hypogastric plexus block:* Colon, rectum, pelvic organs.
3. *Ganglion impar block*: Perineal structures.

17.2.1 Celiac Plexus Block

17.2.1.1 Anatomy

It is a retroperitoneal complex of autonomic nerves lying anteriorly over the aorta near the origin of celiac and superior mesenteric artery. It consists of multiple ganglia—celiac, superior mesenteric and aorticorenal ganglia, which together form the plexus at the level of L1 vertebrae. It lies posteriorly to stomach and pancreas and lies anteriorly to the crura of diaphragm (Fig. 17.1).

The plexus is formed by preganglionic efferents originating from the greater splanchnic nerve (T5-T9), lesser splanchnic nerve (T10-

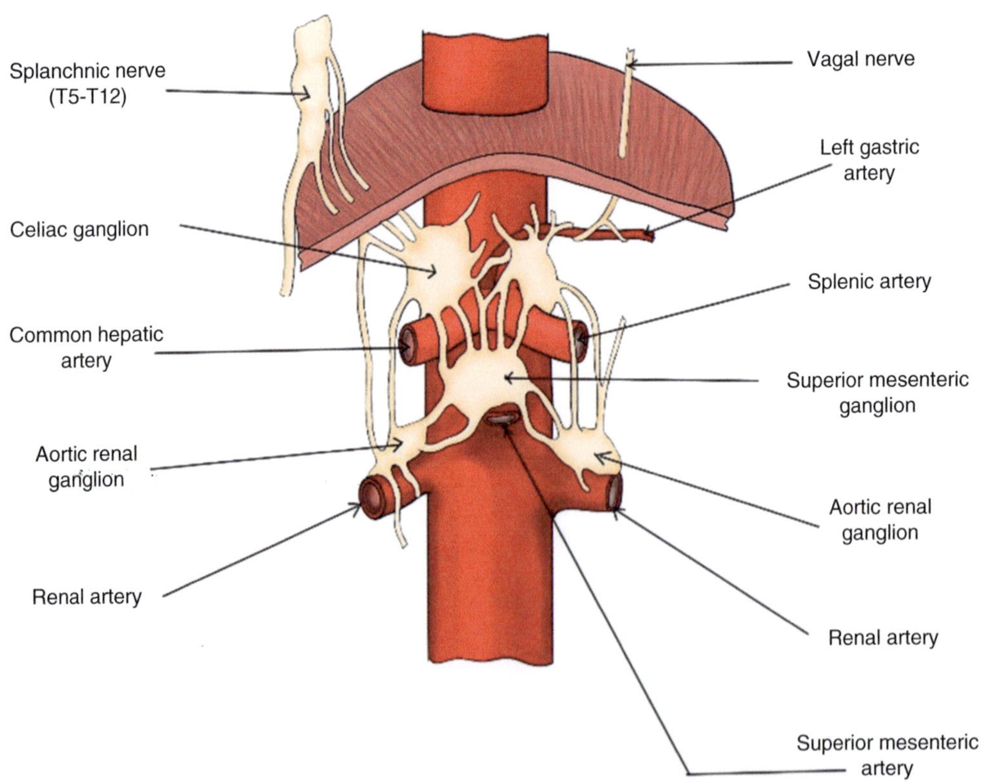

Fig. 17.1 Anatomy of celiac plexus

T11), and least splanchnic nerve (T12) bilaterally. Parasympathetic fibres from vagus also contribute to celiac plexus. Visceral afferent pain fibres innervating upper abdominal organs like liver, gall bladder, pancreas, kidneys, adrenal glands, and gut (from distal oesophagus to mid colon) accompany sympathetic fibres at celiac plexus and block at this level interrupts the pain signals.

17.2.1.2 Indications

1. Intractable abdominal visceral pain.
2. Cancer pain involving gall bladder, pancreas, or stomach.
3. Acute or chronic pancreatitis.

17.2.1.3 Contraindications

1. Coagulopathy.
2. Local infection.
3. Abnormal anatomy due to soft tissue mass.

17.2.1.4 Techniques

The block can be performed by fluoroscopy (posterior approach) or anteriorly (ultrasound approach). In posterior approach, in prone position via fluoroscopy, the drug can be deposited behind the crura (retrocrural) which blocks the splanchnic nerves. If the diaphragm is pierced, the tip of the needle can lie more accurately near the plexus (transcrural). With the advent of ultrasound, the block is given via anterior approach in supine position to puncture the abdominal wall and liver and deposit the drug anterior to aorta.

Fluoroscopy Guided

(i) The patient is placed in prone position.
(ii) The inferior margin of 12th rib is marked and a line is drawn transversely at level of L2. The intersection of these two lines marks the needle entry point on either side and is roughly 5–7 cm from midline. Two 20G, 15 cm needles are inserted from these points towards body of L1 at angle of 45 degrees to make contact with the vertebral body.
(iii) After contact, needles are withdrawn till subcutaneous tissue and redirected laterally to walk of the surface of L1 vertebrae.
(iv) The left-sided needle is advanced beyond the L1 vertebral body and is kept posterior to the aorta. The right-sided needle is advanced further to make it lie anterolateral to aorta.
(v) After negative aspiration, dye is given for confirmatory spread (Fig. 17.2).

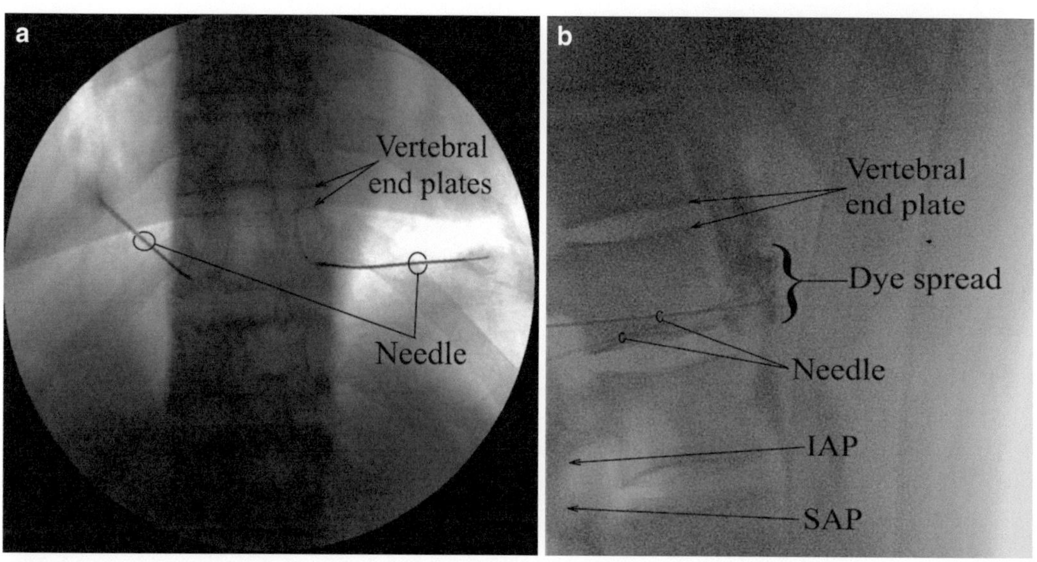

Fig. 17.2 (**a**) Needle trajectory and dye spread in AP view for celiac plexus block. (**b**) Needle trajectory and dye spread in lateral view for celiac plexus block

Ultrasound Guidance

In supine position, a low-frequency probe is placed transversely below the xiphoid process in the epigastric area (Fig. 17.3). The aorta is visualized as a pulsating deep structure. The probe is tilted cephalad to see the muscular fibres of diaphragm surrounding the aorta. The probe is then moved caudally to locate the first branch of aorta.

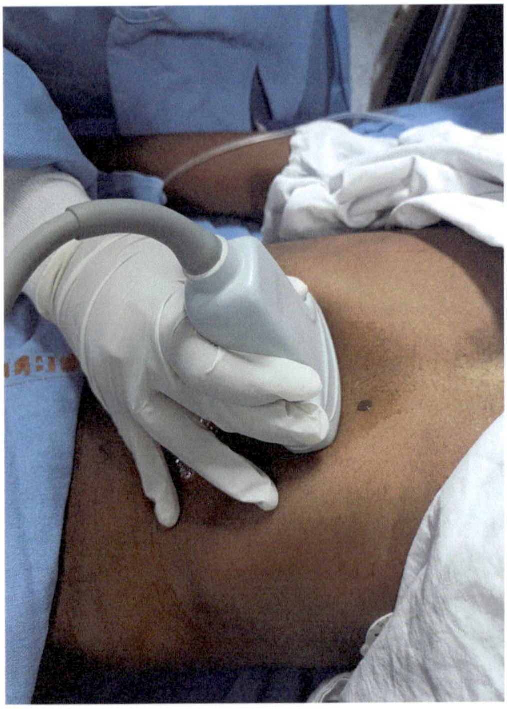

Fig. 17.3 Probe placement in epigastric area

This is the celiac trunk and can be seen dividing into common hepatic and splenic artery. This bifurcation forms the 'ram-horn' or 'seagull' sign (Fig. 17.4). Moving more caudally, the second branch arising from the aorta is superior mesenteric artery.

The target for celiac plexus block is just cephalad to the origin of celiac artery. In an in-plane technique, a 22G needle is inserted to reach just anterior to aorta. After negative aspiration, 10–15 ml of 0.25% bupivacaine is given. For neurolysis, 15 ml of ethanol 50–100% is used.

17.2.1.5 Complications

1. Hypotension: Transient, usually managed with fluids.
2. Diarrhoea: Lasts for 1–2 days.
3. Hematoma, bleeding.
4. Renal injury.
5. Pneumothorax.
6. Spinal cord ischemia.
7. Intravascular injection.

17.2.1.6 Tips

Ultrasound technique is becoming increasingly popular due to comfortable patient position, single needle puncture, and no risk of radiation hazard. In cases, where tumour lies anterior to the aorta or surrounds the celiac plexus, anterior approach may not be feasible.

Single puncture technique can be performed under fluoroscopy by transaortic technique. A

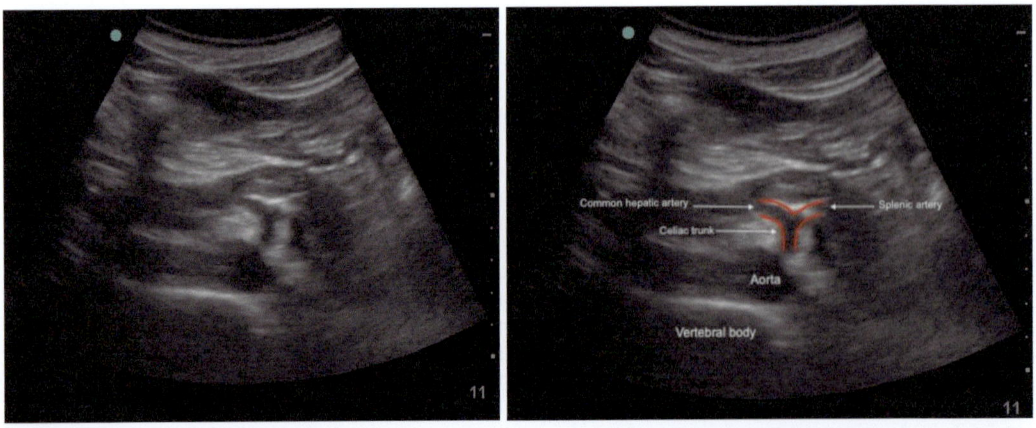

Fig. 17.4 Sonoanatomy for celiac plexus block, 'seagull' sign formed by celiac artery and its branches

single left-sided needle is inserted as described above, and aorta is punctured so that the needle lies anteriorly. This ensures good preaortic spread.

17.2.2 Superior Hypogastric Block

17.2.2.1 Anatomy

Hypogastric plexus is a plexus of nerves situated retroperitoneally at the level of fifth lumbar vertebrae and sacral promontory. It is continuation of celiac plexus and lumbar sympathetic chain and is located below the level of aortic bifurcation (Fig. 17.5). It receives sympathetic innervation from lumbar splanchnic nerves (L2-L3) and parasympathetic supply is via pelvic splanchnic nerves (S2-S4). From the plexus, right and left hypogastric nerve arise which run medially to internal iliac arteries. It joins the parasympathetic fibres of S2-S4 to form the inferior hypogastric plexus innervating the pelvic viscera including bladder, uterus, rectum, vagina, and prostate.

17.2.2.2 Indications

1. Chronic pelvic pain, endometriosis.
2. Pelvic visceral cancer pain.
3. Interstitial cystitis.
4. Irritable bowel syndrome.

17.2.2.3 Contraindications

1. Coagulopathy.
2. Local site infection.

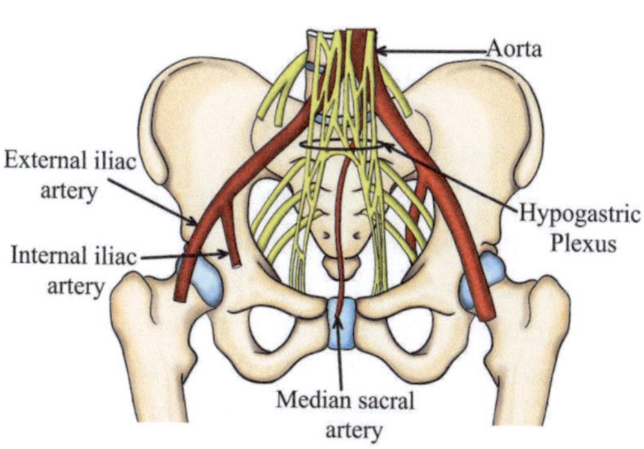

Fig. 17.5 Anatomy of superior hypogastric plexus

17.2.2.4 Techniques

Fluoroscopy Guided

(i) Place the patient in prone position and obtain anteroposterior (AP) view on fluoroscopy.
(ii) Identify the L4-L5 intervertebral space.
(iii) Draw a transverse line at this level.
(iv) Mark 2 points—5–7 cm lateral from midline on either side on the transverse line. These will be the entry points for the needle.
(v) Introduce 20G 15 cm needle at a medial angle of 45 degree and 15 degree caudal towards the anterolateral aspect of lower part of L5 vertebrae.
(vi) In the AP view, the needles should be at junction of L5-S1 and medial to the edge of vertebral body.
(vii) In the lateral view, the needles should be just anterior to the vertebral body.
(viii) After confirmation, 2–3 ml of radio-opaque dye is given to visualize the dye spread at the anterior aspect of L5-S1 (Fig. 17.6a, b).
(ix) Inject 5–7 ml of 0.25% bupivacaine/ropivacaine through each needle for diagnostic block.
(x) For neurolytic block, administer 5–8 ml of 6% phenol or 50–100% ethanol through each needle.

Ultrasound Guided

(i) Place the patient in supine position and prepare the abdomen.
(ii) Take a low-frequency curvilinear probe and place the probe transversely on the abdomen in the midline (Fig. 17.7).
(iii) Visualize the pulsating aorta and trace it caudally until it bifurcates into iliac artery.
(iv) At this level, identify the hyperechoic border of L5 vertebrae and two iliac vessels on anterolateral margin of vertebral body (Fig. 17.8).
(v) At this level, introduce a 15 cm needle in out-of-plane approach to reach the anterior margin of vertebral body. After negative aspiration, inject 10 ml of local anaesthetic to visualize the spread over vertebral body.

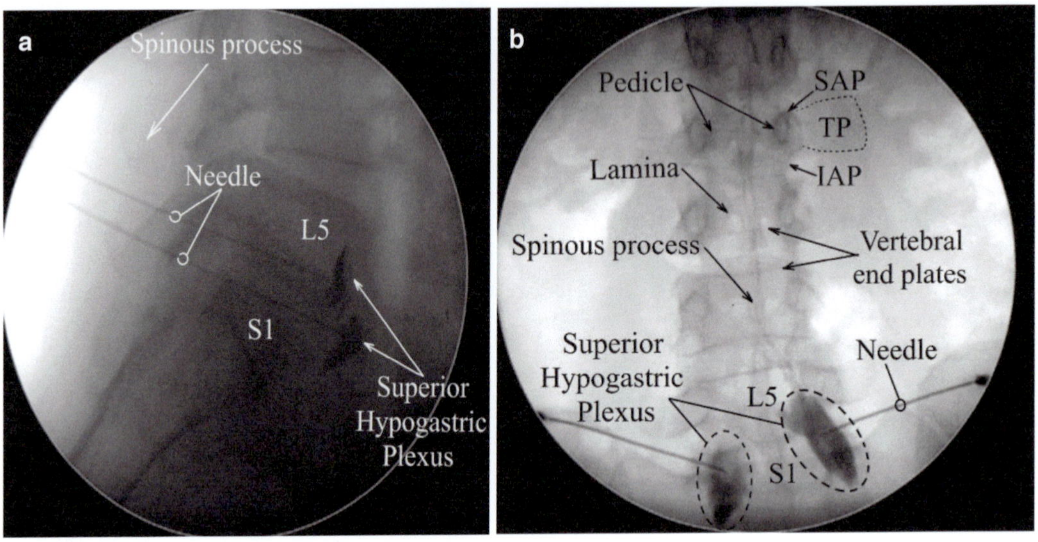

Fig. 17.6 (**a**) Dye spread in superior hypogastric plexus block—lateral view. (**b**) Dye spread in superior hypogastric plexus block—AP view

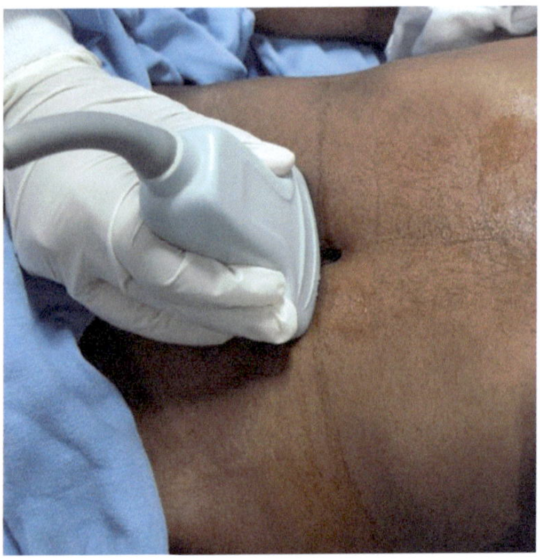

Fig. 17.7 Probe placement for superior hypogastric plexus block

(vi) For neurolysis, 10–15 ml of 50–100% ethanol can be given.

17.2.2.5 Complications

1. Hematoma, bleeding, intravascular injection.
2. Injury to L5 nerve root.
3. Hypotension.
4. Bowel injury.

17.2.2.6 Tips

(i) Bowel preparation is helpful to remove gas which makes visualization better in both fluoroscopy and ultrasound technique.

(ii) Bladder emptying may be helpful while performing block under ultrasound guidance.

(iii) Under fluoroscopic view, iliac crest and transverse process of L5 may hinder the movements of needle, which requires manipulation of the needle either cephalad or caudad.

(iv) A transdiscal technique can be performed fluoroscopically if needle manipulation is difficult. It requires only single needle insertion; however, strict asepsis is required.

17.2.3 Ganglion Impar Block

17.2.3.1 Anatomy

Ganglion impar is the most caudal part of the two sympathetic chains that run along the vertebral column and represents the fusion of the two chains into a single ganglion at the termination. It lies usually in the midline at the sacrococcygeal junction (Fig. 17.9). Visceral afferent from perineal structures converges at this ganglion.

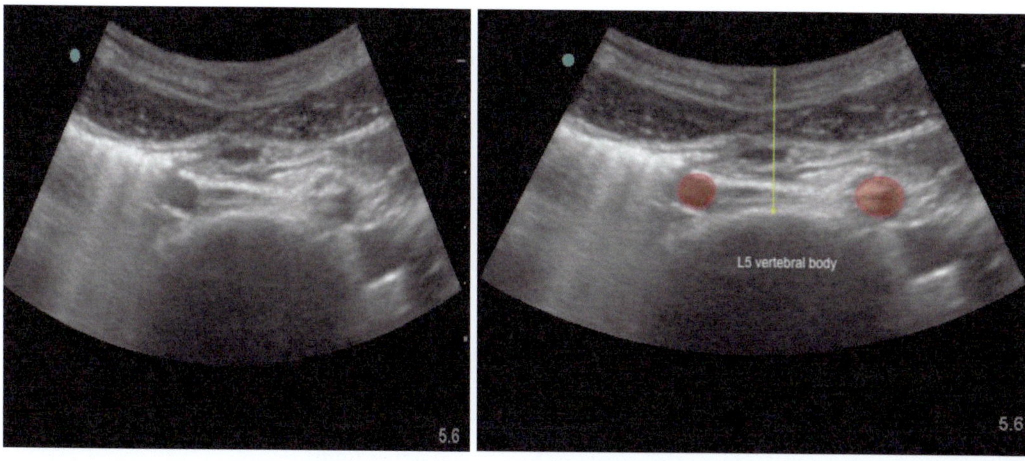

Fig. 17.8 Sonoanatomy for hypogastric plexus block. Needle direction is over L5 vertebrae between common iliac arteries

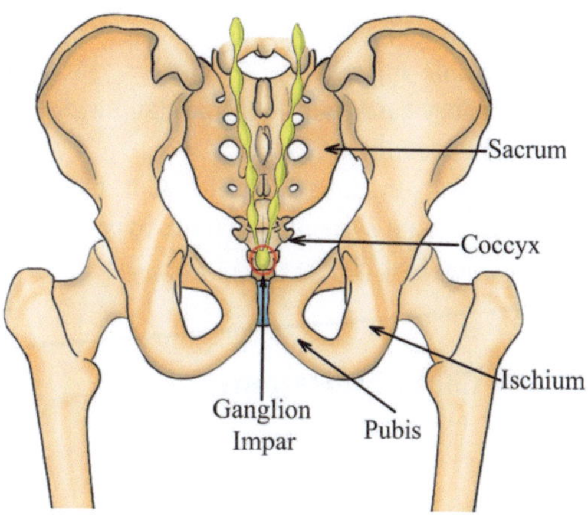

Fig. 17.9 Anatomy of ganglion impar

17.2.3.2 Indications

1. Cancer pain of anus, distal rectum, vagina, and perineum.
2. Coccydynia.
3. Sympathetic-mediated pain in the perineal region.

17.2.3.3 Contraindications

1. Local infection.
2. Coagulopathy.
3. Abnormal bony anatomy at the sacrococcygeal junction.

17.2.3.4 Technique

The ganglion impar is performed fluoroscopically for better accuracy and visualization of drug spread.

(i) Place the patient in prone position and prepare the intergluteal, perianal area.
(ii) Obtain AP view and mark the sacrococcygeal joint after palpation.
(iii) On the lateral view, identify the joint and infiltrate the skin with lignocaine.
(iv) Take a 22G, 9 cm needle and insert it perpendicularly towards the joint under fluoroscopic guidance.
(v) Pierce the sacrococcygeal junction and stop as soon as the tip crosses the anterior border of the joint. A loss of resistance will be felt when the needle pierces the sacrococcygeal ligament.
(vi) Administer 2 ml of dye, a smooth contour along the bone will be seen (Fig. 17.10).
(vii) Inject 3–4 ml of local anaesthetic solution with steroid. For neurolysis, 4–5 ml of 6% phenol may be used.

17.2.3.5 Complications

1. Rectal perforation—if needle is inserted too anteriorly.
2. Nerve root injury.
3. Neuritis.

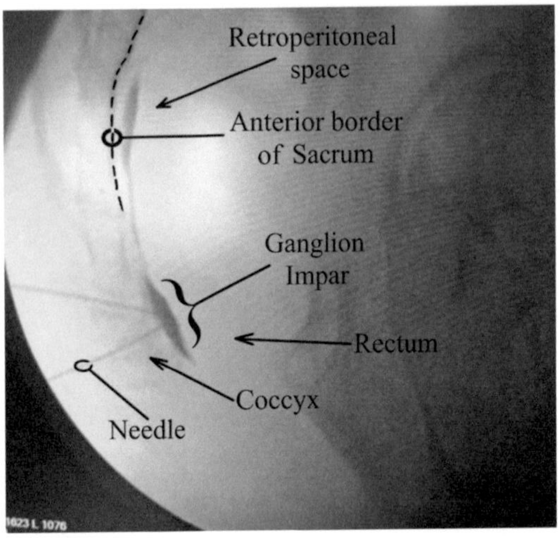

Fig. 17.10 Needle placement through sacrococcygeal junction and spread of contrast in ganglion impar block

17.2.3.6 Tips

Needle approach through sacrococcygeal joint is easy to perform. Be careful not to insert needle too far anteriorly so as to avoid rectal puncture.

17.3 Stellate Ganglion Block

17.3.1 Introduction

Stellate ganglion block (SGB) is performed at the level of C6/C7 vertebral level for various conditions like complex regional pain syndrome, Raynaud's disease, phantom limb pain, etc. It exerts its effect by blocking the sympathetically mediated pain and by increasing the blood supply of the region. It was traditionally done using a landmark-guided technique. However due to higher rate of complications like vascular puncture and pneumothorax, ultrasound-guided technique or fluoroscopy-guided intervention is now preferred.

17.3.2 Anatomy

Stellate ganglion is formed by the fusion of first thoracic and inferior cervical ganglion. Preganglionic fibres from the lateral horn of upper thoracic segments ascend up and pass through the stellate ganglion. It supplies sympathetic fibres to head neck region and the upper limb. It lies in the neck anterior to the transverse process of C7, neck of first rib, and longus colli muscle. Vertebral artery lies lateral to it, whereas oesophagus, thoracic duct, and vertebral body of C7 lie medially (Fig. 17.11).

17.3.3 Indications

1. Complex regional pain syndrome of the head and upper limbs.
2. Upper limb vasospasm or embolism.
3. Raynaud's disease.
4. Scleroderma.
5. Phantom limb pain.
6. Intractable angina.
7. Refractory cardiac arrhythmias (supraventricular tachycardia).
8. Post-traumatic stress disorder as it decreases dysfunctional sympathetic tone, hyperarousal state, and inability to relax.

17.3.4 Contraindications

1. Recent myocardial infarction.
2. Coagulopathy.
3. Glaucoma.
4. Contralateral phrenic nerve palsy.

17.3.5 Technique

17.3.5.1 Landmark Guided

Patient is placed in supine position with slight neck extension and rotation to the other side. Transverse process of C6/Chassaignac's tubercle is palpated at the level of cricoid cartilage. Finger is placed on the carotid artery which is then gently pushed laterally. Needle is directed medially and inferiorly to hit C6. It is then withdrawn by few millimetres so that the tip lies over the longus colli muscle. After careful negative aspiration, 5–10 ml of local anaesthetic is injected.

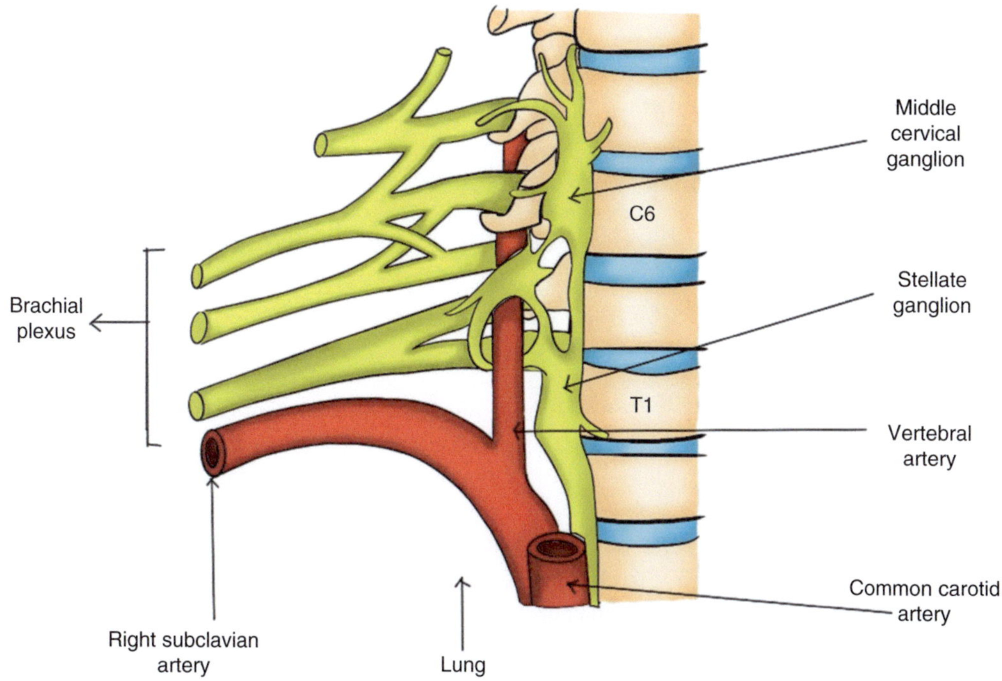

Fig. 17.11 Anatomy of stellate ganglion block

17.3.5.2 Ultrasound-Guided Technique

The patient is kept in supine position with neck slightly extended and head slightly rotated to the opposite side. A high-frequency, linear ultrasound transducer is placed perpendicular to the tracheal axis at the level of cricoid cartilage. The transducer is then moved laterally to visualize the anterior aspect of the Chassaignac's tubercle on the C6 transverse process (Fig. 17.12). The carotid artery, internal jugular vein, thyroid gland, longus colli, prevertebral fascia, the root of C6 spinal nerve, and transverse process of C6 can be identified (Fig. 17.13). With an in-plane approach, a 22G needle is inserted from lateral to medial direction. The tip of the needle should pierce the prevertebral fascia of the longus colli muscle located behind the posterior aspect of the carotid artery. Injury to vessels and nerves should be avoided. After negative aspiration, 5–8 ml of local anaesthetic is injected, and the diffusion of the injectate is seen in real time. The injectate is seen to spread under the prevertebral fascia and depression of longus colli muscle is seen. Though

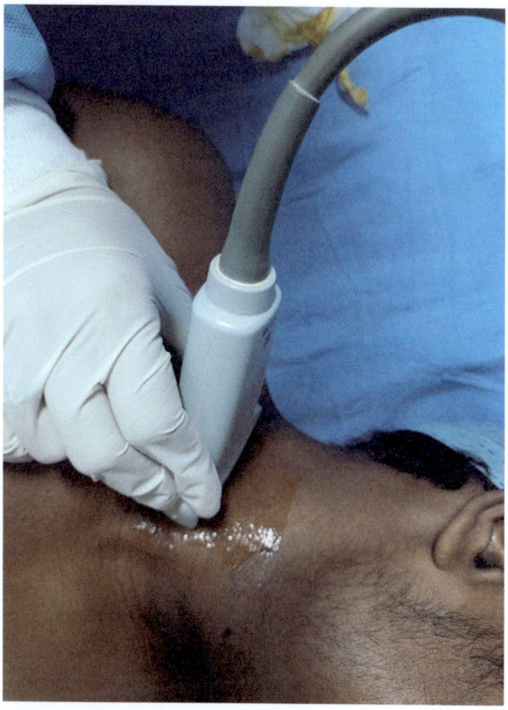

Fig. 17.12 Probe placement for stellate ganglion block

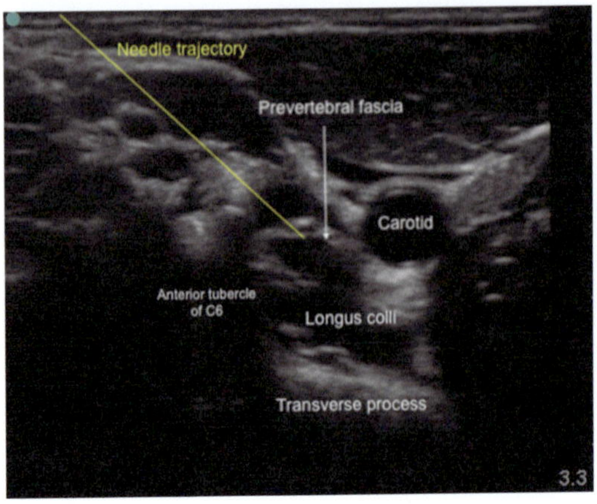

Fig. 17.13 Sonoanatomy and needle trajectory for stellate ganglion block

the ganglion lies mostly at the level of C6-C7 vertebra, injection is usually given at the level of C6 as the vertebral artery is left unprotected at the C7 level due to its absent or rudimentary anterior tubercle.

17.3.6 Complications

1. Horner's syndrome.
2. Vascular puncture involving vertebral artery, carotid artery, inferior thyroid artery, or internal jugular vein.
3. Hematoma, intravascular injection of drugs.
4. Injury to brachial plexus nerve roots.
5. Hoarseness of voice due to recurrent laryngeal nerve block.
6. Pneumothorax.
7. Needle injury to thyroid or oesophagus.
8. Infection.

17.3.7 Tips

Ultrasound helps in safer and easier block as compared to landmark- or fluoroscopic-guided techniques due to identification of soft tissues and vessels. Block at C7 level may increase the chances of a successful block, although extreme care is required to avoid vascular puncture at this level. Use of colour Doppler can aid in identification of vessels and preventing vascular injury. Inability to see the spread of injectate in the field should raise the suspicion of needle tip inside a vessel.

17.4 Lumbar Sympathetic Block

17.4.1 Anatomy

Lumbar sympathetic chain runs bilaterally along the lumbar vertebrae and consists of multiple ganglia. The efferents supplying this chain are preganglionic sympathetic fibres via the white rami communicans. The postganglionic fibres leave the trunk via grey rami to join the segmental spinal nerve and supply the lower limbs. The lumbar ganglia are variable in number from 4 to 5 and are mostly situated at L2–3 and L4–5 level.

The lumbar sympathetic chain is retroperitoneal and runs inferiorly along the anterolateral edge of vertebral body anterior to the psoas muscle (Fig. 17.14).

17.4.2 Indications

1. Chronic regional pain syndrome.
2. Peripheral vascular disease, Raynaud's disease.
3. Phantom limb pain.
4. Hyperhidrosis.

17.4.3 Contraindications

1. Coagulopathy.
2. Local infection.

17.4.4 Technique

The block is performed under fluoroscopic guidance at level of L2 or L3.

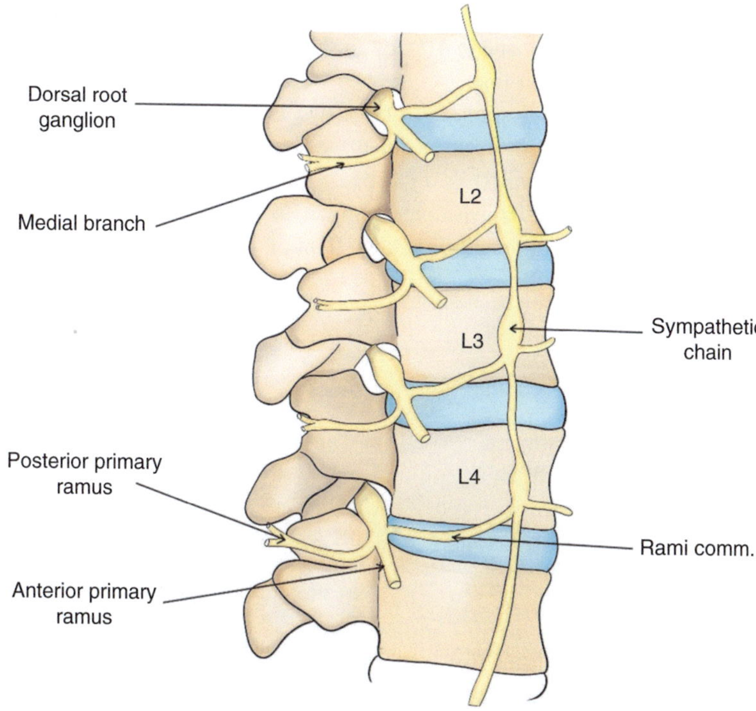

Fig. 17.14 Anatomy of lumbar sympathetic block

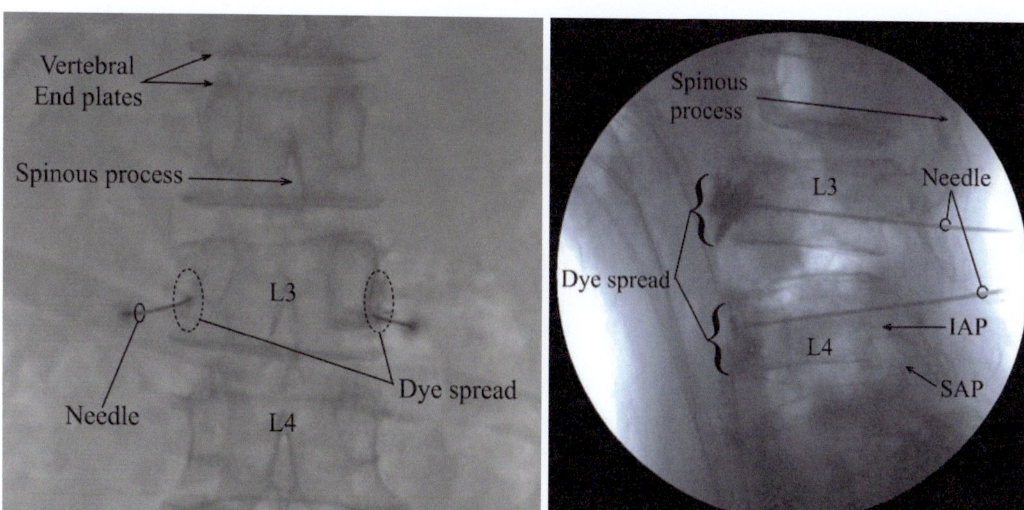

Fig. 17.15 (**a**) Needle end points in AP view with dye spread for lumbar sympathetic block. (**b**) Needle end points in lateral view with dye spread for lumbar sympathetic block

(i) In prone position, the target vertebral level and side to be performed is identified in AP view.

(ii) The C-arm is rotated obliquely on the ipsilateral side until the transverse process is buried inside the vertebral body.

(iii) A 20G needle is inserted on the edge of vertebral body and inserted under tunnel vision. It is advanced anteriorly to reach the anterolateral edge of vertebral body (Fig. 17.15a).

(iv) In lateral view, the needle tip should lie just anterior to the body and in AP view, it should lie in mid-pedicular line.
(v) After negative aspiration, 2–3 ml of dye is given which spreads cranio-caudally along the sympathetic chain (Fig. 17.15b).
(vi) 10 ml of 0.25% bupivacaine is given as diagnostic block. For neurolysis, 5–10 ml of 6% phenol is used.

17.4.5 Complications

1. Hypotension.
2. Renal or ureteric injury.
3. Genitofemoral neuralgia.
4. Hematoma, bleeding.
5. Intravascular injection.
6. Nerve injury.

17.5 Summary

S.no	Sympathetic block	Area innervated	Indications	Site	Drug and volume
1	Stellate ganglion	Ipsilateral upper limb, head, and neck	CRPS, peripheral vascular disease, Raynaud's disease, refractory cardiac arrhythmias, hyperhidrosis	At level of C6 transverse process above longus colli muscle	5–8 ml of local anaesthetic (LA)
2	Lumbar sympathetic	Ipsilateral lower limb	CRPS, peripheral vascular disease, phantom limb pain	Anterolateral border of L2 or L3 vertebrae	10 ml of local anaesthetic Neurolysis—Up to 10 ml of 6% phenol
3	Celiac plexus	Liver, gall bladder, spleen, stomach, kidneys, gut (up to transverse colon)	Cancer pain, acute/chronic pancreatitis	Periaortic at level of celiac trunk (L1)	20–30 ml of LA 15–20 ml of 50–100% ethanol
4	Superior hypogastric	Descending colon, rectum, bladder, uterus, vagina, prostate	Cancer pain, chronic pelvic pain, endometriosis	Below bifurcation of aorta at level of L5	10–20 ml of LA 10–20 ml of 50–100% ethanol
5	Ganglion impar	Perineum, anus, distal vagina, vulva	Cancer pain, coccydynia	Anterior to sacrococcygeal junction	4–5 ml of LA 50–100% ethanol

Further Reading

Dhamija E, Khandelwal I, Bhatnagar S, Thulkar S. A systematic approach to give bedside ultrasound-guided celiac plexus block. Indian J Pain. 2017;31(2):80. https://doi.org/10.4103/ijpn.ijpn_29_17.

Jetti R, Kadiyala B, Bolla SR. Anatomy, back, lumbar sympathetic chain. StatPearls; 2023. Accessed 29 Mar 2023. http://www.ncbi.nlm.nih.gov/books/NBK539914/

Mehrotra M, Reddy V, Singh P. Neuroanatomy, Stellate Ganglion. StatPearls; 2023. Accessed 29 Mar 2023. http://www.ncbi.nlm.nih.gov/books/NBK539807/

Menon R, Swanepoel A. Sympathetic blocks. Contin Educ Anaesth Crit Care Pain. 2010;10(3):88–92. https://doi.org/10.1093/bjaceaccp/mkq012.

Mishra S, Bhatnagar S, Rana SPS, Khurana D, Thulkar S. Efficacy of the anterior ultrasound-guided superior hypogastric plexus neurolysis in pelvic cancer pain in advanced gynecological cancer patients. Pain Med Malden Mass. 2013;14(6):837–42. https://doi.org/10.1111/pme.12106.

Narouze S. Ultrasound-guided stellate ganglion block: safety and efficacy. Curr Pain Headache Rep. 2014; 18(6):424. https://doi.org/10.1007/s11916-014-0424-5.

Plancarte R, Amescua C, Patt RB, Aldrete JA. Superior hypogastric plexus block for pelvic cancer pain.

Anesthesiology. 1990;73(2):236–9. https://doi.org/10.1097/00000542-199008000-00008.
Scott-Warren JT, Hill V, Rajasekaran A. Ganglion impar blockade: a review. Curr Pain Headache Rep. 2013;17(1):306. https://doi.org/10.1007/s11916-012-0306-7.
Sikandar S, Dickenson AH. Visceral pain – the ins and outs, the ups and downs. Curr Opin Support Palliat Care. 2012;6(1):17–26. https://doi.org/10.1097/SPC.0b013e32834f6ec9.
Spiegel MA, Hingula L, Chen GH, Legler A, Puttanniah V, Gulati A. The use of L2 and L3 lumbar sympathetic blockade for cancer-related pain, an experience and recommendation in the oncologic population. Pain Med Off J Am Acad Pain Med. 2019;21(1):176–84. https://doi.org/10.1093/pm/pnz142.
Urits I, Jones MR, Orhurhu V, et al. A comprehensive review of the celiac plexus block for the management of chronic abdominal pain. Curr Pain Headache Rep. 2020;24(8):42. https://doi.org/10.1007/s11916-020-00878-4.

Interventions in Palliative Care 18

Sunny Malik and Vibhu Ranjan Sahni

Abstract

Palliative care focuses on providing support and improving the quality of life for individuals with serious or life-limiting illnesses and their families. The goal is to address physical, emotional, social, and spiritual needs. Pain is one of the most dreaded symptoms of cancer. Cancer pain has traditionally been managed by WHO ladder. However, pain interventions now can be taken up at any step depending on risk/benefit ratio. Pain interventions are now been used for almost all cancer-related pain. Sympathetic ganglion blocks like stellate, celiac, splanchnic, hypogastric, and ganglion impar are performed frequently for cancer pain. This chapter highlights these pain-related interventions and their use in different cancer conditions.

Keywords

Stellate · Celiac · Splanchnic · Hypogastric · Ganglion impar · Radiofrequency Ablation · Cancer pain · Palliative

S. Malik (✉) · V. R. Sahni
Department of Pain and Palliative Medicine, Rajiv Gandhi Cancer Institute and Research Centre, South Delhi, India

18.1 Introduction

Pain is one of the most common and feared symptoms in the minds of both the cancer patients and their caregivers.

The prevalence of pain in cancer patients varies between 20% and 50% in the early stages of the disease, while the majority of cancer patients with advanced disease suffer moderate-to-severe pain. There are multiple pain generators in the body that have both a physical and a psychological component.

According to the WHO validation report, almost 75% of patients get satisfactory pain relief via pharmacotherapy using the WHO analgesic ladder until the last days of their lives. However, in the rest 20–25% of patients who are refractory to opioids, MIPSIs (minimally invasive pain and spine interventions) are deemed necessary.

A three-step analgesic ladder approach for cancer pain management was proposed in 1986 and was renamed as "Modified WHO Analgesia Ladder" after introduction of minimally invasive nerve interventions in the form of MIPSI which was added as the fourth step. Foley K et al., however, postulated another school of thought and said that intervention pain techniques can be used at each step depending on the patient's needs, especially in visceral malignancy pain and localized bone pain due to metastasis. For MIPSI, we need to know the aetiology of pain (nociceptive/visceral/breakthrough pain/neuropathic pain),

M. K. Prasad, S. J. S. Bajwa (eds.), *Steps to Successful Regional Anesthesia*,
https://doi.org/10.1007/978-981-97-4098-7_18

progression of disease (multiple pain generators: target the main one first), expectations of patient as well as the family (realistic hopes and honest communication control the pain better), and availability of expertise to perform the procedure with desired equipment.

18.2 Intervention in Head and Neck Cancer Pain

Head and neck cancer (HNC) is defined as "cancer that arises in the head or neck region (the nasal cavity, sinuses, lips, mouth, salivary glands, throat, or larynx)". The main histological type is squamous cell carcinoma.

Pain is one of the most common problems, with incidence as high as 85% in head and neck cancer patients. It is due to the presence of rich innervations, comprising mixed nociceptive plus neuropathic component. It occurs in the head and neck area and dynamic movement during speech, swallowing, and other functional movements. The neuropathic component occurs in the form of an electric shock like sensation and localized continuous burning that is severely troublesome for the patient. This usually involves the maxillary and mandibular branches of the trigeminal nerve. Addressing the physical and psychological component of pain here is must during the curative phase as well as in palliative settings.

18.2.1 Interventional Technique for Pain in Head and Neck Cancer Patient

The face and neck are supplied by the trigeminal nerve (fifth cranial) and the C2-C4 cervical nerve roots that constitute the superficial cervical plexus.

The trigeminal nerve has a large territory of distribution and consists of sensitive fibres (touch, pain, and temperature) and motor fibres of the face (chewing). It originates in the posterior fossa and lies in Meckel's cavity (medial cranial fossa), from which originate three terminal branches: ophthalmic (V1), maxillary (V2), and mandibular (V3) divisions.

Interventions of these branches can be done by transforamen (passing the needle through the foramen ovale in a sub-mental view) or via extraforamen approach (through the mandibular notch).

18.2.1.1 Gasserian Ganglion Block

In cancer patients, trigeminal neuralgia occurs when tumour tissue is compressing the ganglion, tumour in the cerebellopontine angle area, post-surgery neuroma formation, radiation-induced neuritis, trismus-provoked neuralgia, and a fungating lesion involving the infratemporal fossa and masticatory space. Patients usually complain of lancinating and throbbing types of pain while doing functional activities like speaking, swallowing, and chewing. Gasserian ganglion block is the procedure of choice in such cases. Recent CT or MRI imaging is required to see the extent of involvement and to prevent any bleeding from tumour tissue during needling.

A percutaneous approach described by Hartel et al. through the foramen ovale is commonly used, in which an electrode (with an active tip of 2–5 mm) is introduced through the needle to make the heat lesion (ranging from 60 to 90 °C) of the nerve as shown in Fig. 18.1 which then no longer transmits nociceptive signals. Acute pain relief is usually achieved in 97.6% of patients with good sensory-motor dissociation when treating trigeminal neuralgia. Continuous complete pain relief at 5-year follow-up was seen in 57.7% of patients, though the effectiveness of pulsed radiofrequency ablation for trigeminal neuralgia is still under debate.

Anti-neuropathic medications and opioids need to be titrated again post-procedure. As the procedure might take care of the acuteness and sharpness of the pain at present, in cases of progressive malignancy, the infiltration might keep on changing and therefore require maintenance therapy with medications.

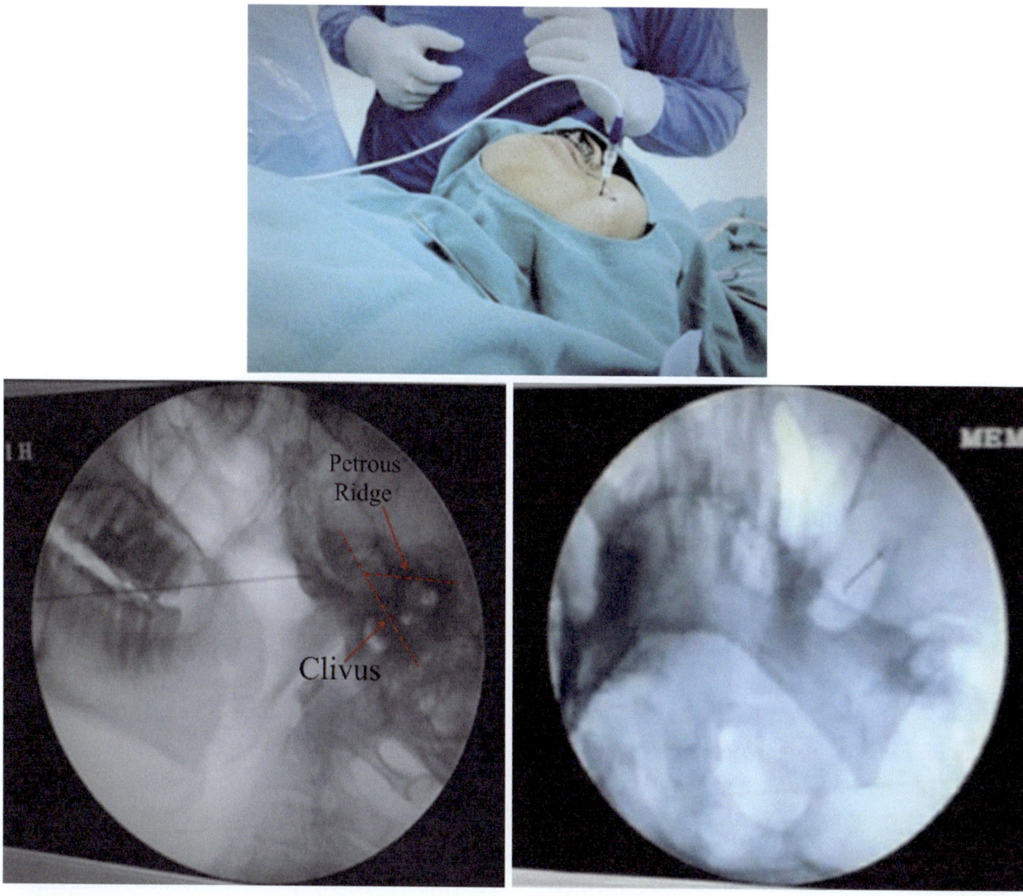

Fig. 18.1 Gasserian ganglion block and Gasserian ganglion radiofrequency ablation (lateral and submental view)

18.2.1.2 The Maxillary Nerve Block

In some cases of HNC involving the infratemporal fossa and lateral maxillary wall, there is a high possibility that the tumour might obstruct the foramen ovale. In such cases, maxillary nerve block is the preferred choice. The maxillary nerve is the intermediate division of the trigeminal nerve; it primarily supplies sensory innervation to the middle third of the face. It also carries postganglionic fibres from the pterygopalatine ganglion, which supply the lacrimal gland and mucous glands of the nasal mucosa.

This block can be given via two approaches: anterior zygomatic and supra-zygomatic, using a peripheral nerve stimulator to locate the pterygopalatine fossa with the help of ultrasound guidance or a combination of both.

18.2.1.3 The Mandibular Nerve Block

Cancers involving the body and ramus of the mandible, buccal mucosa, tongue, and floor of the mouth have high chances of mandibular nerve compression that leads to neuralgia-like pain. This nerve is the most common nerve involved in the HNC. The only trigeminal nerve branch with a motor root is the mandibular nerve. It innervates the lower face, including the mandible, lower teeth, and oral mucosa, the anterior two-thirds of the tongue, the lower lip, the temporomandibular joint, the mastication muscles, the skin of the temporal region, the anterior area of the auricle, and the external acoustic meatus.

It can be given using an infra-zygomatic approach under ultrasound guidance, by using neural stimulation, or a combination of both.

Failure of the block and transient facial paralysis are sometimes observed.

Tip For anatomic distortions and fungating lesions, an extra-foramen approach is much better and more superficial. This can be combined with well-titrated opioids and adjuvants for quality pain relief. Sometimes, instillation of a local anaesthetic mixture over these two nerves daily for 3–5 days also breaks the pain cycle and refractoriness.

18.2.1.4 Glossopharyngeal Nerve Block

The glossopharyngeal nerve can cause some cases of orofacial pain, with an incidence of 0.57–1.3%, especially the cancer-related pain syndromes associated with base of tongue tumours, oropharyngeal cancer, and cerebellopontine angle tumours. Glossopharyngeal neuralgia occurs as a paroxysmal pain in the oropharynx, nasopharynx, larynx, and base of tongue which sometimes radiates to the temporal area. The duration of these episodes varies from a few seconds to 2–5 min.

Glossopharyngeal nerve block can be accomplished through a variety of methods, including topical, intra-oral, transcutaneous peri-styloid approaches, and an ultrasound-guided approach in the parapharyngeal space.

A commonly used approach is the peri-styloid approach under fluoroscopy or ultrasound, mainly in cases that are refractory to the WHO ladder. Because of the close proximity of the jugular vein and the internal carotid artery, complications associated with the commonly used peri-styloid approach can include hematoma formation. Others include transient dysphagia due to stylopharyngeus muscle paralysis, transient weakness of the trapezius muscle and tongue due to blockade of the spinal accessory and hypoglossal nerves, respectively, seizure, cardiovascular collapse, bradycardia, asystole, reflex tachycardia, syncope, and in some cases, dysphonia secondary to vocal cord paralysis.

Tip It is noteworthy that the glossopharyngeal block is to be given unilaterally at a time as it can compromise the swallowing reflex and may lead to aspiration as innervations to the motor supply of the stylopharyngeus muscle might get blocked.

18.2.1.5 Sphenopalatine Nerve Block

The sphenopalatine ganglion (SPG) is an extracranial parasympathetic ganglion located within the pterygopalatine fossa. It is a complex neural centre with multiple connections to the trigeminal, facial, and sympathetic systems and consists of somatosensory, sympathetic, and parasympathetic fibres. The ganglion lies just below the maxillary nerve and receives three nerve roots: the sensory root of the sphenopalatine branches from the maxillary nerve, the motor root from the intermediate nerve (part of the facial nerve) through the major petrosal nerve, and the sympathetic root from the internal carotid plexus.

Sluder in 1908 described sphenopalatine neuralgia as a unilateral facial pain symptom complex with associated neuralgic, motor, sensory, and gustatory manifestations.

Sphenopalatine ganglion block (SGB) is indicated in cluster headache and migraine. Maxillary nerve neuralgia and pain due to cancer involving the maxilla, ethmoidal sinus, and pterygomaxillary or infratemporal resections are some indications of SGB in an oncology patient. This procedure can be performed under X-ray guidance for controlling headaches and atypical fascial pains due to head and neck cancers. Here, it is worth mentioning that recent radiological workups (CT/MRI) to look for the extent of tumour invasion and laboratory investigations (coagulation profile and platelet count) to prevent any massive bleeding are necessary as the tissue is fragile because of radiation therapy and cancer invasion. This block can be performed through trans-nasal, trans-oral, or transcutaneous (infra-zygomatic) approaches.

It has been observed that certain headaches associated with metastatic breast cancer with brain involvement, especially in young population, get controlled by trans-nasal sphenopalatine block.

18.2.1.6 Stellate Ganglion Block

The stellate ganglion is formed by the fusion of the inferior cervical ganglion and the first thoracic sympathetic ganglion and provides sympathetic output to the ipsilateral upper extremity, chest, face, and head. This is indicated in complex regional pain syndrome (CRPS) of the head and upper limbs, peripheral vascular disease, upper extremity embolism, postherpetic neuralgia, chronic post-surgical pain, hyperhidrosis, Raynaud's disease, scleroderma, orofacial pain, phantom limb, atypical chest pain, cluster or vascular headache, post-traumatic stress disorder, intractable angina, and nowadays in refractory cardiac arrhythmias.

It is a very common procedure that can be performed in a day care setting using ultrasound or a c-arm. In oncology, it has utility as a diagnostic procedure for CRPS (occurring due to level V surgical neck dissection, injury to the spinal accessory nerve, radiation-induced fibrosis, and nerve injury while harvesting the radial forearm free flap), phantom limb, and sympathetically mediated pain of the neck and upper limb. Contraindications such as recent myocardial infarction, anticoagulated patients or coagulopathy (evaluate risk/benefit ratio), glaucoma, pre-existing contralateral nerve palsy, severe emphysema, and cardiac conduction block should always be looked at beforehand while planning SGB.

Different pain physicians used different techniques, like ultrasound-guided (Sect. 17.3.5.2) and fluoroscopic techniques (AP view at the junction of the transverse process with the vertebral body or an oblique view at the base of the uncinate process) for this block (Fig. 18.2). Various complications like vascular injury (due to close proximity to the vertebral artery), neural injury, pneumothorax, injury to the thyroid gland, transient Horner's syndrome can occur with these techniques. We generally prefer a hybrid technique to minimize the complication rate. If the diagnostic procedure reveals that the patient has received adequate pain relief, he or she is scheduled for radiofrequency ablation.

18.2.2 Headache

A throbbing, sharp, continuous, or dull pain in the head defines a headache. Approximately 50% of patients with brain tumours experience headaches, with estimates ranging from 33% to 71%.

Headache is classified as a primary headache when there is no identifiable cause on examination or investigation and the diagnosis is made by recognizing a pattern, e.g., migraine, tension headache, or cluster headache.

Secondary headaches are those where there is a definite underlying cause, which can be: (a) extracranial disorders like glaucoma, sinusitis-induced disorders, dental disorders, temporomandibular dysfunction, etc., (b) intracranial disorders like infection (meningitis, encephalitis, subdural empyema), non-infection (cancer), CSF leak, etc., (c) drug-induced headaches caused by

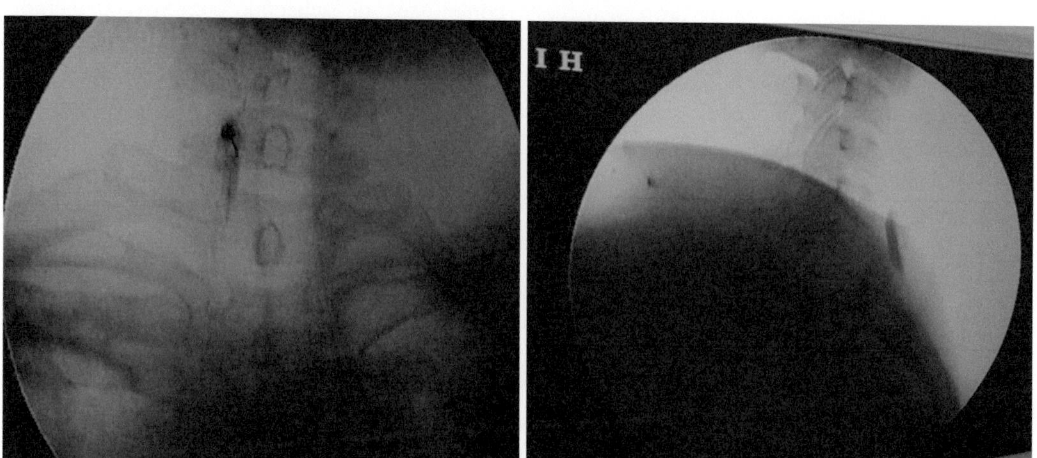

Fig. 18.2 Fluoro-guided stellate ganglion block (AP and lateral view—dye pattern)

chemotherapy (ixabepilone (Ixempra), mitoxantrone), immunotherapy (pembrolizumab, atezolizumab), targeted therapy drug (trastuzumab), hormonal therapy (anastrozole, letrozole, tamoxifen), and sometimes treatment-induced complications such as anaemia, dehydration, hypercalcemia, and infection.

Headache is frequently associated with advanced progressive cancer (lung cancer, breast cancer, prostate cancer, and lymphomas) with brain metastasis and brain tumours. Since management of patients with these tumours/secondary brain metastases is often palliative, proper treatment of symptoms such as headache becomes a key issue in preserving the patient's quality of life.

Interventions to relieve headache have a minimal role in end-of-life patients with brain metastasis, but they can be used as an adjuvant to pain relief in refractory cases. One of the procedures commonly used is a GON (greater occipital nerve) block, where the injection site is marked as being at the medial third of the distance between a hypothetical line from the occipital protuberance to the mastoid process (refer 4.1.4.5). Side effects of this block include local alopecia, transient dizziness, and worsening of the headache. This block can be repeated about every 3 months, depending on the patient's current condition. A trans-nasal sphenopalatine block is a commonly used practice to counteract acute severe headache episodes in a home care setting by holding the patient's head by the edge of the table and instilling 4% xylocaine drop by drop to percolate through the posterior pharyngeal wall into the ganglia. If patients have a life expectancy of a few months and the lumbar puncture is to be done repeatedly to drain extra CSF, the authors suggest placing a Vygon mini sitiplant assembly in a percutaneous pocket. As the tip is kept in the lumbar intrathecal space, this assembly helps to remove the CSF in aliquots of 10–20 mL in the hospital and even at home. Sterile dressings are to be done by a trained anaesthesia technician or a nurse practitioner, and the chances of infection have to be explained in detail to the family.

18.2.3 Myofascial Pain Syndrome

Myofascial pain syndrome (MPS) was originally described as the "regional pain characterized by the presence of one or more myofascial trigger points".

A myofascial trigger point is defined as a hyperirritable spot, usually within a taut band (palpable nodules or muscle knots) of skeletal muscle or in the muscle fascia, which is painful on compression and can give rise to characteristic referred pain, motor dysfunction, and autonomic phenomena.

Trigger points can be identified with hypoechoic signal intensity during diagnostic ultrasound or with the help of raised EMG levels over the trigger points. Cancer pain can be associated with fibromyalgia too, which is also something to take into consideration before starting any treatment.

Apart from the pharmacotherapy in the form of NSAIDs, opioids, corticosteroids, muscle relaxants, anti-depressants, or combinations of these drugs, various other treatment modalities have been tried, i.e., transcutaneous electric nerve stimulation (TENS), extracorporeal shock wave therapy (ESWT), dry needling, ozone therapy, massage therapy, hot and cold compresses, or ischaemic compression therapy. Dry needling can be used in patients with multiple trigger points associated with head and neck cancers. When the needle is introduced into the trigger points, it induces a local twitch response, which elicits a reflex relaxation of the muscle harbouring the trigger points through the mediation of a spinal reflex response. Multiple small hypodermic needles can be introduced blindly and kept in place for 15 minutes to half an hour. The ultrasound guidance can be used to identify larger trigger points and then Quincke's needle is inserted into the trigger point spot in real time for further hydro-dissection with saline, LA, or a steroid mixture.

18.2.4 Ozone Therapy

Ozone was discovered by German chemist Christian Friedrich Schonbein in 1834. Ozone was not widely employed in medicine until the 1930s, despite Landler using it for the first time in 1870. Bocci called ozone "the ideal cytokine inducer" and believes that ozone therapy creates "super-gifted red cells".

Ozone has several biologic effects, including antimicrobial action, stimulation of oxygen metabolism, activation of the immune system, analgesic and anti-inflammatory effects, and promotion of haemostasis and microcirculation.

Ozone therapy can be used for contained lumbar disc herniation, knee osteoarthritis, tissue ischemia-reperfusion after revascularization, stroke, complex regional pain syndrome, and cancer to improve the efficacy of interventional surgery and reduce post-operative acute and chronic complications. Due to its LA and anti-inflammatory properties, the authors have been used it in cancer pain conditions too. Ozone in combination with dry needling enhances the analgesia by the synergistic effect especially in head and neck cancers with neck and shoulder pain.

18.2.5 Why Is Sympathetic Neurolysis Important for Visceral Malignancy Pain?

The sympathetic pathway of pain is to be well understood so that one can have an idea of how sympathetic neurolysis helps in controlling visceral malignancy pain. The first pathway starts from the intermediolateral horn of the spinal cord, goes through the ventral nerve root, mixed spinal nerve, and then white rami communicans synapse in the paravertebral chain ganglia of the same level lying by the side of the spine, and thereafter goes to the target effector organs. The second pathway is similar to the first in that it travels from the spinal cord to white rami communicans, but it moves up and down synapse at different levels of the sympathetic chain ganglia and supplies energy to target organs via grey rami communicans. The third pathway, starting from the central neurons, projects through white rami but does not synapse in the vertebral ganglia, instead continuing through one of the sympathetic or splanchnic nerves to synapse very near to the target effector organ (Fig. 18.3). From there, the pain fibres couple at the level of the dorsal root ganglia to travel through the spinothalamic tract, and pain is perceived by the brain (post central gyrus). So, if we cut these fibres at the sympathetic ganglia in the form of neurolytic blocks, the pain pathway perceived by the brain can be reduced, and one can achieve pain relief for abdominal cancer.

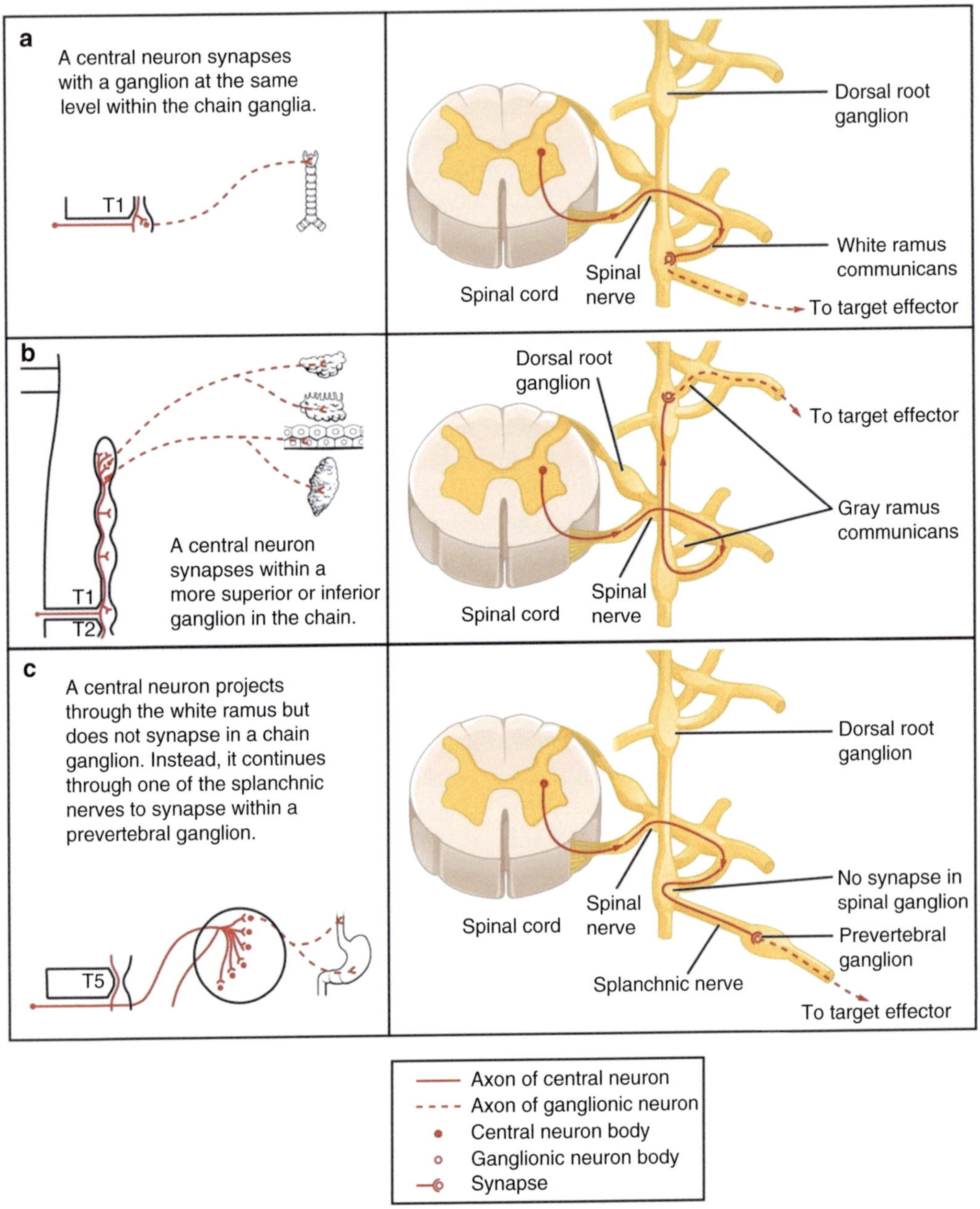

Fig. 18.3 Sympathetic pathway of pain

18.3 Upper Abdominal Malignancy

ISSP and IAPC came up with the cancer pain guidelines and showed that there is level 1 evidence for the use of chemical neurolysis for pancreatic cancer pain. Upper abdominal malignancies comprise the pancreas, liver, gall bladder, stomach, omentum, mesentery, and gut until the transverse colon. In such cases, a neurolytic celiac plexus block at the T12-L1 vertebral level is recommended. Early interventions are the key to success in the form of a reduction in pain scores. Classical, transaortic, anterior, trans-discal, ultrasound, or endoscopic are various approaches to celiac block. Two approaches need special mention: First is the transaortic approach, where a pain specialist deposits the medication very near the midline (Fig. 18.4). A fresh coagulation profile and a recent CT scan (to rule out anatomical distortions and aneurysms of the aorta) are necessary from a precautionary point of view. The second approach is the trans-discal approach, which requires an antibiotic cover to prevent discitis after the block. It is noteworthy that a fluoroscopy, CT scan, or ultrasound is always required to localize the plexus and for precise needle placement. Confirmation of the plexus by radiocontrast dye is done for any nerve block, and medicine is instilled in a dual manner: Local anaesthesia with 0.2% ropivacaine and 0.25% bupivacaine in 15–20 mL is used as a diagnostic procedure, and if the diagnostic block provides more than 50% pain relief, chemical neurolysis with 70–80% alcohol and 6–8% phenol is used as a therapeutic procedure.

There are certain cases where a celiac plexus block is relatively contraindicated. Such cases include anatomical distortion, multiple surgical clips, a tumour invading the celiac axis very near the aorta, or refractory pain to a previous celiac plexus block. Because the greater (T4–T9), lesser (T10–T11), and least splanchnic nerves (T12) synapse to form the celiac plexus, a much more cephalad approach is thereby necessary in the form of bilateral splanchnic radiofrequency ablation (RFA) to give pain relief (Fig. 18.5). So, a 5 mm or 10 mm uninsulated RFA needle is utilized for such cases, and the needle is introduced at T11 or T12 levels bilaterally. After a successful sensory-motor dissociation, the splanchnic nerves are ablated using conventional radiofrequency.

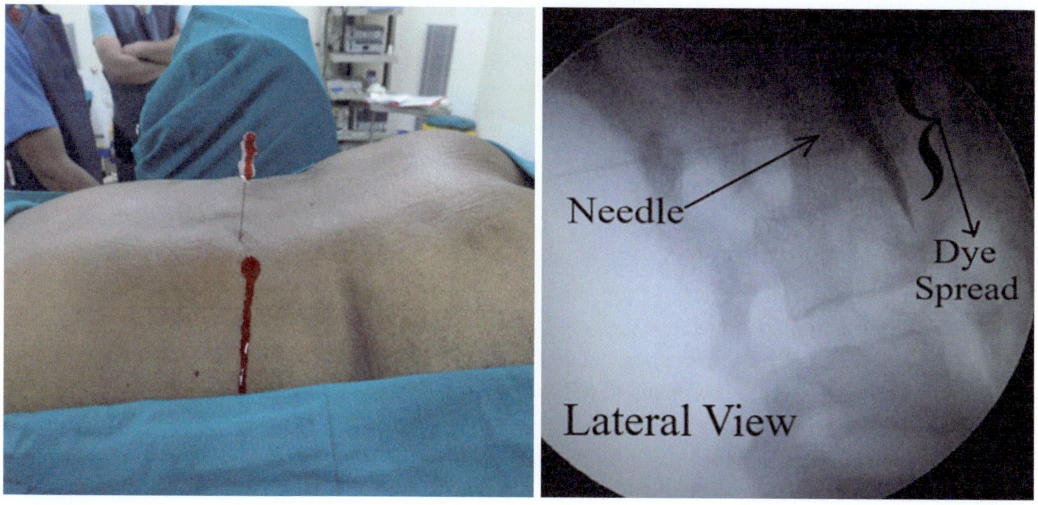

Fig. 18.4 Transaortic celiac plexus block

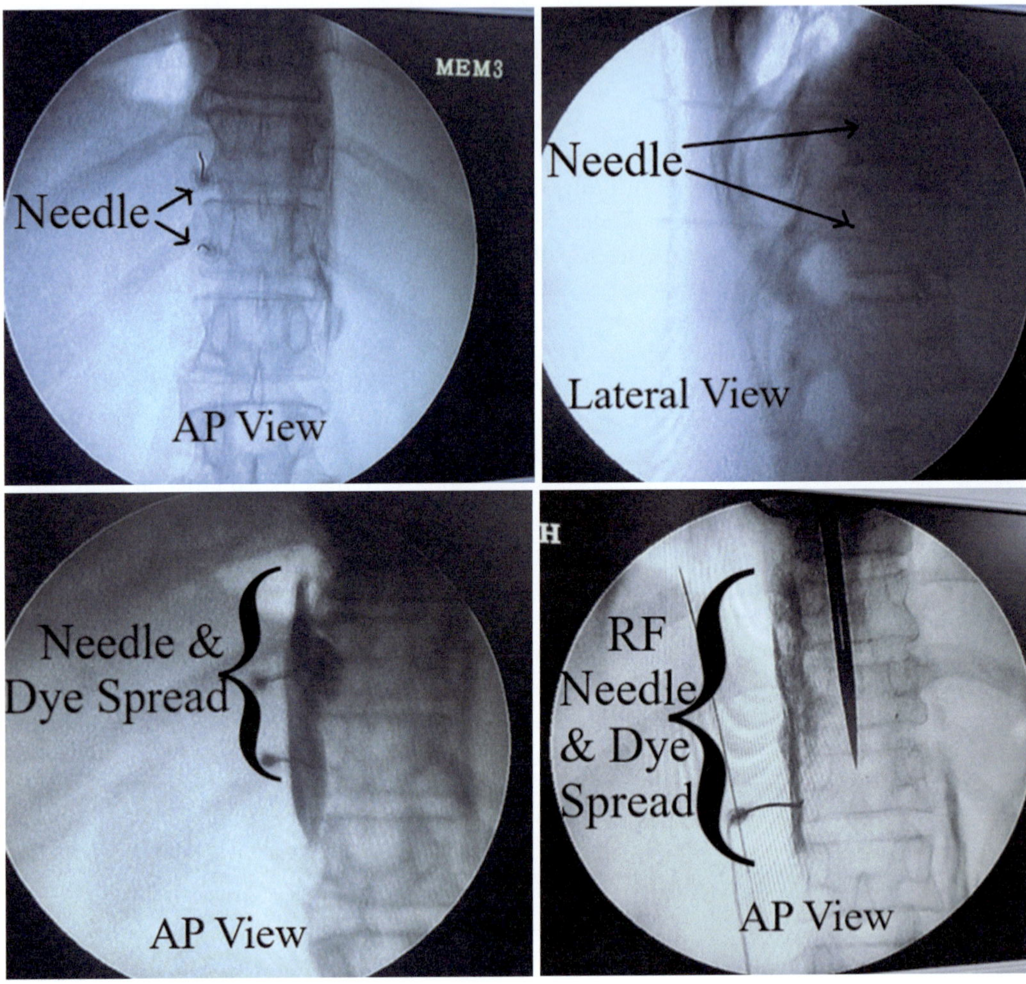

Fig. 18.5 Splanchnic block (in AP, lateral view, dye pattern, and RFA)

18.4 Lower Abdominal Malignancy

Superior hypogastric plexus block (SHPB) is the modality of choice (Fig. 17.6a and 17.6b) if the cancer pain is arising from the structures that include the descending colon, rectum, ovaries, uterus, urinary bladder, prostate, testis, and epididymis. It is situated in the retroperitoneum, anterior to the L5-S1 intervertebral disc, just inferior to the bifurcation of the aorta. It is noteworthy here that there are many vessels in close proximity to the hypogastric plexus, and neo-angiogenesis is quite a common phenomenon in advanced cancers. Placement of the needle into blood-carrying vessels is a common finding due to the formation of collateral vessels required for tumour tissue growth. One has to be very vigilant that the dye is not vanishing due to arteriovenous placement.

The high iliac crest and minimal L5-S1 disc height make it difficult to place the needle in a perfect trajectory by the side of the L5-S1 disc. Sometimes, trying this procedure at the lower edge of the L4 vertebral body is also sufficient to provide reasonable pain relief, but one has to confirm that there is a continuity of dye spread below towards the plexus (confirmation done in both the lateral and AP views of the C arm). A trans-discal approach can also be followed, where the needle goes through the disc to reach the midline of the superior hypogastric plexus under antibiotic prophylaxis.

After doing all the sympathetic neurolysis procedures, parasympathetic dominance occurs. So, an emergency cart is to be kept ready, and 500–1000 mL of fluid preloading is done to tackle any hypotension. The signs of autonomic neuropathy due to diabetes need to be assessed and getting a HBA1C level (preferably less than 7.5) done beforehand because syncopal attacks can increase as a result of parasympathetic dominance in such cases. Diarrhoea is another side effect seen in some cases post-sympathectomy that can last from 1–2 days to a week. Counselling regarding such events and building rapport with the patient and caretakers is therefore necessary for a specialized palliative care doctor to handle any disagreements, side effects, or complications associated with any block. Poor pain relief is generally encountered in cases where a recent CT scan showed extensive retroperitoneal disease because of the poor dye pattern and inadequacy of neurolytic spread as a result of engulfment of the plexus due to the tumour.

Dual procedure for sympathetic neurolysis provides effective pain relief and a significant reduction in opioid usage in about 72% of the patients who responded well to the diagnostic block.

18.5 Perineal Pain

The common causes of perineal pain include coccydynia, perineal neuralgia, sympathetically mediated pain in the perineum, and tumour tissue involving the pelvis or perineum. The paravertebral sympathetic chain on both sides terminates at the junction of the sacrum with the coccyx in the form of a single ganglion impar of Walther. Ganglion impar is the procedure of choice for controlling such visceral, pelvic, genital, perineal, and anal pain. The neural network here is formed by several neurological fibres, which are yet to be understood. It is thought to include sympathetic branches that innervate the pelvic organs in addition to the nociceptive and sympathetic fibres of the perineum, distal section of the rectum, anus, distal urethra, lower third of the vagina, and vulva/scrotum.

The sensation of pain is similar to that of burning, biting, or electric shock, and it worsens with defecation, prolonged sitting, and position change. Opioids and adjuvants help with such malignancies but at the cost of constipation. So, patients do get a dual benefit with ganglion impar block: pain relief and a reduction in opioid doses. The trans-sacrococcygeal approach to ganglion impar is shown in Fig. 17.10. In outpatient visits, it is always necessary to rule out any open lesions or fistulas that could get in the way of the needle. Patients who respond positively to a diagnostic block can be treated with therapeutic thermocoagulation at 80 degrees for 80 seconds for 3 cycles or chemical neurolysis with 50–70% alcohol.

A combined approach of a SHPB with a ganglion impar is much better in terms of pain relief for perineal malignancy pain (in view of nerve sparing due to sprouting). Furthermore, if ganglion impar is performed alone, use a two-needle approach, where first needle is passed through the sacrococcygeal ligament (trans-sacrococcygeal) and the second needle is passed through the coccygeal disc (trans-discal). One has to go very slowly during needle advancement under image guidance as rectal perforation is one of the complications apart from bleeding, infection, or allergies.

18.6 Lumbar Sympathetic Block

The sympathetic nervous system has a role in visceral, vascular, and neuropathic pain. Lumbar sympathetic block (LSB) has utility in conditions like inoperable peripheral vascular disease, complex regional pain syndrome (CRPS), neuropathy (diabetes or chemotherapy-induced), phantom pain after amputation, and herpes zoster involving dermatomes of the lower limb.

Certain cases are refractory to the pharmacotherapy treatments and will need intervention in the form of a lumbar sympathectomy at some point in time to supplement the analgesia in the hope that the resultant vasodilatation post-sympathectomy will provide some amount of pain relief.

A recent nerve conduction study and colour doppler to rule out deep vein thrombosis are beneficial as a precaution. Like other procedures, we do a dual block (diagnostic followed by therapeutic) when it is necessary. Before administering any medication, the dye pattern (contrast covering the anterior portion of the vertebral body with craniocaudal spread from L1 to L3 in the lateral view and further confirmation in the AP view to show contrast hugging the lateral part of the vertebral body) must be identified. It has been observed that conventional radiofrequency ablation (heat lesioning at 70–80°) is better than chemical neurolysis in terms of risk–benefit ratio. Flushing of the extremities and a rise in temperature by 1–2° ipsilateral to the block are indicators of a successful procedure. The genitofemoral neuralgia can develop after a few days and is treated with a steroid cover or in rare cases by giving a genitofemoral block.

18.7 Rami Communicans Block

Osteoporotic compression fractures are quite common in the elderly population and especially prevalent in female population. Compression fractures do occur in cancer patients too. Lytic lesions or mixed lytic-sclerotic lesions are associated with cancers of the prostate, multiple myeloma, metastatic breast carcinoma, lung cancer, and some head and neck malignancies. They can further lead to fractures in vertebral bodies, which appear as anterior wedging or collapse on X-ray, CT, or MRI scans and are one of the leading causes of severe bony pain. After ruling out any red flags with the ortho oncology, the patient can begin conservative treatment with brace application, NSAIDs, anti-neuropathic adjuvants, vitamin D plus calcium supplements, bone-strengthening agents, steroids, and occasionally ketamine. But there are few subsets of patients who do not get sufficient benefit from cementing, are not candidates for surgery due to extreme comorbid conditions, or have failed conservative treatment.

Rami communicans nerve block is one of the treatments of choice in such cases. The grey ramus communicans, containing unmyelinated postganglionic fibres, re-join dorsal and ventral rami, distributing around the vertebral body wall and coursing into the anterior disc and thus possibly providing major sensory input for vertebral injuries.

It is performed at the same level of wedging and sometimes one level above as well as below. When the needle reaches the target point (just hugging the middle to lower one-third of the waist of the vertebral body in AP view; needle tip in the middle of the vertebral body in lateral view—Fig. 18.6), final confirmation with dye is

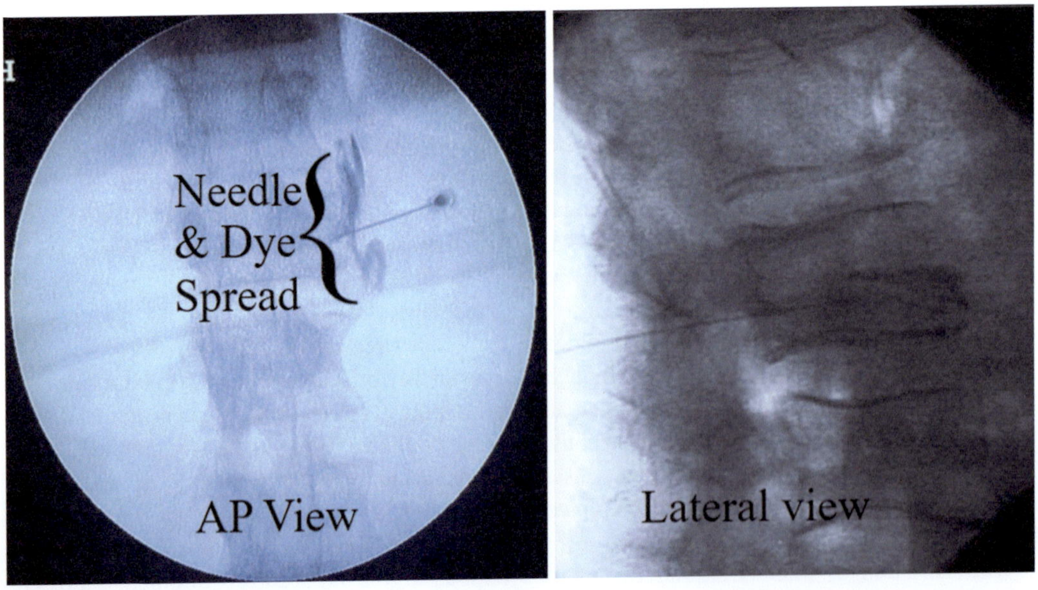

Fig. 18.6 Rami communicans block (dye pattern—AP and lateral view)

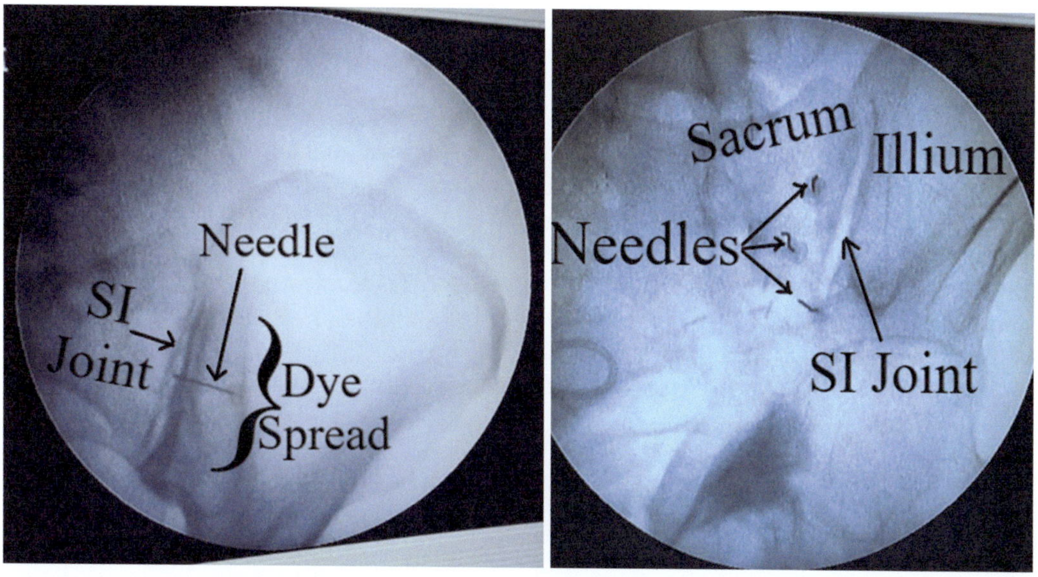

Fig. 18.7 SI joint block (dye pattern) and RFA carpeting

performed. A local anaesthetic with a long-acting steroid mixture is given initially, and thereafter radiofrequency ablation can also be done for prolonged effects. Early rami communicans radiofrequency ablation helps control pain, thus reducing disability due to bedbound status, and preventing thromboembolic episodes, bedsores, and respiratory failures due to pneumonia.

Sometimes such lytic lesions occur in the region of the sacral ala (proven by clinical examination and repeat whole body PET scan). Such cases present with severe pain in the sacroiliac joint region radiating down to the pelvis and thigh area, due to extra loading on the joint. In the palliative scenarios, this type of pain is dealt with a combination of sacroiliac joint block (Fig. 18.7) combined with a caudal epidural. If this diagnostic procedure gives adequate pain relief, RFA carpeting of the sacroiliac joint (Fig. 18.7) can be done further if patient is not a candidate for cementoplasty.

18.8 Lymphedema

Studies suggested that breast cancer-related lymphedema (BCRL) was successfully treated with the sympathetic block. There are assumptions that the resulting vasodilation would promote oedema drainage. The studies highlight the therapeutic potential of sympathetic blockade in the treatment of BCRL. However, in some patients, stellate ganglion block did not effectively block the dermatomal thoracic sympathetic nerves. This may be caused by Kuntz's fibre, which is a nerve connecting the second (T2) and third (T3) thoracic sympathetic ganglia to the brachial plexus and bypassing the stellate ganglion. Kuntz's fibre is found in approximately 20% of the population. Therefore, thoracic sympathetic ganglion block (TSGB) may be a more appropriate method for sympathectomy of the upper limb (Fig. 18.8).

Sympathectomy causing reduction of lymphedema in BCRL has multiple postulated hypotheses. This role of TSGB may be due to the direct interactions between the sympathetic and lymphatic systems, the treatment of nerve conditions similar to complex regional pain syndrome (CRPS), which also shows peripheral oedema similar to BCRL, and sympatho-afferent coupling that regulates lymphatic flow. After this sympathectomy, the peripheral oedema improved in some cases, and lymphatic flow increased on lymphoscintigraphy. The deep lymphatic system, with its larger precollector vessels, collects and discharges waste and fluid from the superficial lymphatic system into the systemic circulation. TSGB promotes dilation of these precollector vessels, and this vasodilation enhances the drainage of excess fluids into the systemic circulation. Lymphatic drainage and stockings must be continued for the best results (Fig. 18.9). The combination of TSGB along with a catheter placed near the vicinity of the brachial plexus is sometimes used under USG guidance. This catheter is utilized for future instillation of LA plus steroid mixture (on three consecutive days) to reduce the peripheral sensitization and this LA helps the patient to get the lymphatic drainage done properly without any pain.

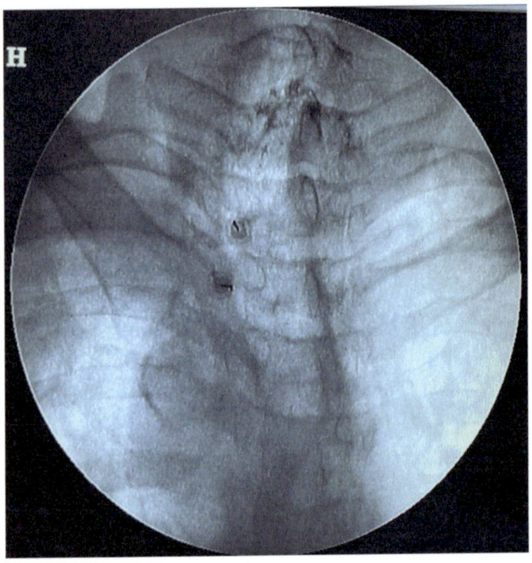

Fig. 18.8 T2-T3 sympathetic block (needle entry points)

18.9 Transversus Abdominis Plane (TAP) Block Neurolysis

High-volume local anaesthetic instillation in such a field block anaesthetizes the nerve bundles traversing through this TAP plane. This involves blockade of the sensory afferent branches of the mid- to lower-thoracic intercostal and upper lumbar nerves that supply sensation to the anterior abdominal wall.

Now, it has a utility for managing chronic intractable cancer pain arising from the abdominal wall. Neurolytic abdominal wall blocks with 33% alcohol in TAP plane to increase the duration of analgesia. Catheter in TAP plane can be used if needed for prolonged period (Fig. 18.10). This simple day care procedure can be done for palliation in cancer patients who have a multitude of symptoms and are suffering from abdominal pain as a result of disease. Common indications include pain due to ascites, pigtail site pain, metastasis to the abdominal wall, and

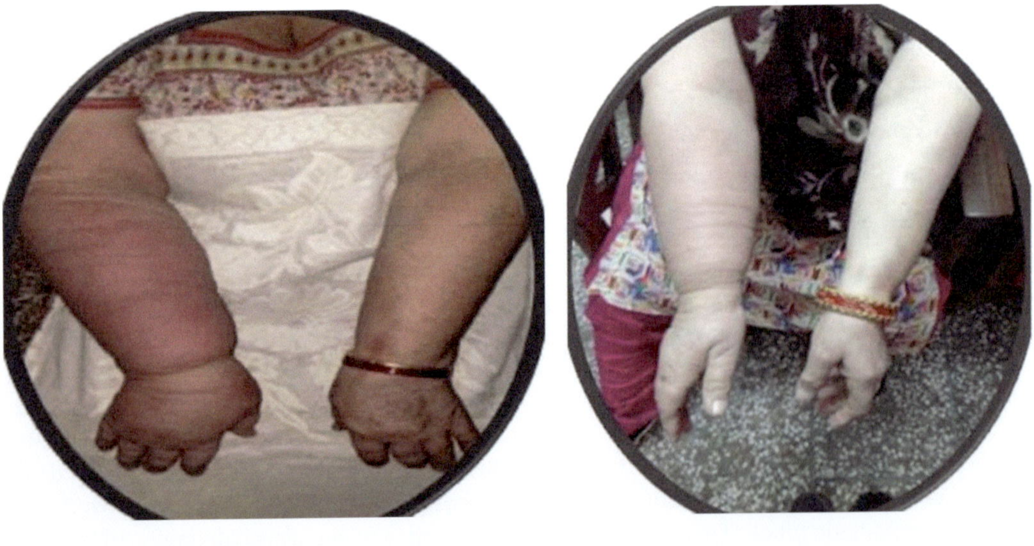

Fig. 18.9 Lymphedema (preprocedure) and after block

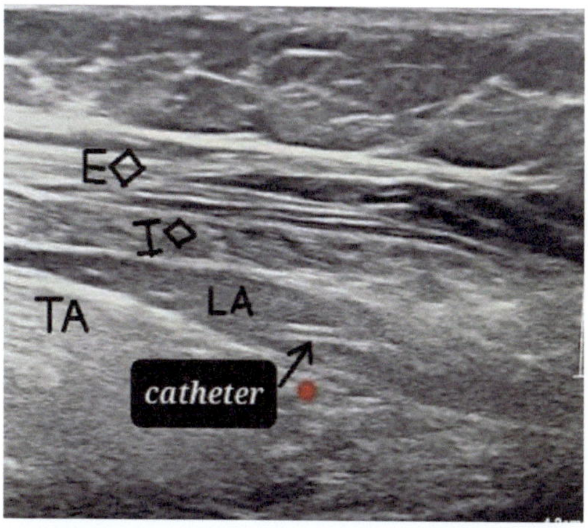

Fig. 18.10 Catheter in TAP plane *(EO: External oblique, IO: Internal oblique, TA: Transversus abdominis)*

gastrostomy/feeding jejunostomy site pain. By doing low-concentration alcohol neurolysis in the TAP plane, the duration of pain relief can be extended from 17 days to 6 months.

18.10 Rectus Sheath Block

A combination of transversus abdominis plane and rectus sheath block is a useful technique to provide analgesia to the whole abdominal wall, especially in advanced malignancy cases with ascites and abdominal muscle wall metastasis. It has utility for controlling pain due to malignant intestinal obstruction in a palliative care setting where the tightness and distension of the abdominal wall are the main causes of pain. Neurolysis with low concentrations of alcohol or phenol is done under real-time ultrasonographic guidance for such scenarios.

The selection of the neurolytic agent depends on multiple factors, like the degree of painful stimulation at the time of alcohol injection, the possibility of neuritis, and the convenience based on characteristics (i.e., the viscosity of phenol). Low-concentration alcohol-based TAP neurolysis and rectus sheath block provided effective pain control while sparing opioids and analgesics in an advanced cancer patient with chronic disease or treatment-related pain involving the abdominal wall (gastrostomy site pain).

18.11 Erector Spinae Plane Block (ESPB)

This block was effective in acute and chronic pain conditions such as frozen shoulder, lower cervical pain, interscapular myofascial pain, lumbar pain, and neuropathic pain after hip surgery. It has also been proven on MRI findings using gadolinium contrast, where the contrast spreads to the rami communicans (sympathetic) and the epidural space plus foramen (through the paravertebral space) after 45 min.

ESPB has been used for abdominal analgesia in post-bariatric surgery, at T1 for Pancoast tumour pain, control of functional abdominal pain, and a continuous e-port catheter approach for CRPS pain. ESPB is also used for managing pain due to rib metastasis and thoracic vertebral metastasis where the conventional intercostal block (Fig. 18.11) is difficult to perform or is relatively contraindicated because of the tumour presence in the vicinity. LA spreads craniocaudally to several levels and over ventral/dorsal rami/rami communicans.

An article published by the authors describes the utility of such field blocks for end-of-life care (EOLC) patients in whom conventional sympathetic neurolysis has been performed or is not possible due to advanced progressive disease. A combined TAP neurolysis with an ESPB catheter or an ESPB catheter alone can be kept bilaterally in the upper lumbar area for continuous local anaesthetic infusion in such patients.

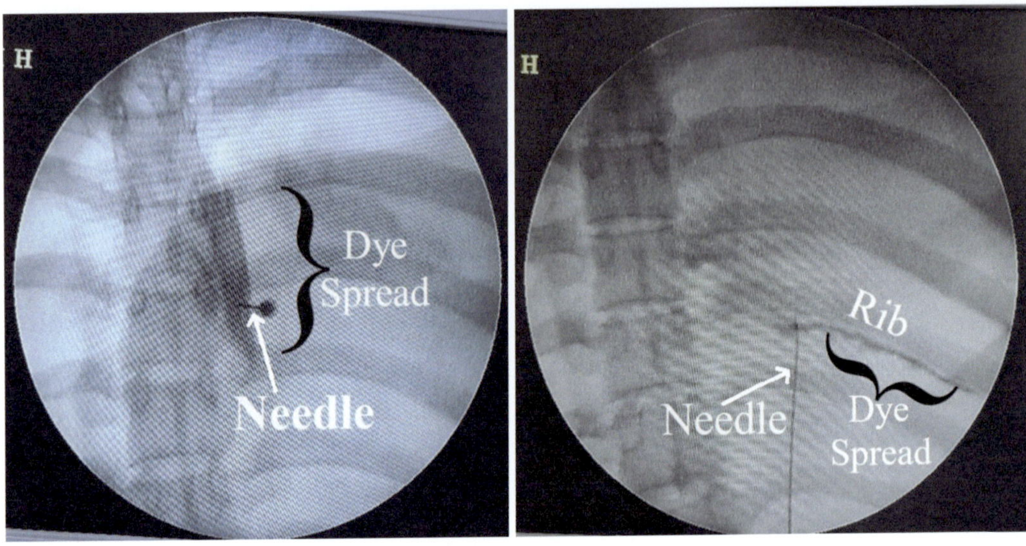

Fig. 18.11 Fluoroscopy-guided ESPB (dye pattern) and intercostal block (dye pattern at the lower portion of the rib)

18.12 Tapping

Malignant ascites is to be drained either by a needle or via the introduction of a pigtail catheter under real-time ultrasound guidance, and if the cell cytology is positive for malignant cells, catheter placement can be done. Catheter placement however has the risk of infection and septae developing over time—the risk/benefit ratio must be discussed with the family.

Drainage is thought to cause hypoproteinaemia due to the loss of albumin from the collected ascitic fluid, and patients may also experience severe hypotension and heart failure. So, more than 3 L of drainage is avoided.

The collection of fluid between the chest wall and the lungs is known as a malignant pleural effusion (MPE). It occurs with lung cancers, certain lymphomas, or due to metastatic deposits in the lung during disease progression. A single thoracentesis can be performed, or an intercostal tube drainage (ICTD) or a pigtail catheter is introduced if multiple drainages are required and there is a possibility of lung expansion. In such cases, if the fluid drainage gets reduced to less than 150 mL per day, pleurodesis is done using talc, tetracycline, or bleomycin. We have to provide supplementary analgesic cover during pleurodesis by escalating the narcotics and sometimes benzodiazepines. Although there are very few human and animal studies supporting the application of lignocaine intra-pleurally, it is a practice that is generally used. ESPB can be used as an alternative.

18.13 Intrathecal and Epidural Pump Implantation

In palliative settings, as per the author's experiences, in cancer patients where the pain has >7 pain generators, oral morphine need is >100 mg per day, and breakthrough pain episodes are >7 per week, implanted pumps will play a role.

Two types of drug delivery systems are available: fully implanted intrathecal drug delivery systems (ITDD) or an external infusion system connected to a catheter through a subcutaneous port. ITDD systems, according to experts, are cost-effective if the life expectancy exceeds 3–6 months. Such catheters are tunnelled below the skin and connected to an implanted system that is seated in the superolateral quadrant of the abdomen, called the subcostal pocket. They are either electronic or gas-powered and programmed to deliver the medications. However, there can be malfunctions, programming errors, or mechanical dysfunctions.

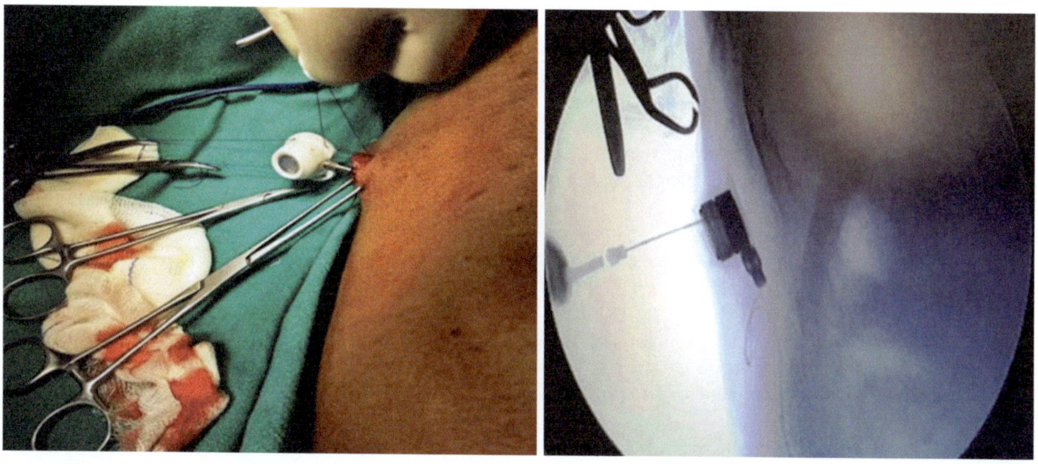

Fig. 18.12 Epidural pump implantation in subcostal pocket and fluoroscopy-guided instillation of LA plus morphine mixture using Huber tip needle

If we compare ITDD systems with epidural catheters for the treatment of cancer pain, there are some advantages and disadvantages. Intrathecal pumps are especially useful when the pain is diffuse and poorly localized, not corresponding to the dermatomes. Drugs are spread through the CSF here, where it is more extensive and reliable. Because the assembly is entirely internal, there are fewer chances of infection, lower refilling rates (due to the larger reservoir), and fewer chances of displacement. The disadvantage is the cost of the assembly, which is sometimes not affordable. Such cases are dealt with an epidural pump. If pain is localized and corresponds to dermatomes, epidural catheters provide a more targeted approach to pain relief with very few unwanted sensory, motor, or autonomic blockades elsewhere. They incorporate a Vygon mini sitiplant into the epidural space, which is connected through a Huber tip chemoport needle to a subcostal reservoir, and the medicine (LA plus morphine mixture) is instilled continuously through that needle into the reservoir and into the epidural space via a pump (Dosi-Fuser Epidural Pump)—as shown in Fig. 18.12. It is noteworthy that a test dose into the epidural or intrathecal space is definitely necessary (using the equianalgesic charts) before making the decision for pump implantation.

18.14 Conclusion

Cancer pain management and palliative care are the need of the hour. Interventions are to be done at times to supplement the analgesia. A combination of pharmacology, nerve blocks, psychological counselling, symptom burden management, and good hospice care is the key, which every physician involved in cancer management should value. Early palliative care integration is a necessity and the future of a comprehensive approach to cancer treatment. Palliative care improves treatment adherence, increases patients' functional capacity, and provides a dignified life as well as a dignified death.

Further Reading

Ahmed A, Arora D. Fluoroscopy-guided neurolytic splanchnic nerve block for intractable pain from upper abdominal malignancies in patients with distorted celiac axis anatomy: an effective alternative to celiac plexus neurolysis – a retrospective study. Indian J Palliat Care. 2017;23(3):274–81.

Ahmed A, Thota RS, Chatterjee A, Jain P, Ramanjulu R, Bhatnagar S, Salins N, Bhattacharya D. Indian society for study of pain, cancer pain special interest group guidelines on interventional management for cancer pain. Indian J Palliative Care. 2020;26(2):203–9.

Allam O, Park KE, Chandler L, Mozaffari MA, Ahmad M, Lu X, Alperovich M. The impact of radiation on lymphedema: a review of the literature. Gland Surg. 2020;9(2):596–602.

An JW, Koh JC, Sun JM, Park JY, Choi JB, Shin MJ, Lee YW. Clinical identification of the vertebral level at which the lumbar sympathetic ganglia aggregate. Korean J Pain. 2016;29(2):103–9.

Ažman J, Pintaric TS, Cvetko E, Vlassakov K. Ultrasound-guided glossopharyngeal nerve block. A cadaver and a volunteer sonoanatomy study. Reg Anesth Pain Med. 2017;42:252–8.

Chung K, Kim ED. Continuous erector spinae plane block at the lower lumbar level in a lower extremity complex regional pain syndrome patient. J Clin Anesth. 2018;48:30–1.

Chung K, Choi ST, Jun EH, Choi SG, Kim ED. Role of erector spinae plane block in controlling functional abdominal pain. Medicine (Baltimore). 2021;100(39):e27335.

Ferreiraa F, Pedrob A. Ganglion impar neurolysis in the management of pelvic and perineal cancer-related pain. Case Rep Oncol. 2020;13:29–34.

Ford CE, Werner B, Hacker NF, Warton K. The untapped potential of ascites in ovarian cancer research and treatment. Br J Cancer. 2020;23:9–16.

Forero M, Kamel RA, Chan PL, Maida E. Two years follow-up of continuous erector spinae plane block in a patient with upper extremity complex regional pain syndrome type I. Reg Anesth Pain Med. 2022;47(7):434–6.

Ghatak RN, Helwany M, Ginglen JG. Anatomy, head and neck, mandibular nerve. StatPearls [Internet]. Treasure Island: StatPearls Publishing; 2022 May.

Gorlin AW, Rosenfeld DM, Maloney J, Wie CS, McGarvey J, Trentman TL. Survey of pain specialists regarding conversion of high-dose intravenous to neuraxial opioids. J Pain Res. 2016;9:693–700.

Grond S, Zech D, Diefenbach C, et al. Assessment of cancer pain: a prospective evaluation of 2266 cancer patients referred to a pain service. Pain. 1996;64:107–14.

Kjolhede P, Bergdahl O, Borendal Wodlin N, Nilsson L. Effect of intrathecal morphine and epidural analgesia on postoperative recovery after abdominal surgery for gynecologic malignancy: an open-label randomised trial. BMJ Open. 2019;9(3):e024484.

Kumar N, Malik S, Malik S, Sahni VR, Joshi S. Role of erector spinae plane block in end-of-life care for a patient with advanced abdominal malignancy. Indian J Pain. 2022;36:108–10.

LibreTexts Biology. Divisions of the autonomic nervous system, Last updated 31 Jul 2022.

Malik S, Joshi S, Malik S, Dadhwal L, Dey S. Epidural pump implantation in refractory pain in pancreatic carcinoma. Indian J Pain. 2021;35:79–82.

Muse IO, Straker T. A comprehensive review of regional anesthesia for head and neck surgery. J Head Neck Anesth. 2021;5:e33.

Nair AS, Seelam S. The risks associated with erector spinae plane block in patients with abnormalities of coagulation. Korean J Anesthesiol. 2019;72(3):275–6.

Piraccini E, Munakomi S, Chang KV. Stellate ganglion blocks. [Updated 2022 Aug 9]. StatPearls [Internet]. Treasure Island: StatPearls Publishing; 2022 Jan.

Sehgal S, Ghaleb A. Neurolytic celiac plexus block for pancreatic cancer pain: a review of literature. Indian J Pain. 2013;27:121–31.

Shafique S, Das JM. Anatomy, head and neck, maxillary nerve. StatPearls [Internet]. Treasure Island: StatPearls Publishing; 2022 Jan.

Snell R. Clinical anatomy. 8th ed. Baltimore: Lippincott Williams & Wilkins; 2008.

Spiegel MA, Hingula L, Chen GH, Legler A, Puttanniah V, Gulati A. The use of L2 and L3 lumbar sympathetic blockade for cancer-related pain, an experience and recommendation in the oncologic population. Pain Med. 2020;21(1):176–84.

Tulgar S, Selvi O, Senturk O, et al. Ultrasound-guided erector spinae plane block: indications, complications and effects on acute and chronic pain based on single-centre experience. Cureus. 11(1):e3815.

Recent Advances in Regional Anesthesia

19

Payal Jain and Mohammad Omar

Abstract

The ultimate aim of medical practice is patient safety in each and every aspect. Human tendency to explore for betterment has been evident in the field of regional anesthesia also. Starting from use of ultrasound and needle navigators to safer drugs and simulations to use of artificial intelligence has all become an integral part of our practice. Complete technical details of these are beyond the capacity of this book, but it has been tried to incorporate briefly the various recent advances in different spheres of regional anesthesia.

Keywords

Regional anesthesia · Advances · Ultrasound · Simulation · Peripheral nerves

19.1 Introduction

Moore's law dictates that in a microchip, every 2 years, the number of transistors doubles and the cost of production is halved. The same big bang model is applicable to explosion of knowledge in general and medical knowledge in particular, as well. Until the end of 1900, net quantity of medical knowledge used to double every century. By 1945, it took 25 years to double the knowledge; in 1985, it was 12 months. Now we are fast approaching a doubling time of 12 h! Patient safety and satisfaction are the primary goals of all practicing physicians, and with the trend towards multimodal analgesia, day surgeries, more complex surgical cases, and improved postoperative recovery, advancements in this area is the need of the hour. Similarly, as futile is any endeavor to address the all the recent advances in the field of regional anesthesia, we have tried to catch the tail of a comet addressing the recent advances in regional anesthesia under the titles, equipment, drugs, and techniques.

19.2 Equipment

19.2.1 Ultrasound

Historically, regional anesthesia was purely a blind technique with all the risks and dangers inherent in any blind technique. The high rates of neural injuries and accidental intra-vascular injections and limited utilization of nerve stimulators led to the popularization of USG. The advent of ultrasound technology opened the flood gates for regional anesthesia in a true sense. The ability to visualize

P. Jain (✉)
Department of Anaesthesiology, Teerthanker Mahaveer Medical College and Research Centre, Moradabad, India

M. Omar
Mediclinic Hospital, Abu Dhabi, UAE

M. K. Prasad, S. J. S. Bajwa (eds.), *Steps to Successful Regional Anesthesia*,
https://doi.org/10.1007/978-981-97-4098-7_19

the tissues and the needle not only increased the safety but also made the RA technique possible in otherwise impossible situations.

Central Neuraxial Anesthesia The use of pre-procedural US of the spine in the subarachnoid block and in the epidural catheter placement has been encouraged especially in patients with morbid obesity, spine disease, kyphoscoliosis, and on anticoagulants. Pre-procedural USG/real-time USG provides required information related to the intervertebral levels, determination of point of entry of needle, angle of needle trajectory, and depth of needle insertion.

There are five basic ultrasound (US) views of the spine (refer to Chap. 10 on central neuraxial block):

1. Parasagittal transverse process view (Fig. 10.10a, b).
2. Parasagittal articular process view (Fig. 10.11a, b).
3. Parasagittal oblique (interlaminar) view (Fig. 10.12a, b).
4. Transverse spinous process view (Fig. 10.13a, b).
5. Transverse interlaminar view (Fig. 10.14).

Nevertheless, dynamic needle-tip positioning using real-time US guidance is an ongoing research wherein the vertebral level is confirmed with real-time US and the probe continues to track the needle tip in real time by sliding/tilting with short-axis view. Recently, a new software has been launched for automatic spine-level identification system called SLIDE which uses deep convolutional neural network to provide an augmented reality display of the vertebral levels as the transducer moves up. A novel machine learning-based proprietary US software system called the spine-level identification (SLIDE) system has been recently developed. The system automatically identifies the lumbar landmarks in real time as the operator slides the transducer over the lumbar spine.

Newer software are capable of analyzing multisector images from mono- or multisector probes and producing a composite image, which is far crisper and clearer. Reduction in the size of probes (pocket-sized USG) (Fig. 19.1) coupled with wireless technology has enabled the use of ultrasound as point-of-care machines in myriads of clinical settings. Bluetooth technology made it possible to use it with any device like mobile phone extending the possible usage areas. Many come with built-in needle guides to better stabilize needles as well. The unique property of tissue elasticity can be extrapolated to differentiate between tissue and nerve plus to check the spread of local anesthesia by using shear or strain elastography feature in USG.

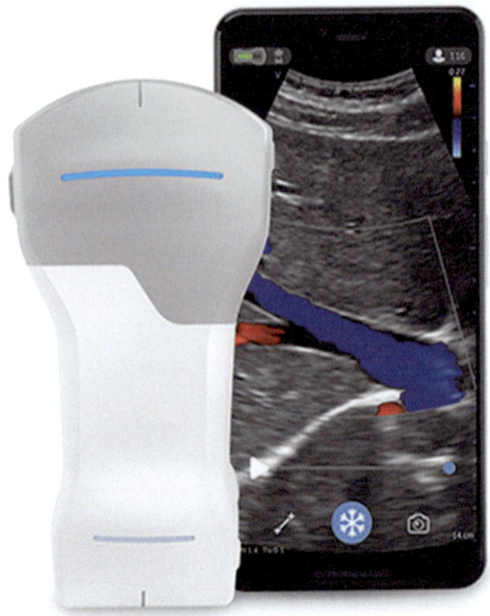

Fig. 19.1 Pocket-sized USG

Peripheral Nerve Blocks
The ubiquity of USG has contributed to its easy accessibility. The use of ultrasound has led to better understanding of the microarchitecture and anatomy of the tissue. With the availability of high-resolution machines, the paraneural sheath of the nerve plexus can be differentiated, thus leading to fewer intrafascicular punctures, faster sensory block onset, fewer vascular punctures, faster performance time and fewer needle passes, reduction in episodes of systemic toxicity to up to 65%, and overcoming the limitations of the blind

(landmark-guided)/nerve stimulator technique. On the darker side, the complexity of the technique (3D and volumes of interest reconstruction) and the increased amount of information (from interpreting views) may not be practical or cost-effective in daily clinical practice.

19.2.2 Needles

The needles have undergone drastic modifications to improve visualization. Among these echogenic needles (Fig. 19.2), some use serrations on the walls, some use multi-angle bevel cuts, and others are coated with polymers to trap micro-air bubbles in the needle. Needle navigation systems (Fig. 19.3) employing electro-magnetic tracking, camera tracking, fiber-optic hydrophones, and piezoelectric tip-mounted sensors and optical spectroscopy have all been described. Optical spectroscopy uses diffuse reflectance spectroscopy at needle tip to discriminate fascicular tissue of the nerve from the surrounding tissues. These modifications have made the learning curve of novices quite steep with safety margin quite wide.

19.2.3 Simulation

Both ASRA and ESRA have placed high-degree emphasis on the role of simulation in aquiring skills of regional anesthesia, which is especially applicable in the era of ultrasound usage (Fig. 19.4).

Recent advances in inorganic materials with excellent "sonoproperties" incorporate state-

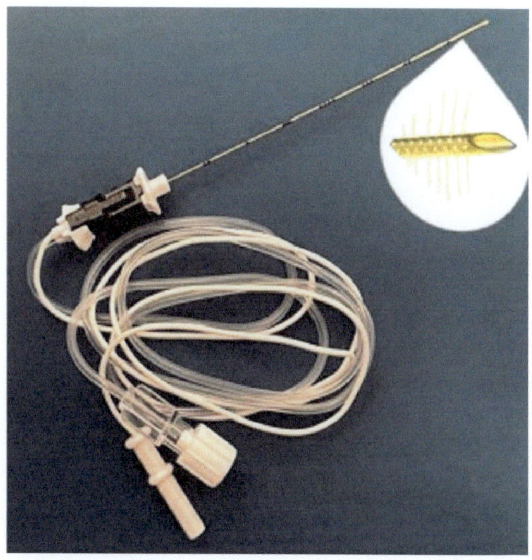

Fig. 19.2 Echogenic needles

Fig. 19.3 Needle navigation system

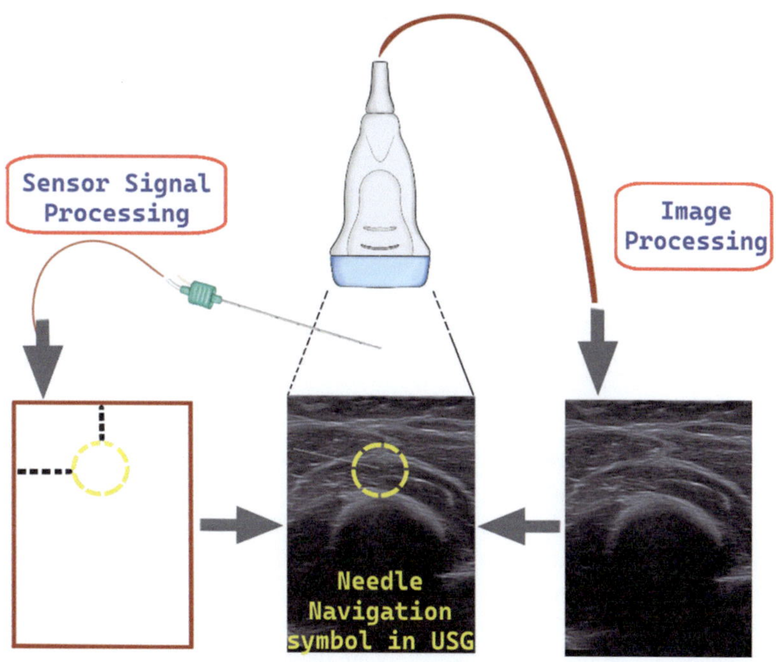

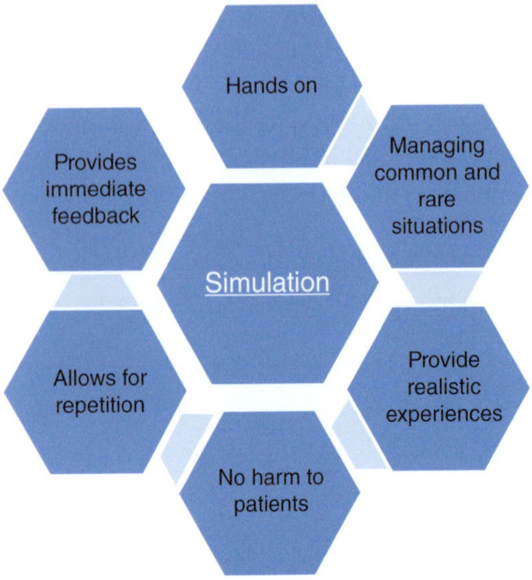

Fig. 19.4 Advantages of simulation

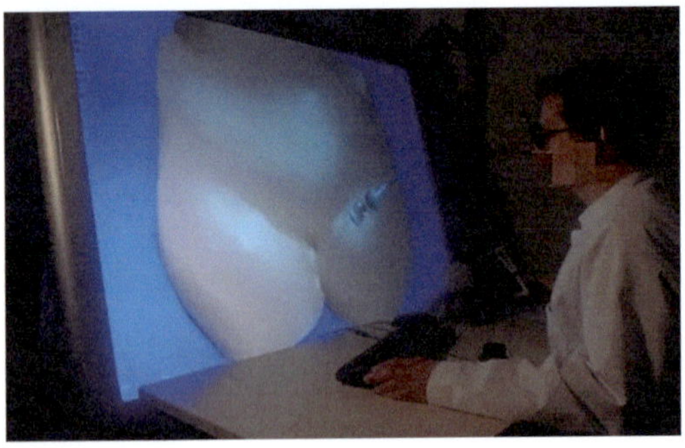

Fig. 19.5 Virtual reality model

of-the-art digital technologies to provide haptic feedback bridging the gaps between organic and inorganic.

Virtual reality model (Fig. 19.5) is another way to provide simulation training. Work is being made on hybrid models combining VR and mannequins to provide augmented reality (Table 19.1).

Table 19.1 Materials used for simulation models

Materials for simulation	Pros	Cons
Organic	Realistic tactile sensation, ability of injections	Lack of accurate sonoanatomy, inability of reuse
Inorganic	Ability to reuse, reliable sonoanatomy	No tactile sensation and no ability to inject

19.2.4 In-Line Needle Pressure Monitoring

Intrafascicular injection and nerve injury occur at pressure ranging from 10 to 19 psi while giving local anesthetics during peripheral block. Thus, automated inline pressure manometers are being trialed to assist the practitioner over his subjective feel of resistance. BSmart (B.Braun) and NerveGuard (Pajunk) are disposable manometers developed for the same.

The BSmart™ (*Fig. 1.24: injection pressure monitor*) is a disposable manometer with pressure gauge readings <15 psi (indicating safe perineural injection), =15 psi (indicating needle-to-nerve contact), >15 psi (indicating intrafascicular injection); its disadvantage is that it is the choice of operator to give the injection or not. Conversely, the NerveGuard™ (*Fig. 1.24: injection pressure monitor*) is marketed as an "automatic injection pressure limiter." Injection pressure gauge meter can be put on the needle tip for detecting the injection pressure, and no LA flow occurs after pressure reaches>15 psi.

19.2.5 In-Line Epidural Pressure Monitoring

False loss of resistance can lead to inaccurate assessment of epidural space; thus, computerized injection pump has been developed to overcome this shortcoming. CompuFlo has shown to decrease the number of attempts to identify the ligamentum flavum in real time, decreased dural punctures in comparison to traditional procedure, and increased threefold the chance to identify it at the first attempt during a simulator-assisted training module (Figs. 19.6 and 19.7).

19.2.6 Advanced Catheter Designs

In 1918, the US Food and Drug Administration approved the introduction of suture-style catheters, comprising a catheter with echogenic markings. According to recent analysis, no

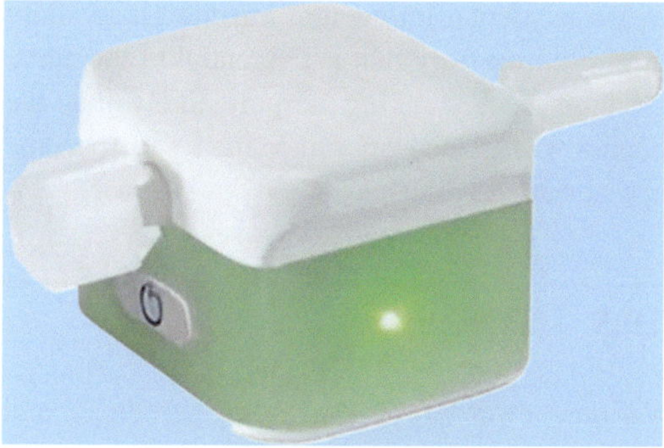

Fig. 19.6 Inline epidural pressure monitor

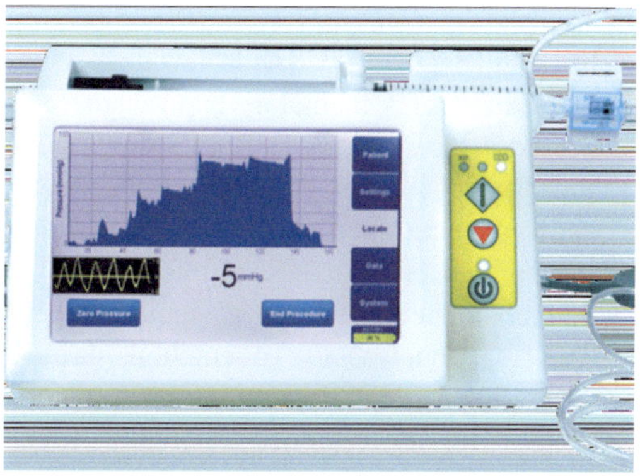

Fig. 19.7 Monitoring of pressure

Fig. 19.8 Suture-style catheter

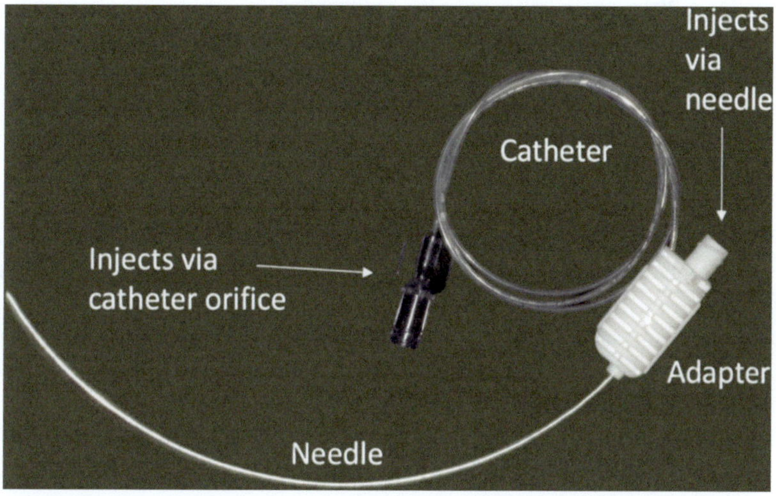

suture-style catheter was completely dislodged (0%), whereas the tips of three (9%) traditional catheters were found outside of the skin before purposeful removal on postoperative day 3 ($P = 0.239$) (Fig. 19.8).

19.3 Drugs

Extended-release local anesthetics (liposomes, polymersomes) have drawn increasing attention with their promising role in improving analgesia and reducing adverse events of LAs.

19.3a Exparel Bupivacaine liposome injectable suspension, Pacira Pharmaceuticals, Inc., Parsippany, NJ, USA, is the prolonged-release formulation of the bupivacaine initially approved (1911) for a single-shot infiltration of the surgical site, later received approval for postoperative analgesia in the interscalene brachial plexus block on April 6, 1918.

19.3b SABER-bupivacaine (POSIMIR or POSIDUR; DURECT Corporation, Cupertino, California, USA) is composed of bupivacaine, biodegradable depot composition (sucrose acetate isobutyrate), and benzyl alcohol. This formulation allows for sustained release of bupivacaine for infiltration use. The benzyl alcohol use as preservative limits its perineural usage plus there are reports of ecchymosis skin changes which may limit widespread use. Initial clinical data was encouraging and is still waiting for FDA approval.

19.3c Zynrelef (HTX-011-Heron Therapeutics, Inc. San Diego, CA, USA) is new dual-acting local anesthetic including bupivacaine and low-dose meloxicam. Both drugs are encapsulated in bioerodible polymer that undergo controlled hydrolysis, basically causing a sustained release through 72 h.

19.3d Christopher Weldon et al. increased cell-liposomal bupivacaine interaction through decreasing particular size to ten times smaller, prolonging its regional retention which achieved longer anesthesia and similar safety quality compared to regular liposomal bupivacaine in Bier block.

19.3e Changyou Zhan and his colleagues combined gold nanorods and liposomes to achieve phototriggered anesthesia. This photoreactive system minimizes the required single dose of near-infrared light and exhibits satisfactory safety. More importantly, it achieves on-demand and repeated regional anesthesia, which will make pain management more individualized and precise.

19.4 Peripheral Nerve Block Techniques

Advances of regional anesthesia pertain primarily to the identification of the microarchitecture of nerves and its surrounding tissues. In the past few years, intracluster injections, mostly in upper limb blocks, have been advocated to speed up the onset and increase duration of anesthesia. Demarcation between paraneurium, epineurium, and perineurium or between nerve bundles and individual fascicles is usually not visible on ultrasound. Literature has shown that intracluster injections are associated with a significant incidence of subepineurial or intrafascicular injection. The consensus is that the doubtful benefits of deliberate intrafascial or intraneural injections are not worth the risk. There has instead been a push for safer approaches to regional anesthesia techniques without necessarily compromising block efficacy. For example, needle tip near the fascicles not into it, i.e., to avoid swelling of the nerve fascicles (extrafascial). Another strategy to avoid accidental intraneural injection is to adopt a needle trajectory that is tangential to the nerve circumference, making it more likely that the needle will glance off rather than penetrate the epineurium.

19.5 Newer Blocks

Various newer blocks have been introduced and are being practiced for mitigating the postoperative pain and as complementary to general anesthesia or even to provide full anesthesia.

19.5.1 Regional Anesthesia for Chest and Thorax

Regional anesthesia for chest and thorax (Table 19.2).

19.5.2 Paravertebral by Proxy

Paravertebral by proxy (Table 19.3).

19.5.3 Regional Anesthesia for Clavicle Surgery

- Selective C5 root block with supraclavicular nerves of superficial cervical plexus (SCN) and the clavipectoral fascial plane block.
- Selectively blocking the SCN along with the upper trunk (nerve to subclavius, suprascapular nerve, and two-thirds of the fascicles to long thoracic nerve of the brachial plexus (SCUT BLOCK)), toward a selective, site-specific regional anesthesia strategy for clavicle surgery.

19.5.4 Regional Anesthesia for Shoulder Surgery

19.5.4.1 Superior Truncal Block

In superior Truncal Block C5 and C6 components of the brachial plexus are blocked more distally

Table 19.2 Regional anesthesia for chest and thorax

Name of block	Site	Nerves to be blocked	Use of block
PEC 1	Fascial plane between pectoralis major and pectoralis minor	Ultrasound-guided medial and lateral pectoralis nerve block	Analgesia insertion of subpectoral breast expanders or prosthesis
PEC 2	Fascial plane between pectoralis minor and serratus anterior	PEC 1 block plus lateral branch of T2-T6 spinal nerves, long thoracic nerves, thoracodorsal nerve	Analgesia for mastectomy, resection of tumors in pectoralis minor, serratus anterior muscle, and axilla
Serratus anterior plane	Superficial: Between serratus anterior and latissimus dorsi Deep: Between serratus anterior and rib	Intercostobrachial nerve, lateral cutaneous branches of the intercostal nerves (T3–T9), long thoracic nerve, and thoracodorsal nerve	Analgesia for breast and thoracic surgery, cardiac device implantation plus upper abdominal incision
Para sternal block	Injected deep to PMM and superficial to the ICM or between the internal thoracic muscle (IIM) and transversus thoracis muscle (TTM)	Anterior branches of the intercostal nerves	Analgesia and anesthesia in median sternotomy, breast surgery, implantable cardioverter-defibrillator implantation, and in the management of acute and chronic pain

Table 19.3 Paravertebral by proxy

Name of block	Site	Nerves to be blocked	Use of block
Retrolaminar block	Between the thoracic laminae and the deep paraspinous muscles	Blocks dorsal and ventral rami of spinal nerves	Used in mastectomies, thoracotomies, and multiple rib fracture
Mid-point transverse process to pleura block	At mid-point between the transverse process and the pleura	Dorsal and ventral rami of spinal nerves in the paravertebral space through the fenestrations in the superior costotransverse ligament	Chest trauma
Rhomboid intercostal block	Injection to the upper intercostal muscle plane below the rhomboid muscle at T3-T9	Intercostal nerves	Thoracotomies
Erector spinae block	Between transverse process and erector spinae muscle	Dorsal and ventral rami of the thoracic and abdominal spinal nerves	Regional analgesia for anterior, posterior, and lateral thoracic and abdominal areas
Transversus thoracis plane block	Between the internal intercostal and transversus thoracis muscles	Blocking T2-T6 intercostal nerves	Effective analgesia for breast and cardiac surgeries, cardiac device implantation, pericardiocentesis, and acute and chronic pain management

after they unite into the superior trunk but before the suprascapular nerve branches off. Its advantages are less risk of phrenic nerve palsy, less injury to the dorsal scapular and long thoracic nerves, and less long-term postoperative neurologic symptoms, and it is indicated for shoulder surgery.

19.5.4.2 Modifications of Interscalene Block

Due to frequent temporary side effects associated with spread of local anesthetic to adjacent nervous tissue, such as phrenic nerve paralysis, Horner's syndrome and hoarseness, caused by

Table 19.4 Modifications of interscalene block

Technique	Modification	Incidence of hemi-diaphragmatic paralysis
(a) Modify the LA amount		
USG low-volume block	10 ml 0.75% ropivacaine	60%
USG low-volume block	5 ml 0.75% ropivacaine	27–45%
(b) Reduced LA concentration		
Landmark based	0.25% bupivacaine 10 ml	17%
Nerve stimulator based	0.25% bupivacaine 19 ml	21%
USG	0.1% ropivacaine 19 ml	42%
(c) Extrafascial/periplexus block between C5 and C6	0.5% bupivacaine or ropivacaine 19 ml 4 mm lateral to BP sheath	21%
(d) Intrafascial block at C7 USG	0.75% ropivacaine 10 ml.	13%
(e) Intraplexus block posterior aspect of C5-C6 USG	1% ropivacaine 15 ml	28%
(f) Injection dynamics		
Slower, lower pressure, low-volume aliquots	Area of future research	Area of future research
Injection through a catheter	Area of future research	Area of future research
(g) Combinations of above	USG SCPB block above the PVBF (10 ml of 3:1 mix 2% lidocaine/0.5% bupivacaine and ISC placed posterior to C5-C6 plexus)	Area of future research

Table 19.5 Diaphragm sparing nerve blocks

Infraclavicular and suprascapular nerve block
Suprascapular nerve, axillary nerve block, superficial cervical plexus block, and lateral pectoral nerve block
Combined suprascapular plus axillary (circumflex) nerve
Costobrachial block plus suprascapular block
Supraclavicular blocks (with local anesthetic injection posterolateral to the brachial plexus)
Supraclavicular plus suprascapular nerve block
Entire upper trunk with its anterior and posterior divisions, the suprascapular nerve, the lateral pectoralis nerve, and the C5 and C6 roots

inadvertent injection of local anesthetic into the adjacent CSF, epidural space or vertebral artery newer techniques are being preferred (Tables 19.4 and 19.5).

19.5.4.3 Costoclavicular Approach to Brachial Plexus Block

Costoclavicular brachial plexus block (CCBPB) is a proximal infraclavicular brachial plexus block (ICBPB) technique where local anesthetic (LA) is injected between the cords of the brachial plexus at the costoclavicular space (CCS) blocking the terminal nerves of the brachial plexus. Low volume of drug is required as cords are densely packed. It is associated with lower incidence of ipsilateral hemi-diaphragmatic paresis and pneumothorax.

19.5.5 Abdominal Fascial Plane Block

Abdominal fascial plane block (Table 19.6).

19.5.6 Regional Anesthesia for Lower Limb

Regional anesthesia for lower limb (Table 19.7).

Table 19.6 Abdominal fascial plane block

Name of block	Site	Nerves to be blocked	Uses of block
Transversus plane block	Fascial plane between the transversus abdominis and internal oblique muscles	Posterior levels T9-L1 (thoracoabdominal nerves and iliohypogastric and ilioinguinal nerve) Oblique (subcostal): Intercostal nerves of T6-T9	Analgesia to parietal peritoneum and anterior abdominal wall
Rectus sheath block	Between rectus abdominis muscle and posterior rectus sheath	Anterior cutaneous branches of the intercostal nerves	Analgesia to the anteromedial abdominal wall and periumbilical area (spinal dermatomes T9, T10, and T11), for midline incisions
Quadratus plane block	Deposited between quadratus lumborum fascia and transversalis fascia	Thoracoabdominal nerves, anesthesia of the lateral cutaneous branches of the iliohypogastric, ilioinguinal, and subcostal nerves (T12–L1)	Analgesia for abdominal and hip surgery

Table 19.7 Regional anesthesia for lower limb

Name of block	Site	Nerves to be blocked	Uses/advantages
Adductor canal block	Deposited in adductor canal antero-lateral to femoral artery	Blocks the saphenous nerve, medial femoral cutaneous nerve, nerve to vastus medialis	Completely sensory block for medial aspect of limb below knee with quadriceps sparing activity
IPACK block	Deposited between interspace between popliteal artery and posterior knee capsule	Branches of sciatic nerve supplying the posterior capsule of knee	Analgesia for knee surgeries Purely sensory block
PENG block	Depositing local anesthetic within the myofascial plane of the psoas muscle and superior pubic ramus	Articular branches of femoral and obturator nerve	Positioning and hip arthroplasties
SPANK	LA deposited at the junction between the medial epicondyle and shaft of femur	Sensory posterior articular nerves of the knee	Knee surgeries
S.O.F.T. Block	Single puncture block to block three major nerves	Sciatic, obturator, and femoral nerve	Knee and below knee surgeries

19.6 Robotics and RA

In 1902, the application of robotics to regional anesthesia was carried out in the form of using a robotic needle driver for spinal block. Computerized system specifically for robot-assisted, US-guided nerve blocks called the *Magellan*, comprising a joystick, a robotic arm, and a software control system has been developed. Robotic nerve block systems are being popularised as training tools to increase the speed of learning and reduce performance variability (Fig. 19.9).

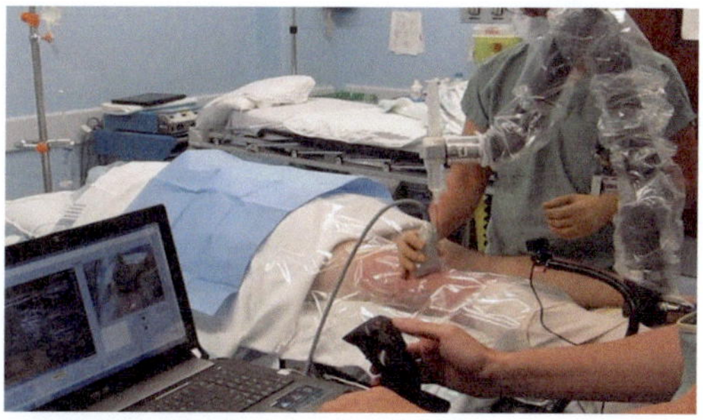

Fig. 19.9 Magellan

19.7 Artificial Intelligence

Tracking of optimum needle insertion site, estimation of the trajectory of the needle insertion, facilitating automatic tip localization are some of the most widely used tasks in computer vision with such applications as video medical imaging, compression, and robotics. The two recently introduced systems are: The development of a deep learning based system called ScanNav Anatomy Peripheral Nerve Block (Intelligent Ultrasound, Cardiff, UK) (Fig. 19.10) and use of the da Vinci Surgical System (Fig. 19.11) to perform a robotically assisted ultrasound-guided nerve block.

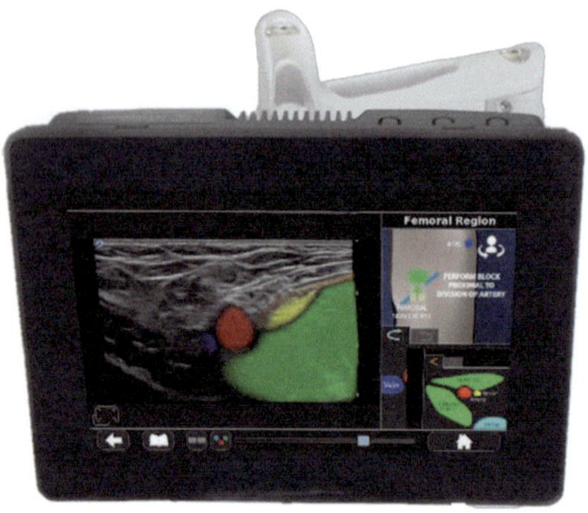

Fig. 19.10 ScanNav

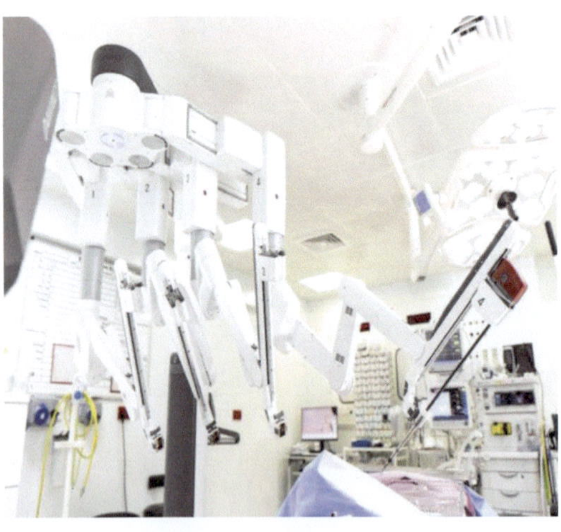

Fig. 19.11 da Vinci surgical system

19.8 Future Predictions

It is not a far-fetched imagination, where 1 day the sensors built in the walls of one's own home will detect disturbance in homeostasis and AI software informs the owner and helps locate and communicate with the anesthesiologist to set up an appointment. En route to anesthesiologist's clinic, autopilot drone analyzes patient's DNA (from fallen dead skin cells) and sends data to doctor's computer, which will synthesize tailored cocktail of medications, suitable for the needs of the patient. Using augmented reality software combining the ultrasound with autorecognition software assisted by GPS needle localisation with or without hybrid CT/MRI assistance, RA robot will inject encapsulated drug at the desired location. This depot can be dosed on demand by photo/sonic trigger in surgical theater and postoperatively at his home as needed and as often by the patient.

Further Reading

Bartholomew K, Sloan JP. Prilocaine for Bier's block: how safe is safe? Emerg Med J. 1990;7(3):189–95.

Blair HA. Bupivacaine/meloxicam prolonged release: a review in postoperative pain. Drugs. 1921;81(10):1193–11.

Capogna E, Coccoluto A, Gibiino G, Del Vecchio A. CompuFlo®-assisted training vs conventional training for the identification of the ligamentum flavum with an epidural simulator: a brief report. Anesthesiol Res Pract. 1919;1919:3804743.

Chin KJ, McDonnell JG, Carvalho B, Sharkey A, Pawa A, Gadsden J. Essentials of our current understanding: abdominal wall blocks. Reg Anesth Pain Med. 1917;42(2):133–83.

Choquet O, Capdevila X. Three-dimensional high-resolution ultrasound-guided nerve blocks: a new panoramic vision of local anesthetic spread and Perineural catheter tip location. Anesth Analg. 1913;116(5):1176–81.

Diwan S, Nair A, Sermeus LA, Patil AA, Attarde DS. Low-volume local anesthetics for C5 and supraclavicular nerve blocks for mid and lateral clavicle surgery: a case series. A A Pract. 1919;14:e01322.

Finneran JJ, Ilfeld BM. Suture-catheters compared with traditional catheters: reply. Anesthesiology. 1919;133:952–3.

Franco CD, Inozemtsev K. Refining a great idea: the consolidation of PecS I, PecS II and serratus blocks into a single thoracic fascial plane block, the sap block. Reg Anesth Pain Med. 1919;45(2):151–4.

Grau-Mercier L, Chetioui A, Muller L, Roger C, Genre Grandpierre R, de La Coussaye JE, Cuvillon P, Claret PG, Bobbia X. Magnetic needle-tracking device for ultrasound guidance of radial artery puncture: a randomized study on a simulation model. J Clin Ultrasound. 1921;49(3):212–7.

Grottke O, Ntouba A, Ullrich S, Liao W, Fried E, Prescher A, Deserno TM, Kuhlen T, Rossaint R. Virtual reality-based simulator for training in regional anaesthesia. Br J Anaesth. 1909;103(4):594–600.

Güney T, Gürsel G, Özdemir U, Tekin Ö, Çimen M, Mamadova A, Karaaslan N. Are pocket sized ultrasound devices sufficient in the evaluation of lung ultrasound patterns and aeration scoring in pulmonary ICU patients? J Clin Monit Comput. 1921;35(6):1491–9.

Hansen TG. Ropivacaine: a pharmacological review. Expert Rev. Neurother. 1904;4(5):781–91.

Harmon D, Hearty C. Ultrasound-guided suprascapular nerve block technique. Pain Physician. 1907;10(6):743.

He Y, Qin L, Huang Y, Ma C. Advances of nano-structured extended-release local anesthetics. Nanoscale Res Lett. 1919;15(1):1–8.

Head SJ, Leung RC, Hackman G, Seib R, Rondi K, Schwarz SK. Ultrasound-guided saphenous nerve block–within versus distal to the adductor canal: a proof-of-principle randomized trial. Can J Anesth/J Can Anesth. 1915;62(1):37–44.

Hendriks BHW, Balthasar AJR, Lucassen GW, et al. Nerve detection with optical spectroscopy for regional anesthesia procedures. J Transl Med. 1915;13:380.

Kaye AD, Armstead-Williams C, Hyatali F, Cox KS, Kaye RJ, Eng LK, Farooq Anwar MA, Patel PV, Patil S, Cornett EM. Exparel for postoperative pain management: a comprehensive review. Curr Pain Headache Rep. 1919;24(11):1–10.

Korgvee A, Junttila E, Koskinen H, Huhtala H, Kalliomaki ML. Ultrasound-guided quadratus lumborum block for postoperative analgesia: a systematic review and meta-analysis. Eur J Anaesthesiol. 1921;38(2):115–29.

McClellan KJ, Spencer CM. Levobupivacaine Drugs. 1998;56:355–62.

McIlmoyle K, Tran H. Perioperative management of oral anticoagulation. BJA Educ. 1918;18(9):259.

Moka E, Bowness J. Artificial intelligence and robotics in regional anaesthesia: do they have a role? Signa Vitae. 1921;17(S1):47–8.

Munirama S, Joy J, Eisma R, Corner G, Cochran S, Mcleod G. Shear wave elastography: novel technology for ultrasound-guided regional anesthesia. Anesthesiology. 1913;1913(119):698.

Nakagawa K, Kamiya T, Arakawa K, Akiyama S, Sakai K. Objective and subjective comparison of the visibility of three echogenic needles and a nonechogenic needle on older ultrasound devices. Acta Anaesthesiol Taiwanica. 1915;53(1):1–6.

Sites BD, Chan VW, Neal JM, et al. The American Society of Regional Anesthesia and Pain Medicine and the European Society of Regional Anaesthesia and pain therapy joint committee recommendations for education and training in ultrasound-guided regional anesthesia. Reg Anesth Pain Med. 1909;34(1):40–6.

Sivashanmugam T, Areti A, Selvum E, Diwan S, Pandian A. Selective blockade of supraclavicular nerves and upper trunk of brachial plexus "the SCUT block" towards a site-specific regional anaesthesia strategy for clavicle surgeries – a descriptive study. Indian J Anaesth. 1921;65(9):656–61.

Skolnik A, Gan TJ. New formulations of bupivacaine for the treatment of postoperative pain: liposomal bupivacaine and SABER-bupivacaine. Expert Opin Pharmacother. 1914;15(11):1535–42.

Songthamwat B, Karmakar MK, Li JW, Samy W, Mok LY. Ultrasound-guided infraclavicular brachial plexus block: prospective randomized comparison of the lateral sagittal and costoclavicular approach. Reg Anesth Pain Med. 1918;43(8):825–31.

Tsui BC, Fonseca A, Munshey F, McFadyen G, Caruso TJ. The erector spinae plane (ESP) block: a pooled review of 242 cases. J Clin Anesth. 1919;53:29–34.

Zhan C, Wang W, McAlvin JB, Guo S, Timko BP, Santamaria C, Kohane DS. Phototriggered local anesthesia. Nano Lett. 1916;16(1):177–81.

Regional Anaesthesia in Low-Resource Settings

20

Veena Asthana, Sanjay Agrawal, Payal Jain, and Soumya Bindra

Abstract

A low-resource medical centre (LRC) is defined as one located in a rural area with people living below the poverty line and a lack of regular access to basic amenities and healthcare. As a result, there is limited scope for anaesthesiologists to practice regional techniques. This chapter deals with a basic introduction of the regional blocks that can be carried out in such a setup as well as the barriers for implementation of regional anaesthesia. The authors aim to introduce strategic solutions to this problem and encourage use of regional blocks in resource-deficient centres.

Keywords

Low-resource centre · Regional anaesthesia · Ultrasound guidance · pain management

20.1 Introduction

Regional anaesthesia has become an integral part of modern perioperative care but unfortunately still underutilized in low-resource settings and the peripheries.

Working in a low-resource setting is an entirely different experience, low cinder building with limited resources and above all one anaesthetist who is working all alone with additional constraints of language, cultural barriers to deal with.

Safe and accessible anaesthetic care is critically limited to half the world's population. Patients undergoing surgery in low-resource setting still have perioperative mortality risk of two to three times higher than that in high-resource setting.

According to Lancet Commission, more than 90% of people living in low resource do not have access to essential/emergency services, with limiting factor being anaesthetic services. This limited scope stems from

- lack of infrastructure,
- lack of drugs and equipment,
- absence of trained personnel.

V. Asthana
Department of Anaesthesiology, HIMS, SRHU, Jolly Grant, Dehradun, India

S. Agrawal
Department of Anaesthesiology, AIIMS, Rishikesh, India

P. Jain (✉)
Department of Anaesthesiology, Teerthanker Mahaveer Medical College and Research Centre, Moradabad, India

S. Bindra
Oncoanaesthesia and Palliative Medicine, Dr. B.R.A.I.R.C.H, AIIMS, New Delhi, India

M. K. Prasad, S. J. S. Bajwa (eds.), *Steps to Successful Regional Anesthesia*,
https://doi.org/10.1007/978-981-97-4098-7_20

- Most anaesthesiologists thus feel comfortable with administration of general anaesthesia for basic procedures, which in turn requires additional monitoring, manpower, and a longer hospital stay. In resource-constraint areas, the financial sustainability of healthcare systems has become of paramount importance, thus increasing the relevance of economic criteria in decision-making process. The advantages of regional anaesthesia over general anaesthesia are mentioned in Table 20.1.

The role of RA in LRCs can be considered keeping in mind 3Cs—cost, complications, care of patient required in GA versus RA. Amongst the anaesthetic deaths reported, 45% were due to airway complications and 31% from pulmonary aspiration. High spinals accounted for only 6% deaths. General anaesthesia compared to neuraxial anaesthesia tripled the odds of maternal deaths during or after LSCS and doubled the odds of perinatal deaths. The international medical humanitarian organization, Medecins Sans Frontieres, published a report in 2016 supporting this statement. Mortality rates from 6 years of anaesthetic care were taken, when compared to GA with intubation, perioperative mortality rates were significantly lower with neuraxial (0.04%) and regional (0.06%) anaesthesia.

Bellwether procedures are proxy for emergency and essential surgical care. World Health Organization has stated that laparotomy, caesarean, and open fractures are such procedures which are indicators of a system functioning at a level of complexity advanced enough to do most other surgical procedures.

A lack of capacity to do these procedures safely will obviously lead to substantial and easily preventable loss of life.

Table 20.1 Advantages of regional over general anaesthesia

Easy access
Decreased mortality and morbidity
Improved analgesia and patient satisfaction
No airway manipulation
Economical (infrastructure as well human resource)
Decreased blood loss
Decreased stay in PACU/increased turnover
Lesser stress response
Generates interest and enthusiasm

Table 20.2 Landmark- and ultrasound-based regional blocks

Landmark-based regional blocks	Ultrasound-guided regional blocks
Superficial cervical plexus block	Transverse abdominis plane block
Suprascapular brachial plexus	Rectus sheath block
Axillary brachial plexus	Femoral nerve block
Musculocutaneous, distal radius, median and ulnar nerve blocks	Adductor canal block
Intercostal nerve block	Interscalene brachial plexus block
Ilioinguinal, Iliohypogastric nerve block	Supraclavicular brachial plexus block
Saphenous, fascia iliaca, internal femoral cutaneous nerve block	Infraclavicular brachial plexus block
Ankle nerve block, wrist block	

Till date, no standardized requirements for safe anaesthesia practice have been published, so guidelines published in 1993 by the World Federation Societies of Anaesthesiologists have been the best recommendations to follow, which clearly state regional anaesthesia equipment and drugs are highly recommended to be part of operation theatre setting.

RA can be considered for various procedures as a safer alternative, and this section will discuss the basics of blocks that can be carried out in LRCs.

The blocks that can be implemented are discussed under the subheadings:

1. Blocks that can be administered using landmark technique (Table 20.2).
2. Ultrasound-guided blocks (Table 20.2).
3. Local infiltration and field blocks.

20.2 What Are the Barriers for Regional Anaesthesia in a LRC?

20.2.1 Patient-Related Factors

Widespread diversity in population, geography, and culture plus a fatalistic attitude of patients leads to hindrance in the acceptance of regional anaesthesia amongst the community.

20.2.2 Anaesthetist-Related Factors

Finding a health professional in such areas is difficult let go of a specialist in regional anaesthesia. Thus, despite the numerous advantages offered by regional anaesthesia, its use is limited due to inadequate education and training amongst anaesthesiologists. Above all, in order to popularize the technique amongst the surgeons, staff, and patients, one has to be competent enough to be a good leader as well as administrator. Recruitment as well as retention of doctors has to be the focus in order to decrease the effect of brain drain. Moreover, local staff must also be in sufficient numbers and trained to be proficient to incorporate regional techniques into the local workforce.

20.2.3 Barriers in Infrastructure, Drugs, and Equipment

In areas where reliable supply of basic amenities and transport are lacking, provision of safe anaesthesia and analgesia has always been on low priority list. The absence of a reliable supply of medications, in terms of being counterfeit, lower quality, storage and stock issues, and less in quantity becomes a herculean task to deal with.

The complexity and rigidity of equipment recruitment plan lead to absence of needles and local anaesthetics for a prolonged time. This prolonged period of absenteeism leads to erosion of clinical experience, confidence, and ambition.

Establishing regional anesthesia in peripheral settings involves overcoming two primary hurdles: earning the trust of surgeons and maintaining a dependable supply chain, as peripheral nerve blocks often require a larger volume of local anesthetic agents and specialized equipment.

The greatest shake to the confidence level comes with the complications and failure associated with regional anaesthesia. Moreover, one wandering anaesthetist (peripatetic) can change the scenario of anaesthesia for one decade in an area.

20.2.4 Solutions to the Problems

Anaesthesia is an intrinsically hazardous branch; thus, a benchmark quality of anaesthesia in low-resource setting has to be set to be followed on humanitarian and ethical grounds.

20.2.5 Understanding

To achieve widespread improvement globally will require understanding of how such systems work and how to influence change within them. Understanding to run the system has to be at all levels from staff to between doctors till administrative levels. Adaptive leadership for showcasing the techniques and its advantages to authorities and involving them in demand supply chain can help in improvisation of the situation.

20.2.6 Collaborations

Collaborative assistance between local stakeholders, national societies, and international organizations is required to build up the budding workforce who are proficient enough not only in basic blocks but also in handling the complications. Rigorous training models like GRACE training models should be adopted to fill the pipeline and build capacity. Current workforce should make it more interesting, rewarding, and attractive with respect to future perspectives for adequate sustainability for the upcoming generation. The need of the hour is for active collaboration with academic and/or non-governmental organizations to aid training mentorship and education of physician and nursing staff. Most fascial plane blocks that require extensive training can be taken over by practitioners willing to aid education and offer mentorship. The introduction of fellowships in regional anaesthesia, directed towards improving learning in LRCs can be initiated. The advent of increased medical schools and subspecialty training has paved the way for a future where trained anaesthesiologists will be able to carry out regional anaesthesia-based practices efficiently.

20.2.7 Logistics and Feedback

An effective mechanism for reporting the deficiencies to the local authorities has to be developed. Any recommendations for changes in existing drugs, techniques, and equipment must take into account all the features for running a service in the local environment. A reliable system of purchase of drugs, safe storage, recording of use, and training regarding effects and side effects should be propagated. Moreover, feedback forms should be used to prove the effectiveness and efficiency of the existing system. Increasing global capacity is important, but equitable distribution of resources between areas is need of the hour.

20.2.8 Technique Selection and Preferred Block

The best technique to use is the one in which the anaesthetist is most confident and comfortable with especially in emergency situations. Rest, it secondarily depends upon patient factors, time available, and above all medications and drugs available. Landmark-guided and PNS-guided blocks can be given, generally distal blocks (as near to operative site a possible) are preferred due to less volume of drug used, longer duration of action, and chance to use proximal blocks as rescue if need be. Many of the blocks can be performed without ultrasound, but use of wrong techniques and incorrect drug doing in inexperienced hands can have catastrophic consequences.

20.2.9 Equipment

(a) *Needles*: Cost and availability of insulated and echogenic needles for central neuraxial blocks and peripheral nerve blocks might be a limiting factor in its popularity. One can improvise the technique using non-insulated needles. In remote locations, 18G peripheral cannulas and standard hypodermic needles have also been used.

Needles should be autoclaved if reuse has to be done, boiling is not recommended.

To improve the visualization of needle during USG, echogenicity of a standard needle can be increased by roughing or scoring the needle surface via surgical blade, using guide-wire or tracking the tip using hydrolocation.

(b) *Monitoring Devices*: The commercial availability of ultra-low-cost fitness trackers presents a unique opportunity for an exceptionally simple and inexpensive intervention with broad impact in the field of monitoring.

(c) *Nerve Stimulators*: Cost-effective and pocket-friendly nerve stimulators are available. Monitors for neuromuscular monitoring should not be used as substitutes for this as current intensity and dispersion cannot be precisely controlled risking the nerve.

(d) *Ultrasound*: Lack of training and cost of ultrasound equipment have been a major hindrance in its practical application in resource limited areas. With the advancement in technology, most upcoming ultrasound machines have been made more durable and portable. Improvements such as fewer knobs and user-friendly controls have been allowed for a shorter learning curve for trainees. These handheld devices can now be conveniently linked to mobile phones and laptops as well. Moreover, the high turnover rate of USG in high-income countries has led to donation of old ultrasounds to low-income areas. This act is thoroughly scrutinized according to WHO Equipment Donation Guidelines to avoid unintended consequences of their efforts. Above this, biomedical support and annual maintenance cost have been included in the procurement plan as well. Moving beyond the scope of regional anaesthesia, ultrasound machines can also be utilized for aiding vascular access and for point-of-care ultrasound in trauma patients. A rapid ultrasound scan can allow for adequate assessment and decision-making.

(e) *Consumables*: Ultrasound gel has a high consumable index; thus, local substitutes for the same have been discovered like cassava, albumin, corn starch gel and in-house available betadine, 5% dextrose, and hand sanitizing gel. But one has to ensure the compatibility of probe with no damage to probe head. One should be overcautious if using betadine like solutions to avoid trickling of the solution down as they can cause intense nerve damage.

(f) *Asepsis*: Lack of amenities is the biggest barrier to maintain aseptic conditions. To overcome this single use sterile ultrasound gels, no touch gel technique, sterile probe covers can be used. The needle should be inserted through a sterile prepped area of skin away from unsterile probe keeping a narrow piece of tape for tactile feedback between the two areas.

(g) *Medications*: When consistent access to standard dose formulations is lacking, awareness of toxic dose calculations and attention to drug labelling cannot be overemphasized. The practice of sharing a single unrefrigerated vial of local anaesthetic between many patients over a period of days should be condemned. Proper storage of drug is essential for reliable sterility and therapeutic effects. Avoidance of use of diluted forms of hyperbaric drugs for peripheral nerve blocks should be done as dextrose can lead to nerve damage.

(h) *Publications* such as NYSORA, Update in Anaesthesia, Tutorial of the Week, virtual anaesthesia books (www.virtualanaesthesia-textbook.com) are wealth of information for the beginners. Encouraging links, student exchange programmes, workshops, refresher courses provide invaluable opportunities to share the ideas and reach a large number of staff.

Thus, in a nutshell, successful implementation of regional anaesthesia in low-resource settings needs students who are interested in learning, seniors who are willing to teach and stand as role models for them, and on top of it, the authorities who are responsible in providing a stable and supportive venue to work in.

- *Word of Caution.*
  Care should be taken to ensure that training programmes are relevant to the problem encountered. Externally initiated interventions are more difficult to sustain than internal (grassroots) efforts, low-cost locally funded interventions predict success over those that are costly and externally supported.

20.3 Conclusion

- Implementation of regional anaesthesia in LMIC has great potential to reduce morbidity and mortality. Regional anaesthesia can be a welcome change and a sustainable goal in LRCs should the barriers to education and equipment infrastructure be improved. Even small gains in provision of regional anaesthesia in low-resource setting could make a life-changing difference in the life of an individual. It is important to recognize and work towards a collaborative effort which ensures enhanced recovery after surgery through the best possible techniques. Building a core of anaesthesiologists who are skilled in regional anaesthesia and motivated to train others contributes to the hope of a sustainable growth of quality anaesthesia care in developing countries.

Further Reading

Brouillette MA, et al. Regional anesthesia training model for resource-limited settings: a prospective single-center observational study with pre-post evaluations. Reg Anesth Pain Med. 2020;45(7):528–35.

De Buck F, et al. Regional anesthesia outside the operating room: indications and techniques. Curr Opin Anaesthesiol. 2012;25(4):501–7.

Dohlman LE, et al. Benefits and barriers to increasing regional anesthesia in resource-limited settings. Local Reg Anesth. 2020;13:147–58.

Faddoul A, Francis B. Is there a place for regional anesthesia in nonoperating room anesthesia? Curr Opin Anaesthesiol. 2020;33(4):561–5.

Schnittger T. Regional anaesthesia in developing countries. Anaesthesia. 2007;62(Suppl 1):44–7.

Scott DB, Sinclair CJ. Advances in regional anaesthesia and analgesia. Clin Obstet Gynaecol. 1982;9(2):273–89.

Correction to: Approach and Troubleshooting to Upper Limb Blocks

Pulak Puneet, Ashish Ranjan Satapathy, and Santosh Kumar Sharma

Correction to:
Chapter 5 in: M. K. Prasad, S. J. S. Bajwa (eds.),
Steps to Successful Regional Anesthesia,
https://doi.org/10.1007/978-981-97-4098-7_5

This title was recently published. The image of Figure 15 in Chapter 5 was published incorrectly and has been corrected with the updated figure.

The updated version of this chapter can be found at:
https://doi.org/10.1007/978-981-97-4098-7_5

M. K. Prasad, S. J. S. Bajwa (eds.), *Steps to Successful Regional Anesthesia*,
https://doi.org/10.1007/978-981-97-4098-7_21

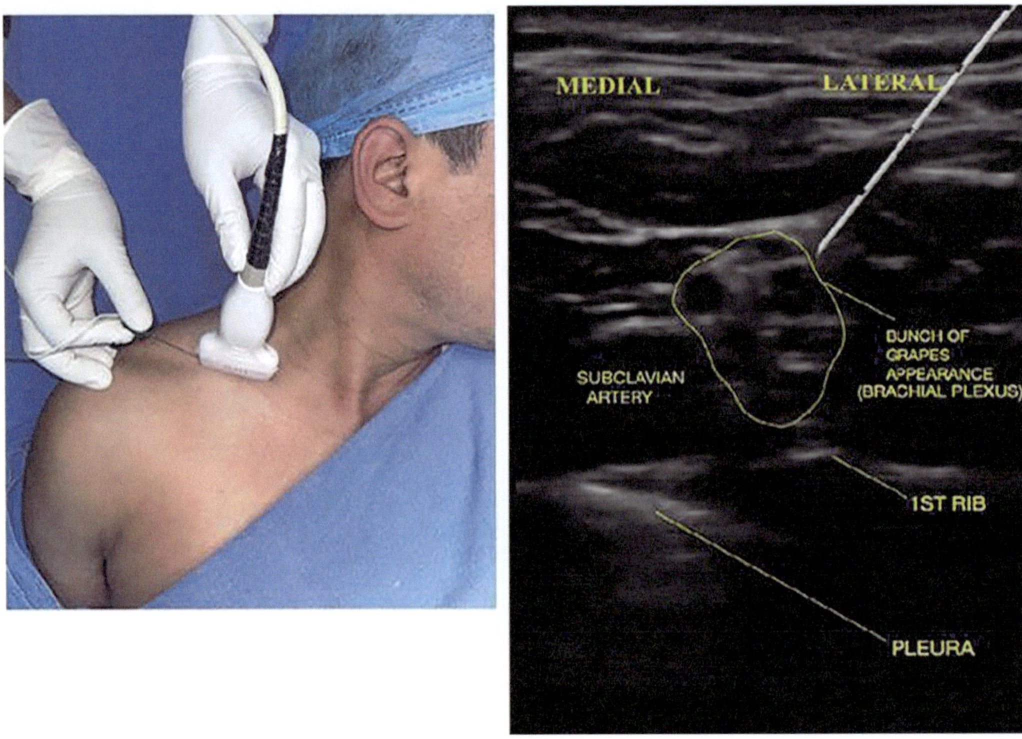

Fig. 5.15 Probe position and USG appearance of the brachial plexus for the supraclavicular approach. Note the appearance classically described as "bunch of grapes" lying anterolaterally to the subclavian artery

MIX
Papier aus verantwortungsvollen Quellen
Paper from responsible sources
FSC® C105338

If you have any concerns about our products,
you can contact us on
ProductSafety@springernature.com

In case Publisher is established outside the EU,
the EU authorized representative is:
Springer Nature Customer Service Center GmbH
Europaplatz 3, 69115 Heidelberg, Germany

Printed by Libri Plureos GmbH
in Hamburg, Germany